WeightWatchers momentum

Complete Food Companion®

WEIGHT WATCHERS, *POINTS*, Food Companion, *POINTS*finder, and the Wave Logo are the registered trademarks of Weight Watchers International, Inc. Momentum and the Diamond Logo are trademarks of Weight Watchers International, Inc. The *POINTS*® Weight-Loss System is proprietary to Weight Watchers International, Inc. Patent Nos. 6,040,531; 6,436,036; and 6,663,564.

©2009 Weight Watchers International, Inc.
All rights reserved.   Printed in U.S.A.

NEW 2010 EDITION

Meal planning and grocery shopping are now more convenient than ever!

New and updated for 2010, **Weight Watchers® Complete Food Companion®** is our most complete food guide yet!

In this book you will find:

- **COMPLETE A-Z FOOD LIST:** a general alphabetical listing of just about every food you can think of. Use it to check **POINTS®** values, plan your meals, make grocery lists, or get great new ideas to help keep your menus exciting.

- **NEW!! COMPLETE FILLING FOODS LIST:** a comprehensive listing of the foods that fill you up and help keep hunger at bay. Use this list to help make sure you're including these foods in your menus.

- **NEW!! Set_POINTS_ FOOD LIST:** food categories with a set **POINTS** value to make estimating **POINTS** values less stressful while eating away from home. If you don't want to fuss over exactly how much you're eating, this **SetPOINTS** food list is what you need.

- **BRAND NAME FOODS LIST:** thousands of brand-name food products, with their **POINTS** values, organized by food category. Comparison shopping is made simple with this extensive list.

- **WEIGHT WATCHERS® FOOD PRODUCTS LIST:** a list of all the products under the Weight Watchers brand name.

- **INDEX:** an alphabetical list of all the food categories, along with their page numbers, making it even simpler to find what you want.

A note about *POINTS* values:

The *POINTS* values for all of the foods in this book were calculated by Weight Watchers International, Inc. using the most current calorie, fat, and fiber information available from manufacturers and the United States Department of Agriculture (USDA). However, since product formulations and nutrition information may change during the year, it's a good idea to continue to use the nutrition labels on products and your *POINTSfinder*® slide or *POINTS* calculator to check *POINTS* values of foods.

Filling Foods and **SetPOINTS** values:

Food Lists include more than just *POINTS* values. In the lists you'll also find:

- Filling Foods identified by a ◆ green diamond
- **SetPOINTS** values in ( ) parentheses following the *POINTS* values

Table of Contents

Complete A-Z Food List 7

Complete Filling Foods List 75

Set*POINTS* Food List 91

Brand Name Foods List 95

    Baking Mixes, Ingredients & Doughs 96

    Beverages 108

    Bread & Baked Goods 146

    Breakfast, Cereals & Cereal Bars 182

    Candy, Cookies & Desserts 204

    Condiments, Sauces & Gravies 261

    Dairy & Eggs 281

    Fish & Seafood 314

Fruit 319

Jams, Spreads, Salsa & Dips 331

Meat & Poultry 345

Oils, Dressings & Seasonings 368

Pasta, Rice & Grains 385

Prepared Foods, Salads & Sides 397

Snacks 443

Soups, Stews & Chilis 494

Soy and Meat Substitutes 511

Vegetables 518

Weight Watchers® Food Products List 539

Index...547

Smart Ziploc® snack solutions!

Ziploc® BRAND

Portion control can be a challenge, but Ziploc® Brand products can help. They come in a variety of sizes that allow for endless combinations.

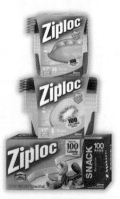

www.ziploc.com

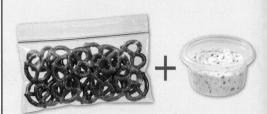

Dunk pretzels in cream cheese, spiced up with fresh herbs!

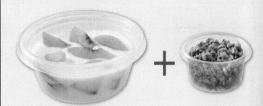

Top off a yogurt and peach parfait with crunchy granola!

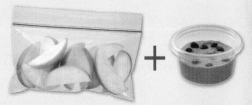

Dress up apples with peanut butter and cranberries!

©2009 S.C. Johnson & Son, Inc. All Rights Reserved. 727682

SC Johnson
A FAMILY COMPANY

Complete
A-Z Food List

POINTS® values help you make
smart food choices.

Use this list to find the *POINTS* values
for thousands of non-branded food items.

Complete A-Z Food List

A

	POINTS VALUE
All-fruit spread (spreadable fruit), 1 1/2 Tbsp	1
Almond butter, 1 Tbsp	3
Almond float, 1/2 cup	2
Almonds	
1 Tbsp sliced	1
23 nuts (1 oz)	4
1 cup sliced	19
1 cup whole	19
Ambrosia, 1/2 cup	2
Antelope, cooked, 1 oz	1
Apple	
baked, 1 large	7
candied, 1 large	10
caramel, 1 large	9
dried, 1/4 cup (3/4 oz)	1
♦ fresh, 1 small (2 1/2" diameter)	1 (2)
♦ fresh, 1 medium (2 3/4" diameter)	1 (2)
♦ fresh, 1 large (3 1/4" diameter)	2 (2)
Apple brown Betty, 1 cup	5
Apple cider, 1/2 cup	1
Apple crisp, 3/4 cup	8
Apple juice, 1/2 cup	1
Apple kuchen, 1 piece (30" square)	10
Apple streusel, 1/2 cup	4
♦ **Applesauce,** unsweetened, 1 cup	2
Apricots	
♦ canned or frozen, unsweetened, 1 cup	1 (2)
dried, 6 halves (3/4 oz)	1
♦ fresh, 3 medium (4 oz)	1 (2)

	POINTS VALUE
Armadillo, cooked, 1 oz	1
Arrowroot powder, 1 tsp	0
Arroz con gandules, 1 cup	8
Arroz con pollo, 3 oz chicken with 1 1/2 cup rice	13
♦ **Artichoke hearts,** cooked, 1 cup	1
Artichokes	
♦ cooked, 1 medium	0
marinated, 1/2 cup	3
stuffed, 1 (7 3/4 oz)	14
♦ **Arugula,** 1 cup	0
♦ **Asparagus,** cooked or uncooked, 1 cup or 12 spears	0
♦ **Avocado,** 1/4 medium (2 oz)	2

B

	POINTS VALUE
Baba au rhum, 1 (3 1/4 oz)	8
Baba ganosh, 1/4 cup	3
Bacon	
♦ **Canadian-style,** cooked, 1 slice (1 oz)	1 (5)
cooked, crisp, 1 slice	1
cooked, crisp, 3 slices	4
reduced-fat, cooked, crisp, 3 slices	3
turkey, cooked, crisp, 3 slices	2
Bacon bits, imitation, 1 tsp	0
Bacon fat, 1 Tbsp	3
Bagel	
any type, 1 mini (2 1/2" diameter)	1
any type, 1 small (3" diameter or 2 oz)	3
any type, 1/2 large (4 1/2" diameter or 2 oz)	3

	POINTS VALUE
Bagel with cream cheese and lox, 1 large (6 1/2 oz)	12
Bahamian macaroni and cheese, 1 cup	9
Bahamian style peas and rice, 1 cup	7
Baked Alaska, 1 piece (2" wedge or 1/12 of 9" cake)	5
Baking mix, buttermilk, 3 Tbsp	2
Baking powder, 1 tsp	0
Baking soda, 1 tsp	0
Baklava	
1 piece (2" square)	4
store-bought, 1 piece (2 oz)	5
Banana	
1 cup sliced	2 (2)
1 small (6 to 6 7/8" long)	1 (2)
1 medium (7 to 7 7/8" long)	2 (2)
1 large (8 to 8 7/8" long)	2 (2)
1 extra large (9" or larger)	2 (2)
Banana bread, with or without nuts, 1 slice (5" x 3/4")	5
Banana chips, 1 oz	3
Banana split, 3 scoops (1 1/2 cups) ice cream, 1 banana, 3 Tbsp syrup, and 1/2 cup whipped cream	19
Bananas Foster, 2 scoops (1 cup) ice cream, 1/2 banana and 1/3 cup sauce	16
Barley	
cooked, 1 cup	3 (6)
uncooked, 1/4 cup	3 (6)
Bay breeze, 1 (5 1/2 fl oz)	3
Bean and lentil stew (Dal maharani), 1 cup	6
Bean curd skin, 1 skin (25" x 26")	1

	POINTS VALUE
Beans	
black, and rice, 1 cup	4
black, cooked, 1/2 cup	2 (5)
black, with rice mix, prepared according to package directions, 1 cup	4
cannellini, canned, 1/2 cup	1 (5)
garbanzo, canned, 1/2 cup	1 (5)
garbanzo, cooked, 1/2 cup	2 (5)
garbanzo, dry, 1 pound	35 (5)
green, cooked, 1 cup	0
kidney, cooked, 1/2 cup	1 (5)
kidney, dry, 1 pound	30 (5)
lima, cooked, 1/2 cup	1 (5)
lima, dry, 1 pound	30 (5)
navy, cooked, 1/2 cup	2 (5)
navy, dry, 1 pound	30 (5)
pinto, cooked, 1/2 cup	2 (5)
pinto, dry, 1 pound	31 (5)
red, and rice, 1 cup	5
red, and rice mix, prepared according to package directions, 1 cup	5
soy, cooked, 1/2 cup	3 (5)
soy, dry, 1 pound	45 (5)
wax, cooked, 1 cup	0
white, cooked, 1/2 cup	2 (5)
white, dry, 1 pound	30 (5)
Beans, baked	
1/2 cup	5
canned, 1/2 cup	2
deli, 1/2 cup	3
fast-food, 1 serving (6 oz)	4
vegetarian, canned, 1/2 cup	2

Complete A-Z Food List

	POINTS VALUE	
Beans, refried		
1/2 cup	3	
black, canned, 1/2 cup	1	
black, low-fat or fat-free, canned, 1/2 cup	1	
◆ fat-free, canned, 1/2 cup	2	(5)
regular, canned, 1/2 cup	2	
with sausage, canned, 1/2 cup	5	
Beans and franks, 1 cup	11	
Bear, cooked, 1 oz	2	
Beaver, cooked, 1 oz	1	
Beef		
brisket, cooked, 1 slice (2 oz)	6	
brisket, cooked, 3 oz	9	
brisket, lean, trimmed, cooked, 1 slice (2 oz)	2	
brisket, lean, trimmed, cooked, 3 oz	4	
brisket, lean, trimmed, raw, 1 oz	1	
brisket, raw, 1 oz	2	
chuck, arm pot roast, cooked, 3 oz	6	
chuck, arm pot roast, trimmed, cooked, 3 oz	6	
chuck, blade roast, cooked, 3 oz	7	
chuck, blade roast, trimmed, cooked, 3 oz	7	
corned, canned, 1 slice (2 oz)	3	
corned, cooked, 3 oz	6	
corned, raw, 1 oz	1	
cube steak, cooked, 3 oz	4	
◆ cube steak, trimmed, cooked, 1/2 cup (2 oz)	3	(5)
◆ cube steak, trimmed, cooked, 3 oz	4	(5)

	POINTS VALUE	
filet mignon, cooked, 3 oz	7	
filet mignon, cooked, 1 small (4 oz)	10	
◆ filet mignon, trimmed, cooked, 3 oz	4	(5)
◆ filet mignon, trimmed, cooked, 1 small (4 oz)	6	(5)
flank steak, cooked, 1 slice (2 oz)	2	
flank steak, cooked, 3 oz	4	
◆ flank, lean only, trimmed, cooked, 1 slice (2 oz)	2	(5)
◆ flank, lean only, cooked, 3 oz	4	(5)
◆ heart, cooked, 1 oz	1	(5)
KC strip, cooked, 3 oz	5	
KC strip, cooked, 1 small (4 oz)	7	
◆ KC strip, trimmed, cooked, 3 oz	4	(5)
◆ KC strip, trimmed, cooked, 1 small (4 oz)	5	(5)
◆ kidney, cooked, 1 oz	1	(5)
◆ liver, cooked, 1 slice or 1/2 cup (2 oz)	2	(5)
New York steak, cooked, 3 oz	6	
New York steak, cooked, 1 small (4 oz)	8	
◆ New York steak, trimmed, cooked, 3 oz	4	(5)
◆ New York steak, trimmed, cooked, 1 small (4 oz)	5	(5)
porterhouse steak, cooked, 3 oz	7	
◆ porterhouse steak, trimmed, cooked, 3 oz	6	(5)
rib eye, trimmed, cooked, 3 oz	5	
rib, small end, trimmed, cooked, 3 oz	5	
rib, large end, cooked, 3 oz	7	
rib, large end, trimmed, cooked, 3 oz	7	
round steak or roast, cooked, 3 oz	5	
◆ round steak or roast, trimmed, cooked, 3 oz	4	(5)

		POINTS VALUE			POINTS VALUE
◆	rump roast, trimmed, cooked, 1 slice (2 oz)	2 (5)		80% lean/20% fat, cooked, 1 patty (3 oz)	5
◆	rump roast, trimmed, cooked, 3 oz	3 (5)		80% lean/20% fat, cooked, 12 oz (1 pound raw)	21
	shortribs, cooked, 3 oz	11		85% lean/15% fat, raw, 1 oz	2
	shortribs, trimmed, cooked, 1 piece (3 oz)	6		85% lean/15% fat, cooked, 1/2 cup (2 oz)	3
	sirloin, cooked, 3 oz	5		85% lean/15% fat, cooked, 1 patty (3 oz)	5
◆	sirloin, trimmed, cooked, 1 slice (2 oz)	2 (5)		85% lean/15% fat, cooked, 12 oz (1 pound raw)	19
◆	sirloin, trimmed, cooked, 3 oz	3 (5)		90% lean/10% fat, raw, 1 oz	1
◆	steak, lean, cooked (round or loin cuts with all visible fat trimmed), 1 small (4 oz)	5 (5)		90% lean/10% fat, cooked, 1/2 cup (2 oz)	3
	steak, regular, cooked, 1 small (4 oz)	10		90% lean/10% fat, cooked, 1 patty (3 oz)	4
	strip sirloin, cooked, 3 oz	5		90% lean/10% fat, cooked, 12 oz (1 pound raw)	23
	strip sirloin, cooked, 1 small (4 oz)	7	◆	95% lean/5% fat, raw, 1 oz	1 (5)
◆	strip sirloin, trimmed, cooked, 3 oz	3 (5)	◆	95% lean/5% fat, cooked, 1/2 cup (2 oz)	2 (5)
◆	strip sirloin, trimmed, cooked, 1 small (4 oz)	4 (5)	◆	95% lean/5% fat, cooked, 1 patty (3 oz)	3 (5)
	T-bone steak, cooked, 3 oz	7	◆	95% lean/5% fat, cooked, 12 oz (1 pound raw)	13 (5)
	T-bone steak, cooked, 1 small (4 oz)	9		regular, 75% lean/25% fat cooked, 12 oz (1 pound raw)	22
◆	T-bone steak, trimmed, cooked, 3 oz	5 (5)		regular, 75% lean/25% fat, cooked, 1/2 cup	4
◆	T-bone steak, trimmed, cooked, 1 small (4 oz)	7 (5)		regular, 75% lean/25% fat, cooked, 1 patty (3 oz)	5
	tenderloin, cooked, 1 slice (2 oz)	5		**Beef, jerky or stick,** 1 oz	3
	tenderloin, cooked, 3 oz	7		**Beef, orange-ginger,** 1 cup	11
◆	tenderloin, trimmed, cooked, 1 slice (2 oz)	3 (5)		**Beef, sliced, with gravy**	
◆	tenderloin, trimmed, cooked, 3 oz	4 (5)		canned, 1/2 cup	6
◆	tongue, cooked, 1 oz	2 (5)		frozen, 2 slices with gravy (4 3/4 oz)	2
	Beef, ground				
	80% lean/20% fat, raw, 1 oz	2			
	80% lean/20% fat, cooked, 1/2 cup (2 oz)	4			

Complete A-Z Food List

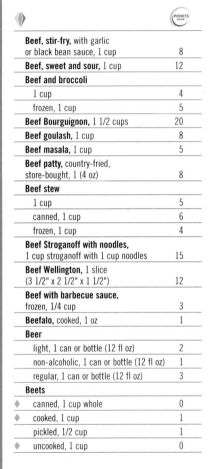

	POINTS VALUE
Beef, stir-fry, with garlic or black bean sauce, 1 cup	8
Beef, sweet and sour, 1 cup	12
Beef and broccoli	
1 cup	4
frozen, 1 cup	5
Beef Bourguignon, 1 1/2 cups	20
Beef goulash, 1 cup	8
Beef masala, 1 cup	5
Beef patty, country-fried, store-bought, 1 (4 oz)	8
Beef stew	
1 cup	5
canned, 1 cup	6
frozen, 1 cup	4
Beef Stroganoff with noodles, 1 cup stroganoff with 1 cup noodles	15
Beef Wellington, 1 slice (3 1/2" x 2 1/2" x 1 1/2")	12
Beef with barbecue sauce, frozen, 1/4 cup	3
Beefalo, cooked, 1 oz	1
Beer	
light, 1 can or bottle (12 fl oz)	2
non-alcoholic, 1 can or bottle (12 fl oz)	1
regular, 1 can or bottle (12 fl oz)	3
Beets	
canned, 1 cup whole	0
cooked, 1 cup	1
pickled, 1/2 cup	1
uncooked, 1 cup	0

	POINTS VALUE
Beignet	
1 (2")	2
from mix, prepared, 1	3
Bellini, 1 (6 fl oz)	2
Benny cake, 1 piece (2" x 3")	3
Berries	
mixed, 1 cup	1
wheat, uncooked, 1/4 cup	2
Beverage mix, sweet and sour, 1/2 cup	2
Bhuna gosht, 1 cup	8
Bialy, 1 (3 oz)	5
Biryani, chicken, 1 cup	9
Biscotti	
chocolate, 1 regular, 2 small, or 8 mini (1 oz)	3
fat-free, 1 regular, 2 small, or 8 mini (1 oz)	2
plain, 8 mini, 2 small, or 1 regular (1 oz)	3
Biscuit	
cheese, 1 (2" diameter)	5
homemade, 1 small (2" diameter)	3
refrigerated, baked, 1 small (2 1/2" diameter) or 1/2 large (1 oz)	2
Biscuit mix, buttermilk, dry, reduced fat, 1 serving (1/4-1/3 cup)	3
Bison, lean, all visible fat trimmed, cooked, 3 oz	3 (5)
Bistec de palomilla (Cuban fried steak), 1 steak (6 oz)	10
Bittermelon (balsam-pear pods), cooked or uncooked, 1 cup	0
Black Russian, 1 (3 fl oz)	5

	POINTS VALUE	
Blackberries, 1 cup	1	(2)
Blanquette of veal, 2 cups	13	
Blintz		
cheese, 1 (4 3/4 oz)	5	
cheese, frozen, 1 (2 1/4 oz)	2	
fruit, frozen, 1 (2 1/4 oz)	2	
potato, frozen, 1 (2 1/4 oz)	2	
Blood pudding (blood sausage), 1 oz	3	
Bloody Mary, 1 (5 fl oz)	2	
Blueberries, 1 cup	1	(2)
Bok choy, uncooked, 1 cup	0	
Bologna, beef or pork, 1 slice (1 oz)	2	
Borscht		
1 cup with 2 Tbsp sour cream	4	
low-calorie, store-bought, 1 cup	0	
store-bought, 1 cup	2	
Boston brown bread, 1 slice (3 3/4" x 1/2")	2	
Boudin, store-bought, 2 oz	2	
Bouillabaisse, 2 cups	7	
Bouillon		
any type except court, 1 cup	0	
court, 1 cup	3	
cube, beef, chicken, or vegetable, 1/2 cube	0	
granules, beef, 1 tsp	0	
Boysenberries, fresh or frozen, unsweetened, 1 cup	1	(2)
Bran		
corn, uncooked, 1/4 cup	0	
oat, uncooked, 1/4 cup	1	
rice, uncooked, 1/4 cup	2	
wheat, uncooked, 1/4 cup	0	

	POINTS VALUE	
Brandy, 1 jigger (1 1/2 fl oz)	2	
Brandy Alexander, 1 (3 fl oz)	6	
Bratwurst, cooked, 2 oz	5	
Brazil nuts, 8 nuts (1 oz shelled)	5	
Bread		
any type (white, wheat, rye, Italian, French, pumpernickel), 1 slice (1 oz)	2	
cocktail (party-style), any type, 2 slices (3/4 oz)	1	
high fiber (3 g or more dietary fiber per slice), 1 slice (1 oz)	1	
Indian (Navajo) fry, 1 (5" diameter)	6	
reduced-calorie, any type, 2 slices (1 1/2 oz)	1	
Bread crumbs, dried		
plain, 3 Tbsp	2	
plain, 1/4 cup	2	
seasoned, 3 Tbsp	2	
seasoned, 1/4 cup	3	
Bread crumbs, panko		
1 Tbsp	0	
1/2 cup	2	
Bread crumbs, whole-wheat, 1/3 cup	1	
Breadfruit, uncooked, 1 cup	4	(2)
Breadsticks		
any type, 2 long (7 1/2" x 1/2"), 3/4 oz	2	
any type, 4 short (5" x 1/2"), or 3/4 oz	2	
soft, 1 (1 1/3 oz)	2	
Breakfast powder, instant, 1 envelope (35.5 g)	3	
Brioche, 1 slice (1 oz)	3	
Broccoli, cooked or uncooked, 1 cup	0	
Broccoli rice casserole, 1 cup	5	

Complete A-Z Food List

	POINTS VALUE
Broccoli stir fry, 1 cup	3
◆ **Broth, any type,** 1 cup	0
Broth, beef with tomato juice, 1 cup	2
Brownie	
1 (2" square)	5
fat-free, store-bought, 1 (1 1/2 oz)	2
low-fat, store-bought, 1 (1 1/2 oz)	3
Brunswick stew, 1 1/2 cups	5
Bruschetta, 1 slice (3 oz)	3
◆ **Brussels sprouts,** cooked or uncooked, 1 cup	0
Bubble & squeak, 1 cup	3
Bubble tea (milk tea), 1 cup	2
Buffalo wings	
3 (4 1/2 oz)	9
frozen (prepared without fat), 3 (3 oz)	4
◆ **Buffalo,** water, cooked or raw, 1 oz	1 (5)
Bulgogi (beef stir fry), 1 cup	5
Bulgur	
◆ cooked, 1 cup	2 (6)
◆ uncooked, 1/4 cup	2 (6)
Burgoo, 1 cup	4
Burrito	
bean, 1 small (6")	5
bean, 1 large (8")	8
bean, fast food, 1	7
bean and cheese, reduced-fat, store-bought, 1 (5 1/2 oz)	5
bean and cheese, store-bought, 1 (5 oz)	6
beef and bean, store-bought, 1 (5 oz)	8
beef and cheese, 1 small (6")	5
beef and cheese, 1 large (8")	8

	POINTS VALUE
beef or chicken and cheese, reduced-fat, store-bought, 1 small or 1/2 large (4 oz)	4
breakfast (egg, cheese and bacon, ham, or sausage), store-bought, 1 (3 1/2 oz)	5
chicken, store-bought, 1 (5 oz)	6
chicken and cheese, 1 small (6")	5
chicken and cheese, 1 large (8")	7
vegetable, 1 small (made with 6" tortilla)	5
vegetable, 1 large (made with 10" tortilla)	10
Butter	
light, 2 tsp	1
light, 1 Tbsp	2
regular, 1 tsp	1
regular, 1 cup	48
whipped, 1 tsp	1
whipped, 1 Tbsp	2
Butter chicken, 1 cup	8

C

	POINTS VALUE
Cabbage	
◆ all varieties, cooked or uncooked, 1 cup	0
stuffed, 2 (2" x 2 1/2")	6
Cake	
angel food, 1 slice (1/16 of 10" tube)	2
carrot, with cream cheese icing, 1/12 of 9" layer cake, or 3" square	16
coffee, 3" square, or 1/12 of 9" tube	8
coffee, fat-free, store-bought, 2 oz	3
coffee, store-bought, 2 oz	6
fat-free, store-bought, 1 slice (3 1/2 oz)	4

	POINTS VALUE
fruit, 1 slice (2 1/2" x 1 3/4" x 1/2"), or 2 oz	4
honey, 1 slice (5" x 3" x 1")	7
Passover sponge, 1/12 of 9" tube	3
pineapple upside-down, 2 1/2" square	5
pineapple upside-down, 1/8 of 10" skillet cake	10
pound, 1 slice (5" x 3" x 1")	8
pound, store-bought, 1 slice (2 1/2 oz)	6
snack, creme-filled, store-bought, 2 (2 1/4 oz)	5
sponge, 1/12 of 9" tube	3
sugar-free, store-bought, 1 slice (2 1/2 oz)	5
with icing, 1/12 of 9" layer cake or 3" square	12
with icing, store-bought, 3 oz	7
Cake mix, banana, dry, 1/3 cup	4
Cake mix, light, prepared, without icing, 1/12 of 9" cake	4
Calamari	
fried, 1/2 cup	11
♦ grilled, 1/2 cup	1 (5)
Calzone, ham and cheese, 1 (5 1/4" x 6")	12
Candy	
caramels, 1 oz	2
chocolate, any type, 1/2 bar, 2 assorted pieces, or 2 Tbsp chips (1 oz)	3
corn, 1 oz	2
cotton, 1 1/2 oz	3
gumdrops, 1 oz	2
hard, 1 oz	2
jelly beans, 10 (1 oz)	2

	POINTS VALUE
Cannelloni	
cheese, frozen, with tomato sauce, 7 oz	6
cheese, with meat sauce, 2 shells with 1/2 cup sauce	15
cheese, with tomato sauce, 2 shells with 1/2 cup sauce	12
meat, with cream sauce, 2 shells with 1/2 cup sauce	17
meat, with tomato sauce, 2 shells with 1/2 cup sauce	14
spinach and cheese, with cream sauce, 2 shells with 1/2 cup sauce	15
spinach and cheese, with tomato sauce, 2 shells with 1/2 cup sauce	12
Cannoli, 1 (3 1/2" long)	9
Cantaloupe	
♦ 10 balls or 1 cup	1 (2)
♦ 1 small (1 pound)	2 (2)
♦ 1 medium (5" diameter)	3 (2)
♦ 1/4 large (6 1/2" diameter)	1 (2)
Cape Cod, 1 (5 1/2 fl oz)	3
Capers, 1 Tbsp	0
Capon, cooked, with skin, without bone, 1 oz	2
Caponata (eggplant appetizer)	
1/4 cup	1
store-bought, 1/4 cup	2
Cappuccino	
♦ made with fat-free milk, 1 small (8 fl oz)	1
♦ made with fat-free milk, 1 tall (12 fl oz)	2
♦ made with fat-free milk, 1 grande (16 fl oz)	2
made with low-fat milk, 1 small (8 fl oz)	2

Complete A-Z Food List

	POINTS VALUE
made with low-fat milk, 1 tall (12 fl oz)	3
made with low-fat milk, 1 grande (16 fl oz)	3
made with whole milk, 1 small (8 fl oz)	2
made with whole milk, 1 tall (12 fl oz)	3
made with whole milk, 1 grande (16 fl oz)	4
ready-made, from machine, any flavor, 1 cup	2
Cappuccino mix, any flavor, 4 tsp	2
Caraway seeds, 1 Tbsp	0
Cardoon, 1 cup	0
Caribou, cooked, 1 oz	1
Carne asada, 4 oz	10
Carne guisado (Cuban beef stew),	
1 cup	5
7 oz	11
Carnitas, 1 cup	9
Carob, without sugar, 1 tsp	0
Carrots	
cooked, 1 cup	1
uncooked, 1 small, medium, or large, 1 cup, or 10 baby	0
Carrots and parsnips, 1 cup	4
Casaba melon, 1 cup	1 (2)
Cashew butter, 1 Tbsp	2
Cashew chicken, 3 oz chicken with 1/3 cup sauce	7
Cashews, 14 (1 oz)	4
Cassava (yucca), uncooked, 1 cup	6
Cassoulet, 1 cup	11

	POINTS VALUE
Cauliflower	
cooked or uncooked, 1 cup	0
1 small head (4" diameter)	1
1 medium head (5-6" diameter)	2
1 large head (6-7" diameter)	4
Cavatelli with sausage & broccoli, 1 cup	5
Caviar (fish roe)	
any type, 1 oz	2 (5)
spread, store-bought, 2 Tbsp	3
Celeriac	
cooked, 1 cup	0
uncooked, 1 cup	1
Celery, cooked or uncooked, 1 cup	0
Cereal, hot	
cream of rice, cooked, 1 cup	3
cream of wheat, cooked, 1 cup	2
farina, cooked, 1 cup	2
farina, uncooked, 1/4 cup	3
grits, corn, cooked, 1 cup	3
grits, corn, uncooked, 1/4 cup	3
in a cup, 1 (2 oz)	4
oatmeal, cooked, regular or instant, 1 cup	2
oatmeal, instant, flavored, 1 packet	3
oatmeal, uncooked, 1/4 cup	1
Cereal, granola	
1/2 cup	4
homemade, 1/2 cup	6
low-fat, 1/2 cup	3

	POINTS VALUE
Cereal, ready-to-eat	
any type (other than those listed here), 1 cup	2
bran flakes, 3/4 cup	1
bran flakes, 1 cup	2
fortified, 1 cup	2
frosted, 1 cup	3
nuggets, 1/2 cup	3
puffed, 1 cup	1
raisin bran, 3/4 cup	2
raisin bran, 1 cup	3
shredded wheat, 1 biscuit	1
wheat germ, 2 Tbsp	1
Cereal bar	
fat-free, 1 (1 1/2 oz)	2
regular, 1 (1 1/4 oz)	3
Ceviche, 1/2 cup	2
Challah bread, 1 slice (5" x 3" x 3/4")	2
Chalupa (pork & bean dish), 1 cup	6
Champagne, 1 small glass (4 fl oz)	2
Chana dal, 1 cup	4
Channa masala, 1 cup	7
Chapati, 1 piece (5" diameter)	2
Char shiu bao (roast pork bun), 1 (2 oz)	4
Chard, Swiss, cooked or uncooked, 1 cup	0
Cheese, blue, 1/4 cup (crumbled)	3
Cheese, brie, 1 oz	3
Cheese, camembert, 1 wedge (1 1/3 oz)	3
Cheese, Cheddar	
1 slice (1 oz)	3
fat-free, shredded, 1/4 cup	1
Cheese, colby, 1 slice (1 oz)	3

	POINTS VALUE
Cheese, cottage	
fat-free, 1 cup	3
fat-free, with fruit, 1 cup	4
low-fat (1%), 1 cup	3
low-fat (1%), with fruit, 1 cup	5
reduced-fat (2%), 1 cup	4
regular (4%), 1 cup	5
regular, with fruit, 1 cup	5
Cheese, cream	
fat-free, 1/4 cup	1
fat-free, 8 oz	5
light, 1 Tbsp	1
regular, 1 Tbsp	1
regular, 8 oz	22
soy, 2 Tbsp	2
whipped, 1 Tbsp	1
Cheese, feta, 1/4 cup crumbled or 1 1/3 oz	3
Cheese, farmer, 1 oz	2
Cheese, fontina	
1 cup diced	14
1 cup shredded	11
1 slice (1 oz)	3
Cheese, goat	
hard type, 1 oz	3
semisoft type, 1 cup	12
semisoft type, 1 oz	3
semisoft type, 1 Tbsp	1
soft type, 1 oz	2
soft type, 1 Tbsp	1
Cheese, gorgonzola, 1 oz	3
Cheese, gouda, 1 oz	3

Complete A-Z Food List

	POINTS VALUE
Cheese, gruyere, 1 slice (1 oz)	3
Cheese, hard or semisoft, fat-free	
1 cube (1"), 3 Tbsp grated, or 4 Tbsp shredded (1 oz)	1
1 slice (3/4 oz)	1
Cheese, hard or semisoft, low-fat	
1 cube (1"), 3 Tbsp grated, or 4 Tbsp shredded (1 oz)	2
1 slice (3/4 oz)	1
Cheese, hard or semisoft, regular (except soy)	
1 cube (1"), 3 Tbsp grated, or 4 Tbsp shredded (1 oz)	3
1 slice (3/4 oz)	2
Cheese, hard or semisoft, regular, soy	
1 cube (1"), 3 Tbsp grated, or 4 Tbsp shredded (1 oz)	2
1 slice (3/4 oz)	1
Cheese, havarti, 1 oz	3
Cheese, Mexican	
queso anejo, 1 cup crumbled	13
queso asadero, 1 cup shredded	11
queso chihuahua, 1 cup shredded	11
Cheese, Monterey, 1 slice (1 oz)	3
Cheese, mozzarella	
fat-free, shredded, 1 oz	1
part skim, 1 oz	2
whole milk, 1 cup shredded	8
Cheese, muenster, 1 slice (1 oz)	3
Cheese, Neufchatel (reduced-fat cream cheese), 1 Tbsp (1/2 oz)	1

	POINTS VALUE
Cheese, Parmesan	
2 Tbsp grated	1
1/4 cup grated	3
1 cup grated	11
1 oz	3
Cheese, pasteurized process, Swiss, 1 oz	2
Cheese, pot, 1 cup	3
Cheese, provolone, 1 slice (1 oz)	3
Cheese, ricotta	
fat-free, 1/2 cup	2
part-skim, 1/2 cup	4
whole milk, 1/2 cup	6
whole milk, 1 cup	11
Cheese, Romano, 1 oz	**3**
Cheese, Roquefort, 1 oz	3
Cheese, squares, mini, regular, 1 oz	3
Cheese, Swiss, 1 cup shredded	11
Cheese ball, store-bought, 2 Tbsp	2
Cheese puffs, hot, 2 (1/2 oz each)	2
Cheese spread	
American, process, 2 Tbsp	2
pasteurized process, American, 1 oz	2
Cheese sticks, breaded, prepared without fat, store-bought, 2 (1 oz)	2
Cheese straws, 2 (2" long each)	2
Cheese twists or balls, 1 1/2 cups (1 oz)	4
Cheeseburger on bun	
fast food, small, 1	7
fast food, large, 1	13
fast food, double, 1	11

	POINTS
fast food, double, with bacon, 1	19
microwave, frozen, 1 (4 3/4 oz)	9
microwave, with bacon, 1	11
plain, without mayonnaise, lettuce, and tomato, 1	11
Cheesecake	
any type, fast food, 1 serving	8
frozen, 1 slice (4 oz)	9
with or without fruit topping, 1/16 of 10" cake	10
Cherries	
chocolate-covered, 2 (1 oz)	2
dried, 1/4 cup (1 1/2 oz)	2
fresh, 1 cup	1 (2)
maraschino, 1	0
Chestnuts, European	
uncooked, 6 (2 oz)	2
roasted, 10 (3 oz)	3
Chicken, blackened, 1 breast (3 oz)	7
Chicken, broiler or fryer, roasted, with skin (without bone), 1/2 (10 1/2 oz)	18
Chicken, buffalo wings	
3 (4 1/2 oz)	9
frozen (prepared without fat), 3 (3 oz)	4
Chicken, canned, 1/2 cup (4 oz)	4 (5)
Chicken, fried	
frozen, 3 oz	7
skinless, frozen, 3 oz	5
Chicken, ground	
cooked, 1/2 cup	3 (5)
cooked, 1 patty (3 oz)	5 (5)
cooked, 12 oz (1 pound raw)	20 (5)

	POINTS
Chicken, nugget-style	
fried, fast food, 6	8
pieces, fried, 6 (2" x 3/4" each)	8
pieces, frozen, 6 (2" x 3/4" each)	6
pieces, frozen, fat-free, 3 (3 oz)	2
Chicken, sesame, 1 cup	9
Chicken, sweet and sour, 1 cup	10
Chicken, skinless, fried, frozen, 1 3 oz	5
Chicken a la king, 1 cup	12
Chicken adobo, 1 thigh (4 oz)	6
Chicken and broccoli, 1 cup	2
Chicken and dumplings	
canned, 1 cup	5
cooked, with skin, 3 oz chicken with 2 dumplings	8
cooked, without skin, 3 oz chicken with 2 dumplings	7
frozen, 1 cup	5
Chicken and meatball fricassee, 2 cups	9
Chicken asopao, 1 cup with 1 piece chicken	8
Chicken breast	
barbecued, with skin and bone, 1 (4 1/2 oz)	6
cooked, without skin and bone, 1 (3 oz)	3 (5)
cooked, without skin (with bone), 1 (4 1/2 oz)	3 (5)
cooked, with skin, without bone, 1 (3 oz)	4
cooked, with skin and bone, 1 (4 1/2 oz)	5
fillet, breaded, frozen, prepared without fat, 3 oz	5
fillet, grilled, 1 (3 oz)	2 (5)

Complete A-Z Food List

Chicken breast (cont'd)	POINTS VALUE	
five spice, with skin and bone, 1 (4 1/2 oz)	7	
fried, with skin and bone, 1 (4 1/2 oz)	11	
fried, with skin, without bone, 1 (5 1/2 oz)	10	
frozen, stuffed with long grain and wild rice, 1 (6 oz)	5	
grilled, on bun, 1 (6 1/4 oz)	9	
patty, breaded, fat-free, prepared without fat, 1 (2 1/2 oz)	1	
stuffed with vegetables and cheese, frozen, 1 (6 oz)	6	
Chicken cacciatore, 1/2 breast or 1 thigh and leg (6 1/2 oz)	10	
Chicken cordon bleu		
1 piece (5 1/2 oz)	13	
frozen, 1 (6 3/4 oz)	10	
Chicken cutlet, pan-fried, 4 oz	7	
Chicken drumstick		
barbecued, with skin and bone, 1 (1 1/2 oz)	2	
cooked, with skin and bone, 1 (1 1/2 oz)	2	
cooked, with skin, without bone, 1 (1 oz)	1	
◆ cooked, without skin and bone, 1 (1 oz)	1	(5)
◆ cooked, without skin, with bone, 1 (1 1/2 oz)	1	(5)
fried, with skin and bone, 1 (1 1/2 oz)	5	
fried, with skin, fast food, 1	4	
◆ **Chicken giblets,** cooked, 1/2 cup chopped or diced	3	(5)
◆ **Chicken gizzard,** cooked, 1 oz	1	(5)
◆ **Chicken heart,** cooked, 1 oz	1	(5)
Chicken hekka, 1 cup	6	

	POINTS VALUE	
Chicken in barbecue sauce, frozen, 1/4 cup	3	
Chicken in the pot, without skin, 2 cups	10	
Chicken jalfrezi, 1 cup	6	
Chicken Kiev		
1 (4" x 8")	18	
frozen, 1 (6 oz)	8	
Chicken leg		
five spice, 1 leg (thigh and drumstick, with skin and bone)	9	
roasted, with skin and bone, 1 leg (3 1/2 oz)	4	
◆ **Chicken liver,** cooked, 1/2 cup (2 oz)	2	(5)
Chicken marsala, 4 oz chicken without bone, with sauce	15	
Chicken mole, 1 cup	8	
Chicken paprika, 1 breast or thigh with 1/2 cup sauce	7	
Chicken parmigiana		
patty, store-bought, 1 patty with sauce(5 oz)	6	
with sauce, 5 oz with 1/2 cup sauce	10	
without sauce, 5 1/2 oz	8	
Chicken patty, fried, frozen, 1 (2 1/2 oz)	4	
Chicken pilaf (Kotta pilafi), 13 1/2 oz	11	
Chicken sausage, cooked, 1 1/2 oz	2	
Chicken stew, canned, 1 cup	5	
Chicken stir-fry		
prepared without fat, 1 cup	3	
with garlic or black bean sauce, 1 cup	7	
Chicken subgum chow mein, 1 cup	4	
Chicken tetrazzini, 1 1/2 cups	14	

	POINTS VALUE
Chicken thigh	
barbecued, with skin and bone, 1 (1 oz)	5
cooked, with skin and bone, 1 (3 oz)	4
cooked, with skin, without bone, 1 (2 oz)	4
◆ cooked, without skin and bone, 1 (2 oz)	3 (5)
◆ cooked, without skin (with bone), 1 (3 oz)	3 (5)
fried, with skin and bone, 1 (3 oz)	7
fried, with skin, fast food, 1	8
Chicken tikka, 4 oz	5
Chicken wing	
cooked, with skin and bone, 1 (1 1/2 oz)	3
fried, with skin, fast food, 1	6
Chicken with cashews, 1 cup	9
◆ **Chicory (curly endive),** 1 cup	0
Chiffon pie, 1/8 of 9" one-crust pie	9
Chile beef (Neua pad prik), 1 cup	6
Chili	
bean, in a cup, 1 (2 oz)	3
low-fat, canned, 1 cup	5
turkey, with beans, canned, 1 cup	4
turkey, without beans, canned, 1 cup	3
vegetarian, low-fat or fat-free, canned, 1 cup	3
with beans, canned, 1 cup	6
without beans, canned, 1 cup	4
without beans, frozen, 1 cup	12
Chili con carne	
with beans, 1 cup	8
without beans, 1 cup	8
Chili con queso	
1/4 cup	5
canned, 1/4 cup	2
frozen, 1/4 cup	5

	POINTS VALUE
Chili dog on roll, 1 (8 1/3 oz)	10
Chili fish (Macher jhol), 1 fillet (6 oz)	12
Chili mac, canned, 1 cup	5
Chili rellenos, beef and cheese, without sauce, 2 (7 1/2 oz)	18
Chimichanga	
beef, 1 (3" x 3 1/2")	11
beef or chicken, with beans, frozen, 1 (6 1/2 oz)	8
chicken, 1 (3" x 3 1/2")	9
Chinese pepper steak, 1 cup	5
Chinese vegetables	
with beef, 1 cup	6
with chicken, 1 cup	5
with pork, 1 cup	7
with shrimp, 1 cup	4
with tofu, 1 cup	4
◆ with peas, prepared without oil, 1 cup	2
Chips, bagel	
1 oz	3
fat-free, 1 oz	2
◆ **Chitterlings,** cooked, 1 oz	2 (5)
Chocolate	
any type, 1/2 bar, 2 assorted pieces, or 2 Tbsp chips (1 oz)	3
drink, 1 cup	3
mousse, 1 cup	12
spread, 2 Tbsp	4
Chocolate martini, 1 (4 fl oz)	7
Cholent, 1 cup	4
Chop suey	
beef, 1 cup	5
chicken, 1 cup	4

Complete A-Z Food List

	POINTS VALUE	
Chop suey (cont'd)		
pork, 1 cup	4	
vegetable, 1 cup	4	
Chow fun		
beef, 1 cup	7	
chicken, 1 cup	7	
pork, 1 cup	7	
shrimp, 1 cup	7	
Chow mein		
beef, 1 cup	5	
beef, chicken, or pork, canned, 1 cup	1	
chicken, 1 cup	4	
pork, 1 cup	5	
Chruscik, 1 (6 g)	1	
Chuleta, 1 pork chop (6 oz)	10	
Chutney, any type, 2 Tbsp	1	
Cinnamon bun, 1 large (4 oz)	6	
Cioppino, 2 cups	13	
Clams, baked, 6 (2 1/2 oz)	7	
Clams, fried, 1 cup	11	
Clementine		
♦ 2 small (3 oz each)	1	(2)
♦ 1 large (6 oz)	1	(2)
Club soda, 1 can or bottle (12 fl oz)	0	
Cobbler, fruit,		
any type, 1 cup	10	
frozen, 4 1/2 oz	6	
Cocoa, hot, instant		
fat-free, sugar-free,1 envelope (17 g)	1	
fat-free, sugar-free,1 Tbsp	0	
fat-free, sugar-free, prepared, 6 fl oz	1	

	POINTS VALUE
regular, prepared, 6 fl oz (1 oz packet with 6 fl oz water)	2
Cocoa, unsweetened, 3 Tbsp	0
Coconut, packaged, shredded	
1 tsp	0
1 cup	8
Coconut cream, canned, 1/4 cup	15
Coconut custard pie, 1/8 of 9" one-crust pie	9
Coconut meat	
dried, without sugar, 1 oz	4
uncooked, 1 cup shredded	7
Coconut milk	
canned, 1/4 cup	3
light, 1/4 cup	1
Coconut rice	
Indian, 1 cup	5
Thai, 1 cup	8
Coconut shrimp, 4 jumbo (7 1/3 oz)	16
Coffee, black, without sugar, 1 cup	0
Coffee drink	
Jamaican, store-bought, 1 cup	2
with milk, canned, 1 (10 fl oz)	4
Coffee mix, flavored, sugar-free or with sugar, prepared, 1 cup	1
Coffee substitute or cereal beverage, powder, 1 tsp	0
Cognac, 1 jigger (1 1/2 fl oz)	2
Colcannon, 1 cup	7
Coleslaw, 1/2 cup	4
♦ **Collards,** cooked or uncooked, 1 cup	0
Conch, cracked, 1 (6" long x 3")	9

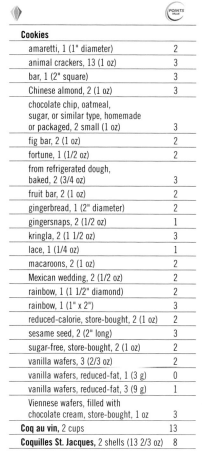

Cookies	POINTS VALUE	
amaretti, 1 (1" diameter)	2	
animal crackers, 13 (1 oz)	3	
bar, 1 (2" square)	3	
Chinese almond, 2 (1 oz)	3	
chocolate chip, oatmeal, sugar, or similar type, homemade or packaged, 2 small (1 oz)	3	
fig bar, 2 (1 oz)	2	
fortune, 1 (1/2 oz)	2	
from refrigerated dough, baked, 2 (3/4 oz)	3	
fruit bar, 2 (1 oz)	2	
gingerbread, 1 (2" diameter)	2	
gingersnaps, 2 (1/2 oz)	1	
kringla, 2 (1 1/2 oz)	3	
lace, 1 (1/4 oz)	1	
macaroons, 2 (1 oz)	2	
Mexican wedding, 2 (1/2 oz)	2	
rainbow, 1 (1 1/2" diamond)	2	
rainbow, 1 (1" x 2")	3	
reduced-calorie, store-bought, 2 (1 oz)	2	
sesame seed, 2 (2" long)	3	
sugar-free, store-bought, 2 (1 oz)	2	
vanilla wafers, 3 (2/3 oz)	2	
vanilla wafers, reduced-fat, 1 (3 g)	0	
vanilla wafers, reduced-fat, 3 (9 g)	1	
Viennese wafers, filled with chocolate cream, store-bought, 1 oz	3	
Coq au vin, 2 cups	13	
Coquilles St. Jacques, 2 shells (13 2/3 oz)	8	

Corn	POINTS VALUE	
◆ baby (ears), 1 cup	1	(6)
breaded, prepared without fat, 6 (3 oz)	4	
cream-style, 1 cup	3	
◆ kernels, cooked, 1 cup	2	(6)
Corn bread		
1 piece (2" square)	3	
dressing, 1 cup	8	
Mexican, 1 piece (1/12 of 10" round or 3 1/3 oz)	7	
Corn cake, sweet, 1/2 cup	8	
Corn casserole, 1/2 cup	8	
Corn chips, 30 small or 10 large (1 oz)	4	
Corn dog, 1 (2 3/4 oz)	5	
Corn flake crumbs, 1/2 cup	3	
Corn nuts, 1/2 cup	4	
Corn on the cob		
◆ 1 small (5 1/2")	1	(6)
◆ 1 medium (7")	1	(6)
◆ 1 large (8")	2	(6)
Corn on the grill, with butter, 1 (4 oz)	4	
Corn pudding, home-prepared, 1 cup	6	
Corned beef, canned, 1 slice (2 oz)	4	
Cornish hen		
cooked, with skin, 1/2 (4 1/2 oz)	9	
◆ cooked, without skin, 1/2 (3 3/4 oz)	3	(5)
Cornmeal		
◆ cooked, 1 cup	2	(6)
◆ dry, 2 Tbsp	1	(6)
mix, self-rising, 2 Tbsp (3/4 oz)	1	

Complete A-Z Food List

	POINTS VALUE	
Cornstarch		
2 Tbsp	1	
1 cup	10	
Cosmopolitan, 1 (3 1/2 fl oz)	4	
Couscous (semolina)		
cooked, 1 cup	3	
in a cup, 1 (2 oz)	4	
uncooked, 1/4 cup	3	
Couscous, whole-wheat		
cooked, 1 cup	3	(6)
uncooked, 1 tsp	0	(6)
uncooked, 1 Tbsp	1	(6)
uncooked, 1/4 cup	3	(6)
Crab, deviled, 1/2 cup	4	
Crab cakes, 2 (2 1/4 oz each, or 3" round)	4	
Crab puffs, 6 (1 1/2" rounds)	5	
Crab Rangoon		
1 large (4 1/2") or 5 mini	5	
frozen, 8 (5 1/4 oz)	9	
Crabapple, 1 cup (slices)	2	(2)
Cracker meal, 1/4 cup	2	
Crackers		
any type (other than those listed here), 1 oz	3	
arare, 50 (1 oz)	2	
cheese squares, mini, reduced-fat, 1 oz	3	
fat-free, 7 (3/4 oz)	1	
graham, 2 (2 1/2" square)	1	
graham, chocolate-coated, 2 (2 1/2" square)	3	
graham, mini, any variety, 3/4 oz	2	
oyster, 1 cup	4	

	POINTS VALUE	
saltines, 4	1	
saltines, 6	2	
snack, 1 oz	3	
snack, with filling (cheese, wheat, rye, toast, or wafer crackers with cheese, peanut butter, or cream cheese filling), 6 (1 1/2 oz)	5	
Cranberries		
dried, 1/4 cup (1 oz)	2	
fresh, 1 1/2 cups (5 oz)	1	(2)
Cranberry juice cocktail		
low-calorie, 1 cup	1	
regular, 1/2 cup	1	
Cranberry sauce, canned, 1/4 cup	2	
Crawfish pie, 1/8 of 9" pie	13	
Cream		
clotted (English double devon cream), 2 Tbsp	4	
half and half, 2 Tbsp	1	
light, 2 Tbsp	2	
Cream pie		
with or without fruit, 1/8 of 9" one-crust pie	9	
with or without fruit, frozen, 1 slice (4 3/4 oz)	10	
Cream puff, 1 (2 oz)	7	
Cream, sour		
fat-free, 1/4 cup	1	
light, 2 Tbsp	1	
light, 3 Tbsp	1	
reduced-fat, 2 Tbsp	1	
regular, 1 Tbsp	1	
regular, 1 cup	14	

	POINTS VALUE
Cream, whipped	
aerosol, 1/4 cup	1
dairy or nondairy, frozen, 2 Tbsp	1
dairy or nondairy, frozen, 1/4 cup	1
homemade, no sugar added, 1/4 cup	3
Cream, whipping	
heavy, 2 Tbsp	3
heavy, 1/2 cup	12
light, 2 Tbsp	3
Creamed chipped beef, 1 cup	11
Creamed chipped chicken, 1 cup	11
Creamed chipped turkey, 1 cup	11
Creamer	
fat-free, 1 Tbsp	0
fat-free, 1/4 cup	1
fat-free, liquid, flavored, 2 Tbsp	1
nondairy, liquid, 2 Tbsp	1
nondairy, powder, 1 Tbsp	1
Creme brulee, 3/4 cup	11
Creme caramel, 1 cup	7
Creme fraiche, 2 Tbsp	3
Creole	
chicken, without rice, 1 cup	6
shrimp, store-bought, 1 cup	5
shrimp, without rice, 1 cup	4
Crepes	
1 (6" diameter)	2
chicken, 2 (10 1/2 oz)	12
seafood, 2 (11 oz)	11
Suzette, 2 (4 3/4 oz)	10
Crispbreads	
1 (3/4 oz)	1
5 thin (3/4 oz)	1

	POINTS VALUE	
Croissant		
chocolate filled, 1 (5" long)	6	
plain, 1 (5" long)	5	
Croque monsieur, 1 (6 1/2 oz)	11	
Croquettes		
beef, 2 (2 1/2 oz each)	10	
chicken, 2 (2 1/2 oz each)	9	
Croutons		
homemade, 1/2 cup	3	
packaged, fat-free, 1/2 cup	2	
packaged, regular, 1/2 cup	3	
Cruller		
1 (2 oz)	6	
French, glazed, 1 (3" diameter)	4	
glazed, 1 (4" diameter)	6	
glazed, 1 long (approximately 5 1/4" x 2 1/2" x 1 1/2" high)	8	
Crumbs, graham cracker, 2 Tbsp (1/2 oz)	1	
Crumpet, 1 (3" diameter)	3	
◆ **Cucumber,** 1 cup	0	
Cupcake, creme-filled, store-bought, 1 (1 3/4 oz)	4	
Currants		
dried, 1/4 cup (1 1/2 oz)	2	
◆ fresh, 1 1/2 cups	1	(2)
Curry		
African, fish, 1/2 cup	6	
African, shrimp, 1/2 cup	6	
beef, 1 cup	10	
Bengali fish, 1 fillet (4 1/2 oz) and 1 cup vegetables	10	
chicken, 1 cup	10	

Complete A-Z Food List

Curry (cont'd)

	POINTS VALUE
green chicken (Gaeng Kheow Wan Gai), 1 cup	7
lamb, 1 cup	10
Curry goat, 4 oz	5
Curry paste	
green, 1/4 cup	1
panang, 1/4 cup	1
Thai, 1 Tbsp	1
Custard, 1 cup	8
Custard pie, 1/8 of 9" one-crust pie	8

D

	POINTS VALUE
Daikon, cooked or uncooked, 1 cup	0
Daiquiri, 1 (3 fl oz)	2
Daiquiri mix, 1/2 cup	3
Dairy shake, reduced calorie, 1 packet (3/4 oz)	2
Dandelion greens, cooked or uncooked, 1 cup	0
Danish	
fast food, 1	8
store-bought, 1 (2 1/4 oz)	6
Date-nut bread, 1 slice (5" x 1/2")	5
Dates	
dried, 5 medium or 1/4 cup	2
fresh, 2 (3/4 oz)	1 (2)
Dhansak, 1 cup	6
Dim sum	
bean curd roll with shrimp and vegetables, 1 (5" long x 2" wide)	2
bean curd roll with vegetables, 1 (5" long x 1.5" wide)	2

	POINTS VALUE
sesame seed balls, 1 (3" x 3")	5
Dip	
any type (other than those listed here), 2 Tbsp	2
artichoke, baked, 1/4 cup	6
bean, fat-free, 1/2 cup	1
black bean, fat-free, 2 Tbsp	0
Mexican 7-layer, 1/2 cup	3
spinach, 1/4 cup	5
Dolma	
4 (3 1/2 oz)	4
store-bought, 4 (3 1/2 oz)	3
Donair, 4 oz meat with onion, tomato and 2 Tbsp sauce	14
Doro wat, 1 cup	7
Doughnut	
any type (other than those listed here), store-bought, 1 (2 oz)	5
cake-type, 1 (3 1/2" diameter)	6
cake-type, sugared or glazed, 1 (3 1/2" diameter)	6
cake-type, with icing, 1 (3 1/2" diameter)	6
holes, yeast, glazed, 2 (1 oz)	2
mini, chocolate-covered, store-bought, 3-4 doughnuts (2 oz)	7
mini, powdered, sugar-covered, store-bought, 3-4 doughnuts (2 oz)	6
with creme filling, 1 (3 1/2" x 2 1/2" oval)	8
yeast, glazed, 1 (4" diameter)	6
yeast, with jelly filling, 1 (3 1/2" x 2 1/2" oval)	7

	POINTS VALUE
Dressing, salad, creamy	
fat-free, 2 Tbsp	1
reduced-calorie, reduced-fat, or light, 2 Tbsp	2
regular, 2 Tbsp	4
Dressing, salad, Italian-type (other than creamy Italian)	
fat-free, 2 Tbsp	0
reduced-calorie, reduced-fat, or light, 2 Tbsp	1
regular, 2 Tbsp	4
Dressing, salad, ginger, 2 Tbsp	2
Dressing, salad, mayonnaise or mayonnaise-type	
fat-free, 1/4 cup	1
reduced-calorie, reduced-fat, or light, 2 tsp	1
regular, 1 tsp	1
regular, 1/2 cup	25
Drink mix, fruit powdered, prepared, 1 cup	2
Duck a l'orange, 1/4 duck with 2 Tbsp sauce	13
Duck with fruit sauce, 1/4 duck with skin and 1/2 cup sauce	13
Duck, domestic	
cooked, with skin, 1/4	13
cooked, without skin, 2 oz	3
cooked, without skin, 1/4 (4 oz)	5
Duck, tea smoked, 2 oz	3
Dumplings	
beef or pork, fried, 4 (6 1/2 oz)	6
beef or pork, steamed, 4 (5 3/4 oz)	6
chicken, fried, 4 (6 1/2 oz)	4

	POINTS VALUE	
chicken, steamed, 4 (5 3/4 oz)	4	
potato, 6 (1" diameter)	2	
shrimp, fried, 4 (6 1/2 oz)	4	
shrimp, steamed, 4 (5 3/4 oz)	4	
vegetarian, fried, 4 (3 1/2" x 2" wide)	3	
vegetarian, steamed, 4 (3 1/2" x 2" wide)	3	

E

	POINTS VALUE	
Eclair, 1 (5 1/4 oz)	9	
Edamame		
◆ in pods, 1 cup	1	(5)
◆ shelled, 1/2 cup	2	(5)
Egg, whole		
◆ cooked or raw, 1	2	(5)
deviled, 2 stuffed halves	4	
fried, 1 large	2	
◆ hard-boiled, 1	2	(5)
◆ poached, 1	2	(5)
scrambled, 2 or 1/2 cup	5	
scrambled, fast food, 2	5	
Egg curry, 1 cup	2	
Egg foo yung		
beef, 1 (3" diameter)	4	
chicken, 1 (3" diameter)	4	
pork, 1 (3" diameter)	5	
shrimp, 1 (3" diameter)	4	
Egg roll		
beef, 1 (4 1/2" long)	5	
chicken, 1 (4 1/2" long)	4	
chicken, store-bought, 1 (3 oz)	3	
pork, 1 (4 1/2" long)	5	

Complete A-Z Food List

Egg roll (cont'd)

	POINTS VALUE
pork, store-bought, 1 (3 oz)	3
shrimp, 1 (4 1/2" long)	4
shrimp, store-bought, 1 (3 oz)	3
vegetable, store-bought, 1 (3 oz)	3
Egg roll snacks	
pork or shrimp, store-bought, 3 oz	3
vegetable, store-bought, 3 oz	3
Egg roll wrapper, 1 (1/2 oz)	1
Egg substitute	
fat-free, 1/4 cup	1 (5)
regular, 1/4 cup	2 (5)
Egg white, chicken	
1	0 (5)
3	1 (5)
Eggnog	
homemade, with or without liquor, 1/2 cup	4
reduced-calorie, store-bought (without liquor), 1/2 cup	3
store-bought (without liquor), 1/2 cup	5
Eggplant	
breaded and baked (without oil), 2 slices (3" diameter)	1
breaded and fried, 2 slices (3" diameter)	3
cooked or uncooked, 1 cup	0
Eggplant parmesan, frozen, 5 oz	4
Eggplant parmigiana	
with sauce, 3" x 4" with 1/2 cup Italian tomato sauce	13
without sauce, 3" x 4"	11

	POINTS VALUE
Eggs Benedict, 2 English muffin halves with 2 eggs and 1/4 cup Hollandaise sauce	16
Eiderduck, 3 1/2 oz	2
Elderberries, 1 cup	1 (2)
Elk, cooked or raw, 1 oz	1 (5)
Empanadas, 2 (3" diameter)	5
Emu, cooked, 1 oz	1
Enchilada de camarones, 1 cup	5
Enchilada meal	
beef (2 enchiladas, beans & rice), 1 (11 1/2 oz)	7
cheese (2 enchiladas, beans & rice), 1 (11 1/2 oz)	7
chicken (2 enchiladas, beans & rice), 1 (11 1/2 oz)	7
Enchiladas	
beef, 2 (10 1/2 oz)	12
cheese, 2 (8 1/2 oz)	10
chicken, 2 (10 1/2 oz)	9
pork, 2 (10 1/2 oz)	12
sour cream, 1 (5 1/2 oz)	8
Endive	
1 cup	0
head, 1	0
English muffin	
light, any type, 1 (2 oz)	1
regular, any type, 1 (2 oz)	2
Enjera, 1 (9" diameter)	1
Escargots, 6 snails with 2 Tbsp butter	7
Escarole, 1 cup	1

	POINTS VALUE
Etouffee	
crawfish, 1 cup	8
crawfish or shrimp, store-bought, 1 cup	6
mix, 2 Tbsp	1
shrimp, 1 cup	9

F

	POINTS VALUE	
Fadge, 1 piece (3 1/4 oz)	2	
Fajitas		
beef, 2 (9 oz)	11	
beef or chicken, kit, frozen, prepared, 2 (7 1/2 oz)	5	
chicken, 2 (8 3/4 oz)	8	
pork, 2 (10 1/2 oz)	13	
shrimp, 2 (9 oz)	8	
vegetarian, 1 (5 1/2 oz)	4	
Falafel		
in pita, 1 large pita with 4 falafel patties	10	
patties, 4 (2" diameter each)	7	
patties, from mix, prepared, 2	4	
Fattoush, 2 cups	5	
Fennel, 1 cup	1	
Fettuccine Alfredo		
1 cup	16	
frozen, 1 cup	7	
Fettuccine with broccoli and chicken in Alfredo sauce, frozen, 1 cup	9	
Fiddlefern (fiddlehead greens), 1 cup	0	
Figs		
dried, 1	1	
fresh, 2 medium (2 1/4")	0	(2)
fresh, 1 large (2 1/2")	1	(2)

	POINTS VALUE	
Fillo (phyllo) dough, frozen		
1 sheet (2/3 oz)	1	
1 1/2 sheets (1 oz)	2	
Fish		
anchovies, canned in oil, drained, 6 (3/4 oz)	1	
arctic char, cooked, 3 oz	4	(5)
bass, striped, cooked, 1 fillet (6 oz)	5	(5)
bluefish, cooked, 1 fillet (6 oz)	6	(5)
carp, cooked, 1 fillet (6 oz)	7	(5)
catfish, cooked, 1 fillet (6 oz)	6	(5)
cod, cooked, 1 fillet (6 oz)	4	(5)
dried, 1 oz	2	
eel, cooked, 1 oz	2	(5)
flounder, cooked, 1 fillet (6 oz)	4	(5)
grouper, cooked, 1 fillet (6 oz)	4	(5)
haddock, cooked, 1 fillet (6 oz)	4	(5)
halibut, cooked, 1 fillet or steak (6 oz)	5	(5)
herring, cooked, 1 oz	1	(5)
lox, 1 oz	1	(5)
mackerel, canned in water, drained, 1/2 cup	3	(5)
mackerel, cooked, 1 fillet (6 oz)	8	(5)
mahimahi (dolphinfish), cooked, 1 fillet (6 oz)	4	(5)
perch, cooked, 1 fillet (6 oz)	4	(5)
pike, cooked, 1 fillet (6 oz)	4	(5)
pollack, cooked, 1 fillet (6 oz)	4	(5)
pompano, cooked, 1 fillet (6 oz)	9	(5)
rockfish, cooked, 1 fillet (6 oz)	4	(5)
salmon, canned, drained, 1/2 cup (4 oz)	4	(5)
salmon, cooked, 1 fillet (6 oz)	9	(5)

Complete A-Z Food List

	POINTS VALUE	
sardines, canned in oil, drained, 5 (2 oz)	3	
sardines, canned in tomato sauce, drained, 2 oz	3	(5)
sardines, canned in tomato sauce, drained, 1 can (13 oz)	16	(5)
skate, uncooked, 3 1/2 oz	2	(5)
smelt, cooked, 1 oz	1	(5)
snapper, cooked, 1 fillet (6 oz)	5	(5)
sole, cooked, 1 fillet (6 oz)	4	(5)
swordfish, cooked, 1 fillet or steak (6 oz)	6	(5)
tilapia, cooked, 1 fillet (6 oz)	4	(5)
trout, cooked, 1 fillet (6 oz)	8	(5)
trout, rainbow, cooked, 1 fillet (6 oz)	6	(5)
tuna, canned in oil, drained, 1/2 cup (4 oz)	5	
tuna, canned in water, drained, 1/2 cup (4 oz)	3	(5)
tuna, cooked, 1 fillet or steak (6 oz)	5	(5)
whitefish, smoked, 2 oz	1	(5)
whiting, cooked, 6 oz	4	(5)
Fish, baked, stuffed, 6 1/2 oz	8	
Fish, blackened, 1 fillet (6 oz)	12	
Fish, fried		
breaded with flour, 1 fillet (6 oz)	12	
without flour, 1 fillet (6 oz)	14	
Fish, gefilte, 1 piece (1 1/2 oz)	1	
Fish, molee, 1 cup	11	
Fish, stuffed, frozen, 1 (5 oz)	5	
Fish, whitefish and pike		
small, store-bought, 2 (1 oz)	2	
large, store-bought, 1 (1 1/4 oz)	2	
Fish amandine, 1 fillet (6 oz)	13	

	POINTS VALUE
Fish and brewis, 1 cup	13
Fish and chips, 5 oz fish fillet with 20 chips (French fries)	15
Fish fillet	
battered, prepared without fat, 1 (3 oz)	5
breaded, prepared without fat, 2 (3 3/4 oz)	7
grilled, with garlic butter, 1 (3 3/4 oz)	3
grilled, with lemon pepper, 1 (3 3/4 oz)	3
light, breaded, prepared without fat, 3 3/4 oz	3
Fish portions, from minced fish, breaded or battered, prepared without fat, 3 oz	5
Fish sticks, breaded, frozen, 4 (2 1/2 oz)	4
Fish Veronique, 1 fillet (6 oz)	11
Flan, 3/4 cup	8
Flanken, 2 slices (4 oz)	8
Flatbreads, 3/4 oz	1
Flauta	
beef, 1 (6" x 1 1/4")	12
chicken, 1 (6" x 1 1/4")	10
pork, 1 (6" x 1 1/4")	11
Flax seed, 1 Tbsp	1
Flour	
potato, 1 tsp	0
potato, 2 Tbsp	1
soy, full fat, 2 Tbsp	1
wheat, whole-grain, 1 tsp	0
wheat, whole-grain, 2 Tbsp	1
wheat, whole-grain, 1 cup	8
white, 1 tsp	0

	POINTS VALUE
white, 2 Tbsp	1
white, 1 cup	9
Focaccia bread	
1 piece (2 1/4 oz)	6
store-bought, 2 oz	3
Fondue, cheese, 1/2 cup fondue with 2 oz bread	12
Frankfurter	
beef or pork, fat-free, 1 (1 3/4 oz)	1
beef or pork, light, 1 (1 3/4 oz)	2
beef or pork, regular, 1 (2 oz)	5
beef or pork, with cheese, 1 (2 oz)	5
chicken, 1 (2 oz)	3
turkey, 1 (2 oz)	3
turkey, fat-free, 1 (1 1/2 oz)	1
turkey, light, 1 (2 oz)	2
Frankfurter on roll, plain, 1 (4 oz)	8
Frankfurter roll or bun	
1 (2 oz)	3
light, 1 (1 1/2 oz)	1
Franks in blankets, frozen, 6 (3 oz)	9
French fries	
homemade, 20 (4 1/2" long), 5 1/2 oz	10
fast food, 1 medium serving	6
fast food, 1 large serving	10
fast food, 1 extra large serving	12
frozen, baked (prepared without fat), 15 (3 oz)	3
French toast	
2 slices (4 1/2 oz)	7
frozen, baked, 2 slices (4 oz)	5

	POINTS VALUE
French toast sticks	
fast food, 5 pieces	11
frozen, 3 (2 1/2 oz)	6
Fritters	
corn, 3 (2 1/2" x 2" each)	5
vegetable, 1 cup	10
Frog legs, fried, 2 (2 oz)	4
Fromage frais (soft cheese with fruit), 3 1/2 oz	3
Frosting, store-bought, reduced-fat or regular, 2 Tbsp	3
Fructose, high, corn syrup, 1 Tbsp	1
Fruit, candied, 2 Tbsp	1
Fruit, dried, mixed, 1/4 cup (1 1/2 oz)	1
Fruit butter, 1 Tbsp	1
Fruit cocktail, canned, unsweetened, 1/2 cup	1
Fruit compote, 1/2 cup	3
Fruit juice bar, frozen, without sugar, 1 (2 3/4 oz)	1
Fruit juice cup, frozen, 1 cup	3
Fruit spread, all spreadable fruit, 1 1/2 Tbsp	1
Fruit-flavored pieces, 1 package (1 oz)	2
Fruit-flavored roll, leather	
1 small (1/2 oz)	1
1 large (3/4 oz)	2
Fudge, with or without nuts, 1 piece (1" x 2"), or 1 oz	3
Funnel cake, 1/2 (8" diameter)	12

Complete A-Z Food List

G

	POINTS VALUE
Garlic bread	
1 slice (1 1/2 oz)	5
garlic, frozen, 1 piece (1 1/2 oz)	4
Gelatin, fruit-flavored	
prepared, 1/2 cup	2
sugar-free, mix, 1 package (10 g)	1
sugar-free, mix, 1 oz	2
sugar-free, prepared, 1/2 cup	0
Gelatin, unflavored, sugar-free	
1 packet	0
1 oz	2
Gelatin-fruit mold, 1/2 cup	2
General Tso's chicken, 1 cup	15
Giardeniera (vegetable medley, without olives, packed in vinegar), 5 pieces	0
Gin, 1 jigger (1 1/2 fl oz)	2
Gin and tonic, 1 (6 fl oz)	3
Gin gimlet, 1 (2 1/2 fl oz)	2
Ginger, crystallized, 1 1/2 oz	3
Ginger chicken, 1 cup	7
Ginger fish, 1 cup	8
Gingerbread, 3"	9
Gnocchi	
any type, frozen, 1 cup	7
cheese, 1 cup	11
potato, 1 cup	4
potato, dry, 1 cup	3
potato, refrigerated, 1 cup	5
spinach, 1 cup	12

	POINTS VALUE	
Goat, cooked, 1 oz	1	
Goat masala, 1 cup	5	
Gobo (burdock), 1/2 cup (2 oz)	1	
Goose		
cooked, with skin, without bone, 2 oz	4	
without skin and bone, 2 oz	3	
Gooseberries, 1 cup	1	(2)
Gordita, beef, 1 (3" diameter)	10	
Gosht shaha korma, 1 cup	14	
Graham cracker crumbs, 2 Tbsp (1/2 oz)	1	
Graham crackers, 2 (2 1/2" square)	1	
Granola bar		
any type (other than chocolate-covered and reduced-calorie), 1 (1 oz)	3	
chocolate-covered, 1 (1 1/4 oz)	4	
reduced-calorie, 1 (1 oz)	2	
Grape juice, 1/2 cup	2	
Grape leaves, 1 cup	0	
Grapefruit		
1 small (approximately 3 1/2" diameter)	1	(2)
1 medium (approximately 4" diameter)	1	(2)
1 large (approximately 5" diameter)	2	(2)
sections, juice pack, 1 cup	2	(2)
Grapefruit juice, 1/2 cup	1	
Grapes, 1 cup	1	(2)
Gravy		
beef, canned, 1/4 cup	1	
brown, 1/4 cup	2	
chicken, canned, 1/4 cup	1	
cream, 1/4 cup	4	
fat-free, canned, 1/2 cup	1	

	POINTS VALUE
giblet, 1/4 cup	2
sausage, 1/4 cup	4
sausage, canned, 1/4 cup	2
Sicilian, 1/2 cup	2
turkey, canned, 1 cup	1
Green bean casserole, 1 cup	5
Green rice, 1 cup	6
Greens	
beet, collard, dandelion, kale, mustard, and turnip, cooked or uncooked, 1 cup	0
seasoned with bacon or salt pork, 1 cup	4
Grenadine, 1 Tbsp,	1
Greyhound, 1 (5 1/2 fl oz)	3
Guacamole, homemade or store-bought, 1/4 cup	2
Guava	
1 cup	1 (2)
1 medium	1 (2)
Guava duff, 1 wedge (4 1/2" x 2") with 1/2 cup sauce	18
Guinea hen, cooked, 1 oz	1
Gum, chewing	
sugarless, 1 piece	0
with sugar, 1 piece	0
Gumbo	
base (seasoning mix), 1 1/2 Tbsp	1
chicken, 1 cup	6
seafood, 1 cup	5
seafood, with rice, store-bought, 1 cup	4
with rice mix, 1/4 cup	3
Gyoza, 3 (1 3/4 oz)	3
Gyro, 1 (6")	15

H

	POINTS VALUE
Halvah	
1 piece (2" x 1 3/4" x 1")	5
store-bought, 1 1/2 oz	6
Ham	
cooked, lean, 1/2 cup (cubed or shredded) 2 oz	2
cooked, lean, 1 slice (2 oz)	2
cooked, regular, 1 slice or 1/2 cup cubed or shredded (2 oz)	3
glazed with pineapple, 4 oz ham with 1/2 pineapple slice	6
Hamantaschen, 1 piece (3" diameter)	3
Hamburger dinner in a box, prepared, 1 cup	7
Hamburger on bun	
small, fast food, 1	6
large, fast food, 1	12
microwave, 1 small	3
plain (without mayonnaise, lettuce, and tomato), 1 (3 oz cooked hamburger on 1 1/2 oz bun)	9
Hamburger roll or bun	
1 (2 oz)	3
light, 1 (1 1/2 oz)	1
Haroset, 1/4 cup	1
Hash	
corned beef, canned, 1 cup	9
roast beef, canned, 1 cup	9
Haupia (coconut pudding), 2" square	3
Hazelnut and chocolate spread, 1 Tbsp	2

Complete A-Z Food List

	POINTS VALUE
Hazelnuts, 20 nuts (1 oz shelled)	4
◆ **Hearts of palm (palmetto),** 1 cup	0
Herring	
fillets, store-bought, 1/4 cup	3
chopped, 1/4 cup	4
in cream sauce, store-bought, 1/4 cup	3
in wine sauce, store-bought, 1/2 cup	2
pickled, 1/2 cup	2
Hibachi	
chicken, 1 cup	8
shrimp, 1 cup	5
steak, 1 cup	10
vegetables, 1 cup	4
Highball	
made with sweetened mixer, 6 fl oz	4
made with unsweetened mixer, 6 fl oz	3
◆ **Hominy,** cooked or canned, whole, 1 cup	2
Honey	
1 Tbsp	1
1 cup	20
Honey roll, 1 (2 oz)	5
Honeybun, glazed, 1 (4" x 3" oval)	6
Honeydew melon	
◆ 1 cup	1 (2)
◆ 1/8 small (5 1/4" diameter) or 1/8 medium (6-7" diameter)	1 (2)
Hot chocolate, homemade	
with whipped topping, 1 cup	7
without whipped topping, 1 cup	6
Hot cross buns, 1 (2 1/3 oz)	5

	POINTS VALUE
Hot dog	
beef or pork, fat-free, 1 (1 3/4 oz)	1
beef or pork, light, 1 (1 3/4 oz)	2
beef or pork, regular, 1 (2 oz)	5
beef or pork, with cheese, 1 (2 oz)	5
chicken, 1 (2 oz)	3
turkey, 1 (2 oz)	3
turkey, fat-free, 1 (1 1/2 oz)	1
turkey, light, 1 (2 oz)	3
Hot dog on roll, plain, 1 (4 oz)	8
Hot dog roll or bun	
1 (2 oz)	3
light, 1 (1 1/2 oz)	1
Huevos rancheros, 2 eggs on 2 tortillas	14
Huli huli chicken	
breast (with skin and bone), 1 (7 1/4 oz)	12
drumstick (with skin and bone), 1 (2 oz)	3
thigh (with skin and bone), 1 (3 oz)	5
Hummus	
1/4 cup	3
store-bought, 1/4 cup	2
Hunan beef, 1 cup	9
Hungarian goulash, 1 cup	8
Hush puppies	
2 (2 1/4 oz)	4
frozen (prepared without fat), 3 (2 oz)	2
mix, 1/4 cup	3

I

	POINTS VALUE
Ice cream	
fat-free, sweetened with sugar, 1 scoop or 1/2 cup	2
fat-free, without sugar, 1 scoop or 1/2 cup	2
fried, 1 scoop or 1/2 cup	11
green tea, 1 scoop or 1/2 cup	3
light, sweetened with sugar, 1 scoop or 1/2 cup	3
light, without sugar, 1 scoop or 1/2 cup	2
premium, 1 scoop or 1/2 cup	7
regular, 1 scoop or 1/2 cup	4
Ice cream bar	
chocolate-covered with crisp rice, with sugar, 1 (2 oz)	5
chocolate-covered, with crisp rice, without sugar, 1 (1 1/2 oz)	3
Ice cream cone, plain or sugar, 1 small (10 g)	1
Ice cream sandwich	
1 (5" x 1 3/4" x 3/4")	3
reduced-calorie, 1 (3 1/3 fl oz)	3
Ice cream soda, 12 fl oz	9
Ice cream sundae	
1 large (6 1/2 oz)	11
1 scoop (1/2 cup) ice cream with syrup, nuts, & whipped topping (4 1/2 oz)	8
cone, 1 (3 1/2 oz)	8
Ice pop, fruit-flavored, 1 (1 3/4 fl oz)	1
Ices	
fruit, 1/2 cup	3
Italian, restaurant-prepared, 1/2 cup	1

	POINTS VALUE
Imperial roll, 1 (4 1/2" long)	4
Irish brown stew, 1 cup	7
Irish coffee, 6 fl oz with 2 Tbsp whipped cream	4
Irish soda bread, 1/12 of 8" round loaf	6
Italian casserole (ground beef, pasta & cheese over rolls)	
1 cup	14
1/8 of 10" round casserole	16
Italian toast snacks, store-bought, 4 (1 oz)	3

J

	POINTS VALUE	
Jackfruit, uncooked, 1/2 cup	1	(2)
Jalapeño bread, 1 slice (1 1/2 oz)	2	
Jalapeño poppers, 1 (1 1/2 oz)	4	
Jalapeños, stuffed (prepared without fat), store-bought, 2	4	
Jam, 1 Tbsp	1	
Jamaican akee (ackee), canned, drained, 3 1/2 oz)	4	
Jamaican rice & peas, 1 cup	6	
Jambalaya, chicken or fish, with rice, 1 1/2 cups	9	
Jambalaya mix, 1/4 cup	3	
Japanese curry, 1 cup	4	
JapChae, beef, chicken, or pork, 1 cup	7	
Jelly, 1 Tbsp	1	
Jerk chicken breast, 1 (large breast, without skin)	5	
Jerusalem artichokes (sunchokes), 1 cup	2	

Complete A-Z Food List

	POINTS VALUE
Jicama	
1 small or medium	1
1 large	2
1 slice	0
1 cup	0
Johnny cake, 1 piece (2 1/2" square)	4
Juice	
apple, 1/2 cup	1
carrot, canned, 1/2 cup	1
clam, canned, 1/2 cup	0
clam-tomato, 1 cup	2
coconut, 12 fl oz	3
cranberry cocktail, low-calorie, 1 cup	1
cranberry cocktail, regular, 1/2 cup	1
fruit (combined), 1/2 cup	1
grape, 1/2 cup	2
grapefruit, 1/2 cup	1
lemon, fresh, 1 Tbsp	0
lemon, fresh, 1 cup	1
lime, fresh, 1 Tbsp	0
lime, fresh, 1 cup	1
orange, 1/2 cup	1
orange-grapefruit, 1/2 cup	1
pineapple, 1/2 cup	1
prune, 1/2 cup	2
tangerine, 1/2 cup	1
tomato, canned, 1/2 cup	0
tomato, canned, 1 cup	1
vegetable, mixed, 1/2 cup	0
vegetable, mixed, 1 cup	1

K

	POINTS VALUE	
Kabobs		
beef, 2 skewers (4 1/2 oz)	8	
chicken, 2 skewers (4 1/2 oz)	5	
fish, 2 skewers (4 1/2 oz)	5	
lamb, 2 skewers (4 1/2 oz)	8	
Kahlua pig, 3 oz	4	
Kasha (buckwheat groats)		
cooked, 1 cup	2	(6)
uncooked, 1/4 cup	2	(6)
Kasha varnishkes, 1 cup	5	
Kashmiri (lamb meatballs), 6 (3 1/2 oz)	11	
Kataifi, 1 piece (2" long)	6	
Katsu		
ahi, 2 slices (4 1/2" x 1/2" x 3/4" thick)	6	
chicken, 2 slices (4 1/2" x 1 1/2" x 3/4" thick)	6	
pork, 2 slices (4 1/2" x 1 1/2" x 3/4" thick)	7	
Ketchup		
1 Tbsp	0	
1/4 cup	1	
Key lime pie, 1/8 of 9" one-crust pie	13	
Khal bi, 4 oz	8	
Kheer, 1/2 cup	6	
Kho-phat (Thai fried rice), 1 cup	8	
Kibbe		
baked, 3 pieces (1 1/2" squares)	3	
uncooked, 1/2 cup	4	

	POINTS VALUE
Kielbasa, 1 oz	2
♦ **Kim chee,** 1/2 cup	0
King ranch chicken casserole, 1 cup	8
Kishke, 1 small piece (3/4 oz)	2
Kiwifruit	
♦ 1 cup	1 (2)
♦ 1 medium (2 1/2 oz)	0 (2)
♦ 1 large (4 oz)	1 (2)
Knish	
potato, 1 (3 1/2" square)	6
potato, store-bought, 1 (3 3/4 oz)	11
Knockwurst, 2 oz	5
Kofta (vegetable balls without sauce), 2	5
Kohlrabi	
♦ cooked, 1 cup	1
♦ uncooked, 1 cup	0
Kolache	
fruit-filled, 1 (3" diameter)	4
without filling, 1 (3" diameter)	4
Korean barbecue beef, 4 oz	7
Korean barbecue chicken thighs, 1 (5 oz)	12
Korean barbecue short ribs, 4 oz	8
Korma	
chicken, 1 cup	14
lamb, 1 cup	15
vegetable, 1 cup	11
Kreplach	
boiled, 2 pieces (4" x 3" x 3" each)	6
fried, 2 pieces (4" x 3" x 3" each)	7
Kroppkakor (potato dumpling), boiled or fried, 1 (2" wide)	3

	POINTS VALUE
Kugel	
lukschen, with fruit, 1 piece (3" x 3 1/4")	7
lukschen, without fruit 1 piece (3" x 3 1/4")	5
noodle, store-bought, 1/2 cup	3
potato, 1 piece (3" x 3 1/4")	4
potato, store-bought, 1/2 cup	4
♦ **Kumquats,** 8 medium (3 oz)	1 (2)
Kung Pao	
beef, 1 cup	10
chicken, 1 cup	8
pork, 1 cup	9
shrimp, 1 cup	9

L

	POINTS VALUE
Ladyfingers, store-bought	
2 small (1/2 oz)	1
1 large (1/2 oz)	1
Lamb	
♦ lean (other than those listed here, with all visible fat trimmed), cooked, 1 slice, 1 chop, or 1/2 cup cubed or shredded, (2 oz)	3 (5)
leg, cooked, 1 slice (2 oz)	3
♦ leg, cooked, trimmed, 1 slice (2 oz)	3 (5)
♦ leg, cooked, trimmed, 3 oz	4 (5)
leg, cooked, 3 oz	5
leg, cooked, 1 slice (2 oz)	3
♦ leg, cooked, trimmed, 3 oz	4 (5)
loin, cooked, 3 oz	6
loin, cooked, 1 slice (2 oz)	4
♦ loin, cooked, trimmed, 1 slice (2 oz)	4 (5)

Complete A-Z Food List

Lamb (cont'd)	POINTS VALUE	
loin, cooked, trimmed, 3 oz	4	(5)
regular, cooked, 1 slice, 1 chop, or 1/2 cup cubed or shredded, (2 oz)	4	
rib, cooked, 3 oz	8	
shoulder, cooked, 1 slice (2 oz)	5	
shoulder, cooked, 3 oz	7	
Lamb, ground		
cooked, 1/2 cup	4	
cooked, lean, 3 oz	3	(5)
Lamb biryani, 1 cup	14	
Lamb masala, 1 cup	6	
Lamb stew, 1 cup	5	
Lambsquarters, cooked, 1 cup	1	
Lard, 1 Tbsp	3	
Lasagna		
chicken, 1 cup	6	
vegetable, 1 cup	5	
vegetarian, with cheese, 10 oz	10	
vegetarian, with cheese and spinach, 10 1/2 oz	9	
with meat, 4" x 2 1/2" or 1 cup	6	
with meat sauce, 1 cup	6	
Latte		
made with fat-free milk, 1 small (8 fl oz)	2	
made with fat-free milk, 1 tall (12 fl oz)	2	
made with fat-free milk, 1 grande (16 fl oz)	3	
made with low-fat milk, 1 small (8 fl oz)	3	
made with low-fat milk, 1 tall (12 fl oz)	4	
made with low-fat milk, 1 grande (16 fl oz)	5	

	POINTS VALUE	
made with whole milk, 1 small (8 fl oz)	3	
made with whole milk, 1 tall (12 fl oz)	5	
made with whole milk, 1 grande (16 fl oz)	6	
Lau lau (pork and fish in taro or spinach leaves), 1	8	
Lavash, 1/4 of 10" cracker	5	
Lechon asado (roast pork), 3 oz	4	
Leeks, cooked, 1 cup	0	
Lefse, 1 (8-10" diameter)	5	
Lemon, 1 medium	0	
Lemon grass chicken, 1 cup	8	
Lemonade, 1 cup	2	
Lentils		
cooked, 1/2 cup	2	(5)
dry, 1 cup	12	(5)
dry, 1 pound	30	(5)
Lettuce, any type, 1 cup	0	
Lettuce wrap		
beef, 2 (each 5" long x 3" wide)	4	
chicken, 2 (each 5" long x 3" wide)	3	
Licorice		
1 oz	2	
1 rope (43" long)	1	
Lime, 1 medium	0	
Limeade, 1 cup	2	
Linguine with red clam sauce, 1 cup linguine with 1/2 cup sauce	6	
Linguine with white clam sauce, 1 cup linguine with 1/2 cup sauce	8	
Liqueur, any type, 1 jigger (1 1/2 fl oz)	3	

	POINTS VALUE	
Liquor (brandy, gin, rum, scotch, tequila, vodka, whiskey), 1 jigger (1 1/2 fl oz)	2	
Litches (lychees)		
dried, 10 nuts	1	
uncooked, 10 medium	1	(2)
Liver, chopped, 1/4 cup	5	
Liver paté, 1 slice (4 1/4" x 1 1/2" x 1/2")	3	
Liver with bacon, 2 slices (4 oz) with 2 slices bacon	10	
Liver with onions, 2 slices (4 oz) with 1/2 cup onions	7	
Lo mein		
beef, 1 cup	8	
chicken, 1 cup	8	
pork, 1 cup	8	
shrimp, 1 cup	8	
vegetable, 1 cup	7	
Lobster, steamed, 1 1/4 -pound lobster or 4 1/2 oz lobster meat	3	(5)
Lobster bisque, 1 cup	4	
Lobster Cantonese, 1 cup	8	
Lobster Newburg, 1 cup	14	
Lobster thermidor, 1 cup	14	
Loganberries, 1 cup	1	(2)
Lollipop, 1 (1 oz)	2	
Lomi lomi salmon, 1/2 cup	1	
Long island iced tea, 1 (8 fl oz)	5	
Logans, 25 (3 oz)	1	(2)
Loquats, 10 medium	1	(2)
Lotus root, cooked or uncooked, 1 cup	1	
Lumpia (Filipino spring roll), 1 (4 1/2" x 1" x 1 1/2")	5	

	POINTS VALUE	
Lumpia wrapper, 1 (1/2 oz)	1	
Luncheon meat		
bologna, beef or pork, 1 slice (1 oz)	2	
bratwurst, 2 oz	5	
canned, 2 oz	5	
chicken roll, 1 slice (1 oz)	1	
fat-free, 2 oz	1	
lean (3 g fat or less per oz), 1 slice (1 oz)	1	
light, canned, 2 oz	3	
liverwurst, 1 oz	3	
regular (4 g fat or more per oz), 1 slice (1 oz)	2	
salami, beef or pork, 1 slice (1 oz)	1	
Lychees (litches)		
dried, 10 nuts	1	
uncooked, 10 medium	1	(2)

M

	POINTS VALUE	
Macaroni		
regular, cooked, 1 cup	4	
regular, dry, 1 cup	7	
regular, dry, 2 oz	4	
regular, dry, 1 pound	34	
whole-wheat, cooked, 1 cup	3	(6)
whole-wheat, dry, 1 cup	6	(6)
whole-wheat, dry, 2 oz	3	(6)
Macaroni and cheese		
1 cup	9	
in a cup, 1 (2 oz)	5	
frozen, 1 cup	6	
package mix, prepared, 1 cup	9	

Complete A-Z Food List

	POINTS VALUE
Madras, 1 (5 1/2 fl oz)	3
Malai kofta (vegetable balls in cream sauce), 2 kofta with 1/2 cup sauce	9
Malanga	
cooked, 3/4 cup	3
cooked, 1 large	4
uncooked, 1 large	6
Malasadas (Portuguese doughnuts), 1 (3" x 2" puff)	3
Mammy-apple (mamey), uncooked, 1 (1 3/4 pounds)	8 (2)
Manapua with char shiu filling, 1 (3 1/4 oz)	5
Mandarin orange (tangerine)	
2 small (2 1/4" diameter)	1 (2)
1 large (3" diameter)	1 (2)
canned, unsweetened, 1 cup	1 (2)
Mandelbrot, 1 slice (3" x 2" x 1/2")	5
Mango	
1 small (8 oz without pit and skin)	2 (2)
1 large (14 1/2 oz without pit and skin)	4 (2)
1 cup	2 (2)
Mango lassi, 1 cup	3
Manhattan	
1 (2 fl oz)	3
dry, 1 (4 fl oz)	5
perfect, 1 (4 fl oz)	5
scotch, 1 (4 fl oz)	5
Manicotti	
cheese, with tomato sauce, frozen, 1 (10 oz)	9

	POINTS VALUE
cheese, without sauce, frozen, 2 (5 1/2 oz)	6
shells, dry, 2 (1 oz)	2
with meat sauce, 2 shells with 1/2 cup sauce	15
with tomato sauce, 2 shells with 1/2 cup sauce	12
Margarine	
fat-free, 1/4 cup	1
reduced-calorie, 2 tsp	1
regular, 1 tsp	1
regular, 1 cup	49
Margarita, 1 (4 fl oz)	5
Margarita mix, 1/2 cup	3
Marmalade, 1 Tbsp	1
Marshmallow, 2 medium	1
Marshmallow crème, store-bought, 2 Tbsp (1/2 oz)	1
Martini, 1 (2 1/2 fl oz)	3
Marzipan, 2 Tbsp	4
Masa harina, 1 cup	9
Masala dosa	
with filling, 1 (6" diameter dosa with 1/3 cup potato filling)	11
without filling, 1 (6" diameter)	10
Matzo, 1 board (1 oz)	2
Matzo brie, 1/4 of 10" round or 1 cup	5
Matzo farfel, store-bought, 1/4 cup	1
Matzo meal	
1 tsp	0
3 Tbsp	2

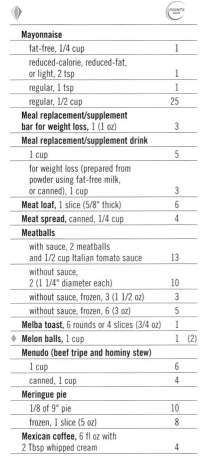

	POINTS VALUE
Mayonnaise	
fat-free, 1/4 cup	1
reduced-calorie, reduced-fat, or light, 2 tsp	1
regular, 1 tsp	1
regular, 1/2 cup	25
Meal replacement/supplement bar for weight loss, 1 (1 oz)	3
Meal replacement/supplement drink	
1 cup	5
for weight loss (prepared from powder using fat-free milk, or canned), 1 cup	3
Meat loaf, 1 slice (5/8" thick)	6
Meat spread, canned, 1/4 cup	4
Meatballs	
with sauce, 2 meatballs and 1/2 cup Italian tomato sauce	13
without sauce, 2 (1 1/4" diameter each)	10
without sauce, frozen, 3 (1 1/2 oz)	3
without sauce, frozen, 6 (3 oz)	5
Melba toast, 6 rounds or 4 slices (3/4 oz)	1
♦ **Melon balls,** 1 cup	1 (2)
Menudo (beef tripe and hominy stew)	
1 cup	6
canned, 1 cup	4
Meringue pie	
1/8 of 9" pie	10
frozen, 1 slice (5 oz)	8
Mexican coffee, 6 fl oz with 2 Tbsp whipped cream	4

	POINTS VALUE
Milk	
buttermilk, dry, 1/4 cup	2
buttermilk, low-fat (1%), 1 cup	2
buttermilk, reduced-fat (2%), 1 cup	3
chocolate, low-fat, 1 cup	3
chocolate, reduced-fat, 1 cup	4
chocolate, regular, 1 cup	4
♦ evaporated, fat-free, 1/2 cup	2
evaporated, low-fat, 1/2 cup	2
evaporated, whole, 1/2 cup	4
♦ fat-free, 1 cup	2
goat, 1 cup	4
♦ instant nonfat dry powder, 1/3 cup	2
low-fat or light (1/2% or 1%), 1 cup	2
oat, any flavor, 1 cup	2
reduced-fat (2%), 1 cup	3
soy, calcium-fortified, flavored, 1 cup	2
♦ soy, calcium-fortified, unflavored, 1 cup	2
sweetened condensed, 1/2 cup	11
sweetened condensed, fat-free, 2 Tbsp	2
whole, 1 cup	4
Milk shake	
any flavor, fast food, 1 medium	10
any flavor, fast food, 1 large	13
Millet	
♦ cooked, 1 cup	4
♦ uncooked, 1/4 cup	3
Mimosa, 1 (6 fl oz)	2
Mince pie, frozen, 1 slice (4 1/4 oz)	7
Mincemeat, store-bought, 1/4 cup	3

Complete A-Z Food List

	POINTS value
Mincemeat pie	
with meat, 1/8 of 9" two-crust pie	12
without meat, 1/8 of 9" two-crust pie	13
Mint, chocolate-covered, 1 (2 1/4" diameter)	3
Miso, 1 tsp	0
Mochi	
1 piece (2" square)	2
butter, 1 piece (2" square)	6
Mojito, 1 (5 1/2 fl oz)	4
Molasses, 1 Tbsp	1
Molé poblano, 1/4 cup	4
Mongolian beef, 1 cup	8
Moo goo gai pan, 1 cup	6
Moo shoo	
chicken, 1/2 cup with 2 pancakes	7
pork, 1/2 cup with 2 pancakes	8
tofu, 1/2 cup with 2 pancakes	7
Moose, cooked, 1 oz	1
Moussaka, 1 piece (3" x 4")	12
Mozzarella	
breaded, frozen (prepared without fat), 2 pieces (1 oz)	3
fried, 2 slices (2 3/4" x 1" x 1/2" each)	9
Muffin	
any type, 1 large (3" diameter)	6
any type, store-bought, 1 large (4 oz)	10
any type, mini, 1 (1 1/4" diameter)	1
any type, mini, store-bought, 2 (2 oz)	6
any type, fast food, 1	9

	POINTS value
breakfast (egg and cheese with sausage, ham, or Canadian bacon on English muffin), frozen, 1 (4 1/2 oz)	7
English, light, any type, 1 (2 oz)	1
English, regular, any type, 1 (2 oz)	2
fat-free, store-bought, 1 small (2 oz)	2
fat-free, store-bought, 1 large (4 oz)	4
Muffuletta, 1 (6")	20
◆ **Mulberries,** 1 cup	1 (2)
Mun doo	
fried, 4 (6 1/2 oz)	4
steamed, 4 (5 3/4 oz)	4
Mung dal, 1 cup	5
Mushroom gravy and charbroiled beef patty, frozen, 1 patty with gravy (5 3/4 oz)	4
Mushrooms	
breaded (prepared without fat), 7 (3 oz)	3
◆ dried, 4 large or 16 small	1
◆ dried, reconstituted, 1 cup	1
◆ fresh, cooked or uncooked, 1 cup	0
marinated, 1/2 cup	3
stuffed, 4 (2 3/4 oz)	3
Mussaman beef curry, 1 cup	19
Mussels Mariniere, 4 mussels with 3 Tbsp sauce	5
Mustard	
1 Tbsp	0
honey, 1 tsp	0
Musubi, spam, 1 (3 1/2"x 2" x1")	6
Mutter paneer, 1 cup	11

POINTS VALUE

N

Naan, 1 piece (7" x 8" diameter)	4
Nachos	
beef, 4 (8 1/2 oz)	13
cheese, 4 (3 oz)	8
cheese and bean, 4 (6 1/2 oz)	9
chicken, 4 (8 1/2 oz)	11
with cheese sauce, 1/2 cup tortilla chips with 1/4 cup cheese sauce	5
Nam prik, 1 Tbsp	1
Napoleon, 1 piece (4 1/2" x 2" x 1 1/2")	14
Nebeyaki udon, 2 cups	5
Nectar, any type, 1/2 cup	1
◆ **Nectarine,** 1 medium (2 1/2" diameter)	1 (2)
Niku jaga, 1 cup	11
Noodles	
cellophane, cooked, 1 cup	4
cellophone, uncooked, 2 oz	4
chow mein, packaged, 1/2 cup	3
drunken, 1 cup	5
egg, cooked, 1 cup	4
egg, no-yolk, uncooked, 2 oz	4
egg, uncooked, 1 cup	3
fried, 1 cup	6
Japanese, soba, cooked, 1 cup	2
Japanese, soba, dry, 2 oz	4
lasagna, dry, 2 1/2 noodles	4
Oriental (bean thread), cooked, 1 cup	4
ramen, fresh, 1/2 cup	5
soba, with sauce, 1 cup	9
Noodles and sauce mix, prepared, 1/2 cup	3

POINTS VALUE

Nuoc cham, 1 Tbsp	0
Nuts	
mixed, 1 oz shelled	4
wheat-based, 1 oz	5

O

Oil	
canola, 1 tsp	1
flaxseed, 1 tsp	1
olive, 1 tsp	1
safflower, 1 tsp	1
sunflower, 1 tsp	1
vegetable, 1 tsp	1
vegetable, 1 cup	57
whale, 1 Tbsp	4
whale, 3 1/2 oz	26
Okonnmiyaki, without sauce & mayonnaise (Japanese style pizza), 1 (8" diameter)	7
Okra	
breaded, frozen (prepared without fat), 3/4 cup	2
◆ cooked or uncooked, 1 cup	0
fried, 1 cup	8
Old fashioned, 1 (2 fl oz)	3
Olive spread, store-bought, 1 Tbsp	2
◆ **Olives,** 10 small or 6 large (1 oz)	1
Omelet	
cheese, 2-egg, 1	8
ham and cheese, 2-egg, 1	9
herb or plain, 2-egg, 1	6
vegetable, 1 2-egg, 1	7

Complete A-Z Food List

	POINTS VALUE
Onion	
♦ cooked, 1 cup	1
♦ uncooked, 1 cup	0
Onion, blooming, 1/4 (16" diameter onion)	6
Onion rings	
breaded, frozen (prepared without fat), 10 large (3-4" diameter)	7
fast food, 1 serving (8-9 onion rings)	7
fried, 4 (4" diameter each)	6
Opossum, cooked, 1 oz	2
Orange	
♦ 1 small (2 3/8" diameter)	0 (2)
♦ 1 medium (2 5/8" diameter)	1 (2)
♦ 1 large (3 diameter)	1 (2)
Orange and apricot drink, 1/2 cup	1
Orange chicken, 1 cup	13
Orange juice, 1/2 cup	1
♦ **Orange sections,** 1 cup	1 (2)
Orange-grapefruit juice, 1/2 cup	1
Oriental potato noodles (dang myeon), 2 oz	4
Osso bucco, 6 oz veal with 1/4 cup sauce	12
♦ **Ostrich,** cooked, 3 oz	3 (5)
Oyster pie, 1 slice (1/8 of 9" pie)	9
Oyster po' boy, 1 (6")	17
Oysters, fried, 10 (5 oz)	7
Oysters Rockefeller, 4 (2 oz)	3

	POINTS VALUE
# P	
Pad si-iew (stir-fried beef with noodles), 1 cup	6
Pad Thai (rice noodles with chicken and shrimp), 1 cup	9
Paella, 1 cup	7
Pajun (Korean green onion & shrimp pancake), 1 (6-8" diameter)	8
Pakora, vegetable, 1 (2" x 3" or 1 3/4 oz)	3
Palak paneer, 1 cup	14
Palak vada (vegetable dumpling)	
fried, 1 (2 1/2" x 1 1/2")	5
steamed, 1 (2 1/2" x 1 1/2")	2
Pan Cubano, 1 (6 1/2" x 3")	8
Panang curry	
with beef, 1 cup	13
with chicken, 1 cup	12
with pork, 1 cup	14
Pancake	
any type, from mix, 1 (4" diameter)	1
any type, frozen, 1 (4" diameter)	2
fast food, 1 serving, without margarine and syrup	9
Chinese, 1 (1 oz)	1
homemade, 1 (4" diameter)	3
mini, frozen, without syrup, 6 (2 1/4 oz)	3
Pancake and sausage on a stick, 1 (2 oz)	5
Pancit canton (sauteed egg noodles), 1 cup	5

	POINTS value
Paneer	
1 (1 oz)	2
fried, 1 oz	2
jalfrezi, 1 cup	5
Panettone, 1/12 of 9" tube or 1 1/2 oz	6
Panini	
chicken, 1 (8 oz)	11
ham & cheese, 1 (7 1/2 oz)	11
vegetable, 1 (13 oz)	10
Papaya	
fresh, 1 small (4 1/2" long x 3" diameter)	1 (2)
fresh, 1 medium (5" long x 3" diameter)	1 (2)
fresh, 1 large (5 1/4" long x 3 1/4" diameter)	1 (2)
fresh, 1 cup	1 (2)
green, 1 cup	1 (2)
Paprikash, 1 1/2 cups chicken mixture with 1/2 cup sauce	9
Paratha, 4" triangle	3
Parsley, fresh or dried, 1 cup	0
Parsnips	
cooked, 1 cup	2
uncooked, 1 medium or 1 cup slices	1
Passion fruit, 3 (2 oz)	0 (2)
Pasta	
brown rice, 2 oz	4 (6)
regular, cooked, 1 cup	4
regular, uncooked, 2 oz	4
regular, uncooked, 1 pound	34
spinach, cooked, 1 cup	4

	POINTS value
spinach, uncooked, 2 oz	4
whole-wheat, cooked, 1 cup	3 (6)
whole-wheat, uncooked, 2 oz	3 (6)
whole-wheat, uncooked, 1 pound	31 (6)
Pasta e fagioli, 1 cup	5
Pasta primavera	
with cream sauce, 1 cup pasta with 3/4 cup sauce	12
with marinara sauce, 1 cup pasta with 3/4 cup sauce	5
Pasta shells, stuffed with ricotta cheese, without sauce, frozen, 1 serving (2-3 pieces)	4
Pasta with garlic and oil, 1 cup	7
Pastelitos de carne (Cuban meat pastry) 1 (2" diameter x 1")	8
Pastitsio, 1 piece (3 1/4" x 3")	13
Pastrami	
beef, 1 slice (1 oz)	3
turkey, 1 slice (1 oz)	1
Pâté	
fish, store-bought, 2 oz	3
meat, store-bought, 1/4 cup (2 oz)	5
Pâté foie gras, canned, 1 Tbsp	2
Peach	
canned, unsweetened, 1 cup	2 (2)
fresh, 1 small (2" diameter or 3 oz)	0 (2)
fresh, 1 medium (2 1/2" diameter or 3 1/2 oz)	0 (2)
fresh, 1 large (2 3/4" diameter or 6 oz)	1 (2)
Peach melba, 1/2 cup ice cream with 2 peach halves and raspberry sauce	7

Complete A-Z Food List

	POINTS VALUE
Peanut brittle	
1 oz	3
store-bought, 4 pieces (1 oz)	3
Peanut butter	
1 Tbsp	2
reduced-fat, 1 Tbsp	2
Peanuts	
40 (1 oz shelled)	4
chocolate-covered, 1 oz	3
honey, reduced-fat, 1/4 cup	2
Pear	
◆ canned, unsweetened, 1 cup	2 (2)
◆ fresh, 1 small (5 oz)	1 (2)
◆ fresh, 1 medium (6 oz)	1 (2)
◆ fresh, 1 large (7 oz)	2 (2)
◆ fresh, prickly, 1 cup	0 (2)
Pear, poached, with 2 Tbsp whipped cream	5
Peas	
◆ black-eyed, cooked, 1/2 cup	1 (5)
◆ black-eyed, dry, 1 pound	30 (5)
◆ chick, cooked, 1/2 cup	2 (5)
◆ chick, dry, 1 pound	35 (5)
◆ cowpeas, cooked, 1/2 cup	1 (5)
◆ green, cooked or uncooked, 1 cup	2 (6)
◆ snow (Chinese pea pods), 1 cup	0 (6)
◆ split, cooked, 1/2 cup	2 (5)
◆ split, dry, 1/4 cup	3 (5)
◆ sugar snap, 1 cup	0 (6)
Peas, Bahamian style, with rice, 1 cup	7

	POINTS VALUE
Pecan pie	
1/8 of 9" one-crust pie	12
frozen, 1 slice (4 1/2 oz)	13
Pecans	
1 cup chopped	21
1 cup halves	20
14 halves (1 oz)	5
Peking duck, 2 oz duck with 1 piece duck skin and 3 pancakes	10
Penne a la vodka, 1 cup pasta with 1/2 cup sauce	7
◆ **Pepper,** any type, 1 small, medium, or large, or 1 cup	0
Pepper, stuffed	
with beef and rice, 1 (8 oz)	8
with beef, in tomato sauce, frozen, 7 oz	4
Pepper steak	
6 oz	14
Chinese, 1 cup	5
Pepperoni, 1 oz	4
◆ **Persimmon,** 1 (2 1/2" diameter, or 6 oz)	2 (2)
Pesarattu, 1/2 of an 8" diameter	7
Petit fours, 2 (1 3/4" x 1 1/2" x 1" each)	5
Petite marmite, 2 cups	7
Pheasant	
breast, raw, without skin and bone, 1/2 breast (6 1/2 oz)	5
cooked, 1 oz	2
leg, raw, without skin and bone, 1 leg	3
Phyllo (fillo) dough, frozen	
1 sheet (2/3 oz)	1
1 1/2 sheets (1 oz)	2

	POINTS VALUE
Picadillo, 1 cup	10
Pickle	
sweet, 1 midget (2 1/8" long)	0
sweet, 1 small (2 1/2" long)	0
sweet, 1 medium (2 3/4" long)	0
sweet, 1 large (3" long)	1
♦ unsweetened, 1 cup or 1 large	0
♦ **Pico de gallo,** 1/2 cup	1
Pignolias (pine nuts)	
1 tsp	0
1 Tbsp	1
1 oz	4
1 cup	20
Pie	
any type, frozen, 1 slice (2 1/2" x 1 3/4" x 1/2")	8
fruit, fast food, 1	8
fruit, one-crust, 1/8 of 9" pie	6
fruit, two-crust, 1/8 of 9" pie	9
individual, 1 (5" x 3 3/4")	9
Pie crust	
any type, 1/8 of 9" one-crust pie	5
any type, 1/8 of 9" two-crust pie	7
refrigerated or frozen, 1/8 of 9" crust	2
graham cracker, 1/8 of 9" crust	5
Pie filling	
canned, fruit, 1/3 cup	2
canned, fruit, light, 1/3 cup	1
Pierogies	
cabbage, 2 (3 1/2" each)	7
cheese, 2 (3 1/2" each)	7
meat, 2 (3 1/2" each)	8

	POINTS VALUE	
potato, 2 (3 1/2" each)	7	
potato and cheese or onion, low-fat, frozen, 3 (4 1/2 oz)	3	
potato and cheese, frozen, 3 (4 oz)	3	
Pigeon, cooked, 1 oz	1	
Pigs' feet, pickled, store-bought, 2 oz	2	
Pigs in blankets, 2 (1 oz)	6	
Pimiento-cheese spread		
reduced-fat, store-bought, 2 Tbsp	2	
regular, store-bought, 2 Tbsp	2	
♦ **Pimientos,** canned, 1 cup	0	
Piña colada		
1 (6 fl oz)	5	
mix, 1/2 cup	3	
Pineapple		
♦ canned, unsweetened, 1 cup	2	(2)
♦ fresh, 1/4 medium or 1 cup	1	(2)
♦ fresh, 2 slices (3 1/2" diameter x 1/2" thick) or 4 oz	1	(2)
Pineapple juice, 1/2 cup	1	
Pistachios		
pistachios, 49 (1 oz shelled)	4	
pistachios, dry roasted, 1 oz shelled	4	
pistachios, 1 cup shelled	16	
Pita		
wheat, 1 small or 1/2 large (1 oz)	1	
white, 1 small or 1/2 large (1 oz)	1	
Pizza, fast food, cheese		
thin crust, 1 slice (1/8 of 12" or 1/12 of 16")	4	

Complete A-Z Food List

	POINTS value
medium crust, 1 slice (1/8 of 12" or 1/12 of 16")	5
thick crust, 1 slice (1/8 of 12" or 1/12 of 16")	7
Pizza, fast food, one-meat topping	
thin crust, 1 slice (1/8 of 12" or 1/12 of 16")	5
medium crust, 1 slice (1/8 of 12" or 1/12 of 16")	6
thick crust, 1 slice (1/8 of 12" or 1/12 of 16")	7
Pizza, frozen	
Canadian-style bacon, 1 slice (5 oz)	7
pepperoni, 1 slice (5 oz)	9
supreme, 1 slice (5 oz)	9
vegetable, 1 slice (5 oz)	6
Pizza, frozen, single serving	
cheese, 1 (6 1/2 oz)	11
pepperoni, 1 (6 3/4 oz)	9
sausage, 1 (6 3/4 oz)	9
supreme, 1 (7 1/4 oz)	11
Pizza, restaurant-type, cheese, thin crust	
1 small slice (1/8 of 12" or 1/12 of 16")	4
1 large slice (1/8 of 16 to 18")	6
Pizza, restaurant-type, cheese, medium crust	
1 small slice (1/8 of 12" or 1/12 of 16")	4
1 large slice (1/8 of 16 to 18")	6
Pizza, restaurant-type, cheese, deep-dish	
1 small slice (1/8 of 12" or 1/12 of 16")	5
1 large slice (1/8 of 16 to 18")	8
Pizza, restaurant-type, cheese, Sicilian, 1 slice (3" x 4")	7

	POINTS value	
Pizza, restaurant-type, one-meat topping, thin crust		
1 small slice (1/8 of 12" or 1/12 of 16")	5	
1 large slice (1/8 of 16 to 18")	7	
Pizza, restaurant-type, one-meat topping, medium crust		
1 small slice (1/8 of 12" or 1/12 of 16")	6	
1 large slice (1/8 of 16 to 18")	9	
Pizza, restaurant-type, one-meat topping, deep-dish		
1 small slice (1/8 of 12" or 1/12 of 16")	7	
1 large slice (1/8 of 16 to 18")	11	
Pizza, restaurant-type, one-meat topping, Sicilian, 1 slice (3" x 4")	9	
Pizza crust dough, refrigerated, frozen or ready-made, 1 oz	2	
Pizza pieces, frozen (prepared without fat), 6	5	
Pizza bagel, mini, any type, 4 (3 oz)	4	
Plantain		
baked or boiled, 1 cup	3	(2)
fried, 1 cup	4	
Plátanos maduros (fried sweet plantains), 1 cup	4	
Plums		
fresh, 2 small (2" diameter)	1	(2)
fresh, 1 medium (2 1/8" diameter)	0	(2)
Poi, 1/2 cup (4 oz)	3	
Poke		
ahi, 1/2 cup	2	
tako, 1/2 cup	2	

	POINTS VALUE
Polenta	
cooked, 1/2 cup	2
dry, 1/4 cup	2
Pomegranate, 1 (3 3/8" diameter)	2 (2)
Pomelo (pummelo), 1 (1 pound)	3 (2)
Popcorn	
buttered, popped, 3 cups	5
butter-flavored, popped, 3 cups	4
caramel-coated, popped, 3 cups	8
cheese-flavored, popped, 2 1/2 cups	4
light, butter-flavored, popped, 3 cups	1
light, caramel-coated, popped, 3 cups	6
light, cheese-flavored, popped, 3 cups	3
light, microwave-popped, 3 cups	1
light, plain, popped, 3 cups	2
movie, without butter, 3 cups	4
regular, plain, air-popped, 3 cups	1
regular, plain, microwave-popped, 3 cups	3
regular, plain, oil-popped, 3 cups	4
regular, plain, popped, packaged, 3 cups	4
reduced-fat (94% fat-free), microwave-popped, 5 cups	1
Popcorn cakes	
any type (other than plain or butter-flavored), 1 (1 1/2 oz)	1
plain or butter-flavored, 2 (2/3 oz)	1
mini, 6 (2/3 oz)	1
Popover, 2 (3" diameter, or 1 1/2 oz each)	4
Poppy seeds	
1 tsp	0
1 Tbsp	1

	POINTS VALUE
Pork	
center loin, lean and fat, cooked, 1 slice (2 oz)	3
center loin, lean and fat, cooked, 3 oz	4
center loin, lean only, cooked, 1 slice (2 oz)	2 (5)
center loin, lean only, cooked, 3 oz	4 (5)
kidney, cooked, 1 oz	1 (5)
leg, cooked, 1 slice (2 oz)	4
leg, cooked, 3 oz	6
leg, trimmed, cooked, 1 slice (2 oz)	3 (5)
leg, trimmed, cooked, 3 oz	4 (5)
loin, lean and fat, cooked, 1 slice (2 oz)	3
loin, lean and fat, cooked, 3 oz	5
loin, trimmed, cooked, 1 slice (2 oz)	2 (5)
loin, trimmed, cooked, 3 oz	4 (5)
shoulder, lean and fat, cooked, 1 slice (2 oz)	3
shoulder, lean and fat, cooked, 3 oz	6
shoulder, lean only, cooked, 1 slice (2 oz)	3
shoulder, lean only, cooked, 3 oz	4
sirloin, lean and fat, cooked, 1 slice (2 oz)	3
sirloin, lean and fat, cooked, 3 oz	5
sirloin, lean only, cooked, 1 slice (2 oz)	3 (5)
sirloin, lean only, cooked, 3 oz	4 (5)
tenderloin, lean only, cooked, 1 slice (2 oz)	2 (5)
tenderloin, lean only, cooked, 3 oz	3 (5)
tenderloin, lean only, cooked, 1 cup	4 (5)
top loin, lean only, cooked, 1 slice (2 oz)	2 (5)
top loin, lean only, cooked, 3 oz	3 (5)

Complete A-Z Food List

	POINTS VALUE
Pork, barbecue, 1 cup	8
Pork, Chinese roast, 1 cup (8 1/2-inch slices)	5
Pork, sweet and sour, 1 cup	12
Pork and beans, canned, 1/2 cup	2
Pork and broccoli, 1 cup	3
Pork hash, 4 (5 3/4 oz)	6
Pork in barbecue sauce, frozen, 1/4 cup	2
Pork stomach, cooked, 3 oz	3
Pork with cashews, 1 cup	10
Pork rinds, 1 oz	4
Pork stir-fry with garlic or black bean sauce, 1 cup	8
Portuguese sweet bread, 3 oz	5
Pot pie	
any type, fast food, 1	19
beef, chicken, or turkey, frozen, 1 (7 oz)	11
chicken, homemade, 8 1/2 oz	10
Pot sticker (filled wontons)	
pork or vegetable, frozen, 1 large or 2 small (1 1/2 oz)	2
vegetarian, fried or steamed, 4 (3 1/2" x 2" each)	3
Potato chips	
baked, 11 (1 oz)	2
fat-free (made with fat substitute), 1 oz	1
reduced-calorie, 14 (1 oz)	3
regular, 14 (1 oz)	4
Potato flakes, dry, 1/3 cup	1
Potato latkes, 2 (3 1/2" diameter)	6
◆ **Potato leaves,** sweet, cooked, 1 cup	0
Potato mix, flavored, prepared, 1/2 cup	2

	POINTS VALUE	
Potato pancake		
1 (3 1/4 oz)	2	
frozen, 1 (2 oz)	1	
mix, 3 Tbsp	2	
Potato puffs (appetizer pastry), frozen, 2 (2 oz)	2	
Potato skins		
2 (4 oz)	5	
with cheese, bacon & sour cream, 2 (7 oz)	9	
Potato starch, 3 Tbsp	2	
Potato tots, frozen (prepared without fat), 9 (3 oz)	3	
Potatoes		
◆ baked, plain, 1 small (3 oz)	1	(6)
◆ baked, plain, 1 large (7 oz)	3	(6)
◆ uncooked, 1/2 cup diced	1	(6)
◆ uncooked, 1 small (4 oz)	1	(6)
◆ uncooked, 1 large (9 oz)	3	(6)
Potatoes, baby		
◆ cooked, 1 (2 oz)	1	(6)
◆ uncooked, 1 (2 1/2 oz)	1	(6)
Potatoes, baked		
with cheese sauce and bacon, fast food, 1	11	
with sour cream and chives, fast food, 1	10	
with vegetables and cheese, fast food, 1	10	
Potatoes, baked, stuffed		
with cheese, 1 (5 1/2 oz)	4	
with cheese and bacon, 1 (9 1/2 oz)	11	

	POINTS value
with sour cream and chives, 1 (5 1/2 oz)	4
with vegetables and cheese, 1 (13 1/2 oz)	9
Potatoes, bliss	
♦ cooked, 1 (2 oz)	1 (6)
♦ uncooked, 1 (2 1/2 oz)	1 (6)
Potatoes, garlic mashed, 1/2 cup	4
Potatoes, hash brown	
1 cup	7
fast food, 1/2 cup	3
patty, frozen (prepared without fat), 1 (1 oz)	1
patty, frozen (prepared without fat), 1 cup	8
Potatoes, home fried, 1 cup	5
Potatoes, mashed	
1/2 cup	2
in a cup, 1 (1 1/2 oz)	3
♦ **Potatoes, new,** cooked, 1 (2 oz)	1 (6)
Potatoes, scalloped, 1/2 cup	4
Potatoes, shoestring, canned, 1 cup	7
Potatoes, sweet	
♦ cooked, 1 cup (7 oz)	3 (6)
♦ cooked, 1 small (3 oz)	1 (6)
♦ cooked, 1 medium (4 1/2 oz)	2 (6)
♦ cooked, 1 large (5") or 7 oz	3 (6)
♦ uncooked, 1 cup cubes	2 (6)
♦ uncooked, 1 small (4 1/2 oz)	2 (6)
♦ uncooked, 1 medium (7 oz)	3 (6)
♦ uncooked, 1 large (8 oz)	4 (6)
Potatoes, sweet, candied, 1/2 cup	4

	POINTS value
Potatoes, white or red	
♦ cooked, 1 cup	2 (6)
♦ cooked, 1 small (2" diameter) or 3 oz	1 (6)
♦ cooked, 1 large (5") or 7 oz	3 (6)
Potatoes au gratin, 1 cup	13
Potatoes O'Brien	
♦ frozen (prepared without fat), 1 cup	1
home-prepared, 1 cup	3
Poutine, 20 French fries with 2 oz cheese and 1/2 cup sauce	17
Pozole, 1 cup	4
Praline, 1 (2 1/2" diameter or 1 1/2 oz)	5
Preserves, 1 Tbsp	1
Pretzels	
Bavarian or hard, 1 (3/4 oz)	2
regular twists, 7 (3/4 oz)	2
rods, 2 (3/4 oz)	2
soft, 1 (2 1/2 oz)	3
soft, Philadelphia, 1 (4 1/2" x 4")	3
small twists, 15 (3/4 oz)	2
sticks, 45 (3/4 oz)	2
yogurt-covered, 7 (1 oz)	3
Profiterole, 1 oz	3
Prune juice, 1/2 cup	2
Prunes, 2 (3/4 oz)	1
Ptarmigan, muscle, uncooked, 3 1/2 oz	3
Pudding	
any flavor (other than those listed here), 1/2 cup	3
any flavor (other than those listed here), 1 cup	7
banana, 1 cup	7

Complete A-Z Food List

Pudding (cont'd)	POINTS VALUE
banana, instant, fat-free, sugar free, with pie filling mix, 1 oz	1
bread, 1 cup	13
butterscotch, instant, fat-free, sugar free, with pie filling mix, 1 oz	1
chocolate, instant, fat-free, sugar free, with pie filling mix, 1 oz	1
from fat-free, sugar-free mix, made with fat-free milk, 1 cup	3
from regular mix, made with fat-free milk, 1 cup	6
Indian, 1 cup	7
plum, 1/2 cup with 1 Tbsp sauce	9
ready-made, 1/2 cup	3
ready-made, reduced-calorie, 1/2 cup	2
rice, 1 cup	8
tapioca, 1 cup	5
Thai tapioca, 1/2 cup	4
vanilla, instant, fat-free, sugar free, with pie filling mix, 1 oz	1
Puff pastry, frozen, baked, 1 oz	4
Pumpkin	
canned, 1 cup	1
fresh, cooked or uncooked, 1 cup	0
Pumpkin bread, 1 slice (3/4" thick)	7
Pumpkin leaves, cooked, 1 cup	0
Pumpkin pie	
1/8 of 9" one-crust pie	9
frozen, 1 slice (5 oz)	7
Pumpkin seeds	
1 tsp	1
1 Tbsp	2
Puris, 4" diameter	2

	POINTS VALUE	
# Q		
Quail		
breast, meat only, raw, 1 breast (2 oz)	2	
cooked, 1 oz	2	
cooked, 3 oz	5	
meat only, raw, 1 (3 1/4 oz)	3	
Quenelles, 8 (2 1/2" x 1 1/2" x 3/4")	12	
Quesadilla		
beef, 1/2 of 6" diameter	7	
cheese, 1/2 of 6" diameter	5	
chicken, 1/2 of 6" diameter	6	
vegetable, 1/2 of 6" diameter	6	
Quiche		
appetizer, frozen, any type, 2 (1 1/2 oz)	3	
crab, frozen, 5 oz	11	
vegetable, 1/8 of 9" pie	8	
vegetable, frozen, 5 oz	9	
Quiche Lorraine		
1/8 of 9" pie	10	
frozen, 5 1/2 oz	10	
Quince, 1 (3 1/4 oz)	1	(2)
Quinoa		
cooked, 1 cup	4	(6)
uncooked, 2 Tbsp	1	(6)
# R		
Rabbit, cooked, 1 oz	1	
Raccoon, cooked, 1 oz	2	
Radicchio, uncooked, 1 cup shredded	0	
Radishes, 1 cup	0	

	POINTS VALUE
Raisins	
1/4 cup (1 1/2 oz)	2
chocolate-covered, 1 oz	2
yogurt-covered, 2 oz	5
Raita, 1/2 cup	1
Rajmah, 1 cup	6
Raspberries, 1 1/2 cups	1 (2)
Ratatouille, 1 cup	4
Ravioli	
beef or chicken, without sauce, frozen, 1 cup	4
beef, breaded, frozen, 6 (4 oz)	5
beef, in meat sauce, canned, 1 cup	5
cheese, breaded, frozen, 6 (4 oz)	7
cheese, with tomato sauce, 8 pieces or 1 cup with 1/2 cup sauce	16
cheese, without sauce, 8 pieces or 1 cup	13
cheese, without sauce, frozen, 1 cup	5
meat, with tomato sauce, 8 pieces or 1 cup with 1/2 cup sauce	14
meat, without sauce, 8 pieces or 1 cup	12
Red snapper Veracruz, 6 oz cooked fillet with 3/4 cup sauce	11
Relish, any type, 1 tsp	0
Rhubarb	
cooked, with sugar, 1 cup	5
cooked or uncooked, 1 cup	0 (2)
Rhubarb pie, 1/8 of 9" two-crust pie	11
Rice, brown	
cooked, 1 cup	4 (6)
uncooked, 1/4 cup	3 (6)

	POINTS VALUE
uncooked, 1 cup	13 (6)
Rice, crisp, and marshmallow treat, store-bought, 1 small (3/4 oz)	2
Rice, Cuban, 1 cup	4
Rice, dirty	
1 cup	9
mix (prepared without fat), 1 cup	3
Rice, fried	
plain, 1 cup	8
with beef, 1 cup	8
with chicken, 1 cup	8
with chicken or pork, frozen, 1/2 cup	2
with pork, 1 cup	8
with shrimp, 1 cup	8
Rice, Spanish	
1 cup	5
canned, 1 cup	2
Rice, sushi, cooked, 1/2 cup	2
Rice, white	
cooked, 1 cup	4
uncooked, 1/4 cup	3
uncooked, 1 cup	13
Rice, wild	
cooked, 1 cup	3 (6)
uncooked, 1 cup	11 (6)
Rice, with pigeon peas (arroz con gandules), 1 cup	8
Rice cakes	
any type (other than plain), 1 (1/2 oz)	1
plain, mini, 6 (3/4 oz)	1
plain, regular, 2 (3/4 oz)	1
Rice crackers, 8 (1/2 oz)	1

Complete A-Z Food List

	POINTS VALUE
Rice drink	
any type (other than those listed here), 1 cup	3
chocolate, 1 cup	4
fat-free, 1 cup	2
Rice mix, flavored, any type, prepared, 1/2 cup	3
Rice pilaf, 1 cup	5
Risotto, 1/2 cup	5
Rob Roy, 1 (4 fl oz)	5
Rocky mountain oysters, 2 slices (1 oz each)	10
Rogan josh, 1 cup	10
Roll	
crescent dinner, store-bought, 1 (1 oz)	2
dinner, 1 (2 oz)	3
hard, 1 (2 oz)	3
high fiber (3 grams or more dietary fiber per roll), 1 (2 oz)	1
light, 1 (2 oz)	1
Ropa vieja, 1 cup	9
Rosettes, 2 (3" x 3" each)	2
Roux, store-bought, 2 Tbsp	5
Rugalach, 1 piece (2 1/2" x 1 1/4")	3
Rum, 1 jigger (1 1/2 fl oz)	2
Runza, 1 (5 1/2 oz)	8
♦ **Rutabaga,** cooked or uncooked, 1 cup	1

S

	POINTS VALUE
Saag gosht, 1 cup	6
Saag paneer, 1 cup	6

	POINTS VALUE
Sachertorte, 1/16 of 9" cake	7
Saganaki, 1 piece (1" x 2" x 1/2" thick)	6
Saimin, 1 cup	2
Sakatini, 1 (4 fl oz)	5
Sake, 1/2 cup	3
Salad	
Caesar, 3 cups	7
carrot and raisin, 1/2 cup	7
chef's, with dressing, 4 cups	8
chef's, without dressing, 4 cups	6
chicken, 1/2 cup	6
chicken, Oriental, 2 cups	7
chicken, store-bought, 1/2 cup	6
chicken macaroni, 1 cup	6
cobb, without dressing, 3 cups	10
conch, 1 cup	2
egg, 1/2 cup	8
fruit, 1 cup	2
Greek, with dressing, 3 cups	9
Greek, without dressing, 3 cups	2
green papaya, with pork and shrimp, 1 cup	3
green papaya, without meat, 1 cup	1
grilled chicken, without dressing, fast food, 1	4
herring, store-bought, 1/4 cup	3
lobster, 1/2 cup	4
♦ mixed greens, 1 cup	0
macaroni, 1/2 cup	6
macaroni, store-bought, 1/2 cup	4
Niçoise, with dressing, 4 cups	18

	POINTS VALUE
Niçoise, without dressing, 4 cups	8
pasta, 1/2 cup	3
pasta, store-bought, 1/2 cup	2
pasta mix, packaged (prepared according to directions), 1/2 cup	4
potato, 1/2 cup	7
potato, German, 1/2 cup	2
potato, hot, with ham, 1 cup	6
potato, store-bought, 1/2 cup	3
potato macaroni, 1/2 cup	10
salmon, kippered (with mayonnaise), store-bought, 2 oz	6
seafood, store-bought, 1/2 cup	6
seaweed, 1/2 cup	1
shrimp, 1/2 cup	3
side, without dressing, fast food, 1	0
spinach, with dressing, 2 cups	7
taco, with shell, without dressing, fast food, 1	16
taco, without shell and dressing, fast food, 1	9
Thai beef, 1 cup	14
Thai chicken, 1 cup	11
Thai seafood, 2 cups	10
three-bean, 1/2 cup	4
three-bean, canned, without oil, 1/2 cup	1
tomato and mozzarella, without dressing, 2 large tomato slices with 2 oz cheese	4
tossed, without dressing, 2 cups	0
tuna, 1/2 cup	7
tuna, store-bought, 1/2 cup	5
tuna macaroni, 1 cup	5

	POINTS VALUE
turkey macaroni, 1 cup	5
Waldorf, 1/2 cup	4
whitefish, store-bought, 1 1/2 oz	5
yogurt and cucumber, 1/2 cup	1
Salisbury steak	
6 oz	11
with gravy, frozen, 1 steak with gravy (4 3/4 oz)	6
Salsa	
black bean & corn, 1/2 cup	1
con queso, store-bought, 2 Tbsp	1
fat-free, 2 Tbsp	0
fat-free, 1/2 cup	0
Salsify (oyster plant), cooked, 1 cup	1
Samosa, 1 (2 1/2" x 2 1/2" x 3" triangle)	3
Sandwich	
bacon, lettuce, and tomato, 1 (9 oz)	12
barbecue beef, frozen, 1 (5 oz)	9
barbecue beef, frozen, microwave, 1 (5 oz)	8
beef, roast, open-faced, with gravy, 1 (6 oz)	9
cheese, restaurant-type, grilled, 1 (4 oz)	13
cheese, with bacon, grilled, 1 (4 3/4 oz)	16
chicken, grilled, fast food, 1	7
chicken, grilled, frozen, 1 (4 1/2 oz)	7
chicken, fried, fast food, 1	11
chicken salad, on reduced-calorie bread, 1 (5 1/4 oz)	8
chicken salad, on regular bread, 1 (5 1/4 oz)	9

Complete A-Z Food List

Sandwich (cont'd)	POINTS VALUE
club, 1 (8 3/4 oz)	15
Cuban, 1/2 (6 1/2" x 3" x 4")	11
egg and cheese, fast food, 1	9
egg salad, 1 (6 oz)	11
fish and cheese, fried, fast food, 1	13
fish fillet, 1 (4 1/2 oz)	8
grinder, 1 (6")	6
ham and cheese, 1 (4 oz)	9
ham and cheese, restaurant-style, grilled, 1 (4 oz)	15
hero, 1 (6")	6
hoagie, 1 (6")	6
lobster roll, 1 (4 1/2 oz)	5
lobster salad, 1 (4 1/2 oz)	7
Monte Cristo, 1 (3 3/4 oz)	6
peanut butter and jelly, 1 (3 1/4 oz)	7
Philly cheese steak, 1 (9 oz)	13
pocket, frozen, 1 (4 1/2 oz)	8
poor boy, 1 (6")	6
Reuben, 1 (8 oz)	17
roast beef, 1 (7 1/2 oz)	8
roast beef, fast food, 1	9
steak, frozen, 1 (2 oz)	5
turkey, 1 (4 oz)	6
shrimp salad, 1 (4 1/2 oz)	7
submarine, 1 (6")	6
toasted cheese, 1 (3 3/4 oz)	8
tuna melt, 1 (5 3/4 oz)	9
tuna salad, 1 (6 1/4 oz)	10
Sandwich spread, pork or beef, 2 Tbsp	2
Sangria, 4 fl oz	2

	POINTS VALUE	
Sashimi		
except mackerel or salmon, 4 pieces (2 oz)	1	(5)
mackerel, 4 pieces (2 oz)	3	(5)
salmon, 4 pieces (2 oz)	2	(5)
Satay		
beef, with peanut sauce, 2 skewers with 1/4 cup sauce	11	
beef, without peanut sauce, 2 skewers (3 oz)	5	
chicken, with peanut sauce, 2 skewers with 1/4 cup sauce	11	
chicken, without peanut sauce, 2 skewers (3 oz)	3	
Sauce		
adobo, store-bought, 1 Tbsp	0	
Alfredo, light, store-bought, 1/2 cup	5	
Alfredo, regular, store-bought, 1/2 cup	10	
barbecue, 1 Tbsp	0	
barbecue, 1/4 cup	1	
béarnaise, 1/4 cup	8	
béarnaise, store-bought, 1/4 cup	10	
béchamel (white), 1/4 cup	3	
black bean, 1 tsp	0	
Bolognese meat, 1/2 cup	6	
brown, Chinese, 1/4 cup	1	
cheese, 1/4 cup	2	
cheese, store-bought, 1/4 cup	3	
chili, 1 Tbsp	0	
chili, green, 1/4 cup	0	
chili, red, 1/4 cup	1	
Chinese brown, 1/4 cup	1	

Complete A-Z Food List

	POINTS VALUE
clam, red, 1/2 cup	3
clam, red, store-bought, 1/2 cup	1
clam, white, 1/2 cup	5
clam, white, store-bought, 1/2 cup	3
cocktail, store-bought, 1/4 cup	1
cranberry, 1/4 cup	2
curry, Hawaiian-style, 1/4 cup	5
donair, 2 Tbsp	2
duck, 1 Tbsp	1
enchilada, canned, 1/2 cup	1
hoisin, 1 tsp	0
hollandaise, 1/4 cup	8
hollandaise, store-bought, 1/4 cup	4
horseradish, store-bought, 2 Tbsp	3
kung pao, 2 Tbsp	1
marinara, 1/2 cup	3
marinara, store-bought, 1/2 cup	1
meat, 1/2 cup	5
mole, store-bought, brown, 2 Tbsp	1
mole, store-bought, green, 2 Tbsp	4
mornay, 1/4 cup	3
oyster, 1 tsp	0
pasta, bottled, any type, 1/2 cup	2
pasta, bottled, any type, reduced-fat, 1/2 cup	1
peanut, spicy, 2 Tbsp	4
peanut, Thai, canned, 2 Tbsp	2
pesto, 2 Tbsp	4
pesto, store-bought, 2 Tbsp	3
pizza, store-bought, 1/4 cup	1
plum, 1 Tbsp	1
puttanesca, 1/2 cup	11

	POINTS VALUE
remoulade, 2 Tbsp	4
Sloppy Joe, store-bought, 1/4 cup	1
sofrito, 1/2 cup	6
soy (shoyu),1 Tbsp	0
spaghetti, bottled, any type, 1/2 cup	2
spaghetti, bottled, any type, reduced-fat, 1/2 cup	1
Spanish, 1/2 cup	2
steak, 1 Tbsp	0
sweet and sour, dehydrated, dry, 2 Tbsp	1
taco 1 Tbsp	0
tahini, 2 Tbsp	5
tamari, 1 Tbsp	0
teriyaki, 1 Tbsp	0
teriyaki, 1/4 cup	1
tartar, 1 Tbsp	2
tartar, fat-free, 1/4 cup	1
◆ tomato, canned, 1/2 cup	0
tomato, Italian, 1/2 cup	3
tzatziki, 1/2 cup	1
Vietnamese spring roll dipping, 2 Tbsp	0
white, medium, 1/4 cup	2
white, thin, 1/4 cup	2
wine, 1/4 cup	2
Worcestershire, 1 Tbsp	0
Sauerbraten, 3 oz beef with 2 Tbsp gravy	6
◆ **Sauerkraut,** 1 cup	0
Sausage	
beef or pork, cooked, 1 link or patty (1 oz)	3
chicken, cooked, 1 1/2 oz	2
chicken, raw, 2 oz	2

Complete A-Z Food List

Sausage (cont'd)	POINTS VALUE
chorizo, 1 link (5 1/2" long)	12
low-fat (1 g fat or less per oz), 2 oz	2
mini, 6 (2 oz)	5
turkey, raw, 3 oz	3
Sausage biscuit	
fast food, 1	12
frozen, 2 small (2 oz)	6
frozen, 1 large (2 oz)	6
Sausage in brioche, 1 slice (2" thick)	15
Sausage on a roll, plain, 1 (5 1/4 oz)	12
Scallion pancake, 1 (5" diameter)	6
Scallions, 1 cup	0
Scallops, fried, 20 small (3 1/2 oz)	5
Schaum torte	
with whipped cream, 1/10 of a 10" pan	8
without whipped cream, 1/10 of a 10" pan	3
Schav, canned, 1 cup	0
Schmaltz, 1 Tbsp	3
Schnapps, any flavor, 1 jigger (1 1/2 fl oz)	3
Scone	
1 small (1 1/2 oz)	3
1 regular (2 1/2 oz)	6
Scotch, 1 jigger (1 1/2 fl oz)	2
Scrapple, 1 slice (4 1/2" x 3/4" x 3/8" thick, or 2 oz)	3
Screwdriver, 1 (6 fl oz)	3
Sea breeze, 1 (5 1/2 fl oz)	3
Seafood cakes (Haw Mok Thalay), 3/4 cup	8
Sechuan pork hotpot, 1 cup	5

	POINTS VALUE	
Seitan		
dry mix, prepared, 2 oz	1	
slices, 2 slices (2 oz)	1	
Seltzer, plain or flavored, unsweetened, 1 can or bottle (12 fl oz)	0	
Sesame candy, 1 piece (2" x 1")	2	
Sesame noodles, 1 cup	5	
Sesame seeds		
1 tsp	0	
1 Tbsp	1	
Sesame sticks, store-bought, 1/3 cup (1 oz)	4	
Seven & seven (7 & 7), 1 (5 1/2 fl oz)	3	
Shabu shabu, 4 oz beef, 2 oz tofu, and 1 1/2 cups vegetables	9	
Shallots		
uncooked, 1 cup	2	
uncooked, 1 small or medium	0	
Shark, cooked, 1 steak (6 oz)	5	
Sharon fruit, 3 oz	1	(2)
Shawarma, chicken		
1/2 cup	6	
1 thigh (without skin and bone) 2 oz	5	
Shellfish		
abalone, cooked, 3 oz	2	(5)
clam, cooked, 1/2 cup (2 oz)	2	(5)
clams, fried, frozen (prepared without fat), 3 oz	7	
clams, stuffed, frozen (prepared without fat), 3 oz	2	
conch, cracked, 1 (6" long x 3")	9	
conch, fritters, 2 (1 3/4 oz)	2	

		POINTS VALUE
◆	crab, cooked, 1/2 cup	1 (5)
◆	crab, imitation, 1/2 cup (3 oz)	2 (5)
	crab, stuffed, frozen, 1 (3 oz)	3
◆	crabmeat, canned, 1/2 cup	1 (5)
◆	crabmeat, canned, 1 cup	3 (5)
◆	crayfish, cooked, 1/2 cup	1 (5)
◆	crayfish, cooked, 16 (2 oz)	1 (5)
◆	lobster, cooked, 1/2 cup (2 oz)	1 (5)
◆	mussel, cooked, 1/2 cup (2 oz)	2 (5)
◆	oyster, canned or cooked, 1/2 cup	2 (5)
◆	oyster, cooked, 6 medium (2 oz)	1 (5)
◆	oyster, raw, 6 medium (3 oz)	1 (5)
◆	scallops, cooked, 10 small or 4 large (2 oz)	1 (5)
	scallops, fried, frozen (prepared without fat), 3 1/4 oz	4
	shrimp, butterfly, breaded, frozen (prepared without fat), 3 1/2 oz	5
◆	shrimp, canned, 1/2 cup	1 (5)
◆	shrimp, cooked, 1/2 cup (2 oz)	1 (5)
	squid, fried, 3 oz	4
◆	squid, cooked, 3 oz	2 (5)
Shells, stuffed with cheese, no sauce, frozen, 2 (4 1/2 oz)		6
Shepherd's pie, 1 cup		9
Sherbet, 1/2 cup		2
Sherry, dry or sweet, 1/2 cup		3
Shish kabob, 2 small skewers (4 1/2 oz)		8
Shortcakes, store-bought, 2 (1 oz each)		4
Shortening, 1 cup		53
Shoyu chicken, 1 thigh (3 1/4 oz)		6

	POINTS VALUE
Shrimp	
barbecued, 4 large shrimp with 1/4 cup sauce	11
broiled, stuffed, 6 large (6 oz)	18
fried, 10 (5 oz)	8
fried, stuffed, 6 large (9 1/2 oz)	9
popcorn, breaded, frozen (prepared without fat), 1 cup	5
stir-fry, with garlic or black bean sauce, 1 cup	7
sweet and sour, 1 cup	10
Shrimp and broccoli, 1 cup	2
Shrimp Cantonese, 1 cup	8
Shrimp po' boy, 1 (6")	18
Shrimp puffs, 6 (1 1/2" rounds)	5
Shrimp remoulade, 6 small shrimp with 1/4 cup remoulade sauce	9
Shrimp scampi, 9 medium (3 1/2 oz)	10
Shrimp toast, 1 piece (1 oz)	3
Shumai, fried or steamed, 2 (2" diameter)	3
Singapore sling, 6 fl oz	4
Sloppy Joe, 1 (6 oz)	7
Smoothie, 1 cup	2
Snack mix	
Oriental, low-fat, store-bought, 1/2 cup	2
reduced-fat, store-bought, 1/2 cup	3
store-bought, 1/2 cup	2
Snack pack	
cheese and breadstick, 1 package (1 oz)	3
cheese and pretzel, 1 package (1 oz)	2
Snow cone, 1 (8 fl oz)	2
Soba noodles with sauce, 1 cup	9

Complete A-Z Food List

	POINTS VALUE
Soft drink	
club soda, 1 can or bottle (12 fl oz)	0
diet, any flavor, 1 can or bottle (12 fl oz)	0
seltzer, plain or flavored, unsweetened, 1 can or bottle (12 fl oz)	0
sweetened with sugar, any flavor, 1 can or bottle (12 fl oz)	3
Sombrero, 1 (3 fl oz)	5
Sopaipillas, 2 (4" x 3" each)	3
Sorbet, any flavor, 1 scoop or 1/2 cup	2
Soufflé	
cheese, 1 cup	5
fruit, 1/2 cup	4
Soup	
asparagus crab, 1 cup	2
avgolemono, 1 cup	4
bean and bacon, canned (made with water), 1 cup	3
♦ bean and ham, canned (made with water), 1 cup	5
beef noodle mix in a cup, 1 (2 oz)	4
♦ beef, canned (made with water), 1 cup	1
♦ beef vegetable, canned (made with water), 1 cup	1
♦ black bean, 1 cup	2
♦ black bean, canned (made with water), 1 cup	2
♦ black bean in cup, 1 (2 oz)	4
♦ bouillon, any type, 1 cup	0
broccoli cheese, 1 cup	7
broccoli cheese, canned (made with fat free milk), 1 cup	3

	POINTS VALUE
broccoli cheese, canned (made with low-fat milk), 1 cup	3
broccoli cheese, canned (made with whole milk), 1 cup	4
broccoli cheese, low-fat, canned (made with fat free or low-fat milk), 1 cup	3
♦ broth, any type, 1 cup	0
♦ cabbage, 1 cup	1
Cheddar cheese, 1 cup	9
Cheddar cheese, canned (made with fat free milk), 1 cup	3
Cheddar cheese, canned (made with low-fat milk), 1 cup	3
Cheddar cheese, canned (made with whole milk), 1 cup	4
cherry, 1 cup	7
chicken, with matzo balls, 1 cup soup with 2 (1 1/2") matzo balls	3
♦ chicken, without matzo balls (broth only), 1 cup	0
chicken, with tortilla strips and shredded cheese, 1 cup	4
chicken and stars, canned (made with water), 1 cup	1
chicken enchilada, 1 cup	5
chicken noodle, 1 cup	3
chicken noodle, canned (made with water), 1 cup	1
chicken noodle, in a cup, 1 (1 oz)	2
chicken noodle mix, prepared, 1 cup	1
♦ chicken vegetable, in cup, 1	2
chicken with rice, canned (made with water), 1 cup	1

Food	POINTS VALUE
chicken with wild rice, canned (made with water), 1 cup	1
corn chowder, canned, condensed, made with fat free milk, 1 cup	4
corn chowder, canned, condensed, made with low-fat milk, 1 cup	4
corn chowder, canned, condensed, made with whole milk, 1 cup	5
corn chowder, in a cup, 1 (1 oz)	2
cream of broccoli, 1 cup	6
cream of broccoli, canned (made with fat free milk), 1 cup	3
cream of broccoli, canned (made with low-fat milk), 1 cup	3
cream of broccoli, canned (made with whole milk), 1 cup	4
cream of broccoli, low-fat, canned (made with fat free milk), 1 cup	3
cream of broccoli, low-fat, canned (made with low-fat milk), 1 cup	3
cream of celery, canned (made with fat free milk), 1 cup	3
cream of celery, canned (made with low-fat milk), 1 cup	3
cream of celery, canned (made with whole milk), 1 cup	4
cream of celery, canned, condensed, 1 can (10.75 oz)	5
cream of celery, low-fat, canned (made with fat free milk), 1 cup	2
cream of celery, low-fat, canned (made with low-fat milk), 1 cup	3
cream of chicken, canned (made with fat free milk), 1 cup	4

Food	POINTS VALUE
cream of chicken, canned (made with low-fat milk), 1 cup	4
cream of chicken, canned (made with whole milk), 1 cup	5
cream of chicken, canned, condensed, 1 can (10.75 oz)	7
cream of chicken, low-fat, canned (made with fat free milk), 1 cup	3
cream of chicken, low-fat, canned (made with low-fat milk), 1 cup	3
cream of mushroom, 1 cup	9
cream of mushroom, canned (made with fat free milk), 1 cup	4
cream of mushroom, canned (made with low-fat milk), 1 cup	4
cream of mushroom, canned (made with whole milk), 1 cup	5
cream of mushroom, canned, condensed, 1 can (10.75 oz)	7
cream of mushroom, low-fat, canned (made with fat free milk), 1 cup	3
cream of mushroom, low-fat, canned (made with low-fat milk), 1 cup	3
cream of potato, 1 cup	2
cream of potato, canned (made with fat free milk), 1 cup	2
cream of potato, canned (made with low-fat milk), 1 cup	3
cream of potato, canned (made with whole milk), 1 cup	3
cream of tomato, 1 cup	4
egg drop, 1 cup	1
escarole, canned, ready-to-serve, 1 cup	1
French onion au gratin, 1 cup	7

Complete A-Z Food List

Soup (cont'd)	POINTS VALUE
gazpacho, 1 cup	3
◆ gazpacho, canned (made with water), 1 cup	1
◆ gazpacho, canned, ready-to-serve, 1 cup	1
hot and sour, 1 cup	2
hot and spicy chicken, 1 cup	3
Italian wedding, 1 cup	5
knefla, 1 cup	5
◆ lentil, 1 cup	3
◆ lentil, in a cup, 1 (2 oz)	4
◆ lentil with ham, canned, ready-to-serve, 1 cup	3
lobster bisque, canned (made with fat free milk), 1 cup	2
lobster bisque, canned (made with low-fat milk), 1 cup	3
lobster bisque, canned (made with whole milk), 1 cup	3
Manhattan clam chowder, 1 cup	4
◆ Manhattan clam chowder, canned (made with water), 1 cup	1
matzo ball, canned (ready-to-serve), 1 cup	3
minestrone, 1 cup	4
minestrone, in a cup, 1 (1 1/2 oz)	2
minestrone, low-fat, canned (made with water), 1 cup	2
◆ miso, 1 cup	2
mulligatawny, 1 cup	6
mushroom barley, 1 cup	3
New England clam chowder, 1 cup	4

	POINTS VALUE
New England clam chowder, canned (made with fat free milk), 1 cup	3
New England clam chowder, canned (made with low-fat milk), 1 cup	3
New England clam chowder, canned (made with whole milk), 1 cup	4
New England clam chowder, low-fat, canned (made with fat free milk), 1 cup	3
New England clam chowder, low-fat, canned (made with low-fat milk), 1 cup	3
◆ onion mix (dry), 1/4 envelope	0
◆ onion mix, prepared, 1 cup	0
Oriental, mix in a cup, 1 (1 oz)	2
oxtail, 1 cup	1
oxtail, Hawaiian-style, 1 cup	7
oyster stew, canned (made with fat free milk), 1 cup	2
oyster stew, canned (made with low-fat milk), 1 cup	3
oyster stew, canned (made with whole milk), 1 cup	3
pasta with vegetables, canned (made with water), 1 cup	1
Persian noodle, store-bought, 1 cup	3
Persian pomegranate, store-bought, 1 cup	4
pigeon pea and dumpling, 1 1/2 cups	7
Portuguese bean, 1 cup	5
potato leek, in a cup, 1 (1 oz)	2
potato, frozen, 1	2
pozole (pork and hominy), canned (ready-to-serve), 1 cup	3
ramen noodle mix, 1	8

	POINTS VALUE
ramen noodle mix, low-fat, 1 (3 oz)	4
ramen, in a cup, low-fat, 1 (2 oz)	3
red beans and rice, in a cup, 1 (2 oz)	3
Sambhar (Indian lentil soup), 1 cup	2
Scotch broth, 1 cup	5
shark fin, 1 cup	2
split pea, 1 cup	3
split pea, frozen, 1 package (7 1/2 oz)	2
split pea, in a cup, 1 (2 oz)	3
split pea with ham, canned (made with water), 1 cup	4
Thai chicken coconut, 1 cup	8
Thai coconut ginger, canned (ready-to-serve), 1 cup	5
tomato, 1 cup	2
tomato, canned (made with fat free milk), 1 cup	3
tomato, canned (made with low-fat milk), 1 cup	3
tomato, canned (made with whole milk), 1 cup	4
tomato, canned (made with water), 1 cup	2
tortilla, 1 cup	6
turkey noodle, canned (made with water), 1 cup	1
turtle, 1 cup	2
vegetable, 1 cup	2
vegetable, canned (made with water), 1 cup	1
vegetable beef, canned (made with water), 1 cup	1
vegetable beef mix, prepared, 1 cup	1

	POINTS VALUE
vegetarian vegetable, in a cup, 1 (3 oz)	3
vichyssoise, 1 cup	2
Vietnamese beef noodle, 1 cup	2
wonton, 1 cup with 4 wontons	4
yogurt and cucumber, 1 cup	2
Sour apple martini, 1 (3 fl oz)	5
Soursop (guanabana), 1/2 cup pulp	1 (2)
Souse, chicken, 1 leg and thigh with skin (4 1/2 oz)	8
Souvlaki	
chicken, 1 large or 2 small skewers (4 1/2 oz)	5
chicken, in pita bread, 1 (6 1/2 oz)	7
lamb, 1 large or 2 small skewers (4 3/4 oz)	8
lamb, in pita bread, 1 (6 1/2 oz)	8
Soy beverage drink	
1 cup	3
reduced-fat, 1 cup	3
Soy cheese, hard or semisoft, fat-free	
1 cube (1"), 3 Tbsp grated, or 4 Tbsp shredded (1 oz)	1
1 slice (3/4 oz)	1
Soy cheese, hard or semisoft, regular	
1 cube (1"), 3 Tbsp grated, or 4 Tbsp shredded (1 oz)	2
1 slice (3/4 oz)	1
Soy milk, calcium-fortified	
flavored, 1 cup	2
unflavored, 1 cup	2
Soy sour cream, 1 oz	1

Complete A-Z Food List

	POINTS VALUE
Soy yogurt	
flavored, 3/4 cup (6 oz)	3
♦ plain, 3/4 cup (6 oz)	2
Soybean nuts, 1/4 cup (1 oz)	3
Spaetzle, 1/2 cup	5
Spaghetti	
regular, cooked, 1 cup	4
regular, uncooked, 2 oz	4
spinach, cooked, 1 cup	4
spinach, uncooked, 2 oz	4
♦ whole wheat, cooked, 1 cup	3 (6)
♦ whole-wheat, uncooked, 2 oz	3 (6)
Spaghetti, in tomato sauce, with cheese, canned, 1 cup	3
Spaghetti, in tomato sauce, with meatballs, canned, 1 cup	5
Spaghetti bolognese, 1 cup spaghetti with 1/2 cup sauce	10
Spaghetti carbonara, 1 cup	11
Spaghetti with marinara sauce, 1 cup spaghetti with 1/2 cup sauce	6
Spaghetti with meat sauce, 1 cup spaghetti with 1/2 cup sauce	9
Spaghetti with tomato sauce and meatballs, 1 cup spaghetti, 1/2 cup sauce and 2 meatballs	16
Spanakopita	
1 (3" square) or 1 cup	8
frozen, 2 pieces (1 oz each)	4
Spareribs	
barbecued, 4 small (4" long each)	8
barbecued, 6 (6 1/4 oz)	12
Chinese, barbecued, 2 (4" long each)	4

	POINTS VALUE
♦ **Spinach,** cooked or uncooked, 1 cup	0
Spinach soufflé, home-prepared, 1 cup	6
Spoon bread, 1/2 cup	4
Sports drink, 1 cup	1
Spring roll	
beef or pork, 1 (4 1/2" long)	5
chicken, 1 (4 1/2" long)	4
fresh, Vietnamese, 1 (1 3/4 oz)	2
fried, Vietnamese, 1 (4" long)	4
shrimp, 1 (4 1/2" long)	4
Thai, 1 (4" long)	4
Sprinkles, any type, 1 Tbsp	1
Sprouts	
♦ alfalfa, 1 cup	0
♦ bean, 1 cup	0
Spumoni, 1/2 cup	7
Squab, (pigeon)	
meat only, raw, 1 (6 oz)	6
without skin and bone, cooked, 1 oz	1
Squash	
♦ spaghetti, cooked or uncooked, 1 cup	0
♦ summer, cooked or uncooked, 1 cup	0
♦ winter, cooked, 1 cup	1
♦ winter, uncooked, 1 cup	0
♦ **Squash leaves,** 1 cup	0
Squirrel, cooked, 1 oz	1
♦ **Starfruit (carambola),** 2 large (4 1/2" long)	0 (2)
Steak, blackened, 6 oz	17
Steak, chicken fried	
with cream gravy, 6 oz with 1/4 cup cream gravy	17

	POINTS VALUE
without gravy, 6 oz	13
Steak au poivre, 6 oz steak with 1 Tbsp sauce	14
Sticky rice with mango, 1 cup sliced mangoes with 1/2 cup sticky rice	9
Stir-fried beef with garlic or black bean sauce, 1 cup	8
Stir-fried chicken with garlic or black bean sauce, 1 cup	7
Stir-fried pork with garlic or black bean sauce, 1 cup	8
Stir-fried shrimp with garlic or black bean sauce, 1 cup	7
Stir-fried vegetables	
prepared with oil, 1 cup	3
with beef, 1 cup	4
with chicken, 1 cup	2
with pork, 1 cup	3
without sauce, 1 cup	0
Strawberries, fresh, 1 1/2 cups whole or sliced	1 (2)
Strawberry shortcake, 1/12 of 9" cake or 1 filled individual shortcake	7
Stromboli, 1 slice (1" thick) or 2 oz	4
Strudel, any type, 1 piece (5 1/2" x 2")	9
Stuffing	
1/2 cup	4
bread, from mix, prepared, 1/2 cup	4
Succotash, cooked, 1 cup	4
Sugar apple (sweetsop)	
1/3 cup	1 (2)
1/2 (2 3/4 oz)	1 (2)

	POINTS VALUE
Sugar, brown	
1 Tbsp unpacked	1
1 cup packed	17
Sugar, white	
1 Tbsp	1
1 cup	15
Sugar substitute, 1 tsp	0
Suimono, 1 cup	1
Sukiyaki with sauce, 2 cups with 1/4 cup sauce	12
Summer squash casserole, 1 cup	9
Sunflower seeds	
1 tsp	0
1 Tbsp	1
Sunomono, 1/2 cup	0
Sushi	
Alaskan roll, 2 pieces (1" high x 1 3/4" diameter)	3
California roll, 4 large pieces (1" high x 1-3/4" diameter, or 1 oz each)	3
cone, 1	2
inari, 1	2
kappa maki (cucumber roll), 6 small (1" diameter, 1" thick)	2
kappa maki (cucumber roll), 4 medium (1 1/2" diameter, 3/4" thick)	2
maki (vegetables and rice rolled with seaweed), 6 small pieces (1" diameter, 1" thick)	2
maki (vegetables and rice rolled with seaweed), 4 medium pieces (1 1/2" diameter, 3/4" thick)	2
nigiri (sliced raw fish over rice), 6 small pieces (1" diameter, 1" thick)	2

Complete A-Z Food List

◈ *Sushi (cont'd)* ⓅOINTS

nigiri (sliced raw fish over rice), 4 medium pieces (1 1/2" diameter, 3/4" thick)	2
nigiri uni (sea urchin), 4 pieces (2" long, 3/4" wide)	2
nigiri, albacore (white tuna), 4 pieces (2" long, 3/4" wide)	2
nigiri, amaebi (sweet shrimp), 4 pieces (2" long, 3/4" wide)	2
nigiri, conch, 4 pieces (2" long, 3/4" wide)	2
nigiri, ebi (cooked shrimp), 4 pieces (2" long, 3/4" wide)	2
nigiri, hamachi (yellow tail), 4 pieces (2" long, 3/4" wide)	2
nigiri, hirame (fluke), 4 pieces (2" long, 3/4" wide)	2
nigiri, hokigai (surf clam), 4 pieces (2" long, 3/4" wide)	2
nigiri, ikura (salmon roe), 4 pieces (2" long, 3/4" wide)	2
nigiri, kani (crab), 4 pieces (2" long, 3/4" wide)	2
nigiri, maguro (tuna), 4 pieces (2" long, 3/4" wide)	2
nigiri, masago (smelt roe), 4 pieces (2" long, 3/4" wide)	2
nigiri, saba (mackerel), 4 pieces (2" long, 3/4" wide)	2
nigiri, sake (fresh salmon), 4 pieces (2" long, 3/4" wide)	2
nigiri, smoked salmon, 4 pieces (2" long, 3/4" wide)	2
nigiri, suzuki (sea bass), 4 pieces (2" long, 3/4" wide)	2

◈   ⓅOINTS

nigiri, suzume, 4 pieces (2" long, 3/4" wide)	2
nigiri, tai (red snapper), 4 pieces (2" long, 3/4" wide)	2
nigiri, tairagai (scallops), 4 pieces (2" long, 3/4" wide)	2
nigiri, tako (octopus), 4 pieces (2" long, 3/4" wide)	2
nigiri, tobiko (flying fish roe), 4 pieces (2" long, 3/4" wide)	2
nigiri, unagi (fresh water eel), 4 pieces (2" long, 3/4" wide)	2
nigri, ika (squid), 4 pieces (2" long, 3/4" wide)	2
nori maki (raw fish and rice rolled with seaweed), 6 small pieces (1" diameter, 1" thick)	2
nori maki (raw fish and rice rolled with seaweed), 4 medium pieces (1 1/2" diameter, 3/4" thick)	2
Philadelphia roll, 2 large pieces (1" high x 1 3/4" diameter)	3
rainbow roll, 6 small (1" diameter, 1" thick)	2
rainbow roll, 4 medium (1 1/2" diameter, 3/4" wide)	2
shrimp tempura roll, 6 pieces (1 1/2" diameter x 1" thick)	8
spider roll, 6 pieces (2" diameter x 1" thick)	9
tamago-yaki (omelet roll), 2 pieces (3/4" wide)	3
tuna roll, 6 small (1" diameter, 1" thick)	2
tuna roll, 4 medium (1 1/2" diameter, 3/4" thick)	2

	POINTS VALUE
tuna roll, spicy, 6 pieces (2" diameter x 1" thick)	5
unagi maki, 6 small (1" diameter, 1" thick)	2
unagi maki, 4 medium (1 1/2" diameter, 3/4" thick)	2
uni maki, 6 small (1" diameter, 1" thick)	2
uni maki, 4 medium (1 1/2" diameter, 3/4" thick)	2
vegetable tempura roll, 6 pieces (1 1/2" diameter x 1" thick)	4
yellow tail roll, 6 small (1" diameter, 1" thick)	2
yellow tail roll, 4 medium (1 1/2" diameter, 3/4" thick)	2
◆ **Swamp cabbage,** (skunk cabbage), cooked or uncooked, 1 cup	0
Swedish meatballs	
6 (1" diameter)	9
with noodles, frozen, 1 cup	7
Sweet and sour	
beef, 1 cup	12
chicken, 1 cup	10
pork, 1 cup	12
shrimp, 1 cup	10
◆ **Sweet potato leaves,** cooked, 1 cup	0
Sweet potato pie, 1/8 of 9" pie	9
Sweet roll	
1 large (4 oz)	5
pecan-swirl, store-bought, 2 (2 oz)	5
store-bought, 1 (2 3/4" square)	5
◆ **Sweetbreads,** cooked, 1 oz	1 (5)

	POINTS VALUE	
Sweetsop (sugar apple)		
◆ 1/3 cup	1	(2)
◆ 1/2 (2 7/8" diameter)	1	(2)
Syrup		
chocolate, 1 Tbsp	1	
maple, 1 Tbsp	1	
maple, 1 cup	16	
pancake, low-calorie, 2 Tbsp	1	
pancake, regular, 1 Tbsp	1	
Szechuan chicken, frozen, 1 cup	6	

T

	POINTS VALUE
Tabouli, 1/2 cup	4
Taco	
beef, 1 (3 1/2 oz)	5
breakfast, 1 (3 3/4 oz)	5
chicken, 1 (3 1/2 oz)	4
fish, 1 (4 1/4 oz)	4
hard, dinner kit in a box, prepared, 2 (5 1/2 oz)	7
hard, fast food, 1	3
pork, 1 (3 1/2 oz)	4
soft, fast food, 1	3
soft, kit in a box, prepared, 2 (5 1/2 oz)	9
Taco salad shells	
small, store-bought, 2 (1 1/2 oz)	4
large, store-bought, 1 (2 oz)	6
Taco shells, store-bought	
4 miniature (3" diameter) or 3/4 oz	2
2 small (4 1/2" diameter) or 3/4 oz	2
1 large (6 1/2" diameter) or 3/4 oz	2

Complete A-Z Food List

	POINTS VALUE
Taffy, 1 piece (1/2 oz)	1
Tahini, 2 Tbsp	5
Tamale pie, 1 cup	11
Tamales	
2 (4" x 2")	9
beef, canned, 2 (4 oz)	3
beef, frozen, 3 small or 1 large (4 3/4 oz)	7
chicken, canned, 2	3
chicken, frozen, 1 large or 3 small (6 oz)	7
pork, frozen, 3 small or 1 large (4 1/2 oz)	7
◆ **Tamarinds,** 10 (3" x 1")	1 (2)
Tandoori	
chicken breast, without skin, 1 piece (4 1/2 oz)	4
chicken thigh, without skin, 1 piece (3 oz)	4
fish, 3/4 cup	5
shrimp, 3/4 cup	3
◆ **Tangelo,** 1 large (5 oz)	1 (2)
Tangerine (Mandarin orange)	
◆ 2 small (2 1/4" diameter)	1 (2)
◆ 2 medium (2 3/8" diameter)	1 (2)
◆ 1 large (3" diameter)	1 (2)
◆ canned, unsweetened, 1 cup	1 (2)
Tapioca, uncooked, 1 tsp	0
Taquitos	
beef, 1 (5 1/2" x 1 1/2")	4
chicken, 1 (5 1/2" x 1 1/2")	2
frozen, 2 (2 oz)	3
◆ **Taro,** cooked, 1 cup	3
◆ **Taro leaves,** cooked, 1 cup	0

	POINTS VALUE
Tart shell	
1 (4" diameter)	6
store-bought, 4"	5
Tarte aux fruits	
1/8 of 9" tart	8
individual, 1 (4")	11
Tea	
black, decaffeinated or regular, without sugar, 1 cup	0
decaffeinated or regular, sweetened, 1 cup	2
sweetened, 1 Tbsp	2
◆ **Tempeh (fermented soybean cake),** 1/4 cup (1 1/2 oz)	2
Tempura	
batter mix, 1/4 cup	1
shrimp, 4 jumbo (3 3/4 oz)	12
vegetable, 1 cup	8
Teppan yaki (mixed grill of beef, chicken, shrimp and vegetables), 1 1/2 cups	12
Tequila, 1 jigger (1 1/2 fl oz)	2
Tequila sunrise, 1 (5 1/2 fl oz)	4
Teriyaki	
beef, 2 slices (4 oz)	7
chicken, 2 slices (4 oz)	6
fish (other than salmon), 4 oz	5
salmon, 4 oz	7
tofu, 1 cup	4
Texas trash (cereal and nut mix), 1 cup	8
Textured vegetable protein	
◆ 1/3 cup (3/4 oz dry)	1 (5)
◆ 1 oz	2 (5)

	POINTS VALUE
Thai chicken with basil, 1 breast (without skin and bone), 3 oz	5
Thai coffee or tea, 1 cup	7
Thai crisp noodles, 1 cup	8
Thai curry paste, 1 Tbsp	1
Thai grilled beef (Nuea nam tok), 1/2 cup on lettuce leaves	5
Thai paste, 2 Tbsp	2
Tirami-su, 2 1/4" square	10
Toaster pastry	
low-fat, 1 (1 3/4 oz)	4
regular, any type, 1 (1 3/4 oz)	5
Tofu	
firm, regular, 1/5 block, 1/3 cup, or 3 oz	2 (5)
low-fat, 1/5 block, 1/3 cup, or 3 oz	1 (5)
soft, regular, 1/5 block, 1/3 cup, or 3 oz	1 (5)
Tofu, frozen, 1/2 cup	5
Tom Collins, 1 (6 fl oz)	2
Tom yum kung, 1 cup	2
Tomato paste	
canned, 2 Tbsp	0
canned, 1/2 cup	1
Tomato puree, canned, 1/2 cup	1
Tomatoes	
canned, 1 cup	0
dried, not packed in oil, 1/4 cup	0
dried, packed in oil, drained, 1 medium	0
dried, packed in oil, drained, 1/4 cup	1
fresh, 1 small, medium, or large, or 1 cup	0
Tomatoes, green, fried, 2 slices (1 1/2" thick)	4

	POINTS VALUE
Tonkatsu	
beef, 3/4 cup	7
chicken, 3/4 cup	6
pork, 3/4 cup	8
Topping	
caramel, regular or fat-free, 2 Tbsp	2
fruit, 1 Tbsp	1
fudge, fat-free, 1 Tbsp	1
fudge, regular, 1 Tbsp	1
whipped, dairy or nondairy, light or fat-free, aerosol or frozen, 2 Tbsp	1
whipped, dairy or nondairy, light or fat-free, aerosol or frozen, 1/4 cup	1
whipped, dairy or nondairy, light or fat-free, aerosol or frozen, 1/3 cup	1
Tortellini	
beef, chicken, or pork, without sauce, frozen, 1 cup	5
cheese, without sauce, 10 (2/3 cup)	3
cheese, without sauce, frozen, 1 cup	6
meat, without sauce, 10 (2/3 cup)	3
mushroom, without sauce, frozen, 1 cup	6
sausage, without sauce, frozen, 1 cup	7
Tortiere (Canadian meat pie), 1/8 of 9" pie	9
Tortilla, corn	
2 (4" diameter), 1 oz	1
1 (6" diameter), 1 oz	1
1/2 (10" diameter), 1 oz	1
Tortilla, flour	
2 (4" diameter), 1 oz	2
1 (6" diameter), 1 oz	2
1/2 (10" diameter), 1 oz	2

Complete A-Z Food List

◆ *Tortilla, flour (cont'd)*   (POINTS VALUE)

	POINTS VALUE	
fat-free, 2 (4" diameter), 1 oz	0	
fat-free, 1 (6" diameter), 1 oz	0	
fat-free, 1 (10" diameter), 2 oz	2	
Tortilla, whole wheat, 1 medium (7")	1	
Tortilla chips		
12 (1 oz)	3	
baked, low-fat, 12 (1 oz)	2	
reduced-fat, 12 (1 oz)	3	
Tortoni, 2 1/2 oz	7	
Tostada		
beef, 1 (8 1/4 oz)	10	
chicken, 1 (8 1/4 oz)	8	
with beans and cheese, fast food, 1	5	
Tostada shells, store-bought, 2 (1 oz)	2	
Trail mix		
1/4 cup	4	
tropical, 1/4 cup	3	
with chocolate chips, 1/4 cup	5	
Trifle, 1 cup	5	
◆ **Tripe,** beef, cooked, 1 oz	1	(5)
Tuna dinner in a box, prepared, 1 cup	7	
Tuna noodle casserole, 1 cup	9	
◆ **Tuna,** grilled, frozen, 3 oz	2	(5)
Turkey		
breast, cooked, with skin, 1 slice (2 oz)	2	
◆ breast, cooked, without skin, 1 slice or 1/2 cup cubed or shredded (2 oz)	2	(5)
◆ canned , 1/2 cup	4	(5)
◆ dark meat, cooked, without skin, 1 slice or 1/2 cup cubed or shredded (2 oz)	2	(5)
leg, cooked, with skin, 1 slice (2 oz)	3	

	POINTS VALUE	
leg, cooked, with skin, 1 (1 1/4 pounds)	27	
thigh, cooked, with skin, 1 slice (2 oz)	3	
Turkey, ground		
◆ 93% lean/7% fat, cooked, 1/2 cup (2 oz)	3	(5)
◆ 93% lean/7% fat, cooked, 1 patty (3 oz)	4	(5)
◆ 93% lean/7% fat, cooked, 12 oz (1 pound raw)	16	(5)
◆ regular, cooked, 1/2 cup (2 oz)	3	(5)
◆ regular, cooked, 1 patty (3 oz)	5	(5)
Turkey, with gravy, frozen, 1 cup	4	
Turkey burger, frozen (prepared), 1 (3 oz)	4	
Turkey croquette, breaded, with gravy, frozen, 1 (3 1/2 oz)	6	
Turkey roll, 1 slice (1 oz)	1	
Turkey tetrazzini, 1 1/2 cups	14	
◆ **Turnips,** cooked or uncooked, 1 cup	0	
Turnover, fruit, any type		
1 (3" x 1 1/2")	5	
fast food, 1	7	
Twice-cooked pork, 1 cup	10	
Tyropitas, frozen, 2 (2 oz)	4	
Tzimmes, vegetable, 3/4 cup	2	

U

	POINTS VALUE	
◆ **Urad dal (split matpe beans without skin),** 1 cup	4	

POINTS VALUE

V

Veal

breast, cooked, 3 oz	6	
◆ breast, trimmed, cooked, 3 oz	4	(5)
◆ lean (round or loin cuts with all visible fat trimmed), cooked, 1 slice, 1 chop, or 1/2 cup cubed or shredded (2 oz)	3	(5)
leg, cooked, 3 oz	4	
◆ leg, trimmed, cooked, 3 oz	4	(5)
loin, cooked, 3 oz	6	
◆ loin, trimmed, cooked, 3 oz	3	(5)
regular, cooked, 1 slice, 1 chop, or 1/2 cup cubed or shredded (2 oz)	3	
rib, cooked, 3 oz	5	
rib, trimmed, cooked, 3 oz	4	
shank, cooked, 3 oz	4	
shank, trimmed, cooked, 3 oz	3	
shoulder, cooked, 3 oz	5	
shoulder, trimmed, cooked, 3 oz	4	
sirloin, cooked, 1 slice, 1 chop, or 1/2 cup cubed or shredded (2 oz)	3	
sirloin, cooked, 1 slice, 1 chop, or 1/2 cup cubed or shredded (3 oz)	5	
◆ sirloin, trimmed, cooked, 1 slice, 1 chop, or 1/2 cup cubed or shredded (3 oz)	3	(5)
Veal cutlet, breaded, fried, 4 oz	8	
Veal marsala, 4 oz veal with sauce	13	

Veal parmigiana

with sauce, 5 oz with 1/2 cup tomato sauce	12	
without sauce, 5 1/2 oz	10	
Veal piccata, 2 slices (4 oz)	10	

Veal scaloppine, 2 pieces (4 1/2 oz)	8	
Veal with peppers, 5 oz	11	
Vegetable pulao, 1 cup	3	
Vegetables		
creamed (except creamed corn), 1 cup	2	
fried, 1 cup	4	
in sauce, frozen, 1 cup	1	
◆ mixed, drained, 1/2 cup	0	
packed in oil, drained, 1 cup	3	
pot roasted with pan drippings, 1 cup	2	
sautéed, 1 cup	6	
◆ stir-fry, without sauce, 1 cup	0	
Vegetables, Chinese		
◆ 1 cup	2	
prepared without oil, 1 cup	4	
Vegetarian breakfast link (sausage-type), 2 (1-1/2 oz)	3	
Vegetarian breakfast patty, sausage-type, 1 (1 1/3 oz)	1	
Vegetarian breakfast strips, 4 (1 oz)	3	
◆ **Vegetarian burger, black bean,** frozen, 1 (1 1/2 oz)	2	(5)
◆ **Vegetarian burger, frozen,** 1 (2 3/4 oz)	1	(5)
◆ **Vegetarian burger, frozen, fat free,** 1 (2 3/4 oz)	1	(5)
Vegetarian chicken patty, frozen, 1 (3 oz)	2	
Vegetarian chicken pieces (nugget-style), frozen, 4 (2 3/4 oz)	3	
Vegetarian deli slices, frozen, 3 (2 3/4 oz)	1	
Vegetarian frankfurter, fat free, frozen, 1 small (2 1/2 oz)	1	
Vegetarian frankfurter, fat free, frozen, 1/2 large (2 1/2 oz)	1	

Complete A-Z Food List

Vegetarian frankfurter, regular, frozen, 1 small (3 oz)	2	
Vegetarian frankfurter, regular, frozen, 1/2 large (3 oz)	2	
◆ **Vegetarian ground "meat,"** frozen, 1/2 cup	1	(5)
Vegetarian sausage, frozen, 1 1/2 oz	2	
Vegetarian topping (made with soy), 2 Tbsp	1	
◆ **Venison,** cooked, 1 oz	1	(5)
Vichyssoise, 1 cup	2	
Vienna sausage		
canned, beef and pork, 3 (2" long each)	3	
chicken, canned, 3 (2" long each)	3	
Vietnamese beef balls (Thit bo vien), 6 (1 1/2 oz)	2	
Vietnamese chicken curry, 1 cup	7	
Vindaloo		
chicken, 1 cup	8	
lamb, 1 cup	16	
pork, 1 cup	9	
Vinegar, 1 Tbsp	0	
Vitello tonnato, 2 slices veal (4 oz) with 1/2 cup sauce	16	
Vodka, 1 jigger (1 1/2 fl oz)	2	
Vodka gimlet, 1 (2 1/2 fl oz)	2	

W

Waffle	
any type (other than those listed here), 1 (7" square)	5
any type, frozen, 1 (4" round or square), or 1 1/4 oz	2

any type, made from mix, 1 (4" round or square)	2	
Belgian, frozen, 1 (1 oz)	2	
low-fat, any type, frozen, 2 (4" round or square)	3	
mini, frozen, 4 (1 3/4 oz)	2	
sticks, frozen, 2 small or 1 large (2 oz)	3	
Walnuts		
1 cup chopped, pieces, or chips	21	
14 halves (1 oz)	5	
1 Tbsp	1	
Water chestnuts		
◆ 1 cup	1	
◆ canned, sliced, 1/2 cup	0	
◆ **Water or mineral water,** 1 cup	0	
◆ **Watercress,** 1 cup	0	
◆ **Watermelon,** 1 cup or 1 slice (2")	1	(2)
◆ **Wax gourd (Chinese winter melon),** cooked or uncooked, 1 cup	0	
Wheat germ		
2 Tbsp	1	
3 Tbsp	1	
Whiskey, 1 jigger (1 1/2 fl oz)	2	
Whiskey sour, 1 (3 fl oz)	2	
White Russian, 1 (3 fl oz)	5	
Wiener schnitzel, 1 slice (3 oz)	9	
Wine		
1 small glass (4 fl oz)	2	
dessert, dry, 2 fl oz	1	
dessert, sweet, 2 fl oz	2	
light, 1 small glass (4 fl oz)	1	
non-alcoholic, 1 small glass (4 fl oz)	1	

	POINTS VALUE
Wine cooler, 8 fl oz	2
Wine spritzer, 8 fl oz	2
Wonton skins (wrappers), 5 (3 1/2" squares)	2
Wontons	
boiled, 6 (6 oz)	5
fried, 6 (4 oz)	11

Y

	POINTS VALUE
Yaki-soba	
beef, 1 cup (1/2 cup noodles with 1/2 cup mixed vegetables)	4
chicken, 1 cup (1/2 cup noodles with 1/2 cup chicken & vegetables)	4
pork, 1 cup (1/2 cup noodles with 1/2 cup pork & vegetables)	4
Yakitori, 1 skewer (7 1/2 oz)	5
Yam	
♦ cooked, 3/4 cup	2 (6)
♦ cooked, 1 cup	3 (6)
♦ cooked, 1 large (5"), or 7 oz	3 (6)
sweet, canned, in syrup, 1 cup	3
♦ uncooked, 1 cup cubes	3 (6)
♦ uncooked, 1 large (8 oz)	4 (6)
♦ **Yam patty,** fat-free, frozen, 1 (4 oz)	1 (6)
Yeast, 1 tsp	0
Yogurt	
fat free, flavored (vanilla, lemon, coffee), sweetened with sugar, 1 cup	3
fat free, fruit-flavored, sweetened with sugar, 1 cup	4
♦ fat free, plain, 1 cup	2
light (artificially sweetened), 1 cup	2

	POINTS VALUE
low-fat, flavored (vanilla, lemon, coffee), sweetened with sugar, 1 cup	4
low-fat, fruit-flavored, sweetened with sugar, 1 cup	5
low-fat, plain, 1 cup	3
plain, whole milk, 1 cup	4
Yogurt, frozen	
fat free, no sugar added, 1 scoop or 1/2 cup	2
fat free, sweetened with sugar, 1 scoop or 1/2 cup	2
low-fat, 1 scoop or 1/2 cup	3
Yogurt bar, chocolate-covered, frozen, 1 (2.8 fl oz)	5
Yogurt drink, 1 cup	5
Yorkshire pudding, 1 piece (4" square)	6
Yosenabe, 2 cups	4
♦ **Yucca (cassava),** uncooked, 1 cup	6

Z

	POINTS VALUE
Zabaglione, 1/2 cup	4
Zeppole, 1 (4" diameter)	6
Ziti, baked	
with meat, 1 cup	9
without meat, 1 cup	6
Zucchini	
breaded, prepared without fat, 6 pieces (4 oz)	4
♦ cooked or uncooked, 1 cup	0
Zucchini bread, 1 slice (3/4" thick)	5
Zuppa di pesce, 2 cups	11
Zuppa Inglese, 1/16 of 10" cake	8
Zwieback, 4 (1 oz)	2

Complete
Filling Foods List

Stay ahead of hunger by choosing Filling Foods.

They fill you up and help keep hunger at bay.

Complete Filling Foods List

POINTS VALUE

POINTS VALUE

A

Apple

fresh, 1 small (2 1/2" diameter)	1
fresh, 1 medium (2 3/4" diameter)	1
fresh, 1 large (3 1/4" diameter)	2
Applesauce, unsweetened, 1 cup	2

Apricots

canned or frozen, unsweetened, 1 cup	1
fresh, 3 medium (4 oz)	1
Artichoke hearts, cooked, 1 cup	1
Artichokes, cooked, 1 medium	0
Arugula, 1 cup	0
Asparagus, cooked or uncooked, 1 cup or 12 spears	0
Avocado, 1/4 medium (2 oz)	2

B

Bacon, Canadian-style, cooked, 1 slice (1 oz)	1

Banana

1 cup sliced	2
1 small (6 to 6 7/8" long)	1
1 medium (7 to 7 7/8" long)	2
1 large (8 to 8 7/8" long)	2
1 extra large (9" or larger)	2

Barley

cooked, 1 cup	3
uncooked, 1/4 cup	3

Beans

black, cooked, 1/2 cup	2
cannellini, canned, 1/2 cup	1
garbanzo, canned, 1/2 cup	1
garbanzo, cooked, 1/2 cup	2
garbanzo, dry, 1 pound	35
green, cooked, 1 cup	0
kidney, cooked, 1/2 cup	1
kidney, dry, 1 pound	30
lima, cooked, 1/2 cup	1
lima, dry, 1 pound	30
navy, cooked, 1/2 cup	2
navy, dry, 1 pound	30
pinto, cooked, 1/2 cup	2
pinto, dry, 1 pound	31
soy, cooked, 1/2 cup	3
soy, dry, 1 pound	45
wax, cooked, 1 cup	0
white, cooked, 1/2 cup	2
white, dry, 1 pound	30
Beans, refried, fat-free, canned, 1/2 cup	25

Beef

cube steak, trimmed, cooked, 1/2 cup (2 oz)	3
cube steak, trimmed, cooked, 3 oz	4
filet mignon, trimmed, cooked, 3 oz	4
filet mignon, trimmed, cooked, 1 small (4 oz)	6
flank, lean only, trimmed, cooked, 1 slice (2 oz)	2
flank, lean only, cooked, 3 oz	4

	POINTS VALUE
heart, cooked, 1 oz	1
KC strip, trimmed, cooked, 3 oz	4
KC strip, trimmed, cooked, 1 small (4 oz)	5
kidney, cooked, 1 oz	1
liver, cooked, 1 slice or 1/2 cup (2 oz)	2
New York steak, trimmed, cooked, 3 oz	4
New York steak, trimmed, cooked, 1 small (4 oz)	5
porterhouse steak, trimmed, cooked, 3 oz	6
round steak or roast, trimmed, cooked, 3 oz	4
rump roast, trimmed, cooked, 1 slice (2 oz)	2
rump roast, trimmed, cooked, 3 oz	3
sirloin, trimmed, cooked, 1 slice (2 oz)	2
sirloin, trimmed, cooked, 3 oz	3
steak, lean, cooked (round or loin cuts with all visible fat trimmed), 1 small (4 oz)	5
strip sirloin, trimmed, cooked, 3 oz	3
strip sirloin, trimmed, cooked, 1 small (4 oz)	4
T-bone steak, trimmed, cooked, 3 oz	5
T-bone steak, trimmed, cooked, 1 small (4 oz)	7
tenderloin, trimmed, cooked, 1 slice (2 oz)	3
tenderloin, trimmed, cooked, 3 oz	4
tongue, cooked, 1 oz	2
Beef, ground	
95% lean/5% fat, raw, 1 oz	1
95% lean/5% fat, cooked, 1/2 cup (2 oz)	2

	POINTS VALUE
95% lean/5% fat, cooked, 1 patty (3 oz)	3
95% lean/5% fat, cooked, 12 oz (1 pound raw)	13
Beets	
canned, 1 cup whole	0
cooked, 1 cup	1
uncooked, 1 cup	0
Berries	
mixed, 1 cup	1
wheat, uncooked, 1/4 cup	2
Bison, lean, all visible fat trimmed, cooked, 3 oz	3
Bittermelon (balsam-pear pods), cooked or uncooked, 1 cup	0
Blackberries, 1 cup	1
Blueberries, 1 cup	1
Bok choy, uncooked, 1 cup	0
Borscht	
low-calorie, store-bought, 1 cup	0
store-bought, 1 cup	2
Bouillon	
any type except court, 1 cup	0
cube, beef, chicken, or vegetable, 1/2 cube	0
granules, beef, 1 tsp	0
Boysenberries, fresh or frozen, unsweetened, 1 cup	1
Bran	
corn, uncooked, 1/4 cup	0
oat, uncooked, 1/4 cup	1
rice, uncooked, 1/4 cup	2
wheat, uncooked, 1/4 cup	0

Complete Filling Foods List

	POINTS VALUE
Breadfruit, uncooked, 1 cup	4
Broccoli, cooked or uncooked, 1 cup	0
Broth, any type, 1 cup	0
Brussels sprouts, cooked or uncooked, 1 cup	0
Buffalo, water, cooked or raw, 1 oz	1
Bulgur	
cooked, 1 cup	2
uncooked, 1/4 cup	2

C

	POINTS VALUE
Cabbage, all varieties, cooked or uncooked, 1 cup	0
Calamari, grilled, 1/2 cup	1
Cantaloupe	
10 balls or 1 cup	1
1 small (1 pound)	2
1 medium (5" diameter)	3
1/4 large (6 1/2" diameter)	1
Cappuccino	
made with fat-free milk, 1 small (8 fl oz)	1
made with fat-free milk, 1 tall (12 fl oz)	2
made with fat-free milk, 1 grande (16 fl oz)	2
Cardoon, 1 cup	0
Carrots	
cooked, 1 cup	1
uncooked, 1 small, medium, or large, 1 cup, or 10 baby	0
Casaba melon, 1 cup	1

	POINTS VALUE
Cassava (yucca), uncooked, 1 cup	6
Cauliflower	
cooked or uncooked, 1 cup	0
1 small head (4" diameter)	1
1 medium head (5–6" diameter)	2
1 large head (6–7" diameter)	4
Caviar (fish roe), any type, 1 oz	2
Celeriac	
cooked, 1 cup	0
uncooked, 1 cup	1
Celery, cooked or uncooked, 1 cup	0
Cereal, hot	
cream of rice, cooked, 1 cup	3
cream of wheat, cooked, 1 cup	2
farina, cooked, 1 cup	2
farina, uncooked, 1/4 cup	3
grits, corn, cooked, 1 cup	3
grits, corn, uncooked, 1/4 cup	3
oatmeal, cooked, regular or instant, 1 cup	2
oatmeal, uncooked, 1/4 cup	1
puffed, 1 cup	1
shredded wheat, 1 biscuit	1
Chard, Swiss, cooked or uncooked, 1 cup	0
Cheese, Cheddar, fat-free, shredded, 1/4 cup	1
Cheese, cottage, fat-free, 1 cup	3
Cheese, hard or semisoft, fat-free	
1 cube (1"), 3 Tbsp grated, or 4 Tbsp shredded (1 oz)	1
1 slice (3/4 oz)	1

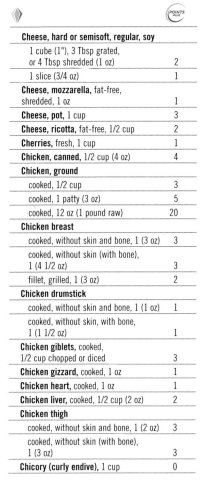

	POINTS VALUE
Cheese, hard or semisoft, regular, soy	
1 cube (1"), 3 Tbsp grated, or 4 Tbsp shredded (1 oz)	2
1 slice (3/4 oz)	1
Cheese, mozzarella, fat-free, shredded, 1 oz	1
Cheese, pot, 1 cup	3
Cheese, ricotta, fat-free, 1/2 cup	2
Cherries, fresh, 1 cup	1
Chicken, canned, 1/2 cup (4 oz)	4
Chicken, ground	
cooked, 1/2 cup	3
cooked, 1 patty (3 oz)	5
cooked, 12 oz (1 pound raw)	20
Chicken breast	
cooked, without skin and bone, 1 (3 oz)	3
cooked, without skin (with bone), 1 (4 1/2 oz)	3
fillet, grilled, 1 (3 oz)	2
Chicken drumstick	
cooked, without skin and bone, 1 (1 oz)	1
cooked, without skin, with bone, 1 (1 1/2 oz)	1
Chicken giblets, cooked, 1/2 cup chopped or diced	3
Chicken gizzard, cooked, 1 oz	1
Chicken heart, cooked, 1 oz	1
Chicken liver, cooked, 1/2 cup (2 oz)	2
Chicken thigh	
cooked, without skin and bone, 1 (2 oz)	3
cooked, without skin (with bone), 1 (3 oz)	3
Chicory (curly endive), 1 cup	0

	POINTS VALUE
Chinese vegetables, with peas, prepared without oil, 1 cup	2
Chitterlings, cooked, 1 oz	2
Clementine	
2 small (3 oz each)	1
1 large (6 oz)	1
Collards, cooked or uncooked, 1 cup	0
Corn	
baby (ears), 1 cup	1
kernels, cooked, 1 cup	2
Corn on the cob	
1 small (5 1/2")	1
1 medium (7")	1
1 large (8")	2
Cornish hen, cooked, without skin, 1/2 (3 3/4 oz)	3
Cornmeal	
cooked, 1 cup	2
dry, 2 Tbsp	1
Couscous, whole-wheat	
cooked, 1 cup	3
uncooked, 1 tsp	0
uncooked, 1 Tbsp	1
uncooked, 1/4 cup	3
Crabapple, 1 cup (slices)	2
Cranberries, fresh, 1 1/2 cups (5 oz)	1
Cream, sour, fat-free, 1/4 cup	1
Cucumber, 1 cup	0
Currants, fresh, 1 1/2 cups	1

Complete Filling Foods List

D

	POINTS VALUE
Daikon, cooked or uncooked, 1 cup	0
Dandelion greens, cooked or uncooked, 1 cup	0
Dates, fresh, 2 (3/4 oz)	1

E

	POINTS VALUE
Edamame	
in pods, 1 cup	1
shelled, 1/2 cup	2
Egg, whole, chicken	
cooked or raw, 1	2
hard-boiled, 1	2
poached, 1	2
Egg substitute	
fat-free, 1/4 cup	1
regular, 1/4 cup	2
Egg white, chicken	
1	0
3	1
Eggplant, cooked or uncooked, 1 cup	0
Elderberries, 1 cup	1
Elk, cooked or raw, 1 oz	1
Endive	
1 cup	0
head, 1	0
Escarole, 1 cup	1

F

	POINTS VALUE
Fennel, 1 cup	1
Fiddlefern (fiddlehead greens), 1 cup	0
Figs	
fresh, 2 medium (2 1/4")	0
fresh, 1 large (2 1/2")	1
Fish	
arctic char, cooked, 3 oz	4
bass, striped, cooked, 1 fillet (6 oz)	5
bluefish, cooked, 1 fillet (6 oz)	6
carp, cooked, 1 fillet (6 oz)	7
catfish, cooked, 1 fillet (6 oz)	6
cod, cooked, 1 fillet (6 oz)	4
eel, cooked, 1 oz	2
flounder, cooked, 1 fillet (6 oz)	4
grouper, cooked, 1 fillet (6 oz)	4
haddock, cooked, 1 fillet (6 oz)	4
halibut, cooked, 1 fillet or steak (6 oz)	5
herring, cooked, 1 oz	1
lox, 1 oz	1
mackerel, canned in water, drained, 1/2 cup	3
mackerel, cooked, 1 fillet (6 oz)	8
mahimahi (dolphinfish), cooked, 1 fillet (6 oz)	4
perch, cooked, 1 fillet (6 oz)	4
pike, cooked, 1 fillet (6 oz)	4
pollack, cooked, 1 fillet (6 oz)	4
pompano, cooked, 1 fillet (6 oz)	9
rockfish, cooked, 1 fillet (6 oz)	4

	POINTS VALUE
salmon, canned, drained, 1/2 cup (4 oz)	4
salmon, cooked, 1 fillet (6 oz)	9
sardines, canned in tomato sauce, drained, 2 oz	3
sardines, canned in tomato sauce, drained, 1 can (13 oz)	16
skate, uncooked, 3 1/2 oz	2
smelt, cooked, 1 oz	1
snapper, cooked, 1 fillet (6 oz)	5
sole, cooked, 1 fillet (6 oz)	4
swordfish, cooked, 1 fillet or steak (6 oz)	6
tilapia, cooked, 1 fillet (6 oz)	4
trout, cooked, 1 fillet (6 oz)	8
trout, rainbow, cooked, 1 fillet (6 oz)	6
tuna, canned in water, drained, 1/2 cup (4 oz)	3
tuna, cooked, 1 fillet or steak (6 oz)	5
whitefish, smoked, 2 oz	1
whiting, cooked, 6 oz	4
Fruit cocktail, canned, unsweetened, 1/2 cup	1

G

	POINTS VALUE
Giardeniera (vegetable medley, without olives, packed in vinegar), 5 pieces	0
Gobo (burdock), 1/2 cup (2 oz)	1
Gooseberries, 1 cup	1
Grape leaves, 1 cup	0
Grapefruit	
1 small (approximately 3 1/2" diameter)	1
1 medium (approximately 4" diameter)	1
1 large (approximately 5" diameter)	2
sections, juice pack, 1 cup	2

	POINTS VALUE
Grapes, 1 cup	1
Greens, beet, collard, dandelion, kale, mustard, and turnip, cooked or uncooked, 1 cup	0
Guava	
1 cup	1
1 medium	1

H

	POINTS VALUE
Ham	
cooked, lean, 1/2 cup (cubed or shredded) 2 oz	2
cooked, lean, 1 slice (2 oz)	2
Hearts of palm (palmetto), 1 cup	0
Hominy, cooked or canned, whole, 1 cup	2
Honeydew melon	
1 cup	1
1/8 small (5 1/4" diameter) or 1/8 medium (6-7" diameter)	1

J

	POINTS VALUE
Jackfruit, uncooked, 1/2 cup	1
Jerusalem artichokes (sunchokes), 1 cup	2
Jicama	
1 small or medium	1
1 large	2
1 slice	0
1 cup	0
Juice, clam, canned, 1/2 cup	0

Complete Filling Foods List

◈   (POINTS VALUE)

K

Kasha (buckwheat groats)

cooked, 1 cup	2
uncooked, 1/4 cup	2
Kim chee, 1/2 cup	0

Kiwifruit

1 cup	1
1 medium (2 1/2 oz)	0
1 large (4 oz)	1

Kohlrabi

cooked, 1 cup	1
uncooked, 1 cup	0

L

Lamb

lean (leg and loin cuts with all visible fat trimmed), cooked, 1 slice, 1 chop, or 1/2 cup cubed or shredded, (2 oz)	3
leg, cooked, trimmed, 1 slice (2 oz)	3
leg, cooked, trimmed, 3 oz	4
leg, cooked, trimmed, 3 oz	4
loin, cooked, trimmed, 1 slice (2 oz)	4
loin, cooked, trimmed, 3 oz	4
Lamb, ground, cooked, lean, 3 oz	3
Lambsquarters, cooked, 1 cup	1

Latte

made with fat-free milk, 1 small (8 fl oz)	2
made with fat-free milk, 1 tall (12 fl oz)	2
made with fat-free milk, 1 grande (16 fl oz)	3
Leeks, cooked, 1 cup	0

◈   (POINTS VALUE)

Lemon, 1 medium	0
Lentils	
cooked, 1/2 cup	2
dry, 1 cup	12
dry, 1 pound	30
Lettuce, any type, 1 cup	0
Lime, 1 medium	0
Litches (lychees), uncooked, 10 medium	1
Lobster, steamed, 1 1/4 -pound lobster or 4 1/2 oz lobster meat	3
Loganberries, 1 cup	1
Lomi lomi salmon, 1/2 cup	1
Logans, 25 (3 oz)	1
Loquats, 10 medium	1
Lotus root, cooked or uncooked, 1 cup	1
Lychees (litches), uncooked, 10 medium	1

M

Macaroni

whole-wheat, cooked, 1 cup	3
whole-wheat, dry, 1 cup	6
whole-wheat, dry, 2 oz	3

Malanga

cooked, 3/4 cup	3
cooked, 1 large	4
uncooked, 1 large	6
Mammy-apple (mamey), uncooked, 1 (1 3/4 pounds)	8

Mandarin orange (tangerine)

2 small (2 1/4" diameter)	1
1 large (3" diameter)	1
canned, unsweetened, 1 cup	1

	POINTS VALUE
Mango	
1 small (8 oz without pit and skin)	2
1 large (14 1/2 oz without pit and skin)	4
1 cup	2
Melon balls, 1 cup	1
Milk	
evaporated, fat-free, 1/2 cup	2
fat-free, 1 cup	2
instant nonfat dry powder, 1/3 cup	2
soy, calcium-fortified, unflavored, 1 cup	2
Millet	
cooked, 1 cup	4
uncooked, 1/4 cup	3
Mulberries, 1 cup	1
Mushrooms	
dried, 4 large or 16 small	1
dried, reconstituted, 1 cup	1
fresh, cooked or uncooked, 1 cup	0

N

	POINTS VALUE
Nectarine, 1 medium (2 1/2" diameter)	1

O

	POINTS VALUE
Okra, cooked or uncooked, 1 cup	0
Olives, 10 small or 6 large (1 oz)	1
Onion	
cooked, 1 cup	1
uncooked, 1 cup	0
Orange	
1 small (2 3/8" diameter)	0
1 medium (2 5/8" diameter)	1
1 large (3 diameter)	1

	POINTS VALUE
Orange sections, 1 cup	1
Ostrich, cooked, 3 oz	3

P

	POINTS VALUE
Papaya	
fresh, 1 small (4 1/2" long x 3" diameter)	1
fresh, 1 medium (5" long x 3" diameter)	1
fresh, 1 large (5 1/4" long x 3 1/4" diameter)	1
fresh, 1 cup	1
green, 1 cup	1
Parsley, fresh or dried, 1 cup	0
Parsnips	
cooked, 1 cup	2
uncooked, 1 medium or 1 cup slices	1
Passion fruit, 3 (2 oz)	0
Pasta	
brown rice, 2 oz	4
whole-wheat, cooked, 1 cup	3
whole-wheat, uncooked, 2 oz	3
whole-wheat, uncooked, 1 pound	31
Peach	
canned, unsweetened, 1 cup	2
fresh, 1 small (2" diameter or 3 oz)	0
fresh, 1 medium (2 1/2" diameter or 3 1/2 oz)	0
fresh, 1 large (2 3/4" diameter or 6 oz)	1
Pear	
canned, unsweetened, 1 cup	2
fresh, 1 small (5 oz)	1
fresh, 1 medium (6 oz)	1

Complete Filling Foods List

◈ *Pear (cont'd)* ⬡ POINTS VALUE

fresh, 1 large (7 oz)	2
fresh, prickly, 1 cup	0
Peas	
black-eyed, cooked, 1/2 cup	1
black-eyed, dry, 1 pound	30
chick, cooked, 1/2 cup	2
chick, dry, 1 pound	35
cowpeas, cooked, 1/2 cup	1
green, cooked or uncooked, 1 cup	2
snow (Chinese pea pods), 1 cup	0
split, cooked, 1/2 cup	2
split, dry, 1/4 cup	3
sugar snap, 1 cup	0
Pepper, any type, 1 small, medium, or large, or 1 cup	0
Persimmon, 1 (2 1/2" diameter, or 6 oz)	2
Pickle, unsweetened, 1 cup or 1 large	0
Pico de gallo, 1/2 cup	1
Pimientos, canned, 1 cup	0
Pineapple	
canned, unsweetened, 1 cup	2
fresh, 1/4 medium or 1 cup	1
fresh, 2 slices (3 1/2" diameter x 1/2" thick) or 4 oz	1
Plantain, baked or boiled, 1 cup	3
Plums	
fresh, 2 small (2" diameter)	1
fresh, 1 medium (2 1/8" diameter)	0
Poi, 1/2 cup (4 oz)	3

◈ ⬡ POINTS VALUE

Polenta	
cooked, 1/2 cup	2
dry, 1/4 cup	2
Pomegranate, 1 (3 3/8" diameter)	2
Pomelo (pummelo), 1 (1 pound)	3
Popcorn	
regular, plain, air-popped, 3 cups	1
reduced-fat (94% fat-free), microwave-popped, 5 cups	1
Pork	
center loin, lean only, cooked, 1 slice (2 oz)	2
center loin, lean only, cooked, 3 oz	4
kidney, cooked, 1 oz	1
leg, trimmed, cooked, 1 slice (2 oz)	3
leg, trimmed, cooked, 3 oz	4
loin, trimmed, cooked, 1 slice (2 oz)	2
loin, trimmed, cooked, 3 oz	4
sirloin, lean only, cooked, 1 slice (2 oz)	3
sirloin, lean only, cooked, 3 oz	4
tenderloin, lean only, cooked, 1 slice (2 oz)	2
tenderloin, lean only, cooked, 3 oz	3
tenderloin, lean only, cooked, 1 cup	4
top loin, lean only, cooked, 1 slice (2 oz)	2
top loin, lean only, cooked, 3 oz	3
Potato leaves, sweet, cooked, 1 cup	0
Potatoes	
baked, plain, 1 small (3 oz)	1
baked, plain, 1 large (7 oz)	3
uncooked, 1/2 cup diced	1

	POINTS VALUE
uncooked, 1 small (4 oz)	1
uncooked, 1 large (9 oz)	3
Potatoes O'Brien, frozen (prepared without fat), 1 cup	1
Potatoes, baby	
cooked, 1 (2 oz)	1
uncooked, 1 (2 1/2 oz)	1
Potatoes, bliss	
cooked, 1 (2 oz)	1
uncooked, 1 (2 1/2 oz)	1
Potatoes, new, cooked, 1 (2 oz)	1
Potatoes, sweet	
cooked, 1 cup (7 oz)	3
cooked, 1 small (3 oz)	1
cooked, 1 medium (4 1/2 oz)	2
cooked, 1 large (5") or 7 oz	3
uncooked, 1 cup cubes	2
uncooked, 1 small (4 1/2 oz)	2
uncooked, 1 medium (7 oz)	3
uncooked, 1 large (8 oz)	4
Potatoes, white or red	
cooked, 1 cup	2
cooked, 1 small (2" diameter) or 3 oz	1
cooked, 1 large (5") or 7 oz	3
Pudding	
banana, instant, fat-free, sugar free, with pie filling mix, 1 oz	1
butterscotch, instant, fat-free, sugar free, with pie filling mix, 1 oz	1
chocolate, instant, fat-free, sugar free, with pie filling mix, 1 oz	1

	POINTS VALUE
from fat-free, sugar-free mix, made with fat-free milk, 1 cup	3
vanilla, instant, fat-free, sugar free, with pie filling mix, 1 oz	1
Pumpkin	
canned, 1 cup	1
fresh, cooked or uncooked, 1 cup	0
Pumpkin leaves, cooked, 1 cup	0

Q

Quince, 1 (3 1/4 oz)	1
Quinoa	
cooked, 1 cup	4
uncooked, 2 Tbsp	1

R

Radicchio, uncooked, 1 cup shredded	0
Radishes, 1 cup	0
Raspberries, 1 1/2 cups	1
Rhubarb, cooked or uncooked, 1 cup	0
Rice, brown	
cooked, 1 cup	4
uncooked, 1/4 cup	3
uncooked, 1 cup	13
Rice, wild	
cooked, 1 cup	3
uncooked, 1 cup	11
Rutabaga, cooked or uncooked, 1 cup	1

Complete Filling Foods List

S

Salad

mixed greens, 1 cup	0
Niçoise, without dressing, 4 cups	8
three-bean, canned, without oil, 1/2 cup	1
tossed, without dressing, 2 cups	0

Salsa

black bean & corn, 1/2 cup	1
fat-free, 2 Tbsp	0
fat-free, 1/2 cup	0

Salsify (oyster plant), cooked, 1 cup — 1

Sashimi

except mackerel or salmon, 4 pieces (2 oz)	1
mackerel, 4 pieces (2 oz)	3
salmon, 4 pieces (2 oz)	2

Sauce, tomato, canned, 1/2 cup — 0

Sauerkraut, 1 cup — 0

Scallions, 1 cup — 0

Schav, canned, 1 cup — 0

Seitan

dry mix, prepared, 2 oz	1
slices, 2 slices (2 oz)	1

Shallots

uncooked, 1 cup	2
uncooked, 1 small or medium	0

Shark, cooked, 1 steak (6 oz) — 5

Sharon fruit, 3 oz — 1

Shellfish

abalone, cooked, 3 oz	2

clam, cooked, 1/2 cup (2 oz)	2
crab, cooked, 1/2 cup	1
crab, imitation, 1/2 cup (3 oz)	2
crabmeat, canned, 1/2 cup	1
crabmeat, canned, 1 cup	3
crayfish, cooked, 1/2 cup	1
crayfish, cooked, 16 (2 oz)	1
lobster, cooked, 1/2 cup (2 oz)	1
mussel, cooked, 1/2 cup (2 oz)	2
oyster, canned or cooked, 1/2 cup	2
oyster, cooked, 6 medium (2 oz)	1
oyster, raw, 6 medium (3 oz)	1
scallops, cooked, 10 small or 4 large (2 oz)	1
shrimp, canned, 1/2 cup	1
shrimp, cooked, 1/2 cup (2 oz)	1
squid, cooked, 3 oz	2

Soup

bean and ham, canned (made with water), 1 cup	5
beef, canned (made with water), 1 cup	1
beef vegetable, canned (made with water), 1 cup	1
black bean, 1 cup	2
black bean, canned (made with water), 1 cup	2
black bean in cup, 1 (2 oz)	4
bouillon, any type, 1 cup	0
broth, any type, 1 cup	0
cabbage, 1 cup	1
chicken, without matzo balls (broth only), 1 cup	0

	POINTS VALUE
chicken vegetable, in cup, 1	2
escarole, canned, ready-to-serve, 1 cup	1
gazpacho, canned (made with water), 1 cup	1
gazpacho, canned, ready-to-serve, 1 cup	1
lentil, 1 cup	3
lentil, in a cup, 1 (2 oz)	4
lentil with ham, canned, ready-to-serve, 1 cup	3
Manhattan clam chowder, canned (made with water), 1 cup	1
miso, 1 cup	2
onion mix (dry), 1/4 envelope	0
onion mix, prepared, 1 cup	0
split pea, 1 cup	3
split pea, frozen, 1 package (7 1/2 oz)	2
split pea, in a cup, 1 (2 oz)	3
split pea with ham, canned (made with water), 1 cup	4
tomato, canned (made with fat free milk), 1 cup	3
tomato, canned (made with water), 1 cup	2
vegetable, 1 cup	2
vegetable, canned (made with water), 1 cup	1
vegetable beef, canned (made with water), 1 cup	1
vegetable beef mix, prepared, 1 cup	1
vegetarian vegetable, in a cup, 1 (3 oz)	3
Soursop (guanabana), 1/2 cup pulp	1

	POINTS VALUE
Soy cheese, hard or semisoft, fat-free	
1 cube (1"), 3 Tbsp grated, or 4 Tbsp shredded (1 oz)	1
1 slice (3/4 oz)	1
Soy cheese, hard or semisoft, regular	
1 cube (1"), 3 Tbsp grated, or 4 Tbsp shredded (1 oz)	2
1 slice (3/4 oz)	1
Soy milk, calcium-fortified, unflavored, 1 cup	2
Soy yogurt, plain, 3/4 cup (6 oz)	2
Spaghetti	
whole wheat, cooked, 1 cup	3
whole-wheat, uncooked, 2 oz	3
Spinach, cooked or uncooked, 1 cup	0
Sprouts	
alfalfa, 1 cup	0
bean, 1 cup	0
Squash	
spaghetti, cooked or uncooked, 1 cup	0
summer, cooked or uncooked, 1 cup	0
winter, cooked, 1 cup	1
winter, uncooked, 1 cup	0
Squash leaves, 1 cup	0
Starfruit (carambola), 2 large (4 1/2" long)	0
Stir-fried vegetables, without sauce, 1 cup	0
Strawberries, fresh, 1 1/2 cups whole or sliced	1
Succotash, cooked, 1 cup	4

Complete Filling Foods List

	POINTS VALUE
Sugar apple (sweetsop)	
1/3 cup	1
1/2 (2 3/4 oz)	1
Swamp cabbage, (skunk cabbage), cooked or uncooked, 1 cup	0
Sweet potato leaves, cooked, 1 cup	0
Sweetbreads, cooked, 1 oz	1
Sweetsop (sugar apple)	
1/3 cup	1
1/2 (2 7/8" diameter)	1

T

	POINTS VALUE
Tamarinds, 10 (3" x 1")	1
Tangelo, 1 large (5 oz)	1
Tangerine (Mandarin orange)	
2 small (2 1/4" diameter)	1
2 medium (2 3/8" diameter)	1
1 large (3" diameter)	1
canned, unsweetened, 1 cup	1
Taro, cooked, 1 cup	3
Taro leaves, cooked, 1 cup	0
Tempeh (fermented soybean cake), 1/4 cup (1 1/2 oz)	2
Textured vegetable protein	
1/3 cup (3/4 oz dry)	1
1 oz	2
Tofu	
firm, regular, 1/5 block, 1/3 cup, or 3 oz	2
low-fat, 1/5 block, 1/3 cup, or 3 oz	1
soft, regular, 1/5 block, 1/3 cup, or 3 oz	1

	POINTS VALUE
Tomato paste	
canned, 2 Tbsp	0
canned, 1/2 cup	1
Tomato puree, canned, 1/2 cup	1
Tomatoes	
canned, 1 cup	0
dried, not packed in oil, 1/4 cup	0
fresh, 1 small, medium, or large, or 1 cup	0
Tripe, beef, cooked, 1 oz	1
Tuna, grilled, frozen, 3 oz	2
Turkey	
breast, cooked, without skin, 1 slice or 1/2 cup cubed or shredded (2 oz)	2
canned , 1/2 cup	4
dark meat, cooked, without skin, 1 slice or 1/2 cup cubed or shredded (2 oz)	2
Turkey, ground	
93% lean/7% fat, cooked, 1/2 cup (2 oz)	3
93% lean/7% fat, cooked, 1 patty (3 oz)	4
93% lean/7% fat, cooked, 12 oz (1 pound raw)	16
regular, cooked, 1/2 cup (2 oz)	3
regular, cooked, 1 patty (3 oz)	5
Turnips, cooked or uncooked, 1 cup	0

U

	POINTS VALUE
Urad dal (split matpe beans without skin), 1 cup	4

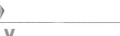

V

	POINTS VALUE
Veal	
breast, trimmed, cooked, 3 oz	4
lean (round or loin cuts with all visible fat trimmed), cooked, 1 slice, 1 chop, or 1/2 cup cubed or shredded (2 oz)	3
leg, trimmed, cooked, 3 oz	4
loin, trimmed, cooked, 3 oz	3
sirloin, trimmed, cooked, 1 slice, 1 chop, or 1/2 cup cubed or shredded (3 oz)	3
Vegetables	
mixed, drained, 1/2 cup	0
stir-fry, without sauce, 1 cup	0
Vegetables, Chinese, 1 cup	2
Vegetarian burger, black bean, frozen, 1 (1 1/2 oz)	2
Vegetarian burger, frozen, 1 (2 3/4 oz)	1
Vegetarian burger, frozen, fat free, 1 (2 3/4 oz)	1
Vegetarian ground "meat," frozen, 1/2 cup	1
Venison, cooked, 1 oz	1

W

	POINTS VALUE
Water chestnuts	
1 cup	1
canned, sliced, 1/2 cup	0
Watercress, 1 cup	0
Watermelon, 1 cup or 1 slice (2")	1
Wax gourd (Chinese winter melon), cooked or uncooked, 1 cup	0

Y

	POINTS VALUE
Yam	
cooked, 3/4 cup	2
cooked, 1 cup	3
cooked, 1 large (5"), or 7 oz	3
uncooked, 1 cup cubes	3
uncooked, 1 large (8 oz)	4
Yam patty, fat-free, frozen, 1 (4 oz)	1
Yogurt, fat free, plain, 1 cup	2
Yucca (cassava), uncooked, 1 cup	6

Z

	POINTS VALUE
Zucchini, cooked or uncooked, 1 cup	0

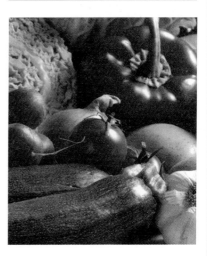

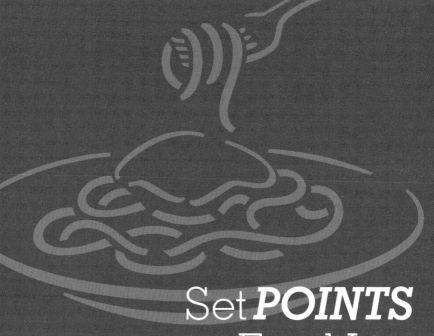

Set *POINTS*
Food List

Use Set*POINTS* values
and listen to your body's signals.

Navigate eating away from home, or have an easier way
of estimating the ***POINTS***® value of a dish, with less stress.

SetPOINTS Food List

LEAN PROTEINS Plain, without sauces, added fat, or breading (trimmed of excess fat after purchase)

5 SetPOINTS values

Egg (white, yolk, whole, or egg substitute)

Fish and shellfish (fresh, frozen, or canned in water)

Poultry (fresh, frozen, or canned chicken or turkey, including ground poultry)

Beef (loin or round cuts, including ground beef with no more than 7% fat)

Lamb (leg or loin cuts, including lean ground lamb)

Pork (Canadian bacon, leg, and loin cuts)

Veal (loin or round cuts)

Organ meats (liver, kidneys, heart, etc.)

Game (buffalo, elk, ostrich, and venison)

Vegetable proteins (dried or canned beans, including black, cannellini, garbanzo, kidney, lima, navy, pinto, soy, fat-free refried beans (canned only); split peas; black-eye peas; lentils; tofu; vegetarian burgers)

GRAINS AND STARCHY VEGETABLES Plain, without sauces, added fat, sugar, or breading

6 SetPOINTS values

Barley

Buckwheat

Bulgur

Corn (fresh, frozen or canned kernels, ears, or on the cob)

Cornmeal

Couscous, whole wheat

Kasha

Pasta, macaroni, and noodles (whole-grain varieties such as whole-wheat, brown rice pasta, etc.)

Peas (fresh, frozen, or canned green, snow, or sugar snap. Does not include dried peas such as split or black-eye)

Potatoes (cooked white, red, or sweet/yams)

Quinoa

Rice (brown or wild)

FRUIT Fresh, frozen, or canned varieties
without added sugar (applesauce not included)

2 Set*POINTS* values

Single fruits only (does not include fruit
combinations such as mixed berries, fruit
salad, or fruit-cocktail type combinations)

Dried fruits and fruit juices are not included

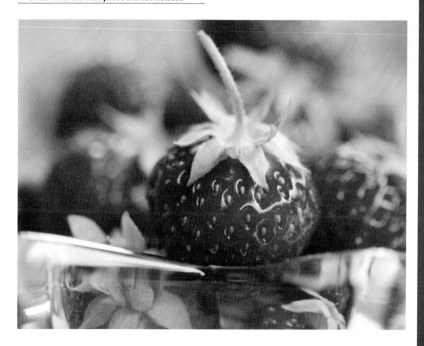

Brand Name Foods List

Find **POINTS**® values for thousands of brand-name foods right here, organized by food category.

Comparison shopping will be simpler when you use this extensive list.

Baking Mixes, Ingredients & Doughs

	POINTS VALUE
Baking Powders	
Calumet	
Baking powder, 1/8 tsp	0
Bread, Biscuit & Popover Mixes & Doughs	
Athens	
Fillo dough, 5 sheets	3
Mini fillo shells, 2	0
Bisquick	
Heart smart baking mix, 1/3 cup	3
Original all purpose baking mix, 1/3 cup	3
Original baking mix (pouch), 1/3 cup	4
Hodgson Mill	
Multi purpose baking mix - gluten free, 1/4 cup	1
Whole wheat insta-bake mix, 1/3 cup	2
Jiffy Mixes	
All purpose baking mix, 1/4 cup	3
Buttermilk biscuit mix, dry, 1/3 cup	3
Tony Chachere's	
Shredded coconut batter mix, 1/4 cup	3
Bread Crumbs	
4C	
Plain bread crumbs, 1 serving (30 g)	2
Seasoned bread crumbs, 1 serving (30 g)	2
Seasoned salt free bread crumbs, 1 serving (30 g)	2
Contadina	
Roasted garlic and savory spices bread crumbs, 1/4 cup	2

	POINTS VALUE
Three cheese bread crumbs, 1/4 cup	2
Unseasoned bread crumbs, 1/4 cup	2
Kellogg's	
Corn flake crumbs, 6 Tbsp	2
Kraft	
Cracker meal, 1/4 cup	2
Lance	
Cracker meal, 1/4 cup	2
Nabisco	
Cracker meal, 1 serving (26 g)	2
Progresso	
Garlic & herb, 1/4 cup	2
Italian style, 1/4 cup	2
Panko crispy bread crumbs - Italian style, 1/4 cup	3
Panko crispy bread crumbs - plain, 1/4 cup	2
Parmesan, 1/4 cup	2
Plain, 1/4 cup	2
Chocolate	
Baker's	
225th anniversary bittersweet chocolate bar, 2 squares	1
Bittersweet chocolate bar, 1/2 square	2
Chocolate melts, 6 wafers	2
German's sweet chocolate bar, 1 serving (13 g)	1
Milk dipping chocolate, 6 wafers	2
Semi sweet (dark) dipping chocolate, 6 wafers	2
Semi-sweet chocolate bar, 1/2 square	2
Semi-sweet chocolate shavings, 1 tsp	0

Baking Mixes, Ingredients & Doughs

	POINTS VALUE
Unsweetened bar, 1/2 square	2
White chocolate bar, 1/2 square	2
Hershey's	
Baking bar, special dark, 1 block	2
Baking bar, unsweetened, 1 block	2
Cocoa, 1 Tbsp	0
M&M's	
Milk chocolate mini baking bits, 1/2 oz (about 1 Tbsp)	2
Semisweet chocolate mini baking bits, 1/2 oz (about 1 Tbsp)	1
Nestle	
Choco bake, 1/2 oz	2
Cocoa for baking, 1 Tbsp	0

Coconut
A Taste of Thai

Coconut milk, 1/3 cup	3
Lite coconut milk, 1/3 cup	1
Dole	
Coconut, 1 cup	7
Port Arthur	
Coconut milk, 1/4 cup	2
Lite coconut milk, 1/4 cup	1
Tree of Life	
Organic shredded coconut, 1 oz	4

Dessert Mix
Aunt Jemima

Easy mix coffee cake, 1/8 package	4
Betty Crocker Classic Cake Mixes	
Gingerbread mix, prepared, 1 slice (1/8 cake)	5

	POINTS VALUE
Pineapple upside down cake mix & topping, prepared, 1 slice (1/6 cake)	9
Pound cake, prepared, 1 slice (1/8 cake)	6
Betty Crocker Warm Delights Dessert Bowl Mixes	
Fudgy chocolate chip mix, 1 package	7
Cherrybrook Kitchen	
Chocolate chip cookie mix, 1 serving (mix for 1 cookie)	2
Sugar cookie mix, 1 serving (mix for 1 cookie)	1
Wheat free/gluten free chocolate chip cookie mix, 1 serving (mix for 1 cookie)	2
Wheat free/gluten free sugar cookies mix, 1 serving (mix for 1 cookie)	1
Dromedary	
Pound cake mix, prepared, 1 serving (1/8 cake)	6
Hodgson Mill	
Brownie mix made with whole wheat flour & milled flaxseed, 3 Tbsp	2
Jiffy Mixes	
Devil's food cake mix, dry, 1 serving (1/5 package)	4
Golden yellow cake mix, dry, 1 serving (1/5 package)	5
Lemon cake mix, dry, 1 serving (1/5 package)	5
White cake mix, dry, 1 serving (1/5 package)	5
Manischewitz	
Angel food cake mix, 3 Tbsp	2
Sponge cake mix, 2 Tbsp	3

Baking Mixes, Ingredients & Doughs

	POINTS VALUE
SuperMoist	
Butter recipe chocolate mix, prepared, 1 slice (1/12 cake)	6
Sweet 'N Low	
Banana snack cake mix, 1 serving (1/5 package)	3
Chocolate chip cookie mix, 3 Tbsp	2
Chocolate snack cake mix, 1 serving (1/5 package)	3
Gingerbread snack cake mix, 1 serving (1/5 package)	3
Lemon snack cake mix, 1 serving (1/5 package)	3
White snack cake mix, 1 serving (1/5 package)	3
Yellow snack cake mix, 1 serving (1/5 package)	3

Extracts & Pastes

	POINTS VALUE
A Taste of Thai	
Green curry paste, 1 tsp	0
Yellow curry paste, 1 tsp	0
Contadina	
◆ Italian paste - tomato paste product with Italian seasonings, 2 Tbsp	1
Del Monte	
◆ Organic tomato paste, 2 Tbsp	0
Eden Selected	
Umeboshi paste, 1 tsp	0
McCormick	
Almond extract, 1/4 tsp	0
Peppermint extract, 1/4 tsp	0
Pure vanilla extract, 1/4 tsp	0

	POINTS VALUE
Odense	
Pure almond paste, 2 Tbsp	4
Thai Kitchen	
Green curry paste, 1 Tbsp	0
Red curry paste, 1 Tbsp	0
Roasted red chili paste, 1 Tbsp	1

Flour

	POINTS VALUE	
Arrowhead Mills		
Gluten - vital wheat, 3 tsp	1	
Long grain brown rice flour, 1/4 cup	2	
Aunt Jemima		
Enriched self-rising flour, 3 Tbsp	2	
Faraon		
Rice flour, 1/4 pack	3	
Gold Medal		
All purpose, 1/4 cup	2	
Better for bread, 1/4 cup	2	
Better for bread - unbleached specialty flour, 1/4 cup	2	
Organic - all purpose, 1/4 cup	2	
Self rising, 1/4 cup	2	
Stone ground wheat, 1/4 cup	1	
Unbleached, 1/4 cup	2	
Hodgson Mill		
100% organic stone ground whole grain whole wheat flour, 1/4 cup	1	
100% soy flour (defatted), 1/4 cup	1	
◆ 100% whole grain stone ground yellow corn meal, 1/4 cup	1	(6)
100% whole grain stone ground white whole wheat flour, 1/4 cup	1	

	POINTS VALUE
100% whole wheat stone ground pastry flour, 1/4 cup	1
Brown rice flour, 1/4 cup	2
Buckwheat flour, 1/4 cup	1
Oat bran flour, 1/4 cup	2
Organic soy flour, 1/4 cup	2
Organic whole grain rye flour, 1/4 cup	1
Organic whole wheat stone ground pastry flour, 1/4 cup	1
Pasta flour, 1/4 cup	2
Stone ground whole grain rye flour, 1/4 cup	1
Whole wheat graham flour, 1/4 cup	1
Manischewitz	
Cake meal, 1/4 cup	3
Martha White	
All purpose bleached, 1/4 cup	2
Self rising bleached, 1/4 cup	2
Pillsbury	
All purpose bleached, 1/4 cup	2
All purpose unbleached, 1/4 cup	2
Bread, 1/4 cup	2
Self rising bleached, 1/4 cup	2
Shake & blend, 1/4 cup	2
Whole wheat, 1/4 cup	1
Wondra	
Flour, 1/4 cup	2
Quick mixing flour for sauce & gravy, 1/4 cup	2
Wondra flour, 1/4 cup	2

	POINTS VALUE
Frosting/Icing	
Betty Crocker Homestyle Frosting	
Fluffy white, mix (box), 3 Tbsp	2
Betty Crocker Rich & Creamy	
Butter cream, 2 Tbsp	3
Caramel (dulce de leche), 2 Tbsp	3
Cherry, 2 Tbsp	3
Chocolate, 2 Tbsp	3
Coconut pecan, 2 Tbsp	3
Cream cheese, 2 Tbsp	3
Creamy white, 2 Tbsp	3
Dark chocolate, 2 Tbsp	3
Lemon, 2 Tbsp	3
Milk chocolate, 2 Tbsp	3
Rainbow chip, 2 Tbsp	3
Sour cream chocolate, 2 Tbsp	3
Triple chocolate fudge chip, 2 Tbsp	3
Vanilla creamy white, 2 Tbsp	3
Betty Crocker Whipped	
Butter cream, 2 Tbsp	2
Chocolate, 2 Tbsp	2
Cream cheese, 2 Tbsp	2
Fluffy white, 2 Tbsp	3
Milk chocolate, 2 Tbsp	2
Strawberry mist, 2 Tbsp	2
Vanilla, 2 Tbsp	2
Whipped cream, 2 Tbsp	2
Cherrybrook Kitchen	
Chocolate frosting mix, 1 Tbsp	1
Vanilla frosting mix, 2 Tbsp	3

Baking Mixes, Ingredients & Doughs

	POINTS VALUE
Jiffy Mixes	
Fudge frosting mix, 1/4 package	3
White frosting mix, 1/4 cup	3
Litehouse	
Blueberry glaze, 3 Tbsp	1
Peach glaze, 3 Tbsp	1
Strawberry glaze, 3 Tbsp	1
Strawberry glaze, 1 1/2 Tbsp	1
Sugar free strawberry glaze, 3 Tbsp	1
Marzetti	
Glaze for blueberries, 3 Tbsp	1
Glaze for peaches, 3 Tbsp	1
Glaze for strawberries, 3 Tbsp	1
Naturally Fresh	
Strawberry glaze, 2 Tbsp	1
Pillsbury Creamy Supreme	
Banana creme, 2 Tbsp	3
Chocolate, 2 Tbsp	3
Chocolate fudge, 2 Tbsp	3
Coconut pecan, 2 Tbsp	4
Cookies & creme, 2 Tbsp	3
Cream cheese vanilla, 2 Tbsp	4
French vanilla, 2 Tbsp	4
Funfetti Easter, 2 Tbsp	4
Funfetti Halloween, 2 Tbsp	4
Funfetti holiday, 2 Tbsp	4
Funfetti pink vanilla, 2 Tbsp	4
Funfetti valentines, 2 Tbsp	4
Funfetti vanilla, 2 Tbsp	4
Lemon creme, 2 Tbsp	4
Milk chocolate, 2 Tbsp	3

	POINTS VALUE
Strawberry creme, 2 Tbsp	4
Vanilla, 2 Tbsp	4
Sweet 'N Low	
Chocolate frosting mix, 2 Tbsp	1
White frosting mix, 2 Tbsp	1

Honey, Syrups & Molasses

Aunt Jemima	
Butter lite syrup, 1/4 cup	2
Butter rich syrup, 1/4 cup	4
Country rich syrup, 1/4 cup	4
Lite syrup, 1/4 cup	2
Original syrup, 1/4 cup	4
Brer Rabbit	
Molasses, blackstrap, 1 Tbsp	1
Molasses, full flavored, 1 Tbsp	1
Molasses, mild flavored, 1 Tbsp	1
DaVinci Gourmet	
Sugar free caramel syrup, 2 Tbsp	0
Sugar free hazelnut syrup, 2 Tbsp	0
Sugar free kahlua coffee liqueur flavored syrup, 2 Tbsp	0
Sugar free raspberry syrup, 2 Tbsp	0
Sugar free vanilla syrup, 2 Tbsp	0
Eden Organic	
Barley malt syrup, 1 Tbsp	1
Grandma's	
Original molasses, 1 Tbsp	1
Robust molasses, 1 Tbsp	1
Hershey's	
Sugar free strawberry syrup, 2 Tbsp	0
Syrup, 2 Tbsp	2

Baking Mixes, Ingredients & Doughs

	POINTS VALUE
Joseph's	
Original sugar free maple flavor syrup, 1 oz	1
Kellogg's Eggo	
Butter pecan flavored syrup, 1/4 cup	4
Syrup buttery, 1/4 cup	3
Syrup lite, 1/4 cup	2
Syrup original, 1/4 cup	5
Syrup, cinnamon French toast flavored, 1/4 cup	3
Log Cabin	
100% pure maple syrup, 1/4 cup	4
Lite syrup, 1/4 cup	2
Original syrup, 1/4 cup	4
Sugar free syrup, 1/4 cup	1
Manischewitz	
Honey clover, 1 Tbsp	1
Orange blossom honey, 1 Tbsp	1
Premium golden honey, 1 Tbsp	1
Wild flower honey, 1 Tbsp	1
Maple Grove	
Sugar free butter flavor pancake syrup, 1/4 cup	1
Sugar free butter flavor syrup, 1/4 cup	1
Maple Mountain	
Sugar free syrup, 2 Tbsp	0
Mrs. Butterworth's	
Lite syrup, 1/4 cup	2
Original syrup, 1/4 cup	4
Sugar free syrup, 1/4 cup	1
Muirhead	
Pomegranate syrup, 1 Tbsp	1

	POINTS VALUE
Nesquik	
Chocolate syrup, 2 Tbsp	2
Strawberry syrup, 2 Tbsp	2
Smucker's	
Sugar free breakfast syrup, 1/4 cup	1
Tree of Life	
Blackstrap molasses, unsulphered, 1 Tbsp	1
Honey, 1 Tbsp	1
Maple syrup, 1/4 cup	4
Vermont Maid	
Sugar free butter lite, 1/4 cup	1
Sugar free syrup, 1/4 cup	1
Walden Farms	
Blueberry syrup, 1/4 cup	0
Chocolate syrup, 2 Tbsp	0
Pancake syrup, 1/4 cup	0

Pie Filling & Mixes

	POINTS VALUE
Betty Crocker Supreme Dessert Bar Mixes	
7 layer bar kit, prepared, 1 bar	5
Almond joy dessert bar mix, prepared, 1 bar	5
Heath dessert bar mix, prepared, 1 bar (1/12 pan)	4
Reese's dessert bar mix, prepared, 1 bar	4
Sunkist lemon bar, prepared, 1 piece (1/16 pan)	3
Comstock/Wilderness	
Apple cranberry, 1 serving (89 g)	2
Berry medley pie filling, 1/3 cup	2
Caramel apple, 1 serving (89 g)	2
Creme key lime, 1/3 cup	4
Creme lemon, 1/3 cup	3

Baking Mixes, Ingredients & Doughs

Comstock/Wilderness (cont'd)	POINTS VALUE
Lite cherry, 1/3 cup	1
More fruit apple, 1/3 cup	1
More fruit blueberry, 1/3 cup	2
More fruit cherry, 1/3 cup	2
More fruit cinnamon 'n spice apple, 1/3 cup	2
More fruit lite cherry, 1/3 cup	1
More fruit peach, 1/3 cup	2
No sugar added cherry, 1/3 cup	1
Original country cherry, 1/3 cup	2
Premium apricot, 1/3 cup	2
Premium blackberry, 1/3 cup	2
Premium dark sweet cherry, 1/3 cup	2
Premium pineapple, 1/3 cup	2
Premium raspberry, 1/3 cup	1
Premium strawberry, 1/3 cup	2
Quick & easy lemon, 1/3 cup	3
Durkee	
Lemon pie filling, 1 Tbsp	1
Jell-O Instant	
Chocolate dirt cup kit mix, 1 serving (1/6 box)	3
Chocolate dirt cup kit, prepared, 1/2 cup	5
Easy southern banana pudding dessert kit, 1 serving (1/12 package)	2
Easy southern banana pudding dessert kit, 1/2 cup	3
Jell-O No Bake	
Cherry cheesecake mix, 1 serving (1/8 package)	4
Cherry cheesecake, prepared, 1 serving (1/9 package)	6

	POINTS VALUE
Chips ahoy, as packaged, 1 serving (60 g)	6
Chips ahoy, prepared, 1 serving (1/6 package)	8
Double chocolate pie mix, 1 serving (1/6 package)	4
Double chocolate pie, prepared, 1 serving (1/6 package)	7
Homestyle cheesecake mix, 1 serving (1/8 package)	5
Homestyle cheesecake, prepared, 1 serving (1/6 package)	8
Oreos and creme mix, 1 serving (62 g)	6
Oreos and crème, prepared, 1 serving (1/6 package)	8
Peanut butter cup mix, 1 serving (1/8 package)	7
Peanut butter cup, prepared, 1 serving (1/8 package)	9
Pumpkin style pie mix, 1 serving (34 g)	3
Pumpkin style pie, prepared, 1 serving (1/6 package)	6
Real cheesecake mix, 1 serving (1/8 package)	5
Real cheesecake, prepared, 1 serving (1/6 package)	8
Strawberry cheesecake mix, 1 serving (1/8 package)	4
Strawberry cheesecake, prepared, 1 serving (1/9 package)	6
Libby's	
Pumpkin pie mix, 1/3 cup	1
Lucky Leaf	
Apple pie filling, 1/3 cup	2
Blueberry pie filling, 1/3 cup	2

Baking Mixes, Ingredients & Doughs

	POINTS VALUE
Cherry pie filling, 1/3 cup	2
Lemon pie filling, 1/3 cup	2
Lite apple pie filling, no sugar added, 1/3 cup	0
Lite cherry pie filling, no sugar added, 1/3 cup	1
Peach pie filling, 1/3 cup	2
Strawberry pie filling, 1/3 cup	1
Payaso	
Flan dessert mix, 1/4 pack	1
Philadelphia	
Ready to eat cheesecake filling, as packaged, 1/8 package	7
Ready to eat cheesecake filling, prepared, 1/8 package	9
Silken Creations	
Dark chocolate, 1/2 cup	2
Strawberry, 1/2 cup	2
Vanilla, 1/2 cup	2

Pie/Pastry Dough & Crusts

	POINTS VALUE
Betty Crocker	
Pie crust mix (box), 1 serving (1/8 of 9" crust)	3
Pizza crust mix (pouch), 1 serving (1/4 crust)	3
Jiffy Mixes	
Pie crust mix, 1 serving (1/16 package)	2
Pizza crust mix, 1 serving (1/5 package)	3
Keebler	
Graham cracker crumbs, 3 Tbsp	1
Ready crust chocolate pie shell, 3-inch, 1	2

	POINTS VALUE
Mrs. Smith's	
9" pie crust, deep dish, 1 serving (1/8 pie crust)	3
9" pie crust, regular, 1 serving (1/8 pie crust)	3
Nabisco	
Nilla pie crust, 1 serving (1/8 pie crust)	3
Nilla wafers crumbs, 2 1/2 Tbsp	2
Oreo basecake - crumbs, 1/4 cup	3
Oreo pie crust, 1/6 pie crust (19 g)	2
Oreo pie crust, 1/6 pie crust (28 g)	3
Nabisco Honey Maid	
Graham pie crust, 1 serving (1/8 pie crust)	3
Oronoque Orchards	
9" pie crust, deep dish, ready to bake, 1 serving (1/8 pie crust)	3
9" pie crust, regular, ready to bake, 1 serving (1/8 pie crust)	2
Pepperidge Farm	
Mini puff pastry shells, 4 shells	4
Puff pastry sheets, 1 serving (1/6 sheet)	4
Puff pastry shells, 1 shell	5
Pillsbury	
All ready pie crust, refrigerated, rolled, 1/8	3
Pie crust mix, 2 Tbsp	3
Pie crusts - frozen 9-inch, 1 serving (1/8 of pie crust)	3
Pillsbury Pet-Ritz	
Deep dish 9-inch, frozen, 1/8	2
Deep dish, frozen, vegetable oil, 1/8	2

Baking Mixes, Ingredients & Doughs

Pillsbury Pet-Ritz (cont'd)	POINTS VALUE
Large 9 5/8-inch, frozen, 1/8	3
Regular 9-inch, frozen, 1/8	2
Ready Crust	
Chocolate pie crust (6 oz), 1/8	2
Graham cracker pie crust (10"), 1 serving (1/10 crust)	3
Graham cracker pie crust (6 oz), 1/8	2
Reduced fat graham cracker pie crust (6 oz), 1/8	2
Shortbread pie crust (6 oz), 1/8	3
Tart graham cracker crusts (4 oz), 1 crust	2

Shortening/Lard
Earth Balance
Natural shortening stick, 1 Tbsp	4

Smart Balance
Vegetable shortening, 1 Tbsp	3

Spectrum Naturals
Organic shortening, 1 Tbsp	3

Spices
Durkee
Basil leaf, 1 serving (0.4 g)	0
Bay leaf, whole, 1 serving (0.44 g)	0
Chili powder, mild, 1/4 tsp	0
Cinnamon, ground, 1/4 tsp	0
Cumin seed, ground, 1/4 tsp	0
Garlic powder, 1/4 tsp	0
Lemon pepper, 1/4 tsp	0
Nutmeg, ground, 1/4 tsp	0
Pepper, black, ground, 1/4 tsp	0

McCormick	POINTS VALUE
Alum, 1/4 tsp	0
Caraway seed, 1/4 tsp	0
Celery flakes, 1/4 tsp	0
Celery seed, 1/4 tsp	0
Chives, 1/4 tsp	0
Cilantro leaves, 1/4 tsp	0
Cream of tartar, 1/4 tsp	0
Cumin seeds, 1/4 tsp	0
Curry powder, 1/4 tsp	0
Dill seed, 1/4 tsp	0
Dill weed, 1/4 tsp	0
Fennel seed, 1/4 tsp	0
Garlic powder, 1/4 tsp	0
Ground allspice, 1/4 tsp	0
Ground black pepper, 1/4 tsp	0
Ground cinnamon, 1/4 tsp	0
Ground cloves, 1/4 tsp	0
Ground cumin, 1/4 tsp	0
Ground ginger, 1/4 tsp	0
Ground mace, 1/4 tsp	0
Ground marjoram, 1/4 tsp	0
Ground mustard, 1/4 tsp	0
Ground nutmeg, 1/4 tsp	0
Ground oregano, 1/4 tsp	0
Ground red pepper, 1/4 tsp	0
Ground sage, 1/4 tsp	0
Ground thyme, 1/4 tsp	0
Ground turmeric, 1/4 tsp	0
Ground white pepper, 1/4 tsp	0
Italian seasoning, 1/4 tsp	0

	POINTS VALUE
Marjoram leaves, 1/4 tsp	0
Mustard seeds, 1/4 tsp	0
Onion powder, 1/4 tsp	0
Oregano leaves, 1/4 tsp	0
Paprika, 1/4 tsp	0
Parsley flakes, 1/4 tsp	0
Pickling spice, 1/4 tsp	0
Poppy seeds, 1/4 tsp	0
Pumpkin pie spice, 1/4 tsp	0
Rosemary leaves, 1/4 tsp	0
Rubbed sage, 1/4 tsp	0
Sesame seeds, 1/4 tsp	0
Tarragon leaves, 1/4 tsp	0
Thyme leaves, 1/4 tsp	0
Whole allspice, 1/4 tsp	0
Whole basil leaves, 1/4 tsp	0
Whole bay leaves, 1/4 tsp	0
Whole cloves, 1/4 tsp	0
Nu-Salt	
Salt substitute, 1 serving (1/6 tsp)	0
Spice Islands	
Basil leaf, 1 serving (0.4 g)	0
Cayenne pepper, 1 serving (0.67 g)	0
Curry powder, 1/4 tsp	0
Dill weed, 1 serving (0.25 g)	0
Sesame seed, whole, 1 serving (0.75 g)	0
Tree of Life	
Bee pollen, 1 tsp	1
Crystallized ginger, 7 pieces	3
Sesame seeds, 1/4 cup	5
Turmeric in brine, 1 Tbsp	0

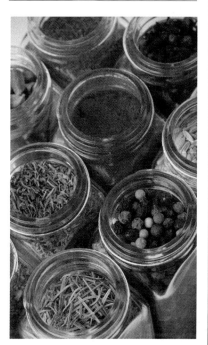

Baking Mixes, Ingredients & Doughs

	POINTS VALUE
Sugar/Sugar Substitutes	
Equal	
Sweetener, 1 packet	0
Estee	
Fructose natural sweetener, 1 packet	0
Fructose natural sweetener, 1 tsp	0
Joseph's	
Maltitol sweetener, 1 serving (1 oz)	1
NatraTaste	
Sugar substitute, 1 packet	0
Sans Sucre	
Cinnamon sugar, 1/2 tsp	0
SPLENDA Sweetener	
SPLENDA no calorie sweetener, 1 packet	0
SPLENDA no calorie sweetener, 1 tsp (granulated)	0
SPLENDA no calorie sweetener, flavor accents, lemon, 1 packet	0
SPLENDA no calorie sweetener, flavor accents, raspberry, 1 packet	0
SPLENDA no calorie sweetener café sticks, 1 stick	0
SPLENDA no calorie sweetener with 1 gram fiber, 1 packet	0
SPLENDA no calorie sweetener, flavors for coffee, caramel, 1 packet	0
SPLENDA no calorie sweetener, flavors for coffee, cinnamon spice, 1 packet	0
SPLENDA no calorie sweetener, flavors for coffee, French vanilla, 1 packet	0
SPLENDA no calorie sweetener, flavors for coffee, hazelnut, 1 packet	0
SPLENDA no calorie sweetener, flavors for coffee, mocha, 1 packet	0

	POINTS VALUE
SPLENDA brown sugar blend, 1/2 tsp	0
SPLENDA sugar blend, 1/2 tsp	0
Sugar in the Raw	
Turbinado sugar, 1 tsp	0
Sugar Twin	
Calorie free sweetener, 1 packet	0
Calorie free sweetener, white, 1 tsp	0
Spoonable brown, 1 tsp	0
Sweet & Slender	
Natural sweetener packets, 1/2 packet	0
Natural sweetener shaker jar, 1/8 tsp	0
Sweet Magic	
Sweet magic, 1 packet	0
Sweet 'N Low	
Brown zero calories sweetener, 1 serving (1/10 tsp)	0
Zero calorie sweetener, 1 packet	0
Zero-calorie liquid sweetener, 10 drops	0
Sweet One	
Granulated sugar substitute, 1 packet	0
SweetLeaf	
Stevia extract powder, 1 serving (1/40 tsp)	0
Steviaclear liquid stevia extract, 2 drops	0
Steviaplus fiber, 1/2 packet	0
Steviatabs, 1 tablet	0
Tree of Life	
Date sugar, 1 tsp	0
Fructose, 1 tsp	0
Turbinado sugar, 1 tsp	0
Yeast	
Gaylord Hauser	
Brewer's yeast, 2 Tbsp (rounded)	2

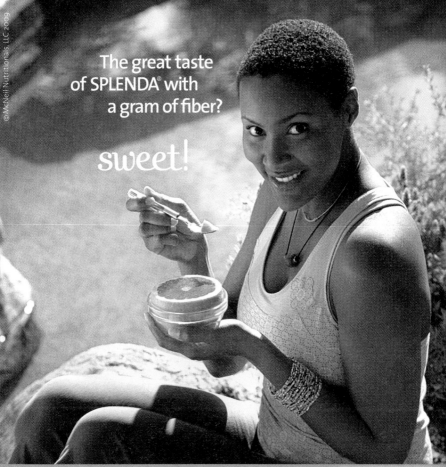

The great taste
of SPLENDA® with
a gram of fiber?

sweet!

©McNeil Nutritionals, LLC 2009

SPLENDA® No Calorie Sweetener with Fiber.
All the sweet taste you want and a gram of healthy fiber in every packet.

imagine life sweeter®

splenda.com

Beverages

POINTS VALUE

Beer

Aguila

Aguila, 1 can or bottle (12 fl oz)	2

Blue Moon

Belgian white, 1 can or bottle (12 oz)	3
Full moon winter ale, 1 can or bottle (12 oz)	4
Harvest moon pumpkin ale, 1 can or bottle (12 oz)	4
Honey moon summer ale, 1 can or bottle (12 oz)	3
Rising moon spring ale, 1 can or bottle (12 oz)	3

Budweiser

Bud dry, 1 can or bottle (12 fl oz)	3
Bud ice, 1 can or bottle (12 fl oz)	3
Bud ice light, 1 can or bottle (12 fl oz)	2
Bud light, 1 can or bottle (12 fl oz)	2
Bud light lime, 1 can or bottle (12 fl oz)	2
Budweiser, 1 can or bottle (12 fl oz)	3
Budweiser select, 1 can or bottle (12 fl oz)	2
Light lime, 1 serving (12 fl oz)	2

Busch

Busch, 1 can or bottle (12 fl oz)	3
Busch ice, 1 can or bottle (12 fl oz)	3
Busch light, 1 can or bottle (12 fl oz)	2
Busch non-alcoholic beer, 1 can or bottle (12 fl oz)	1

Coors

Extra gold lager, 1 can or bottle (12 oz)	3
Light, 1 can or bottle (12 oz)	2
Coors non-alcoholic, 1 can or bottle (12 oz)	1

Cristal

Cristal, 1 can or bottle (12 fl oz)	3

Cusquena

Cusquena, 1 can or bottle (12 fl oz)	3

Fosters

Fosters, 1 can or bottle (12 fl oz)	3

Foster's

Premium ale, 1 can or bottle (12 oz)	3

Frederick Miller

Frederick miller classic chocolate lager, 1 can or bottle (12 fl oz)	4

George Killian's

Irish red, 1 can or bottle (12 oz)	3

Grolsch

Amber ale, 1 can or bottle (12 fl oz)	3
Blonde lager, 1 can or bottle (12 fl oz)	2
Light lager, 1 can or bottle (12 fl oz)	2
Premium lager, 1 can or bottle (12 fl oz)	3

Hamm's

Golden draft, 12 fl oz	3
Hamm's, 12 fl oz	3
Special light, 12 fl oz	2

Henry Weinhard's

Blond, 1 can or bottle (12 fl oz)	3
Blue boar, 1 can or bottle (12 fl oz)	3
Classic dark lager, 1 can or bottle (12 fl oz)	3
Hefeweizen, 1 can or bottle (12 fl oz)	3

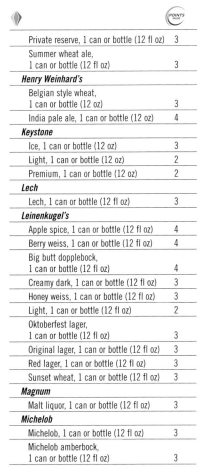

	POINTS VALUE
Private reserve, 1 can or bottle (12 fl oz)	3
Summer wheat ale, 1 can or bottle (12 oz)	3
Henry Weinhard's	
Belgian style wheat, 1 can or bottle (12 oz)	3
India pale ale, 1 can or bottle (12 oz)	4
Keystone	
Ice, 1 can or bottle (12 oz)	3
Light, 1 can or bottle (12 oz)	2
Premium, 1 can or bottle (12 oz)	2
Lech	
Lech, 1 can or bottle (12 fl oz)	3
Leinenkugel's	
Apple spice, 1 can or bottle (12 fl oz)	4
Berry weiss, 1 can or bottle (12 fl oz)	4
Big butt dopplebock, 1 can or bottle (12 fl oz)	4
Creamy dark, 1 can or bottle (12 fl oz)	3
Honey weiss, 1 can or bottle (12 fl oz)	3
Light, 1 can or bottle (12 fl oz)	2
Oktoberfest lager, 1 can or bottle (12 fl oz)	3
Original lager, 1 can or bottle (12 fl oz)	3
Red lager, 1 can or bottle (12 fl oz)	3
Sunset wheat, 1 can or bottle (12 fl oz)	3
Magnum	
Malt liquor, 1 can or bottle (12 fl oz)	3
Michelob	
Michelob, 1 can or bottle (12 fl oz)	3
Michelob amberbock, 1 can or bottle (12 fl oz)	3

	POINTS VALUE
Michelob light, 1 can or bottle (12 fl oz)	2
Michelob ultra, 1 can or bottle (12 fl oz)	2
Michelob ultra brand, 1 can or bottle (12 fl oz)	2
Ultra amber, 1 serving (12 fl oz)	2
Ultra fruit lime cactus, 1 serving (12 fl oz)	2
Ultra fruit pomegranate raspberry, 1 serving (12 fl oz)	2
Ultra fruit Tuscan orange grapefruit, 1 serving (12 fl oz)	2
Mickey's	
Ice, 12 fl oz	3
Mickey's, 12 fl oz	3
Miller	
Genuine draft, 1 can or bottle (12 fl oz)	3
High life, 1 can or bottle (12 fl oz)	3
High life light, 1 can or bottle (12 fl oz)	2
Icehouse, 1 can or bottle (12 fl oz)	3
Icehouse 5.0, 1 can or bottle (12 fl oz)	3
Icehouse light, 1 can or bottle (12 fl oz)	2
Lite, 1 can or bottle (12 fl oz)	2
Lite brewers collection amber, 1 can or bottle (12 oz)	2
Lite brewers collection blonde, 1 can or bottle (12 oz)	2
Lite brewers collection wheat, 1 can or bottle (12 oz)	2
MGD 64, 1 can or bottle (12 oz)	1
Miller chill, 1 can or bottle (12 fl oz)	2

Beverages

Milwaukee's Best

	POINTS VALUE
Milwaukee's best, 1 can or bottle (12 fl oz)	3
Milwaukee's best ice, 1 can or bottle (12 fl oz)	3
Milwaukee's best light, 1 can or bottle (12 fl oz)	2

Molson

Canadian, 1 can or bottle (12 fl oz)	3
Canadian light, 1 can or bottle (12 fl oz)	2
Golden, 1 can or bottle (12 fl oz)	3
Ice, 1 can or bottle (12 fl oz)	3
XXX, 1 can or bottle (12 fl oz)	4

Natural Light

Natural ice, 1 can or bottle (12 fl oz)	3
Natural light, 1 can or bottle (12 fl oz)	2

O'Doul's

O'Doul's amber non-alcoholic beer, 1 can or bottle (12 fl oz)	2
O'Doul's non-alcoholic beer, 1 can or bottle (12 fl oz)	1

Olde English 800

Olde English 800, 1 can or bottle (12 fl oz)	3
Olde English 800 7.5, 1 can or bottle (12 fl oz)	4
Olde English high gravity 800, 1 can or bottle (12 fl oz)	4

Peroni Nastro Azzurro

Peroni nastro azzurro, 1 can or bottle (12 fl oz)	3

Pilsner Urquell

Pilsner urquell, 1 can or bottle (12 fl oz)	3

Red Dog

	POINTS VALUE
Red dog, 1 can or bottle (12 fl oz)	3

Sharp's

Sharp's, 1 can or bottle (12 fl oz)	1

Sheaf Stout

Sheaf stout, 1 can or bottle (12 fl oz)	4

Southpaw

Southpaw light, 1 can or bottle (12 fl oz)	2

Sparks

Sparks, 1 can or bottle (12 fl oz)	5
Sparks light, 1 can or bottle (12 fl oz)	3
Sparks plus 6%, 1 can or bottle (12 fl oz)	5
Sparks plus 7%, 1 can or bottle (12 fl oz)	6

Steel Reserve

Steel reserve six, 1 can or bottle (12 fl oz)	3
Steel reserve triple export 8.1%, 1 can or bottle (12 fl oz)	4

Steel Six

Steel reserve, 1 can or bottle (12 fl oz)	4

Tequiza

Tequiza, 1 can or bottle (12 fl oz)	3

Tyskie

Tyskie, 1 can or bottle (12 fl oz)	3

Winterfest

Winterfest, 1 can or bottle (12 oz)	4

Zima

Pineapple citrus, 1 can or bottle (12 oz)	4
Tangerine, 1 can or bottle (12 oz)	4
Zima, 1 can or bottle (12 oz)	4

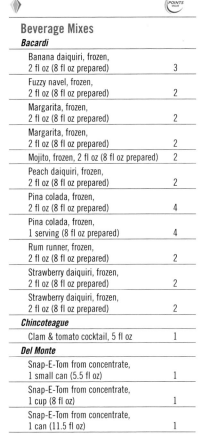

Beverage Mixes
Bacardi

	POINTS VALUE
Banana daiquiri, frozen, 2 fl oz (8 fl oz prepared)	3
Fuzzy navel, frozen, 2 fl oz (8 fl oz prepared)	2
Margarita, frozen, 2 fl oz (8 fl oz prepared)	2
Margarita, frozen, 2 fl oz (8 fl oz prepared)	2
Mojito, frozen, 2 fl oz (8 fl oz prepared)	2
Peach daiquiri, frozen, 2 fl oz (8 fl oz prepared)	2
Pina colada, frozen, 2 fl oz (8 fl oz prepared)	4
Pina colada, frozen, 1 serving (8 fl oz prepared)	4
Rum runner, frozen, 2 fl oz (8 fl oz prepared)	2
Strawberry daiquiri, frozen, 2 fl oz (8 fl oz prepared)	2
Strawberry daiquiri, frozen, 2 fl oz (8 fl oz prepared)	2

Chincoteague

Clam & tomato cocktail, 5 fl oz	1

Del Monte

Snap-E-Tom from concentrate, 1 small can (5.5 fl oz)	1
Snap-E-Tom from concentrate, 1 cup (8 fl oz)	1
Snap-E-Tom from concentrate, 1 can (11.5 fl oz)	1

Seagram's

	POINTS VALUE
Club soda, 8 fl oz	0
Diet tonic water, 8 fl oz	0
Tonic water, 8 fl oz	2
Tonic water with a twist of lime, 8 fl oz	2

Tree of Life

Black cherry concentrate, 8 tsp	2
Concord grape concentrate, 9 tsp	3
Cranberry concentrate, 8 tsp	2
Pomegranate concentrate, 8 tsp	2
Wild blueberry concentrate, 8 tsp	2

Cocoa & Chocolate Drinks
Horizon Organic

Lowfat chocolate milk, 1 cup	3

Nestle

Butterfinger, 1 envelope	2
Chocolate meltdown flavor hot cocoa mix, 1 envelope	3
French vanilla hot cocoa mix, 1 envelope	2
Milk chocolate hot cocoa mix, 1 envelope	2
Mini marshmallows with rich chocolate flavor hot cocoa mix, 1 envelope	2
Nesquik with marshmallows, 1 envelope	3
No sugar added, rich chocolate flavor hot cocoa mix (with calcium), 1 envelope	1
Rich chocolate hot cocoa mix, 1 envelope	2
Smores with marshmallows, 1 envelope	3

Beverages

	POINTS VALUE
Nestle CARB SELECT	
Fat free with marshmallows, hot cocoa mix (with calcium), 1 envelope	1
Fat free, rich chocolate flavor hot cocoa mix, 1 envelope	0
Suchard	
Hot cocoa, 1 serving (t-disc)	3

Coffee
Drenchers

Chocolate raspberry frappe super blend, 9 1/2 fl oz	1
Iced coffee super blend, 9 1/2 fl oz	1
Mocha cappuccino super blend, 9 1/2 fl oz	1

General Foods

Vanilla crème drink mix, 1 1/3 Tbsp	1
Vanilla crème sugar free drink mix, 1 1/3 Tbsp	1

General Foods International Coffee

Café Francais, prepared, 8 fl oz	1
Cafe Vienna, prepared, 8 fl oz	2
Cappuccino café mocha decaffeinated single serve coffee mix, 1 envelope	2
Cappuccino café mocha single serve coffee mix, 1 envelope	2
Cappuccino coolers French vanilla, 1 serving (8 oz)	3
Cappuccino coolers hazelnut, 1 serving (8 oz)	3
Cappuccino French vanilla decaffeinated single serve coffee mix, 1 envelope	2
Cappuccino French vanilla single serve coffee mix, 1 envelope	2

	POINTS VALUE
Crème caramel mix, 1 serving (15 g)	1
French vanilla cafe decaffeinated, 1 serving (14 g)	1
French vanilla cafe, 1 serving (14 g)	1
French vanilla nut coffee mix, 1 1/3 Tbsp	1
Hazelnut Belgian cafe, prepared, 8 fl oz	2
Italian cappuccino, prepared, 8 fl oz	1
Orange cappuccino, 1 serving (13 g)	1
Pumpkin spice coffee mix, 1 1/3 Tbsp	2
Sugar free café Vienna, 1 Tbsp	1
Sugar free decaffeinated French vanilla café, 1 Tbsp	1
Sugar free French vanilla café, 1 Tbsp	1
Sugar free Suisse mocha, 1 Tbsp	1
Sugar free Suisse mocha decaffeinated, 1 Tbsp	1
Suisse mocha (sugar free, fat free), prepared, 1 serving (7 g)	1
Suisse mocha, 1 serving (13 g)	1
Swiss white chocolate, 1 serving (16 g)	2
Viennese chocolate café, 1 serving (13 g)	1

Gevalia

Decaffeinated cappuccino, 1 serving (1 coffee t-disc & 1 milk creamer t-disc)	1
Decaffeinated latte, 1 serving (1 coffee t-disc & 1 milk creamer t-disc)	2

Gevalia Café Collection

Cappuccino, 1 serving (1 coffee t-disc & 1 milk creamer t-disc)	1
Latte, 1 serving (1 coffee t-disc & 1 milk creamer t-disc)	2

	POINTS VALUE

Maxwell House Café Collection

Cappuccino, 1 serving (1 coffee t-disc & 1 milk creamer t-disc)	1
Latte, 1 serving (1 coffee t-disc & 1 milk creamer t-disc)	2

POM Wonderful Products

POMx iced coffee – café au lait, 10.5 oz	4
POMx iced coffee – chocolate, 10.5 oz	3

Starbucks

Doubleshot coffee drink, 8 fl oz	4
Doubleshot coffee drink light, 8 fl oz	2
Doubleshot energy - cinnamon dulce, 8 fl oz	2
Doubleshot energy - coffee, 8 fl oz	2
Doubleshot energy - mocha, 8 fl oz	2
Doubleshot energy - vanilla, 8 fl oz	2
Frappuccino - caramel, 8 fl oz	4
Frappuccino - coffee, 8 fl oz	4
Frappuccino - dark chocolate mocha, 8 fl oz	3
Frappuccino - mocha, 8 fl oz	3
Frappuccino - mocha lite, 8 fl oz	2
Frappuccino - vanilla, 8 fl oz	4
Iced coffee, 8 fl oz	1
Iced coffee light, 8 fl oz	1

Sun Shower

Chocolate raspberry frappe super blend, 9 1/2 fl oz	1
Iced coffee super blend, 9 1/2 fl oz	1
Mocha cappuccino super blend, 9 1/2 fl oz	1

Fruit Juices & Drinks

4C Totally Light

Cranberry pomegranate antioxidant drink mix, 1 serving (8 fl oz prepared)	0
Fruit punch drink mix, 1 serving (8 fl oz prepared)	0

4C Totally Light 2Go

Cranberry pomegranate antioxidant drink mix, 1 serving (8 fl oz prepared)	0
Energy rush - berry, 1 serving (8 fl oz prepared)	0
Energy rush - orange, 1/2 packet	0
Energy rush - citrus, 1 serving (8 fl oz prepared)	0
Fruit punch drink mix, 1 serving (8 fl oz prepared)	0
Just apple mix, 1 serving (1.6 g)	0
Morning orange mix, 1 serving (1.6 g)	0
Reboot - passionfruit/citrus, 1/2 packet	0
Vision - strawberry/kiwi, 1/2 packet	0
Vitamin C-drive - dragonfruit/acai, 1/2 packet	0
Wild berry pomegranate mix, 1 serving (0.99 g)	0

Bright & Early

Orange, 8 fl oz	2
Orange, frozen, 2 fl oz (8 fl oz prepared)	2

Capri Sun

Coastal cooler, 1 pouch	2
Fruit punch, 1 pouch	2
Grape, 1 pouch	2
Mountain cooler, 1 pouch	2

Beverages

Capri Sun (cont'd)

	POINTS VALUE
Orange, 1 pouch	2
Pacific cooler, 1 pouch	2
Red berry, 1 pouch	2
Splash cooler, 1 pouch	2
Strawberry, 1 pouch	2
Strawberry-kiwi, 1 pouch	2
Surfer cooler, 1 pouch	2
Tropical punch, 1 pouch	2
Wild cherry, 1 pouch	2
Wild cherry, 8 fl oz	2

Capri Sun On the Go

Sport lightspeed lemon lime, prepared, 1 serving (8.45 fl oz)	1
Sport thunder punch, prepared, 1 serving (8.45 fl oz)	1

Cascadian Farm

Orange juice frozen concentrate, 2 fl oz	2
Organic apple juice from concentrate, 2 fl oz	2
Organic cranberry cocktail concentrate, 2 fl oz	2
Organic grape juice from concentrate, 2 fl oz	3
Organic raspberry juice from concentrate, 2 fl oz	3

Ceres 100% Pure Fruit Juice Blend

Apricot juice, 8 fl oz	2
Cranberry & kiwi juice, 8 fl oz	2
Guava juice, 8 fl oz	2
Litchi juice, 8 fl oz	2
Mango juice, 8 fl oz	2
Medley of fruits, 8 fl oz	2
Papaya juice, 8 fl oz	2

	POINTS VALUE
Passion fruit juice, 8 fl oz	2
Peach juice, 8 fl oz	2
Pear juice, 8 fl oz	2
Pineapple juice, 8 fl oz	2
Secrets of the valley, 8 fl oz	2
Strawberry juice, 8 fl oz	2
White grape juice, 8 fl oz	3
Youngberry juice, 8 fl oz	2

Crayons

Kiwi strawberry, 8 fl oz	1
Outrageous orange mango, 8 fl oz	1
Redder than ever fruit punch, 8 fl oz	1
Wild watermelon & berries, 8 fl oz	1

Crystal Light

Energy wild strawberry, sugar free, 8 fl oz	0
Fruit punch, sugar free, prepared, 8 fl oz	0
Immunity berry pomegranate, sugar free, 8 fl oz	0
Pineapple-orange mix, sugar free, prepared, 8 fl oz	0
Ruby red grapefruit mix, sugar free, prepared, 8 fl oz	0
Strawberry-kiwi, sugar free, 8 fl oz	0
Strawberry-orange-banana mix, sugar free, prepared, 8 fl oz	0
Tangerine strawberry, sugar free, prepared, 8 fl oz	0

Crystal Light Calcium

Raspberry peach mix, sugar free, prepared, 8 fl oz	0

	POINTS VALUE
Crystal Light On the Go	
Cherry pomegranate, prepared, 1 serving (8.45 fl oz)	0
Fruit punch, prepared, 1 serving (8.45 fl oz)	0
Hydration berry splash, prepared, 1 serving (8.45 fl oz)	0
Hydration lightly lemon, prepared, 1 serving (8.45 fl oz)	0
Raspberry ice mix, 1 serving (8.45 fl oz)	0
Wild strawberry, prepared, 1 serving (8.45 fl oz)	0
Crystal Light Sunrise	
Classic orange mix, sugar free, prepared, 8 fl oz	0
Classic orange on the go, 1 packet	0
Ruby red grapefruit, sugar free, 8 fl oz	0
Strawberry-kiwi mix, sugar free, 8 fl oz	0
Tangerine strawberry, prepared, 8 fl oz	0
Crystal Light Sunrise On The Go	
Orange, prepared, 1 serving (8.45 fl oz)	0
Del Monte	
Pineapple juice from concentrate, 5 1/2 fl oz	2
Pineapple juice from concentrate, 1 cup	3
Dole	
Apple juice, 1 serving (8 fl oz)	2
Apple juice, 1 can (11.5 fl oz)	3
Cranberry grape, 1 serving (8 fl oz)	3
Cranberry grape, 1 can (11.5 fl oz)	5
Cranberry juice cocktail, 1 can (11.5 fl oz)	3

	POINTS VALUE
Grape raspberry, 1 serving (8 fl oz)	3
Grape raspberry, 1 can (11.5 fl oz)	4
Grape raspberry cocktail, frozen concentrate, 1/4 cup	3
Orange, 8 fl oz	2
Orange (no pulp & w/pulp), 1 serving (8 fl oz)	2
Orange (no pulp & w/pulp), 1 can (11.5 fl oz)	3
Orange guava, 8 fl oz	2
Orange pacific passion, 1 can (8.4 oz)	3
Orange peach mango, 8 fl oz	2
Orange peach mango, frozen concentrate, 1/4 cup	2
Orange strawberry banana, 1 small cup	3
Orange strawberry banana, 1 large cup	5
Orange strawberry banana, frozen concentrate, 1/4 cup	3
Orange tropical, 8 fl oz	2
Orange tropical, frozen concentrate, 1/4 cup	3
Orange with calcium, 1 serving (8 fl oz)	2
Orange with double vitamin C, 1 serving (8 fl oz)	2
Orchard peach, 1 bottle (10 fl oz)	3
Paradise blend, 1 serving (8 fl oz)	2
Paradise blend, 1 can (11.5 fl oz)	3
Pineapple citrus, 1 serving (8 fl oz)	2
Pineapple citrus, 1 can (11.5 fl oz)	3
Pineapple juice, canned, 8 fl oz	2
Pineapple juice, reconstituted, 8 fl oz	2
Pineapple juice, reconstituted, 1 can (11.5 fl oz)	2

Beverages

	POINTS VALUE
Pineapple juice, refrigerated, 8 fl oz	3
Pineapple orange, 1 serving (8 fl oz)	2
Pineapple orange banana, 1 serving (8 fl oz)	3
Pineapple orange banana, frozen concentrate, 1/4 cup	3
Pineapple orange strawberry, 1 serving (8 fl oz)	2
Pineapple orange strawberry, frozen concentrate, 1/4 cup	3
Pineapple orange, frozen concentrate, 1/4 cup	2
Pineapple passionfruit mango, 8 fl oz	3
Pineapple peach mango juice, 8 fl oz	3
Pineapple, frozen concentrate, 1/4 cup	2
Pine-grapefruit juice, 1 can (11.5 fl oz)	2
Pine-orange juice, 1 can (11.5 fl oz)	2
Pine-orange-banana juice, 1 can (11.5 fl oz)	2
Pink pine grapefruit drink, 1 can (11.5 fl oz)	2
Pink pine grapefruit drink, 1 serving (8 fl oz)	3
Raspberry kiwi 1 serving (8 fl oz)	2
Ruby red grapefruit juice, 8 fl oz	3
Ruby red grapefruit juice, 1 can (11.5 fl oz)	4
Ruby red grapefruit juice, 1 bottle (10 fl oz)	4
Strawberry kiwi, 1 serving (8 fl oz)	4
Strawberry kiwi juice, 1 serving (8 fl oz)	2
Strawberry splash, 1 can (11.5 fl oz)	3

	POINTS VALUE
Dole Plus	
Apple, 8 fl oz	2
Fruit punch, 8 fl oz	2
Orange, 8 fl oz	2
Drenchers Super Juice	
Endurance grape apple, 8 fl oz	2
Heart healthy tropical passion, 8 fl oz	2
Immunity fruit and veggie berry, 8 fl oz	2
Power protein juice orange crème, 8 fl oz	4
Restore apple/kiwi/mango, 8 fl oz	2
Drenchers Super Juice Beverage Fit N' Lean	
Endurance grape apple, 8 fl oz	0
Heart healthy tropical passion, 8 fl oz	0
Immunity fruit and veggie berry, 8 fl oz	0
Power protein juice orange crème, 8 fl oz	0
Restore apple/kiwi/mango, 8 fl oz	0
Eden Organic	
Apple juice, 8 oz	2
Apple juice concentrate, 2 Tbsp	2
Cherry concentrate, 2 Tbsp	2
Cherry juice (Montmorency tart cherries), 8 oz	3
Five Alive	
Citrus, 8 fl oz	2
Citrus, frozen, 2 fl oz (8 fl oz prepared)	2
Florida's Natural	
Home squeezed orange juice, 8 fl oz	2
Home squeezed orange juice with calcium & vitamin D, 8 fl oz	2

	POINTS VALUE
Orange juice grower's style, 8 fl oz	2
Orange juice original, 8 fl oz	2
Orange juice with calcium & vitamin D, 8 fl oz	2
Ruby red grapefruit juice, 8 fl oz	2
Ruby red grapefruit juice, calcium added, 8 fl oz	2

Fruit 2 Day

Cherry grape, 1 container	2
Mango peach, 1 container	2
Pineapple banana, 1 container	2
Strawberry orange, 1 container	2

Fruitopia

Cherry vanilla groove, 8 fl oz	2
Fruit integration, 8 fl oz	2
Kiwiberry ruckus, 8 fl oz	2
Peach out, 8 fl oz	2
Raspberry dragonfruit reflection, 8 fl oz	2
Starfruit citrus synthesis, 8 fl oz	2
Strawberry passion awareness, 8 fl oz	2

Fruitworks

Blue raspberry freeze, 8 fl oz	1
Red cherry freeze, 8 fl oz	1

Futuro

Tmarinodo mix, 2 tsp	3

Goya

Acerola, 8 fl oz	2
Guanabana, 8 fl oz	2
Guava, 8 fl oz	2
Mango, 8 fl oz	2
Papaya, 8 fl oz	2

	POINTS VALUE
Passion & papaya, 8 fl oz	2
Passion fruit, 8 fl oz	2
Tamarind, 8 fl oz	2

Herdez

Tropical fruit juice, 1 can	3

Hi-C

Blazin' blueberry, 1 box	2
Boppin' strawberry, 1 box	2
Grabbin' grape, 1 box	2
Orange lavaburst, 1 box	2
Smashin' wild berry, 1 box	2
Strawberry kiwi kraze, 1 box	2
Torrential tropical punch, 1 box	2
Wild cherry, 1 box	2

Hi-C Blast

Blue watermelon, 1 pouch	2
Fruit punch, 1 pouch	2
Orange, 1 pouch	2
Raspberry kiwi, 1 pouch	2
Strawberry, 1 pouch	2
Wild blue, 1 pouch	2

Indian Summer

Apple cider, 8 fl oz	2
Apple juice with vitamin C added, 8 fl oz	2
Cherry pomegranate juice, 8 fl oz	3
Natural apple juice, 8 fl oz	2
Red tart cherry juice, 8 fl oz	3

Juicy Juice

Apple-banana, 8 fl oz	2
Apple-raspberry, 8 fl oz	2

Beverages

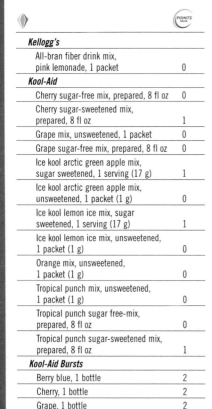

Kellogg's

All-bran fiber drink mix, pink lemonade, 1 packet	0

Kool-Aid

Cherry sugar-free mix, prepared, 8 fl oz	0
Cherry sugar-sweetened mix, prepared, 8 fl oz	1
Grape mix, unsweetened, 1 packet	0
Grape sugar-free mix, prepared, 8 fl oz	0
Ice kool arctic green apple mix, sugar sweetened, 1 serving (17 g)	1
Ice kool arctic green apple mix, unsweetened, 1 packet (1 g)	0
Ice kool lemon ice mix, sugar sweetened, 1 serving (17 g)	1
Ice kool lemon ice mix, unsweetened, 1 packet (1 g)	0
Orange mix, unsweetened, 1 packet (1 g)	0
Tropical punch mix, unsweetened, 1 packet (1 g)	0
Tropical punch sugar free-mix, prepared, 8 fl oz	0
Tropical punch sugar-sweetened mix, prepared, 8 fl oz	1

Kool-Aid Bursts

Berry blue, 1 bottle	2
Cherry, 1 bottle	2
Grape, 1 bottle	2
Lime, 1 bottle	2
Strawberry-kiwi, 1 bottle	2
Tropical punch, 1 bottle	2

Kool-Aid Jammers

Blue raspberry, 1 pouch	2
Cherry, 1 pouch	1
Grape, 1 pouch	2
Green apple, 1 pouch	2
Kiwi strawberry, 1 pouch	2
Orange, 1 pouch	2
Tropical punch, 1 pouch	2

Kool-Aid Jammers 10

Cherry, 1 pouch	0
Kiwi strawberry, 1 pouch	0
Tropical punch, 1 pouch	0

Kool-Aid Magic Twists

Grape illusion mix, sugar sweetened, 1 serving (17 g)	1

Kool-Aid On The Go

Tropical punch, sugar free, prepared, 8 fl oz	0

Kool-Aid Singles

Cherry, prepared, 1 packet (8 fl oz)	1
Grape, prepared, 1 packet (8 fl oz)	1
Orange, prepared, 1 packet (8 fl oz)	1
Tropical punch, prepared, 1 packet (8 fl oz)	1

Libby's Juicy Juice

Apple, 1 small box	1
Apple, 1 box	2
Apple, 1 cup	2
Apple concentrate, 1 serving (2 fl oz)	2
Apple-grape, 1 cup	2
Berry, 1 small box	1
Berry, 1 box	2

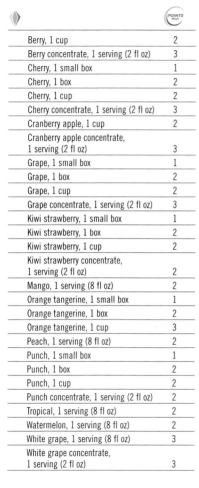

	POINTS VALUE
Berry, 1 cup	2
Berry concentrate, 1 serving (2 fl oz)	3
Cherry, 1 small box	1
Cherry, 1 box	2
Cherry, 1 cup	2
Cherry concentrate, 1 serving (2 fl oz)	3
Cranberry apple, 1 cup	2
Cranberry apple concentrate, 1 serving (2 fl oz)	3
Grape, 1 small box	1
Grape, 1 box	2
Grape, 1 cup	2
Grape concentrate, 1 serving (2 fl oz)	3
Kiwi strawberry, 1 small box	1
Kiwi strawberry, 1 box	2
Kiwi strawberry, 1 cup	2
Kiwi strawberry concentrate, 1 serving (2 fl oz)	2
Mango, 1 serving (8 fl oz)	2
Orange tangerine, 1 small box	1
Orange tangerine, 1 box	2
Orange tangerine, 1 cup	3
Peach, 1 serving (8 fl oz)	2
Punch, 1 small box	1
Punch, 1 box	2
Punch, 1 cup	2
Punch concentrate, 1 serving (2 fl oz)	2
Tropical, 1 serving (8 fl oz)	2
Watermelon, 1 serving (8 fl oz)	2
White grape, 1 serving (8 fl oz)	3
White grape concentrate, 1 serving (2 fl oz)	3

	POINTS VALUE
Lucky Leaf	
Apple juice, 8 fl oz	2
Premium apple juice, 8 fl oz	2
Manischewitz	
Concord grape juice, 8 fl oz	3
Niagara grape juice, 8 fl oz	3
Market Day	
Tropicana orange juice singles, 1 carton (8 fl oz)	2
Minute Maid	
Apple juice, 1 bottle (10 fl oz)	3
Apple juice, 1 box	1
Apple juice, 1 can (15.25 fl oz)	4
Apple juice, 8 fl oz (prepared from concentrate)	2
Apple juice, frozen concentrate, 2 fl oz (8 fl oz prepared)	2
Apple strawberry, 1 box	2
Berry punch, 8 fl oz	2
Berry punch, frozen concentrate, 8 fl oz (prepared)	2
Cherry limeade, 8 fl oz	2
Citrus punch, 8 fl oz	2
Citrus punch, frozen concentrate, 8 fl oz (prepared)	2
Country style 100% orange juice, 8 fl oz	2
Country style orange juice, frozen concentrate, 2 fl oz (8 fl oz prepared)	2
Enhanced juice/heart wise, orange juice, 8 fl oz	2
Enhanced pomegranate blueberry, 8 fl oz	2

Beverages

Minute Maid (cont'd)	POINTS VALUE
Fruit medley, 1 bottle (10 fl oz)	3
Fruit medley, 1 can (11.5 fl oz)	3
Fruit punch, 1 box	2
Fruit punch, 1 can (12 fl oz)	3
Fruit punch, frozen concentrate, 8 fl oz (prepared)	2
Grape, 1 box	2
Grape juice cocktail, frozen concentrate, 8 fl oz (prepared)	2
Grape punch, 8 fl oz	2
Grapefruit juice, frozen concentrate, 8 fl oz (prepared)	2
Home squeezed style orange juice with calcium & vitamin D, 8 fl oz	2
Kids + orange juice, 8 fl oz	2
Lemonade, frozen concentrate, 8 fl oz (prepared)	2
Limeade, 8 fl oz	2
Low acid orange juice, 8 fl oz	2
Low acid orange juice, frozen concentrate, 2 fl oz (8 fl oz prepared)	2
Mixed berry, 1 box	2
Mixed berry, 1 bottle (10 fl oz)	3
Mixed berry, 1 can (11.5 fl oz)	3
Multi-vitamin, 100% orange juice, 8 fl oz	2
Orange juice, 8 fl oz	2
Orange juice with C, E & zinc, 8 fl oz	2
Orange juice with C, E & zinc, frozen concentrate, 2 fl oz (8 fl oz prepared)	2
Orange passion, 8 fl oz	3
Orange tangerine, frozen concentrate, 2 fl oz (8 fl oz prepared)	2

	POINTS VALUE
Orangeade, 1 bottle (16.9 fl oz)	5
Orangeade, 8 fl oz	2
Orangeade, 12 fl oz	5
Original orange juice, 8 fl oz	2
Original orange juice, 1 box	2
Original orange juice with calcium, 8 fl oz	2
Original orange juice with calcium, frozen concentrate, 8 fl oz (prepared)	2
Original orange juice, frozen concentrate, 8 fl oz (prepared)	2
Pink lemonade, frozen concentrate, 8 fl oz (prepared)	2
Pulp free orange juice, 8 fl oz	2
Pulp free orange juice, frozen concentrate, 2 fl oz (8 fl oz prepared)	2
Pure lemon juice, 1 serving	0
Raspberry lemonade, frozen concentrate, 8 fl oz (prepared)	2
Strawberry passion, 1 can or bottle (12 oz)	3
Strawberry raspberry, 8 fl oz	2
Tropical punch, 8 fl oz	2
Tropical punch, frozen concentrate, 8 fl oz (prepared)	2
Minute Maid	
Enhanced pomegranate lemonade, 8 fl oz	2
Light limonada - limeade, 8 fl oz	0
Minute Maid Coolers	
Clear cherry, 1 pouch	2
Fruit punch, 1 pouch	2
Orange strawberry, 1 pouch	2

Beverages

Minute Maid Juices To Go	POINTS VALUE
Apple juice, 8 fl oz	2
Cranberry apple cocktail, 1 can (11.5 fl oz)	4
Cranberry apple raspberry, 8 fl oz	2
Cranberry grape, 8 fl oz	3
Fruit medley, 8 fl oz	3
Fruit punch, 1 bottle (10 fl oz)	3
Grape, 1 bottle (10 oz)	3
Grape, 1 can (11.5 oz)	3
Mixed berry, 1 bottle (10 oz)	3
Mixed berry, 1 can (11.5 oz)	3
Orange juice with calcium, 8 fl oz	2
Orange juice with calcium & vitamin D, 8 fl oz	2
Orange tropical, 1 can (11.5 oz)	4
Ruby red grapefruit, 8 fl oz	3
Strawberry raspberry, 8 fl oz	2

Minute Maid Light	
Cherry limeade, 1 can (12 fl oz)	0
Orange juice beverage, 8 fl oz	1
Orange tangerine, 8 fl oz	0
Orangeade, 8 fl oz	0
Orangeade, 1 can (12 fl oz)	0
Raspberry passion, 8 fl oz	0
Raspberry passion, 1 can (12 fl oz)	0

Minute Maid Premium	
Heart wise 100% orange juice, 8 fl oz	2

Minute Maid Simply	
Pure pressed apple juice, 8 fl oz	3

Musselman's	POINTS VALUE
Apple juice, 8 fl oz	2
Premium apple juice, 8 fl oz	2

No Fear	
No fear, 8 fl oz	3
Sugar free no fear, 8 fl oz	0

Ocean Spray	
100% juice blend white cranberry, 8 fl oz	3
100% juice blend cranberry, 8 fl oz	3
100% juice blend cranberry and concord grape, 8 fl oz	3
100% juice blend cranberry and raspberry, 8 fl oz	3
100% juice blend ruby red grapefruit, 8 fl oz	2
100% juice blend, cranberry & pomegranate, 8 fl oz	3
Cran-grape juice drink, 8 fl oz	3
Cranberry cocktail, 8 fl oz	3
Cranberry grape cocktail, 8 fl oz	3
Cranberry raspberry, 1 serving	3
Grapefruit tangerine juice drink, 8 fl oz	3
Low calorie ruby red grapefruit cocktail, 8 fl oz	1
Ruby red grapefruit juice drink, 8 fl oz	3
White cranberry and peach cocktail, 8 fl oz	3
White cranberry and strawberry cocktail, 8 fl oz	3
White cranberry cocktail, 8 fl oz	3

Beverages

POINTS VALUE

Ocean Spray Cranergy	
Cranberry lift, 8 fl oz	1
Pomegranate cranberry lift, 8 fl oz	1
Raspberry cranberry lift, 8 fl oz	1
Ocean Spray None	
Low calorie cran-raspberry cocktail, 8 fl oz	1
Low calorie cranberry grape cocktail, 8 fl oz	1
Low calorie cranberry juice cocktail, 8 fl oz	1
Low calorie white cranberry cocktail, 8 fl oz	1
Odwalla	
Antioxidance, 8 fl oz	2
Apple juice, 8 fl oz	3
B berrier, 8 fl oz	2
Berries gomega, 8 fl oz	3
Glorious morning orange cranberry juice drink blend, 8 fl oz	2
Grapefruit juice, 8 fl oz	2
Mo' beta fruit juice drink, 8 fl oz	3
Orange juice, 8 fl oz	2
Orange juice from valencias, 8 fl oz	2
Super protein original vitamin fruit juice drink, 8 fl oz	4
Superfood micronutrient fruit juice drink, 8 fl oz	3
Tangerine juice blend, 8 fl oz	2
Wellness fruit juice drink, 8 fl oz	3
Payaso	
Apple juice, 1 bottle (8.45 fl oz)	2
Orange juice, 1 bottle (8.45 fl oz)	3

POM Wonderful Products	
100% wonderful pomegranate juice, 8 fl oz	3
POM blueberry, 8 fl oz	3
POM cherry, 8 fl oz	3
POM mango, 8 fl oz	3
Promise	
Activ super shot, strawberry, 1 bottle	1
Activ super shots, peach, 1 bottle	1
Activ super shots, raspberry, 1 bottle	1
Promise Supershots	
Mixed berry, 1 bottle	1
Peach apricot, 1 bottle	1
Strawberry banana, 1 bottle	1
SoBe	
Adrenaline rush, 1 serving (8 fl oz)	3
Black & blue berry brew, 8 fl oz	2
Cranberry grapefruit elixer, 8 fl oz	2
Liz blizz, 8 fl oz	3
Lizard fuel, 8 fl oz	2
Lizard lava, 8 fl oz	3
Nirvana, 8 fl oz	2
Orange carrot elixer, 8 fl oz	2
Sugar free adrenaline rush, 8 fl oz	0
Tsunami, 8 fl oz	2
SoBe Lean	
Diet cranberry grapefruit, 8 fl oz	0
Diet energy, 8 fl oz	0
Diet mango melon, 8 fl oz	0
Sun Shower Light 'N Healthy	
Defense fruit and veggie berry super juice beverage, 8 fl oz	0

	POINTS VALUE
Heart healthy tropical passion super juice beverage, 8 fl oz	0
Revitalize apple/kiwi/mango super juice beverage, 8 fl oz	0
Stamina grape apple super juice beverage, 8 fl oz	0
Strength orange crème super juice protein beverage, 8 fl oz	0
Sun Shower Super Juice	
Defense fruit and veggie berry, 8 fl oz	2
Heart healthy tropical passion, 8 fl oz	2
Revitalize apple/kiwi/mango, 8 fl oz	2
Stamina grape apple, 8 fl oz	2
Strength protein juice orange crème, 8 fl oz	4
Sunsweet	
Plumsmart light, 8 fl oz	1
Plumsmart plum juice, 8 fl oz	3
Prune juice, 8 fl oz	3
Tang	
Orange (with fruitrition), prepared, 8 fl oz	1
Tangerine strawberry (with fruitrition), prepared, 8 fl oz	1
Wild berry (with fruitrition), prepared, 8 fl oz	1
Tree of Life	
Apple juice, east coast, 8 fl oz	2
Noni juice, 2 Tbsp	0
Tree Top	
100% apple juice, no sugar added, 8 fl oz	2

	POINTS VALUE
Tree Top Trim	
Mango peach, 8 fl oz	1
Pomegranate blackberry, 8 fl oz	1
Strawberry kiwi, 8 fl oz	1
Tangerine pineapple, 8 fl oz	1
Tropicana	
Antioxidant advantage, orange juice with C, E & selenium, 8 fl oz	2
Apple, 8 fl oz	2
Apple, 1 carton (6 fl oz)	2
Apple cranberry, 1 can (11.5 fl oz)	4
Berry punch, 8 fl oz	3
Cranberry, 8 fl oz	3
Cranberry, 1 container (414 ml)	5
Fruit punch, 8 fl oz	4
Fruit punch, 1 can (11.5 oz)	6
Grape, 8 fl oz	2
Grape, 1 container (414 ml)	5
Grape, 1 can (11.5 fl oz)	4
Grape, 1 fl oz	3
Grape punch, 8 fl oz	2
Healthy kids orange juice with A, C, E & D & calcium, 8 fl oz	2
Heart healthy orange juice with omega 3, 8 fl oz	2
Light berry, 8 fl oz	0
Light lemonade, 8 fl oz	0
Light orangeade, 8 fl oz	0
Low acid orange juice, 8 fl oz	2
Orange cranberry frozen concentrate, 1 serving (1/4 cup)	3

Beverages

Tropicana (cont'd)

	POINTS VALUE
Orange juice with fiber, 8 fl oz	2
Orange peach frozen concentrate, 1 serving (1/4 cup)	2
Orange pulp free & with pulp frozen concentrate, 1 serving (1/4 cup)	2
Orange strawberry banana frozen concentrate, 1 serving (1/4 cup)	3
Orangeade, 8 fl oz	3
Orchard berry, 8 fl oz	2
Organic orange juice, 8 fl oz	2
Organic orchard medley, 8 fl oz	2
Peach orchard punch, 8 fl oz	3
Peach papaya, 8 fl oz	2
Pink lemonade, 8 fl oz	2
Strawberry melon, 8 fl oz	2
Strawberry splash punch, 8 fl oz	2
Tropical orange, 8 fl oz	2
Tropical orange pineapple, 8 fl oz	2
Tropical punch, 8 fl oz	2
Tropicana fruit punch, 8 fl oz	2

Tropicana Light 'N Healthy

Orange juice beverage with calcium, 8 fl oz	1
Orange juice beverage with pulp, 8 fl oz	1

Tropicana Pure Premium

Golden grapefruit, 8 fl oz	2
Indian river grapefruit juice, 8 fl oz	2
Orange juice, 1 carton (177 ml)	2
Orange juice, 1 container (296 ml)	3
Orange juice, 1 large container (414 ml)	4
Orange juice, 8 fl oz	2
Orange juice - lots of pulp, 8 fl oz	2

	POINTS VALUE
Orange juice - original, some pulp, 1 container (414 ml)	4
Orange juice - original, some pulp, 8 fl oz	2
Orange juice + calcium & vitamin D- lots of pulp, 8 fl oz	2
Orange pineapple, 8 fl oz	3
Orange strawberry banana, 8 fl oz	3
Orange tangerine, 8 fl oz	2
Orange with calcium & vitamin D, 8 fl oz	2
Peach papaya mango juice, 8 fl oz	3
Pomegranate blueberry, 8 fl oz	3
Raspberry acai, 8 fl oz	3
Ruby red grapefruit, 8 fl oz	2
Sweet grapefruit, 8 fl oz	3
Triple berry, 8 fl oz	2
Tropical orange, 8 fl oz	2
Valencia juice with pulp, 8 fl oz	2
Valencia mango, 8 fl oz	3
Valencia orange, 8 fl oz	2

Tropicana Pure Tropics

Orange peach mango, 8 fl oz	2
Orange pineapple, 8 fl oz	2
Orange, strawberry, banana, 8 fl oz	2

Tropicana Season's Best

Apple, 1 carton (6 fl oz)	2
Apple, 8 fl oz	2
Apple + calcium and vit C, 10 fl oz	3
Apple juice, 1 bottle (10 fl oz)	3
Apple juice, 1 can (11.5 fl oz)	3
Cranberry cocktail, 10 fl oz	3

	POINTS VALUE
Cranberry grape, 8 fl oz	3
Fruit punch + calcium & vits. A, C, E, 10 fl oz	3
Grape juice, 8 fl oz	3
Grapefruit + vit C, 8 fl oz	2
Grapefruit juice, 1 small bottle (7 fl oz)	1
Grapefruit juice, 1 bottle (10 fl oz)	2
Grapefruit juice, 1 cup (8 fl oz)	2
Grapefruit juice, 8 fl oz	2
Orange + vit. C, 8 fl oz	2
Orange juice, 1 bottle (10 fl oz)	2
Orange juice, 1 can (11.5 fl oz)	3
Orange juice, pulp free & with pulp, 8 fl oz	2
Orange pineapple, 8 fl oz	2
Pineapple orange banana + calcium & vits. A, C, E, 10 fl oz	3
Ruby red grapefruit, 8 fl oz	2
Ruby red grapefruit, 10 fl oz	3
Tropicana Twister	
Grape, 8 fl oz	2
Orange, 8 fl oz	3
Strawberry, 8 fl oz	2
Turkey Hill	
Limonade, 1 cup	2
Orangeade, 1 cup	2
Pink lemonade, 1 cup	2
Pomegranate lemonade, 1 cup	2
V8 Splash	
Berry blend, 1 cup	1
Diet berry blend, 1 cup	0

	POINTS VALUE
Diet tropical blend, 1 cup	0
Fruit medley, 1 cup	1
Mango peach, 1 cup	2
Strawberry kiwi, 1 cup	1
Tropical blend, 1 cup	1
V8 V. Fusion	
Acai berry, 8 oz	2
Very Fine	
Apple cranberry juice cocktail, 8 fl oz	3
Apple juice, 8 fl oz	2
Apple strawberry, 8 fl oz	3
Apricot nectar, 10 fl oz	4
Cranberry juice cocktail, 8 fl oz	3
Fruit punch, 8 fl oz	2
Fruit punch 100% vitamin c & 10% calcium, 8 fl oz	3
Grape juice, 8 fl oz	3
Guava nectar, 10 fl oz	4
Orange juice, 8 fl oz	2
Orange tangerine, 8 fl oz	2
Peach nectar, 10 fl oz	3
Pear nectar, 10 fl oz	3
Tropical fusion, 8 fl oz	3
Welch's	
100% apple juice, 1 serving (8 fl oz)	2
100% grape juice (refrigerated), 1 serving (8 fl oz)	3
100% grape juice, 8 fl oz	3
100% grape juice with calcium, 8 fl oz	3
100% grape juice with fiber, 8 fl oz	4
100% juice, fruit punch, 1 serving (8 fl oz)	3

Beverages

Welch's (cont'd)	POINTS VALUE
100% juice, grape juice, 1 serving (8 fl oz)	3
100% juice, orange fusion, 1 serving (8 fl oz)	2
100% juice, strawberry mango splash, 1 serving (8 fl oz)	3
100% juice, white grape mango passion fruit, 1 serving (8 fl oz)	3
100% juice, white grape peach, 1 serving (8 fl oz)	3
100% orange juice, 1 serving (8 fl oz)	2
100% white grape cherry, 1 serving (8 fl oz)	3
100% white grape juice, 1 serving (8 fl oz)	3
100% white grape peach, 1 serving (8 fl oz)	3
100% white grape pomegranate, 1 serving (8 fl oz)	3
Black cherry concord grape 100% juice, 1 serving (8 fl oz)	3
Light berry blend, 1 serving (8 fl oz)	1
Light concord grape, 1 serving (8 fl oz)	1
Light cranberry raspberry, 1 serving (8 fl oz)	1
Light grape, 1 serving (8 fl oz)	1
Light strawberry mango, 1 serving (8 fl oz)	1
Red grape 100% juice, 1 serving (8 fl oz)	3
Strawberry kiwi 100% juice, 1 serving (8 fl oz)	3
Tropical passionfruit 100% juice, 1 serving (8 fl oz)	3

	POINTS VALUE
Welch's Naturals	
Berry, 1 serving (10 fl oz)	2
Berry, 1 serving (11.5 fl oz)	2
Fruit punch, 1 serving (10 fl oz)	2
Fruit punch, 1 serving (11.5 fl oz)	2
Peach pear, 1 serving (10 fl oz)	2
Peach pear, 1 serving (11.5 fl oz)	2
Wilderness	
Apple cider, 8 fl oz	2
Apple juice, with vitamin c added, 8 fl oz	2
Cherry pomegranate juice, 8 fl oz	3
Natural Apple juice, 8 fl oz	2
Red tart cherry juice, 8 fl oz	3

Meal Replacement Drinks
Balanced

	POINTS VALUE
Chocolate, 1 can (11 oz)	4
Vanilla, 1 can (11 oz)	4
Gatorade	
Nutrition shake, chocolate, 1 can	8
Nutrition shake, vanilla, 1 can	8
Kashi GOLEAN	
Chocolate shake mix, 2 scoops	4
Vanilla shake mix, 2 scoops	4
Nestle Carnation	
Instant breakfast mix, chocolate malt, no sugar added, 1 packet	1
Instant breakfast mix, classic chocolate malt, 1 packet	2
Instant breakfast mix, classic French vanilla, 1 packet	3

	POINTS VALUE
Instant breakfast mix, classic French vanilla, no sugar added, 1 packet	1
Instant breakfast mix, dark chocolate powder, 1 packet	2
Instant breakfast mix, rich milk chocolate, 1 packet	2
Instant breakfast mix, rich milk chocolate, no sugar added, 1 packet	1
Instant breakfast mix, strawberry sensation, 1 packet	3
Instant breakfast mix, strawberry sensation, no sugar added, 1 packet	1
Instant breakfast, creamy milk chocolate, 1 can (10.6 fl oz)	5
Instant breakfast, creamy milk chocolate, no sugar added, 1 can (10.6 fl oz)	3
Instant breakfast, French vanilla, 1 can (10.6 fl oz)	5
Instant breakfast, French vanilla, no sugar added, 1 can (10.6 fl oz)	3
Instant breakfast, strawberry crème, 1 can (10.6 fl oz)	5

Milk & Milk Based Drinks
Alba

	POINTS VALUE
Chocolate, prepared, 8 fl oz	1
Double fudge, prepared, 8 fl oz	1
◆ Nonfat dry milk, prepared, 8 fl oz	2
Strawberry, prepared, 8 fl oz	1
Vanilla, prepared, 8 fl oz	1

Borden Eagle Brand

	POINTS VALUE
Low fat sweetened condensed milk, 2 Tbsp	3

Carnation

	POINTS VALUE
◆ Evaporated fat free milk, 2 Tbsp	1
Evaporated lowfat milk, 2 Tbsp	1
Evaporated milk, 2 Tbsp	1
Sweetened condensed milk, 2 Tbsp	3

Eagle Brand

	POINTS VALUE
Fat free sweetened condensed milk, 2 Tbsp	2
Sweetened condensed milk, 2 Tbsp	3

Turkey Hill

	POINTS VALUE
Egg nog (limited edition), 1/2 cup	5

Turkey Hill Cool Moos

	POINTS VALUE
2% reduced fat milk, 1 cup	3
Chocolate, 1 cup	4
Strawberry, 1 cup	3
Whole milk, 1 cup	4

Smoothies
Jell-O Smoothie Snacks

	POINTS VALUE
Mixed berry, 1 container (4 oz)	2
Strawberry banana, 1 container (4 oz)	2

Odwalla

	POINTS VALUE
Blackberry fruit shake fruit smoothie blend, 8 fl oz	3
Blueberry b monster vitamin b fruit smoothie blend, 8 fl oz	3
Citrus c monster vitamin c fruit smoothie blend, 8 fl oz	3
Mango tango fruit smoothie blend, 8 fl oz	3
New super protein latte, 8 fl oz	4

Beverages

Odwalla (cont'd)

	POINTS VALUE
Raspberry cha cha fruit smoothie blend, 8 fl oz	2
Strawberry banana fruit smoothie blend, 8 fl oz	3
Strawberry c monster vitamin c fruit smoothie blend, 8 fl oz	3
Tropical calci-yum monster calcium fruit smoothie blend, 8 fl oz	4

Stonyfield Farm Smoothie

Banana berry, 1 container (10 oz)	5
Peach, 1 container (10 oz)	5
Raspberry, 1 container (10 oz)	5
Strawberry, 1 bottle (6 oz)	3
Strawberry, 1 container (10 oz)	5
Vanilla, 1 container (10 oz)	5
Wild berry, 1 bottle (6 oz)	3

Sun Shower

Defense fruit & veggie superfood smoothie, 8 fl oz	2
Heart healthy fruit superfood smoothie, 8 fl oz	2
Revitalize fruit superfood smoothie, 8 fl oz	2
Stamina fruit superfood smoothie, 8 fl oz	2
Strength protein superfood smoothie, 8 fl oz	4

Sun Shower Superfood Fruit 'N Yogurt Smoothie

Berry blast, 8 fl oz	2
Orange passion, 8 fl oz	2
Pina colada, 8 fl oz	2
Strawberry banana, 8 fl oz	2

Tropicana

Mixed berry fruit smoothie, 11 fl oz	4
Strawberry banana fruit smoothie, 11 fl oz	4
Tropical fruit - fruit smoothie, 11 fl oz	4

V8 Splash

Strawberry banana, 8 oz	2
Tropical colada, 8 oz	2

Weight Watchers Smoothie Drink Mix

Smoothie - creamy chocolate, 1 packet	1
Smoothie – French vanilla, 1 packet	1
Smoothie - white chocolate peppermint, 1 packet	1
Smoothie - wild berry, 1 packet	1

Yoplait Go-Gurt Smoothies

Punch, 1 container (5 oz)	2
Strawberry, 1 container (5 oz)	2
Strawberry banana, 1 container (5 oz)	2
Wild berry, 1 container (5 oz)	2

Yoplait Light

Peach, 1 bottle	1

Yoplait Light Smoothies

Strawberry, 1 container	1
Strawberry banana, 1 container	1

Yoplait Nouriche Super Smoothie

Mixed berry, 1 container	4
Peach, 1 container	4
Raspberry, 1 container	4
Strawberry, 1 container	4
Strawberry banana, 1 container	4

	POINTS VALUE
Yoplait Original Smoothies	
Mixed berry, 1 container	5
Strawberry, 1 container	5
Strawberry banana, 1 container	5

Soft Drinks
4C

Lemonade flavor drink, 1 serving (8 fl oz prepared)	1

4C Totally Light

Lemonade drink mix, 1 serving (8 fl oz prepared)	0
Pink lemonade drink mix, 1 serving (8 fl oz prepared)	0

4C Totally Light 2Go

Lemonade drink mix, 1 serving (8 fl oz prepared)	0
Pink lemonade drink mix, 1 serving (8 fl oz prepared)	0

Barq's

Diet French vanilla crème soda, 8 fl oz	0
Diet red crème soda, 8 fl oz	0
Diet root beer, 8 fl oz	0
Floatz, 8 fl oz	3
French vanilla crème soda, 8 fl oz	2
Frozen root beer, 8 fl oz	1
Red crème soda, 8 fl oz	2
Root beer, 8 fl oz	2

Capri Sun

Lemonade, 1 pouch	2

Carver's

Ginger ale, 8 fl oz	2

	POINTS VALUE
Cascadian Farm	
Lemonade frozen concentrate, 1 serving (1.6 oz)	2
Coca-Cola	
Black cherry vanilla coke, 8 fl oz	2
C2, 8 fl oz	1
Caffeine free classic, 8 fl oz	2
Caffeine free diet coke, 8 fl oz	0
Cherry coke, 8 fl oz	2
Classic, 8 fl oz	2
Diet black cherry vanilla coke, 8 fl oz	0
Diet cherry coke, 8 fl oz	0
Diet coke, 8 fl oz	0
Diet coke sweetened with splenda, 8 fl oz	0
Diet coke with lime, 8 fl oz	0
Diet inca kola, 8 fl oz	0
Diet vanilla coke, 8 fl oz	0
Frozen classic, 8 fl oz	1
Frozen vanilla coke, 8 fl oz	2
Inca kola, 8 fl oz	2
Manzana mia, 8 fl oz	2
Vanilla coke, 8 fl oz	2
With lime, 8 fl oz	2
Zero, 8 fl oz	0
Country Time	
Lemonade large ready to drink pouches, 1 pouch	4
Lemonade, prepared, 8 fl oz	1
Lite lemonade, prepared, 8 fl oz	1
Lite pink lemonade, prepared, 8 fl oz	1
Pink lemonade, prepared, 8 fl oz	1

Beverages

Country Time (cont'd)

	POINTS VALUE
Raspberry lemonade, prepared, 8 fl oz	2
Strawberry lemonade, prepared, 8 fl oz	2

Country Time On the Go

Lemonade yellow, prepared, 1 serving (8.45 fl oz)	1

Crayons

Tickled pink lemonade, 8 fl oz	1

Crystal Light

Hydration pink lemonade, sugar free, 8 fl oz	0
Lemonade mix, sugar free, prepared, 8 fl oz	0
Lemonade, sugar free, 8 fl oz	0
Pink lemonade mix, sugar free, prepared, 8 fl oz	0
Pink lemonade, sugar free, 8 fl oz	0
Raspberry ice, sugar free, 8 fl oz	0
Raspberry lemonade, sugar free, prepared, 8 fl oz	0

Crystal Light On the Go

Lemonade mix, 1 packet	0
Raspberry lemonade, prepared, 1 serving (8.45 fl oz)	0

Crystal Light Sunrise

Classic orange, 8 fl oz	0

Fanta

Apple, 8 fl oz	2
Berry, 8 fl oz	2
Black cherry, 8 fl oz	2
Citrus, 8 fl oz	2
Grape, 8 fl oz	2
Lemon, 8 fl oz	2
Orange, 8 fl oz	2

	POINTS VALUE
Peach, 8 fl oz	2
Pineapple, 8 fl oz	2
Pink grapefruit, 8 fl oz	2
Red tangerine, 8 fl oz	3
Strawberry, 8 fl oz	2
Zero orange, 8 fl oz	0

Fanta Frozen

Banana, 8 fl oz	1
Blue raspberry, 8 fl oz	2
Grape, 8 fl oz	1
Green lemon lime, 8 fl oz	2
Kiwi strawberry, 8 fl oz	1
Master chill cherry limeade, 8 fl oz	1
Orange, 8 fl oz	1
Orange crème, 8 fl oz	1
Peach, 8 fl oz	1
Pina colada, 8 fl oz	1
Pineapple, 8 fl oz	1
Purple berry cherry, 8 fl oz	2
Strawberry, 8 fl oz	2
Strawberry banana, 8 fl oz	1
Super sour apple, 8 fl oz	1
Super sour cherry, 8 fl oz	1
Super sour watermelon, 8 fl oz	2
Watermelon, 8 oz	1
White cherry, 8 fl oz	1
Wild cherry, 8 fl oz	2

Fresca

Fresca, 8 fl oz	0
Fresca black cherry, 8 fl oz	0
Fresca peach, 8 fl oz	0

	POINTS VALUE
Goya	
Lemonade, 8 fl oz	2
Hi-C	
Poppin' lemonade, 1 box	2
Kellogg's	
Special K20 protein water mix, pink lemonade, 1 packet	0
Kool-Aid	
Lemonade mix, unsweetened, 1 packet	0
Lemonade sugar-free mix, prepared, 8 fl oz	0
Soarin' strawberry lemonade sugar-free mix, prepared, 8 fl oz	0
Kool-Aid Jammers	
Lemonade, 1 pouch	2
Manzanita Sol	
Manzanita sol, 8 fl oz	2
Master	
Frozen chill strawberry crème, 8 fl oz	1
Mello Yello	
Cherry, 8 fl oz	2
Diet mello yello, 8 fl oz	0
Frozen mello yello, 8 fl oz	1
Mello Yello, 8 fl oz	2
Melon, 8 fl oz	2
Minute Maid	
Frozen blueberry, 8 fl oz	1
Frozen lemonade, frozen concentrate, 1 1/2 fl oz (8 fl oz prepared)	2
Grape, 1 bottle (10 fl oz)	3
Grape, 1 can (11.5 fl oz)	3
Lemonade, 1 box	2
Lemonade, 8 fl oz	2

	POINTS VALUE
Lemonade, 1 small can (8 fl oz)	2
Lemonade, 1 can (12 fl oz)	3
Pink lemonade, 8 fl oz	2
Pink lemonade, 1 bottle (16.9 fl oz)	4
Pink lemonade, 1 can (8 oz)	2
Pink lemonade, 8 fl oz	2
Raspberry lemonade, 8 fl oz	2
Raspberry lemonade, frozen concentrate, 2 fl oz (8 fl oz prepared)	2
Minute Maid Coolers	
Pink lemonade, 1 pouch	2
Minute Maid Light	
Lemonade, 8 fl oz	0
Lemonade, 1 can (12 fl oz)	0
Minute Maid Premium	
Lemonade iced tea, 8 fl oz	2
Mountain Dew	
Caffeine free, 8 fl oz	2
Code red, 8 fl oz	2
Diet, 8 fl oz	0
Diet caffeine free, 8 fl oz	0
Diet code red, 8 fl oz	0
Live wire, 1 can or bottle (8 fl oz)	2
Mountain dew blue shock freeze, 8 fl oz	1
Mountain dew freeze, 8 fl oz	1
Mountain dew voltage, 8 fl oz	2
Mountain dew voltage freeze, 8 fl oz	1
Regular, 8 fl oz	2
Mr. Pibb	
Diet Mr. Pibb, 8 fl oz	0
Pibb xtra, 8 fl oz	2
Pibb zero, 8 fl oz	0

Beverages

	POINTS VALUE
Mug	
Cream soda, 8 fl oz	2
Diet cream soda, 8 fl oz	0
Diet root beer, 8 fl oz	0
Root beer, 8 fl oz	2
Northern Neck	
Diet ginger ale, 8 fl oz	0
Ginger ale, 8 fl oz	2
Odwalla	
Pure squeezed lemonade, 8 fl oz	2
Strawberry lemonade, 8 fl oz	2
Summertime lime, 8 fl oz	2
Payaso	
Horchata drink mix, 3 tsp	3
Pepsi	
Caffeine free, 8 fl oz	2
Diet, 8 fl oz	0
Diet caffeine free, 8 fl oz	0
Diet pepsi lemon, 8 fl oz	0
Diet pepsi lime, 8 fl oz	0
Diet vanilla, 8 fl oz	0
Diet wild cherry, 8 fl oz	0
Jazz - caramel cream, 8 fl oz	0
Pepsi freeze, 8 fl oz	1
Pepsi max, 8 fl oz	0
Pepsi natural, 8 fl oz	2
Pepsi one, 8 fl oz	0
Regular, 8 fl oz	2
Wild cherry, 8 fl oz	2
Red Flash	
Red Flash, 8 fl oz	2

	POINTS VALUE
Seagram's	
Diet ginger ale, 8 fl oz	0
Diet raspberry ginger ale, 8 fl oz	0
Flavored seltzer - raspberry seltzer naturals, 8 fl oz	0
Flavored seltzer - black cherry seltzer naturals, 8 fl oz	0
Flavored seltzer - lemon lime seltzer naturals, 8 fl oz	0
Flavored seltzer - orange seltzer naturals, 8 fl oz	0
Ginger ale, 8 fl oz	2
Raspberry ginger ale, 8 fl oz	2
Original seltzer, 8 fl oz	0
Sierra Mist	
Diet sierra mist ruby splash, 8 fl oz	0
Sierra Mist, 8 fl oz	2
Sierra mist cranberry splash, 8 fl oz	2
Sierra mist free cranberry splash, 8 fl oz	0
Sierra mist ruby splash, 8 fl oz	2
Sierra mist, diet, 8 fl oz	0
Slice	
Diet orange, 1 (8 fl oz)	0
Grape, 1 (8 fl oz)	2
Orange, 1 (8 fl oz)	2
Peach, 1 (8 fl oz)	2
Strawberry, 1 (8 fl oz)	2
Sprite	
Diet sprite zero, 8 fl oz	0
Frozen sprite, 8 fl oz	1
Sprite, 8 fl oz	2
Sprite remix Aruba jam, 8 fl oz	2

	POINTS VALUE
Steaz Organic Sparkling Green Tea	
Cola, 8 fl oz	2
Ginger ale, 8 fl oz	2
Grape, 8 fl oz	2
Key lime, 8 fl oz	2
Orange, 8 fl oz	2
Raspberry, 8 fl oz	2
Root beer, 8 fl oz	2
Sunkist	
Diet orange soda, 12 fl oz	0
Tab	
Tab, 8 fl oz	0
Tropicana	
Lemonade, 8 fl oz	2
Lemonade, 1 container (414 ml)	4
Tropicana Twister	
Diet orange, 8 fl oz	0
Turkey Hill	
Raspberry lemonade, 1 cup	2
Regular lemonade, 1 cup	2
Strawberry kiwi lemonade, 1 cup	2
Waist Watcher	
Diet black cherry, 8 oz	0
Diet black cherry, 1 can	0
Diet black raspberry, 8 oz	0
Diet black raspberry, 1 can	0
Diet cherry cola, 8 oz	0
Diet cherry cola, 1 can	0
Diet chocolate, 8 oz	0
Diet chocolate, 1 can	0
Diet citrus frost, 8 oz	0

	POINTS VALUE
Diet citrus frost, 1 can	0
Diet grape frost, 8 oz	0
Diet grape frost, 1 can	0
Diet grape, 8 oz	0
Diet grape, 1 can	0
Diet lemon up, 1 can	0
Diet orange dry, 8 oz	0
Diet orange dry, 1 can	0
Diet pomegranate frost, 8 oz	0
Diet pomegranate frost, 1 can	0
Diet raspberry ginger ale, 8 oz	0
Diet raspberry ginger ale, 1 can	0
Diet tonic water, 1 can	0
Diet vanilla cream, 8 oz	0
Diet vanilla cream, 1 can	0

Soy, Rice & Chai Drinks
Azumaya

	POINTS VALUE
◆ Lite plus plain soy beverage, 8 fl oz	1
Lite plus vanilla soy beverage, 8 fl oz	1
Better Than Milk	
Rice original, powder, 2 Tbsp	1
Rice vanilla, powder, 2 Tbsp	1
Soy light, powder, 2 Tbsp	2
Soy original, powder, 2 Tbsp	2
Soy vanilla, powder, 2 3/4 Tbsp	2
Eden Organic	
Edenblend, 8 fl oz	2
Edensoy chocolate, 8 oz	4
◆ Edensoy extra original, 8 oz	3
Edensoy extra vanilla, 8 oz	3
◆ Edensoy light original, 8 oz	2

Beverages

Eden Organic (cont'd)

Edensoy light vanilla, 8 oz	2
Edensoy original, 8 oz	3
Edensoy unsweetened, 8 oz	3
Edensoy vanilla, 8 oz	3

Fearn

Chocolate, 8 fl oz	2
Original, 8 fl oz	2
Soyness, chocolate, 8 fl oz	2
Soyness, original, 8 fl oz	2
Soyness, vanilla, 8 fl oz	2
Vanilla, 8 fl oz	2

General Foods International Coffee

Sugar free chai latte, 1 Tbsp	1

Oregon Chai

Sugar free original chai tea latte, 1/2 cup	0

Pacific Chai

Caffeine free spice chai latte, 4 fl oz	1
Spice chai latte, 2 Tbsp	2
Spice chai latte, organic, 4 fl oz	2
Vanilla chai latte, 2 Tbsp	2
Vanilla chai latte, organic, 4 fl oz	2

Rice Dream

Classic carob, 8 oz	3
Classic original, 8 oz	3
Classic vanilla, 8 oz	3
Enriched chocolate, 8 oz	3
Enriched original, 8 oz	3
Enriched vanilla, 8 oz	3
Heartwise original, 8 oz	2
Heartwise vanilla, 8 oz	2
Horchata original, 8 oz	3

Silk

Chai, 1 cup	3
Chocolate, 1 cup	3
Coffee, 1 cup	3
Coffee soylatte, 1 cup	4
Coffee soylatte, 11 fl oz	6
Cultured soy - black cherry, 1 container	3
Cultured soy - blueberry, 1 container	3
Cultured soy - key lime, 1 container	3
Cultured soy - plain, 8 oz	3
Cultured soy - vanilla, 1 container	3
Light chocolate, 1 cup	2
Light plain, 1 cup	1
Light vanilla, 1 cup	2
Mocha, 1 cup	3
Nog, 1/2 cup	2
Organic plain, 1 cup	2
Organic unsweetened, 1 cup	2
Organic vanilla, 1 cup	2
Plus dha omega-3, 1 cup	2
Plus fiber, 1 cup	1
Pumpkin spice, 1 cup	4
Spice soylatte, 11 fl oz	4
Very vanilla, 1 cup	3

Soy Dream

Classic original, 8 oz	3
Classic vanilla, 8 oz	3
Enriched chocolate, 8 oz	3
Enriched original, 8 oz	2
Enriched vanilla, 8 oz	2

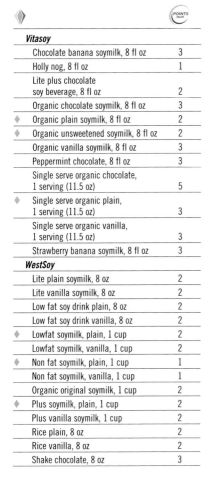

Vitasoy	POINTS VALUE
Vitasoy	
Chocolate banana soymilk, 8 fl oz	3
Holly nog, 8 fl oz	1
Lite plus chocolate soy beverage, 8 fl oz	2
Organic chocolate soymilk, 8 fl oz	3
Organic plain soymilk, 8 fl oz	2
Organic unsweetened soymilk, 8 fl oz	2
Organic vanilla soymilk, 8 fl oz	3
Peppermint chocolate, 8 fl oz	3
Single serve organic chocolate, 1 serving (11.5 oz)	5
Single serve organic plain, 1 serving (11.5 oz)	3
Single serve organic vanilla, 1 serving (11.5 oz)	3
Strawberry banana soymilk, 8 fl oz	3
WestSoy	
Lite plain soymilk, 8 oz	2
Lite vanilla soymilk, 8 oz	2
Low fat soy drink plain, 8 oz	2
Low fat soy drink vanilla, 8 oz	2
Lowfat soymilk, plain, 1 cup	2
Lowfat soymilk, vanilla, 1 cup	2
Non fat soymilk, plain, 1 cup	1
Non fat soymilk, vanilla, 1 cup	1
Organic original soymilk, 1 cup	2
Plus soymilk, plain, 1 cup	2
Plus vanilla soymilk, 1 cup	2
Rice plain, 8 oz	2
Rice vanilla, 8 oz	2
Shake chocolate, 8 oz	3

	POINTS VALUE
Shake vanilla, 8 oz	3
Unsweetened, 1 cup	1
Unsweetened almond soymilk, 1 cup	1
Unsweetened chocolate soymilk, 1 cup	2
Unsweetened original soymilk, 1 cup	1
Unsweetened vanilla soymilk, 1 cup	2
Unsweetened, almond, 1 cup	1
Unsweetened, chocolate, 1 cup	2
WestSoy drink plain, 1 cup	2
WestSoy lite plain, 1 cup	2
WestSoy lite vanilla, 1 cup	2
WestSoy Soy Slender	
Cappuccino, 8 oz	1
Chocolate, 8 oz	1
Sugar free soymilk, cappuccino, 1 cup	1
Sugar free soymilk, chocolate, 1 cup	1
Sugar free soymilk, vanilla, 1 cup	1
Vanilla, 8 oz	1

Sports Drinks
AMP Energy

	POINTS VALUE
Amp energy, 8 fl oz	2
Amp energy with black tea, 8 fl oz	2
Amp energy with green tea, 8 fl oz	2
Amp energy, elevate, 8 fl oz	2
Amp energy, lightning, 8 fl oz	2
Amp energy, overdrive, 8 fl oz	2
Amp energy, relaunch, 8 fl oz	2
Amp energy, sugar free, 8 fl oz	0
Amp energy, traction, 8 fl oz	2

Beverages

	POINTS VALUE
Crayons	
Breakaway berry, 8 fl oz	1
Leaping lemon-lime, 8 fl oz	1
Playoff punch, 8 fl oz	1
Fearn	
Liquid lecithin, 1 Tbsp	4
Natural mint flavor liquid lecithin, 1 Tbsp	4
FRS Healthy Energy	
Diet lemon lime powdered drink mix, 1 packet (makes 8 fl oz with water)	0
Diet orange powdered drink mix, 1 packet (makes 8 fl oz with water)	0
Diet wild berry powdered drink mix, 1 packet (makes 8 fl oz with water)	0
Lemon lime, 1 can (11.5 fl oz)	2
Low cal peach mango, 1 can (11.5 fl oz)	0
Low cal peach mango liquid concentrate, 1 serving (makes 8 fl oz with water)	0
Low calorie - orange, 1 can (11.5 fl oz)	0
Low calorie - orange concentrate, 2 fl oz	0
Low calorie wild berry, 1 can (11.5 fl oz)	0
Orange, 1 can (11.5 fl oz)	2
Orange liquid concentrate, 1 serving (makes 8 fl oz with water)	2
Peach mango concentrate, 1 serving (makes 8 fl oz with water)	0
Gatorade	
All flavors, 8 fl oz	1
Bring it - grape, 8 fl oz	1
G - berry, 8 fl oz	1
G - cool blue, 8 fl oz	1
G - fruit punch, 8 fl oz	1
G - glacier freeze, 8 fl oz	1
G - ice punch, 8 fl oz	1
G - lemon lime, 8 fl oz	1
G - orange, 8 fl oz	1
G - riptide rush, 8 fl oz	1
G2 - grape, 8 fl oz	1
G2 - orange, 8 fl oz	1
G2 - strawberry kiwi, 8 fl oz	1
No excuses - berry, 8 fl oz	1
Powder, all flavors, 1 serving (makes 8 fl oz)	1
Market Day	
Gatorade kid size variety pack, 1 bottle	2
No Fear	
No fear bloodshot, 8 fl oz	2
No fear motherload, 8 fl oz	3
Nutrisoda	
Calm, 1 can	0
Energize, 1 can	0
Flex, 1 can	0
Focus, 1 can	0
Immune, 1 can	0
Radiant, 1 can	0
Renew, 1 can	0
Slender, 1 can	0
Powerade	
Arctic shatter, 8 fl oz	1
Black cherry lime, 8 fl oz	1
Citrus blend, 8 fl oz	1
Flava 23 sourberry, 8 fl oz	1
Flava 23 sourmelon, 8 fl oz	1

	POINTS VALUE
Fruit punch, 8 fl oz	1
Green squall, 8 fl oz	1
Jagged ice, 8 fl oz	1
Lemon-lime, 8 fl oz	1
Mango, 8 fl oz	1
Mountain blast, 8 fl oz	1
NHRA, 8 fl oz	2
Olympic (citrus), 8 fl oz	1
Option black cherry, 8 fl oz	0
Option lemon, 8 fl oz	0
Option strawberry, 8 fl oz	0
Orange, 8 fl oz	1
Strawberry melon, 8 fl oz	1

SoBe

Sobe energy, 8 fl oz	2
Sobe power, 8 fl oz	2
Sobe yumberry pomegranate, 8 fl oz	2

SoBe Lean

Diet blackberry currant, 8 fl oz	0

Steaz Diet Energy

Diet berry, 8 fl oz	1

Steaz Energy

Berry, 8 fl oz	2
Lime, 8 fl oz	2
Orange, 8 fl oz	2

Tea/Iced Tea

4C

Decaffeinated iced tea mix with sugar and natural lemon flavor, 1 serving (8 fl oz prepared)	2

	POINTS VALUE
Green tea with sugar, honey and natural lemon flavor, 1 serving (8 fl oz prepared)	2
Iced tea mix with sugar and natural lemon flavor, 1 serving (8 fl oz prepared)	1
Peach iced tea mix with sugar and natural peach flavor, 1 serving (8 fl oz prepared)	1

4C Light

Decaffeinated low calorie iced tea mix with natural lemon flavor, 1 serving (8 fl oz prepared)	0
Low calorie green tea with honey and lemon, 1 serving (8 fl oz prepared)	0
Low calorie iced tea mix with natural lemon flavor, 1 serving (8 fl oz prepared)	0

4C Totally Light

Iced tea mix, antioxidant green tea, 1 serving (8 fl oz prepared)	0
Iced tea mix, natural decaffeinated natural lemon flavor, 1 serving (8 fl oz prepared)	0
Iced tea mix, natural lemon flavor, 1 serving (8 fl oz prepared)	0
Red tea antioxidant peach - canister, 1/8 container	0

4C Totally Light Tea 2Go

Iced tea mix antioxidant green tea, sugar free, 1 serving (8 fl oz prepared)	0
Iced tea mix naturally decaffeinated natural lemon flavor, 1 serving (8 fl oz prepared)	0

Beverages

	POINTS VALUE
Iced tea mix, green antioxidant with honey and natural lemon flavor, 1 serving (8 fl oz prepared)	0
Red tea antioxidant peach, 1/2 packet	0
Country Time	
Lemonade iced tea classic mix, 1 serving	2
Lemonade iced tea peach mix, 1 serving	2
Lemonade iced tea raspberry mix, 1 serving	2
Crystal Light	
Green tea raspberry, sugar free, prepared, 8 fl oz	0
Iced tea decaffeinated mix, sugar free, prepared, 8 fl oz	0
Iced tea mix, sugar free, prepared, 8 fl oz	0
Lemon tea, sugar free, 8 fl oz	0
Peach iced tea mix, sugar free, prepared, 8 fl oz	0
Peach tea mix, sugar free, prepared, 8 fl oz	0
Raspberry iced tea mix, sugar free, prepared, 8 fl oz	0
Crystal Light On the Go	
Green tea honey lemon, sugar free, prepared, 1 serving (8.45 fl oz)	0
Iced tea mix, sugar free, 1 packet	0
Peach tea mix, sugar free, 1 packet	0
White tea blueberry, 1 serving (8.45 fl oz)	0
Drenchers	
Chai tea latte super blend, 9 1/2 fl oz	2

	POINTS VALUE
Eden Organic	
Lotus root tea, 1 tsp	0
Organic matcha tea, 1 serving (1 g)	0
General Foods	
Instant chai latte flavored tea mix, 1 1/3 Tbsp	2
Kellogg's	
All-bran fiber drink mix, iced tea, 1 packet	0
Special K20 protein water mix, iced tea, 1 packet	0
Special K20 protein water, iced tea, 1 bottle	0
Lipton	
Diet green tea with citrus, 8 fl oz	0
Diet green tea with mixed berry, 8 fl oz	0
Diet iced tea with lemon, 8 fl oz	0
Diet iced tea with lemon flavor - decaf, prepared, 1 serving (8 fl oz)	0
Diet iced tea with lemon flavor, prepared, 1 serving (8 fl oz)	0
Diet iced tea with peach flavor, prepared, 1 serving (8 fl oz)	0
Diet iced tea with raspberry flavor, prepared, 1 serving (8 fl oz)	0
Diet white tea with peach papaya, 8 fl oz	0
Diet white tea with raspberry, 8 fl oz	0
Green tea with citrus, 8 fl oz	2
Green tea with mixed berry, 8 fl oz	1
Iced tea with lemon, 8 fl oz	1
Sparkling berry, 8 fl oz	1
Sparkling diet strawberry kiwi, 8 fl oz	0

	POINTS VALUE
Sparkling strawberry kiwi, 8 fl oz	1
Unsweetened iced tea mix, prepared, 1 serving (8 fl oz)	0
White tea with raspberry, 8 fl oz	1
Lipton Black	
Cold brew, prepared, 1 serving (8 fl oz)	0
Regular, prepared, 1 serving (8 fl oz)	0
Lipton Brisk	
Green tea, 8 fl oz	2
Lemon, 8 fl oz	2
Lemon, no calorie, 8 fl oz	0
Raspberry iced tea, 8 fl oz	2
Sweet tea, 8 fl oz	2
Lipton Green	
Citrus blossom, prepared, 1 serving (8 fl oz)	0
Cranberry pomegranate, prepared, 1 serving (8 fl oz)	0
Green honey, prepared, 1 serving (8 fl oz)	0
Green mint, prepared, 1 serving (8 fl oz)	0
Honey lemon decaf, prepared, 1 serving (8 fl oz)	0
Lemon, prepared, 1 serving (8 fl oz)	0
Mountain berry, prepared, 1 serving (8 fl oz)	0
Orange passionfruit & jasmine, prepared, 1 serving (8 fl oz)	0
Unflavored decaf, prepared, 1 serving (8 fl oz)	0
Unflavored, prepared, 1 serving (8 fl oz)	0

	POINTS VALUE
Lipton PureLeaf	
Diet lemon, 8 fl oz	0
Extra sweet tea, 8 fl oz	2
Green tea with honey, 8 fl oz	1
Lemon tea, 8 fl oz	1
Peach tea, 8 fl oz	2
Raspberry tea, 8 fl oz	2
Sweetened tea, 8 fl oz	1
Unsweetened tea, 8 fl oz	0
White tea with tangerine, 8 fl oz	1
Lipton Pyramid	
Bavarian berry, prepared, 1 serving (8 fl oz)	0
Bedtime story, prepared, 1 serving (8 fl oz)	0
Black pearl, prepared, 1 serving (8 fl oz)	0
Green mandarin orange, prepared, 1 serving (8 fl oz)	0
Red harvest strawberry, prepared, 1 serving (8 fl oz)	0
Tuscan lemon, prepared, 1 serving (8 fl oz)	0
Vanilla caramel truffle, prepared, 1 serving (8 fl oz)	0
White blueberry pomegranate, prepared, 1 serving (8 fl oz)	0
White island mango, prepared, 1 serving (8 fl oz)	0
Lipton To Go	
Apple cranberry white iced tea, 1/2 packet	0
Cherry green iced tea, 1/2 packet	0

Beverages

	POINTS VALUE
Citrus green iced tea, 1/2 packet	0
Green tea blueberry pomegranate, prepared, 1 serving (8 fl oz)	0
Green tea with pink lemonade (defense), prepared, 1 serving (8 fl oz)	0
Green tea with raspberry Lime (revitalize), prepared, 1 serving (8 fl oz)	0
Lemon black iced tea, 1/2 packet	0
Mandarin mango green iced tea, 1/2 packet	0
Peach black iced tea, 1/2 packet	0
Raspberry white iced tea, 1/2 packet	0
Tea with cherry blossom, prepared, 1 serving (8 fl oz)	0
Tea with citrus, prepared, 1 serving (8 fl oz)	0
Tea with honey and lemon, prepared, 1 serving (8 fl oz)	0
Tea with lemon, prepared, 1 serving (8 fl oz)	0
Tea with mandarin and mango, prepared, 1 serving (8 fl oz)	0
White tea with apple cranberry, prepared, 1 serving (8 fl oz)	0
White tea with raspberry, prepared, 1 serving (8 fl oz)	0
Minute Maid	
Enhanced pomegranate flavored tea, 8 fl oz	2
Lemonade iced tea, 8 fl oz	2
Nestea	
100% decaf tea iced tea mix, 2 tsp	0
100% tea iced tea mix, 2 tsp	0

	POINTS VALUE
Brewed unsweetened, 8 fl oz	0
Cool, 8 fl oz	2
Cool lemonade tea, 8 fl oz	2
Cool peach frrreezer, 8 fl oz	2
Cool raspbrrry cooler, 8 fl oz	2
Decaffeinated sweetened tea, 8 fl oz	1
Diet green, 8 fl oz	0
Diet lemon, 8 fl oz	0
Diet nestea sweetened with splenda, 8 fl oz	0
Green, 8 fl oz	2
Green tea concentrate, 1 fl oz	2
Herb tea lemon bliss iced tea mix, 1 Tbsp	0
Honey lemon green tea, 8 fl oz	2
Lemon, 8 fl oz	2
Lemon & sugar iced tea mix, 1 1/3 Tbsp	1
Lemon concentrate, 1 fl oz	2
Lemon iced tea mix, 2 tsp	0
Lemon sweet, 8 fl oz	2
Lemonade tea iced tea mix, 1 1/3 Tbsp	1
Nestea ice lemon green tea, 8 fl oz	2
Nestea ice lime iced tea, 8 fl oz	2
Peach concentrate, 2 Tbsp	2
Peach iced tea, 8 fl oz	2
Raspberry, 8 fl oz	2
Raspberry concentrate, 1 fl oz	2
Sugar free decaf iced tea mix, 2 tsp	0
Sugar free iced tea mix, 2 tsp	0
Sweetened, 8 fl oz	2
Unsweetened, 8 fl oz	0
Unsweetened concentrate, 2 Tbsp	0

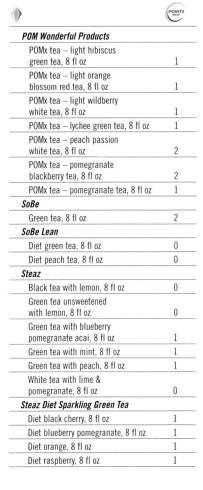

	POINTS VALUE
POM Wonderful Products	
POMx tea – light hibiscus green tea, 8 fl oz	1
POMx tea – light orange blossom red tea, 8 fl oz	1
POMx tea – light wildberry white tea, 8 fl oz	1
POMx tea – lychee green tea, 8 fl oz	1
POMx tea – peach passion white tea, 8 fl oz	2
POMx tea – pomegranate blackberry tea, 8 fl oz	2
POMx tea – pomegranate tea, 8 fl oz	1
SoBe	
Green tea, 8 fl oz	2
SoBe Lean	
Diet green tea, 8 fl oz	0
Diet peach tea, 8 fl oz	0
Steaz	
Black tea with lemon, 8 fl oz	0
Green tea unsweetened with lemon, 8 fl oz	0
Green tea with blueberry pomegranate acai, 8 fl oz	1
Green tea with mint, 8 fl oz	1
Green tea with peach, 8 fl oz	1
White tea with lime & pomegranate, 8 fl oz	0
Steaz Diet Sparkling Green Tea	
Diet black cherry, 8 fl oz	1
Diet blueberry pomegranate, 8 fl oz	1
Diet orange, 8 fl oz	1
Diet raspberry, 8 fl oz	1

	POINTS VALUE
Steaz Organic Sparkling Green Tea	
Green tea with lemon, 8 fl oz	2
Sun Shower	
Chai tea super blend, 9 1/2 fl oz	2
Turkey Hill	
Blueberry oolong tea, 1 cup	2
Decaffeinated iced tea, 1 cup	2
Diet decaffeinated iced tea, 1 cup	0
Diet decaffeinated iced tea, 1 cup	0
Diet decaffeinated orange tea, 1 cup	0
Diet decaffeinated orange tea, 1 cup	0
Diet green tea, 1 cup	0
Diet green tea, mango, 1 cup	0
Diet iced tea, 1 cup	0
Diet mojito tea, 1 cup	0
Diet peach white tea, 1 cup	0
Green tea, 1 cup	1
Green tea mango, 1 cup	2
Iced tea, 1 cup	2
Lemonade, 1 cup	2
Mojito green tea, 1 cup	1
Orange tea, 1 cup	2
Peach green tea, 1/2 cup	2
Peach tea, 1 cup	2
Pomegranate lemonade, 1/2 cup	2
Raspberry tea, 1 cup	2
Southern brew extra sweet tea, 1 cup	2
Tangerine white tea, 1 cup	1
Zero calorie chai spiced tea, 1 cup	0
Zero calorie pomegranate acai white tea, 1 cup	0

Beverages

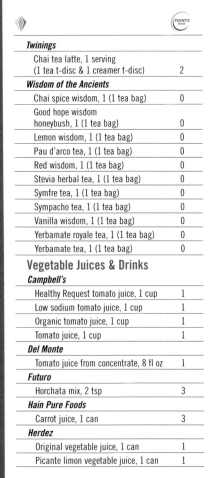

Twinings

	POINTS VALUE
Chai tea latte, 1 serving (1 tea t-disc & 1 creamer t-disc)	2

Wisdom of the Ancients

Chai spice wisdom, 1 (1 tea bag)	0
Good hope wisdom honeybush, 1 (1 tea bag)	0
Lemon wisdom, 1 (1 tea bag)	0
Pau d'arco tea, 1 (1 tea bag)	0
Red wisdom, 1 (1 tea bag)	0
Stevia herbal tea, 1 (1 tea bag)	0
Symfre tea, 1 (1 tea bag)	0
Sympacho tea, 1 (1 tea bag)	0
Vanilla wisdom, 1 (1 tea bag)	0
Yerbamate royale tea, 1 (1 tea bag)	0
Yerbamate tea, 1 (1 tea bag)	0

Vegetable Juices & Drinks

Campbell's

Healthy Request tomato juice, 1 cup	1
Low sodium tomato juice, 1 cup	1
Organic tomato juice, 1 cup	1
Tomato juice, 1 cup	1

Del Monte

Tomato juice from concentrate, 8 fl oz	1

Futuro

Horchata mix, 2 tsp	3

Hain Pure Foods

Carrot juice, 1 can	3

Herdez

Original vegetable juice, 1 can	1
Picante limon vegetable juice, 1 can	1

Odwalla

	POINTS VALUE
Carrot juice, 8 fl oz	1

V8

Calcium enriched V8 juice, 1 cup	1
Essential antioxidants, 1 cup	1
High fiber, 8 oz	0
Low sodium V8, 1 cup	1
Organic V8, 1 cup	1
Spicy hot V8, 1 cup	1
V8 100% vegetable juice, 1 cup	1

V8 V. Fusion

Light peach mango, 8 oz	1
Light strawberry banana, 8 oz	1
Peach mango juice, 8 oz	2
Pomegranate blueberry, 8 oz	2
Strawberry banana juice, 8 oz	2
Tropical orange juice, 8 oz	2

Water

Aquafina

Aquafina, 8 fl oz	0
Aquafina sparkling - citrus twist, 8 fl oz	0

Aquafina FlavorSplash

Lemon, 8 fl oz	0
Peach mango, 8 fl oz	0
Raspberry, 8 fl oz	0
Strawberry kiwi, 8 fl oz	0
Wild berry, 8 fl oz	0

Aquafina Sparkling

Berry burst, 8 fl oz	0

	POINTS VALUE
Dasani	
Dasani, 8 fl oz	0
Dasani with lemon, 8 fl oz	0
Dasani with raspberry, 8 fl oz	0
Dasani with strawberry, 8 fl oz	0
Ethos	
Ethos water, 8 fl oz	0
FIJI Water	
Bottled water, 16 fl oz	0
Fruit 2 0	
Energy raspberry, 8 fl oz	0
Hydration strawberry tangerine, 8 fl oz	0
Immunity berry pomegranate, 8 fl oz	0
Natural cherry, 8 fl oz	0
Natural grape, 8 fl oz	0
Natural lemon, 8 fl oz	0
Natural lime, 8 fl oz	0
Natural orange, 8 fl oz	0
Natural peach, 8 fl oz	0
Natural raspberry, 8 fl oz	0
Natural strawberry, 8 fl oz	0
Relax tropical fruit, 8 fl oz	0
Tropical fruit, 8 fl oz	0
Fruit 2 0 Plus 10	
Natural apple, 8 fl oz	0
Natural berry, 8 fl oz	0
Watermelon kiwi, 8 fl oz	0
Kellogg's	
Special K20 protein strawberry kiwi, 1 bottle	0
Special K20 protein water lemon twist, 1 bottle	0

	POINTS VALUE
Special K20 protein water mix, strawberry kiwi, 1 packet	0
Special K20 protein water tropical blend, 1 bottle	0
Special K20 protein water, mixed berry, 1 bottle	0
Minute Maid	
Just 10 - fruit punch, 1 pouch	0
Minute Maid Fruit Falls	
Berry water beverage, 1 pouch	0
Tropical water beverage, 1 pouch	0
Naturally Fresh	
Mountain spring water, 2 Tbsp	0
Propel	
All flavors, 8 fl oz	0
Berry, 8 fl oz	0
Blueberry pomegranate, 8 fl oz	0
Body - peach mango, 8 fl oz	0
Fit water - berry, 8 fl oz	0
Fit water - grape, 8 fl oz	0
Grape, 8 fl oz	0
Kiwi strawberry, 8 fl oz	0
Lemon, 8 fl oz	0
Mind - black cherry, 8 fl oz	0
SoBe	
Lifewater - black and blueberry-o cal, 8 fl oz	0
Lifewater - blackberry grape, 8 fl oz	1
Lifewater - fuji apple pear-o cal, 8 fl oz	0
Lifewater - goji melon, 8 fl oz	1
Lifewater - orange tangerine, 8 fl oz	1
Lifewater - passionfruit citrus, 8 fl oz	1

Beverages

	POINTS VALUE
Lifewater - pomegranate cherry, 8 fl oz	1
Lifewater - strawberry kiwi, 8 fl oz	1
Lifewater - yumberry pomegranate-o cal, 8 fl oz	0
Lifewater yuzu black currant, 8 fl oz	1
Lifewater - agave lemonade, 8 fl oz	1

Wine & Wine Coolers

Eden

Mirin (rice cooking wine), 1 Tbsp	1

Fanci Food

Cooking wine, burgundy, 2 Tbsp	0
Cooking wine, sherry, 2 Tbsp	1

Little Boomey

Cabernet merlot, 1/2 cup	2
Cabernet sauvignon, 1/2 cup	2
Chardonnay, 1/2 cup	2
Merlot, 1/2 cup	2
Shiraz, 1/2 cup	2
Shiraz cabernet, 1/2 cup	2

Ola

Cooking wine, 1 tsp	0

Regina

Cooking wine, red, 2 Tbsp	0
Cooking wine, sherry, 2 Tbsp	1
Cooking wine, white, 2 Tbsp	0

Sutter Home

	POINTS VALUE
Cabernet sauvignon, 1/2 cup	2
Chardonnay, 1/2 cup	2
Johannisberg riesling, 1/2 cup	2
Merlot, 1/2 cup	2
Pinot grigio, 1/2 cup	2
Pinot noir, 1/2 cup	2
Shiraz, 1/2 cup	2
White merlot, 1/2 cup	2
White zinfandel, 1/2 cup	2
Zinfandel, 1/2 cup	2

Sutter Home Fre

Dealcoholized chardonnay, 1/2 cup	1
Dealcoholized merlot, 1/2 cup	1
Dealcoholized sparkling brut, 1/2 cup	1
Dealcoholized white zinfandel, 1/2 cup	1

Trinity Oaks

Cabernet sauvignon, 1/2 cup	2
Chardonnay, 1/2 cup	2
Merlot, 1/2 cup	2
Pinot grigio, 1/2 cup	2
White merlot, 1/2 cup	2
Zinfandel, 1/2 cup	2

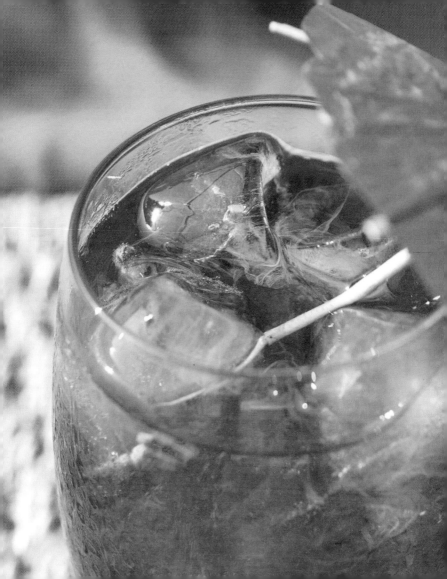

Bread & Baked Goods

Bagels

Alvarado

Sprouted spelt bagel, 1	4
Sprouted wheat bagel, 1	4
Sprouted wheat cinnamon raisin bagel, 1	5
Sprouted wheat onion poppyseed bagel, 1	6
Sprouted wheat sesame seed bagels, 1	6

French Meadow Bakery

Organic spelt bagel, 1	5
Organic sprouted bagels with Ezekiel 4:9 grains, 1	5

Healthy Life Original

100% whole wheat light bagels, 1	2

Market Day

Cinnamon brown sugar bagel-ers, 1	4
Original plain bagel-ers, 1	4

Nature's Own

Cinnamon raisin bagel, 1	6
Honey wheat bagel, 1	4
Original bagel, 1	5

Otis Spunkmeyer

Blueberry, 1 (85 g)	4
Blueberry, 1 (113 g)	5
Cinnamon raisin, 1 (85 g)	4
Cinnamon raisin, 1 (113 g)	5
Onion, 1 (85 g)	4
Onion, 1 (113 g)	5
Plain, 1 (85 g)	4

Pepperidge Farm

100% whole wheat bagels, 1	4
100% whole wheat mini bagels, 1	1
Brown sugar cinnamon mini bagels, 1	2
Cinnamon raisin bagels, 1	5
Everything bagels, 1	5
Mini chocolatey chip bagels, 1	2
Onion bagels, 1	5
Plain bagels, 1	5
Plain mini bagels, 1	2
Sesame bagels, 1	5
Whole grain white bagels, 1	4
Whole grain white mini bagels, 1	2

Thomas'

100 calorie bagel, 1	1
Cinnamon raisin bagel, 1	4
Everything bagel, 1	5
Hearty grains whole wheat bagel, 1	4
Hearty grains double oat golden honey bagel, 1	5
Plain bagel, 1	5
Whole wheat mini, 1	2

Weight Watchers

Original bagel, 1	2
Petite bagels, 1	1

Western Bagel Original Recipe

100% whole wheat, 1	3
Blueberry bagel, 1	4
Cinnamon raisin bagel, 1	4
Egg bagel, 1	4
Everything bagel, 1	5

	POINTS VALUE		POINTS VALUE
Honey wheat bagel, 1	4	Sweet wheat (refrigerated), 1	1
Jalapeño bagel, 1	4	Very blueberry, 1	1
Onion bagel, 1	4	***Western Bagel The Alternative English Muffin***	
Plain/water bagel, 1	4	Plain (refrigerated), 1	1
Pumpernickel, 1	4	Wheat, 1	1
Rye bagel, 1	4	***Western Bagel The Perfect 10 Bagel***	
Sesame bagel, 1	5	The Perfect 10 Bagel, 1	2

Western Bagel Preservative Free Alternative Bagel

	POINTS VALUE		POINTS VALUE
Blueberry, 1	4		

Biscuits

Bisquick Complete Biscuit Mixes

	POINTS VALUE
Cinnamon spice, 1	1
Everything, 1	5
Sweet wheat, 1	1
Whole wheat, 1	4

	POINTS VALUE
Buttermilk, 1/3 cup	3
Cheese garlic, 1/3 cup	4
Honey butter, 1/3 cup	3
Three cheese, 1/3 cup	4

Western Bagel Preservative Free Bagel

Market Day

	POINTS VALUE
Cinnamon raisin, 1	4
Onion, 1	4
Plain, 1	4
Sesame bagel, 1	4

	POINTS VALUE
Homestyle biscuit dough, 1 piece (2.5 oz)	5

Martha White

Western Bagel Preservative Free Bagelettes

	POINTS VALUE
Buttermilk biscuit mix, prepared, 1 serving (1/4 package)	4

Pillsbury

	POINTS VALUE
Plain, 1	2
Whole wheat, 1	2

	POINTS VALUE
Buttermilk, 3	3
Cheddar flaky layers, 1	5
Country biscuits, 3	3
Flaky layer buttermilk, 3	3
Reduced fat biscuits - flaky layers, 1	4

Western Bagel The Alternative Bagel

Pillsbury Golden Layers

	POINTS VALUE
Cinnamon spice, 1	1
Cinnamon spice (refrigerated), 1	1
Country white, 1	1
Country white, 1	1
Country white (refrigerated), 1	1
Roasted onion, 1	1
Roasted onion (refrigerated), 1	1

	POINTS VALUE
Butter tastin flaky, 1	2
Buttermilk flaky, 1	3
Honey butter, 1	3
Original flaky, 1	3

Bread & Baked Goods

Pillsbury Grands!	
Homestyle shortcake biscuits, 1	4
Pillsbury Grands! Flaky	
Butter tastin', 1	4
Buttermilk, 1	4
Original, 1	4
Pillsbury Grands! Homestyle	
Butter tastin', 1	4
Buttermilk, 1	4
Buttermilk, reduced fat, 1	4
Extra rich, 1	5
Original, 1	4
Southern style, 1	4
Wheat, reduced fat, 1	4
Pillsbury Homestyle	
Butter tastin' fluffy, 1	2
Buttermilk fluffy, 1	2
Pillsbury Oven Baked	
Butter tastin', 1	4
Buttermilk, 1	4
Cheddar garlic, 1	4
Extra-large easy split, 1	6
Flaky layers, 1	4
Southern style, 1	4
Pillsbury Perfect Portions	
Butter tastin', 1	4
Buttermilk, 1	4
Buttermilk reduced fat, 1	4
Flaky layers, 1	4

Bread
Alexia
Garlic baguette, 2 pieces	3

Alvarado
California style complete protein bread, 1 slice	1
Diabetic lifestyle bread, 1 slice	1
Essential flax seed bread, 2 slices	2
No-salt sprouted multi-grain bread, 1 slice	1
Sprouted barley bread, 1 slice	1
Sprouted multi-grain bread, 1 slice	1
Sprouted rye seed bread, 1 slice	1
Sprouted sourdough bread, 1 slice	1
Sprouted sourdough French bread, 1 slice	1
Sprouted soy crunch bread, 1 slice	1
Sprouted wheat California style low fat/no cheese pizza bread, 1/8 pizza	4
Sprouted wheat California style original pizza bread, 1/8 pizza	4
Sprouted wheat cinnamon raisin bread, 1 slice	1
Sprouted whole wheat bread, 1 slice	1
Ultimate kids bread, 1 slice	1

Arnold
100% natural soft 100% whole wheat bread, 2 slices	3
100% natural soft honey wheat bread, 2 slices	3
100% natural soft whole grain white bread, 2 slices	3

	POINTS VALUE
Bakery light 7 grain bread, 2 slices	1
Bakery light oatmeal bread, 2 slices	1
Carb counting multi-grain bread, 1 slice	1
Dutch country 100% whole wheat bread, 1 slice	2
Dutch country double fiber bread, 1 slice	1
Real Jewish rye bread - seeded, 1 slice	2
Select 100% whole wheat sandwich thins, 1 slice	1
Select multigrain sandwich thins, 1 slice	1
Select whole grain white sandwich thins, 1 slice	1
Stone ground 100% whole wheat bread, 2 slices	2
Arnold & Brownberry	
Country wheat bread, 1 slice	2
Grains & more double fiber bread, 1 slice	1
Grains & more double omega bread, 1 slice	2
Grains & more double protein bread, 1 slice	2
Natural flax & fiber bread, 1 slice	1
Whole grains 100% whole wheat bread, 1 slice	2
Whole grains 12 grain bread, 1 slice	2
Whole grains grain lover's bread, 1 slice	2
Whole grains healthy multi-grain bread, 1 slice	2
Aunt Jemima	
Easy mix corn bread, 1/8 package	3

	POINTS VALUE
B&M	
Brown bread plain, 2 oz	2
Raisin brown bread, 2 oz	2
Baker's Inn	
100% whole wheat bread, 1 slice	2
9 grain bread, 1 slice	2
Harvest multigrain bread, 1 slice	2
Honey whole wheat bread, 1 slice	2
Seven grain bread, 1 slice	2
White bread made with whole grain, 1 slice	2
Be Happy & Healthy	
Almond cherry, 1/2 slice	5
Apple spice, 1/2 slice	4
Banana, 1/2 slice	4
Cappuccino-chocolate chip, 1/2 slice	5
Carrot, 1/2 slice	5
Chocolate, 1/2 slice	2
Old fashion pound cake, 1/2 slice	6
Orange cranberry, 1/2 slice	2
Pumpkin, 1/2 slice	3
Sweet potato, 1/2 slice	4
Zucchini, 1/2 slice	4
Beefsteak	
Hearty rye bread, 1 slice	1
Light soft rye bread, 2 slices	1
Soft rye bread, 1 slice	1
Betty Crocker	
Banana mix, prepared, 1 slice	4
Banana, no cholesterol/low-fat recipe, prepared, 1 slice	3

Bread & Baked Goods

Betty Crocker (cont'd)

	POINTS VALUE
Cinnamon streusel, no cholesterol/reduced fat recipe, prepared, 1 slice	4
Cranberry orange, no cholesterol/low-fat recipe, prepared, 1 slice	3

Butternut

Honey wheat bread, 2 slices	2
White bread, 1 slice	1

Cobblestone Mill

German pumpernickel bread, 1 slice (1.1 oz)	1
New York Jewish rye bread, 1 slice (1.1 oz)	1
San Francisco sour dough bread, 1 slice (1.1 oz)	1

Cobblestone Mill Hearty Recipe

Potato, 1 slice	2

D'Italiano

Plain, 1 slice	2
Seeded, 1 slice	2

Dromedary

Gingerbread cake & cookie mix, prepared, 2 oz	4
Hot roll mix, prepared, 1 roll	2

Flatout

Healthy grain multi-grain, 1 slice	1
Healthy grain whole grain white, 1 slice	2
Kidz original, 1 slice	1
Light Italian herb, 1 slice	1
Light original, 1 slice	1
Light sundried tomato light, 1 slice	1
Mini harvest wheat, 1 slice	1
Traditional garden spinach, 1 slice	2

	POINTS VALUE
Traditional Italian, 1 slice	2
Traditional original, 1 slice	2
Traditional southwest chipotle, 1 slice	2
Traditional sundried tomato, 1 slice	2

Food for Life

7-sprouted grains, 1 slice (34 g)	1
Cinnamon raisin 7-sprouted grains, 1 slice	1
Ezekiel 4:9 sprouted grain, 1/2 slice	1
Ezekiel 4:9 sprouted grains, 1 slice	1
Ezekiel 4:9 sprouted grain cinnamon raisin, 1/2 slice	1
Genesis 1:29 sprouted grain, 1/2 slice	1
Organic bran for life bread, 1 slice	1
Organic Ezekiel 4:9 cinnamon raisin sprouted grains, 1 slice	1
Organic Ezekiel 4:9 low sodium sprouted grain bread, 1 slice	1
Organic Ezekiel 4:9 sprouted with sesame, 1 slice	1
Organic genesis 1:29 sprouted grains bread, 1 slice	1
Organic low sodium 7-sprouted grains bread, 1 slice	1
Sprouted whole wheat, 1 slice	1

Freihofer's

100% whole wheat, 1 slice	2
12 grain bread, 1 slice	2
Country double fiber 100% whole wheat, 1 slice	1
Country potato, 1 slice	2
Double fiber 100% whole wheat, 1 slice	1

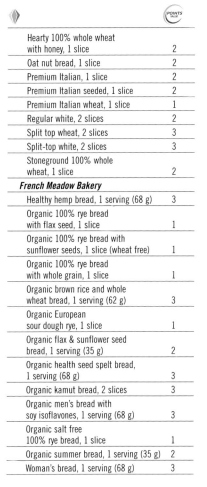

	POINTS VALUE
Hearty 100% whole wheat with honey, 1 slice	2
Oat nut bread, 1 slice	2
Premium Italian, 1 slice	2
Premium Italian seeded, 1 slice	2
Premium Italian wheat, 1 slice	1
Regular white, 2 slices	2
Split top wheat, 2 slices	3
Split-top white, 2 slices	3
Stoneground 100% whole wheat, 1 slice	2
French Meadow Bakery	
Healthy hemp bread, 1 serving (68 g)	3
Organic 100% rye bread with flax seed, 1 slice	1
Organic 100% rye bread with sunflower seeds, 1 slice (wheat free)	1
Organic 100% rye bread with whole grain, 1 slice	1
Organic brown rice and whole wheat bread, 1 serving (62 g)	3
Organic European sour dough rye, 1 slice	1
Organic flax & sunflower seed bread, 1 serving (35 g)	2
Organic health seed spelt bread, 1 serving (68 g)	3
Organic kamut bread, 2 slices	3
Organic men's bread with soy isoflavones, 1 serving (68 g)	3
Organic salt free 100% rye bread, 1 slice	1
Organic summer bread, 1 serving (35 g)	2
Woman's bread, 1 serving (68 g)	3

	POINTS VALUE
Gladiola	
Mexican cornbread mix, prepared, 1 piece (1/6 package)	3
Sweet yellow cornbread mix, prepared, 1 piece (1/6 package)	3
White cornbread mix, prepared, 1 piece (1/6 package)	3
Yellow cornbread mix, prepared, 1 piece (1/6 package)	3
Healthy Life Natural	
All whole grain 100% whole wheat bread, 1 slice	1
All whole grain farmer's 12 grain bread, 1 slice	1
All whole grain flaxseed bread, 1 slice	1
Healthy Life Original	
100% whole grain sugar free rye bread made with caraway seeds, 2 slices	1
100% whole grain sugar free rye bread no seeds, 2 slices	1
100% whole grain sugar free wheat bread, 2 slices	1
100% whole wheat whole grain bread, 2 slices	1
100% whole wheat whole grain flaxseed bread, 2 slices	1
Italian bread, 2 slices	1
Light English muffins, 1	1
Sourdough bread, 2 slices	1
White bread, 2 slices	1
Healthy Life Southern Country Style	
100% whole wheat 1/2 loaf, 2 slices	2
100% whole wheat bread, 1 slice	1

Bread & Baked Goods

Healthy Life Southern Country Style (cont'd)

	POINTS VALUE
Oatmeal 1/2 loaf, 2 slices	3
Whole grain white 1/2 loaf, 2 slices	2

Hodgson Mill

Barley bread mix with soy, 1/4 cup	2
Caraway rye bread mix with soy, 1/4 cup	2
Honey whole wheat bread mix with soy, 1/4 cup	2
Mexican cornbread mix, 1/4 cup (dry)	2
Nine grain bread mix with soy, 1/4 cup	2
Whole wheat gingerbread mix, 1/4 cup	2

Home Pride Butter Top

Wheat bread, 1 slice	1
White bread, 1 slice	1

Maier's

Premium Italian, 1 slice	2
Premium Italian - seeded, 1 slice	2
Premium Italian - wheat, 1 slice	1

Market Day

Cherry braided bread, 1 serving (1/10 loaf)	3
Cream cheese braided bread, 1 slice	3
Stuffed appetizer bread, 1 serving (1/4 loaf)	10

Martha White

Buttermilk cornbread mix, prepared, 1 piece (1/5 package)	3
Cotton pickin' buttermilk cornbread mix, 1 serving (34 g)	3
Golden honey cornbread mix, prepared, 1 piece (1/5 package)	4
Mexican cornbread mix, prepared, 1 piece (1/6 package)	3

	POINTS VALUE
Sweet yellow cornbread mix, prepared, 1 piece (1/6 package)	3
Yellow cornbread mix, prepared, 1 serving (1/5 package)	3

Merita

Autumn grain bread, 1 slice	1
Calcium fortified old fashioned white bread, 1 slice	1

Millbrook

Cracked wheat bread, 1 slice	2
Wheat bread, 2 slices	2

Nature's Own

100% whole grain sugar free bread, 1 slice	1
100% whole wheat bread, 1 slice	1
100% whole wheat specialty bread, 1 slice	2
12 grain specialty bread, 1 slice	1
9 grain specialty bread, 1 slice	2
Butterbread, 1 slice	1
Cinnamon raisin swirl bread, 2 slices	3
Cranberry raisin swirl bread, 2 slices	3
Double fiber wheat bread, 1 slice	0
Double fiber wheat specialty bread, 1 slice	1
Honey wheat, 1 slice	1
Honey wheat berry specialty bread, 1 slice	2
Honey wheat English muffins, 1	3
Honey wheat specialty bread with organic flour, 1 slice	1
Light honey wheat bread, 2 slices	1

	POINTS VALUE
Light wheat, 2 slices	1
Light white, 2 slice	1
Original English muffin, 1	3
Wheat n' fiber bread, 1 slice	1
Nature's Own Whitewheat	
Whitewheat bread, 2 slices	1
Nature's Path	
Carrot raisin manna bread, 1 slice	2
Cinnamon date manna bread, 1 slice	2
Fruit and nut manna bread, 1 slice	2
Millet rice manna bread, 1 slice	2
Multigrain manna bread, 1 slice	2
Sun seed manna bread, 1 slice	3
Whole rye manna bread, 1 slice	2
Whole wheat manna bread, 1 slice	2
Oroweat	
100% whole wheat, 1 slice	1
100% whole wheat English muffin, 1 muffin	2
100% whole wheat sandwich style bread, 1 slice	1
12 grain bread, 1 slice	2
Buttermilk, 1 slice	2
Country white bread, 1 slice	2
Double fiber bread, 1 slice	1
Double fiber English muffin, 1 muffin	1
Extra crispy English muffin, 1 muffin	3
Healthnut bread, 1 slice	2
Honey wheatberry, 1 slice	1
Jewish rye, 1 slice	1
Oatnut bread, 1 slice	2
Oroweat light 100% whole wheat, 2 slices	1

	POINTS VALUE
Potato bread, 1 slice	2
Raisin English muffin, 1 muffin	3
Russian rye, 1 slice	1
Seven grain bread, 1 slice	2
Whole grain and flax bread, 1 slice	2
Otis Spunkmeyer	
Apple spice mini loaf, 1	8
Banana walnut mini loaf, 1	11
Chocolate fudge pecan mini loaf, 1	10
Otis Spunkmeyer Café Collection	
Chocolate marble bread slices, 1 slice	11
Vanilla pound cake, 1 slice	11
Yogurt lemon poppy, 1 slice	10
Paraclete	
Bread, 1 slice	0
Wheat bread, 1 slice	0
Pepperidge Farm	
100% natural German dark wheat bread, 1 slice	2
100% natural honey flax bread, 1 slice	2
100% natural nine grain bread, 1 slice	2
100% natural sprouted wheat bread, 1 slice	2
100% whole grain stone ground 100% whole wheat bread, 1 slice	2
100% whole wheat English muffins, 1	2
100% whole wheat thin sliced bread, 1 slice	1
Breakfast bread apple & grains, 1 slice	1
Breakfast bread blueberry & grains, 1 slice	1
Breakfast bread raisin & grains, 1 slice	2

Bread & Baked Goods

Pepperidge Farm (cont'd)	POINTS VALUE
Brown sugar cinnamon swirl bread, 1 slice	2
Canadian white bread, 1 slice	2
Carb style 7 grain bread, 1 slice	1
Carb style white bread, 1 slice	1
Carb style whole wheat bread, 1 slice	1
Cinnamon swirl bread, 1 slice	2
Deli swirl bread, 1 slice	1
Family size white sandwich bread, 2 slices	3
Farmhouse 12 grain bread, 1 slice	2
Farmhouse country wheat bread, 1 slice	2
Farmhouse harvest 7 grain bread, 1 slice	2
Farmhouse hearty white bread, 1 slice	2
Five cheese garlic bread, 1 slice (2 1/4")	4
Garlic bread, 1 slice (2 1/2")	4
Garlic parmesan bread, 1 slice (2 1/2")	3
Hearth fired artisan rosemary olive oil petite loaves, 1 slice (2")	2
Hearth fired artisan sourdough petite loaves, 1 serving (2")	2
Hot & crusty Italian bread, 1 slice (2" slice)	3
Hot & crusty thin sliced French bread, 2 slices	3
Hot & crusty twin French bread, 1 slice (4")	3
Italian bread, 1 slice	2
Jewish rye party bread, 5 slices	2
Light style white bread, 3 slices	2
Light style oatmeal bread, 3 slices	2

	POINTS VALUE
Light style wheat bread, 3 slices	2
Mozzarella & garlic bread, 1 slice (2 1/4")	3
Natural whole grain 9 grain bread, 1 slice	2
Natural whole grain multigrain bread, 1 slice	1
Oatmeal bread, 1 slice	1
Original English muffins, 1	3
Original white bread, 1 slice	1
Original white thin sliced enriched bread, 3 slices	2
Premium cracked pepper parmesan toast, 1 slice	3
Premium roasted garlic bread, 1 slice (2 1/2")	4
Premium roasted garlic toast, 1 slice	3
Premium Romano and herb toast, 1 slice	3
Premium Romano and herb toast club pack, 1 slice	3
Pumpernickel bread, 1 slice	1
Pumpernickel party bread, 5 slices	2
Raisin cinnamon swirl bread, 1 slice	2
Seeded rye bread, 1 slice	1
Seedless rye bread, 1 slice	1
Small slice whole grain 100% whole wheat bread, 1 slice	1
Small slice whole grain 15 grain bread, 1 slice	1
Small slice whole grain oatmeal bread, 1 slice	1
Texas toast five cheese, 1 slice	3

	POINTS VALUE
Texas toast garlic, 1 slice	3
Texas toast mozzarella Monterey Jack, 1 slice	4
Texas toast parmesan, 1 slice	4
Toasting white bread, 1 slice	1
Very thin sliced soft 100% whole wheat bread, 3 slices	2
Very thin sliced whole grain white bread, 3 slices	2
White sandwich bread, 2 slices	3
Whole grain 100% whole wheat bread, 1 slice	2
Whole grain 15 grain bread, 1 slice	2
Whole grain cinnamon swirl bread, 1 slice	2
Whole grain cinnamon with raisins swirl bread, 1 slice	2
Whole grain double fiber bread, 1 slice	1
Whole grain golden harvest grains bread, 1 slice	2
Whole grain oatmeal bread, 1 slice	2
Whole grain rye with seeds, 1 slice	1
Whole grain soft honey oat bread, 1 slice	2
Whole grain soft honey whole wheat bread, 1 slice	2
Whole grain Texas toast, 1 slice	3
Whole grain white sandwich bread, 2 slices	2
Pepperidge Farm Farmhouse	
Nutty oat bread, 1 slice	2
Premium white rolls with sesame seeds, 1	4

	POINTS VALUE
Soft 100% whole wheat bread, 1 slice	2
Sourdough bread, 1 slice	2
Whole grain white bread, 1 slice	2
Pillsbury	
Cinnamon mini bites, 3 pieces	4
Crusty French loaf, 1 slice (1/5 loaf)	2
Pillsbury Ballard	
Gingerbread, baked, 1 slice (1/8 loaf)	5
Pillsbury Quick Bread & Muffin Mix	
Apple cinnamon mix, baked, 1 slice (1/14 loaf)	3
Banana mix, baked, 1 slice (1/14 loaf)	3
Carrot mix, baked, 1 slice (1/16 loaf)	3
Chocolate chip swirl mix, baked, 1 slice (1/14 loaf)	4
Cinnamon swirl mix, baked, 1 slice (1/14 loaf)	4
Cranberry mix, baked, 1 slice (1/14 loaf)	3
Date mix, baked, 1 slice (1/14 loaf)	3
Lemon poppy seed mix, baked, 1 slice (1/14 loaf)	3
Nut mix, baked, 1 slice (1/14 loaf)	3
Pecan swirl mix, baked, 1 slice (1/14 loaf)	4
Pumpkin mix, baked, 1 slice (1/12 loaf)	3
Roman Meal	
100% whole wheat, 1 slice	1
Round top, 1 slice	1
White bread made with whole grain, 2 slices	2
Whole grain, 1 slice	1

Bread & Baked Goods

	POINTS VALUE
Sara Lee Delightful	
100% multi-grain, 1 slice	0
100% multi-grain, 2 slices	1
100% whole wheat, 1 slice	0
100% whole wheat, 2 slices	1
Wheat, 1 slice	0
Wheat, 2 slices	1
White, 1 slice	1
White, 2 slices	1
Stroehmann	
100% whole wheat double fiber, 1 slice	1
Deli soft rye - no seeds, 1 slice	2
Deli soft rye - seeds, 1 slice	2
Dutch country 100% whole wheat, 1 slice	2
Dutch country 12 grain, 1 slice	2
Dutch country cracked wheat, 1 slice	1
Dutch country potato, 1 slice	2
Soft family 100% whole wheat, 2 slices	3
Soft family honey wheat, 2 slices	2
Soft family whole grain white, 2 slices	3
Split top wheat, 2 slices	3
Sun-Maid	
Raisin bread, cinnamon swirl, 1 slice	1
Raisin English muffins, 1	3
Thomas'	
100 calorie English muffin, 1	1
Cinnamon raisin English muffin, 1	2
Cinnamon swirl toasting bread, 1 slice	2
English muffin toasting bread, 1 slice	2

	POINTS VALUE
Hearty grains double fiber honey wheat English muffin, 1	2
Hearty grains whole wheat English muffin, 1	2
Hearty grains double oat golden honey English muffin, 1	2
Light multi-grain English muffin, 1	1
Original English muffin, 1	2
Sourdough English muffin, 1	2
The original nooks and crannies, 1 muffin	2
Weight Watchers	
100% whole wheat bread, 2 slices	1
English muffin, 1	1
Multi-grain bread, 2 slices	1
Seedless rye, 2 slices	1
Wheat English muffin, 1	1
Wheat sandwich roll, 1	2
Western Bagel English Muffins	
Cinnamon raisin, 1	3
Plain, 1	2
Sourdough, 1	2
Western Bagel The Alternative English Muffin	
Plain English muffin, 1	1
Wonder	
100% whole grain bread, 1 slice	1
Cinnamon swirl bread, 1 slice	2
Kid's white bread, 1 slice	1
Made with whole grain honey wheat bread, 2 slices	3

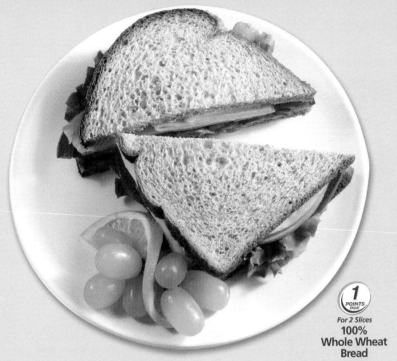

1 POINTS VALUE

For 2 Slices
**100%
Whole Wheat
Bread**

BRILLIANT

wholesomeness.

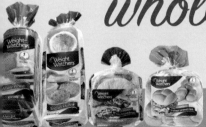

to WeightWatchers.com/bread to learn more about all of our delicious breads.

WeightWatchers
Stop Dieting. Start Living.

IGHT WATCHERS on foods and beverages is the registered trademark of WW Foods, LLC and is used under license by George Weston Bakeries, Inc. WEIGHT WATCHERS for services and *POINTS* are the registered trademarks of Weight Watchers International, Inc. and are used under license by George Weston Bakeries, Inc. ©2009 Weight Watchers International, Inc. All rights reserved. Selection may vary by store.

Bread & Baked Goods

Wonder (cont'd)	POINTS VALUE
White bread, 1 slice	1
White made with whole grain bread, 2 slices	2
Wonder Light	
Italian bread, 2 slices	1
Sourdough bread, 2 slices	1
Wheat bread, 2 slices	1
White bread, 2 slices	1

Breadsticks
Lance

Cheese, 2 packages	1
Garlic, 2 packages	1
Plain, 2 packages	1
Sesame, 2 packages	1

Market Day

Bosco breadsticks, 1 piece (3.1 oz)	5
French breadsticks, 1	2

Pepperidge Farm

Garlic breadsticks, 1	3

Pillsbury

Cornbread twists, 1	3
Garlic flavored, 2	4
Italian garlic with herb, 2	4
Italian parmesan with garlic, 2	4
Original, soft, 2	3

Stella D'oro

Breadsticks, cracked pepper, mini, 1 serving (17 g)	2
Breadsticks, original, 1 (10 g)	1
Breadsticks, original, mini, 1 serving (16 g)	1
Breadsticks, sesame, 1 (11 g)	1

	POINTS VALUE
Breadsticks, sesame, mini, 1 serving (18 g)	2
Breadsticks, sodium free, 1 (10 g)	1

Brownies
Arrowhead Mills

Brownie mix, 1 serving (41 g)	3
Gluten free brownie mix, 1 serving (1/20 package) (25 g)	2
Gluten free brownie mix, prepared, 1 serving (41 g)	4

Betty Crocker

Fudge brownie mix (pouch), prepared, 1	5
Hershey's mini kisses, prepared, 1	4
Ultimate chocolate brownie, prepared, 1	4
Ultimate fudge truffle mix, prepared, 2	4

Betty Crocker Complete Desserts

Triple chocolate hot fudge cake mix, prepared, 1 serving (1/6 package)	9

Betty Crocker Supreme Brownie Mixes

Chocolate chunk supreme, prepared, 1 piece (1/20 pan)	4
Dark chocolate (with Hershey's syrup pouch), prepared, 1 piece (1/20 pan)	4
Dark chocolate fudge, prepared, 1 piece (1/20 pan)	4
Frosted brownie supreme, prepared, 1 piece (1/20 pan)	4
Fudge traditional chewy, prepared, 1 piece (1/20 pan)	4
Hershey's triple chocolate chunk, prepared, 1 (40 g)	4

	POINTS VALUE
Hershey's ultimate fudge, prepared, 1 piece (1/20 pan)	4
Low fat fudge, mix, 1 serving (1/18 package)	3
Original fudge with syrup pouch, prepared, 1 piece (1/20 pan)	4
Peanut butter, prepared, 1 piece (1/20 pan)	4
Triple chunk, prepared, 1 piece (1/20 pan)	4
Turtle, prepared, 1 piece (1/20 pan)	4
Walnut chocolate chunk supreme, prepared, 1 piece (1/20 pan)	4
Walnut supreme, prepared, 1 piece (1/20 pan)	4
Betty Crocker Warm Delights Dessert Bowl Mixes	
Hot fudge brownie mix, 1 package	8
Peanut butter flavored brownie mix, 1 package	9
Cherrybrook Kitchen	
Fudge brownie mix, 1 serving (mix for 1 brownie)	3
Gluten free fudge brownie mix, 1 serving (mix for 1 brownie)	3
Dr. Oetker	
Frosted brownie mix, 1 serving (1/9 package)	4
Eagle Brand Premium Dessert Kits	
Decadent fudge, 1 piece (1 x 1")	5
Entenmann's	
Little bites - brownies, 1 pouch	5

	POINTS VALUE
Erin Baker's Organic Brownie Bites	
Chocolate chip mint, 1	2
Double chocolate, 1	2
Guiltless Gourmet	
Hot chocolate brownie with fudge sauce, 1 serving (1/3 cup mix and 1 Tbsp sauce)	4
Hershey's	
Brownie, 1/2 package	4
Hostess	
Plain brownie bites, 1 pouch	7
Jiffy Mixes	
Fudge brownie mix, dry, 1 serving (1/8 package)	3
Joseph's Sugar Free Cookies	
Pecan walnut brownies, 4	2
Lance	
Fudge brownie with nuts, 1	7
Little Debbie	
Be my valentine iced brownies, 1	5
Christmas tree brownie, 1	5
Cosmic brownie, 1	6
Fall brownies, 1	6
Football brownies, 1	4
Fudge brownies, 1	7
Stars & stripes frosted brownies, 1	6
Triple fudge brownies, 1	2
Martha White	
Chewy fudge, prepared, 1 piece (1/20 of a 8 x 8" pan)	3
Chewy fudge, prepared, 1 piece (1/20 of a 9 x 13" pan)	4

Bread & Baked Goods

Martha White (cont'd)	POINTS VALUE
Moist 'n fudgy, prepared, 1 piece (1/20 of a 9 x 13" pan)	4
Walnut, prepared, 1 piece (1/20 of a 9 x 13" pan)	4
Mrs. Freshleys Snackaway	
Brownie bites, 1 package	1
No Pudge!	
Fat free fudge brownie mix - cappuccino, prepared, 1 square (1/2 package)	2
Fat free fudge brownie mix - mint, prepared, 1 square (1/2 package)	2
Fat free fudge brownie mix - original, prepared, 1 square (1/2 package)	2
Fat free fudge brownie mix - raspberry, prepared, 1 square (1/2 package)	2
Otis Spunkmeyer	
Double chocolate brownie, 1 serving (2 oz)	6
Double chocolate brownie, 1 serving (3.3 oz)	9
Double chocolate with walnuts brownie, 1 serving (3.3 oz)	10
Snickers brownie, 1 serving (3.3 oz)	9
Turtle brownie, 1 serving (3.3 oz)	10
Otis Spunkmeyer Café Collection	
Café au lait brownie, 2 oz	6
Turtle brownie, 2 oz	6
Pillsbury	
Fudge mix (15 oz), baked, 1 piece (1/16 package)	3
Thick 'n fudgy caramel swirl mix, baked, 1 piece (1/12 package)	4
Thick 'n fudgy cheesecake swirl, baked, 1 piece (1/18 package)	3

	POINTS VALUE
Thick 'n fudgy chocolate chunk, baked, 1 piece (1/16 package)	3
Thick 'n fudgy deluxe brownie mix, chocolate frosted, baked, 1 piece (1/16 recipe)	4
Thick 'n fudgy double chocolate mix, baked, 1 piece (1/16 package)	3
Thick 'n fudgy hot fudge swirl mix, baked, 1 piece (1/12 package)	4
Thick 'n fudgy walnut mix, baked, 1 piece (1/12 package)	4
Pillsbury Brownie Batter	
Traditional chocolate fudge brownies, 1 serving (1/12 package)	3
Triple chocolate chunk brownie, 1 serving (1/12 package)	4
Reese's	
Brownie, 1/2 package	4
Vitamuffin Vita Brownie	
Dark chocolate pomegranate brownie, 1	1
Deep & velvety chocolate brownie, 1	1
Weight Watchers	
Chocolate brownie, 1	2

Cakes

Betty Crocker	
Cupcake mix, devil's food, prepared, 2	6
Cupcake mix, yellow, prepared, 2	6
Betty Crocker Classic Dessert Mixes	
Pineapple upside down cake, no-cholesterol recipe, prepared, 1 slice (1/6 cake)	9

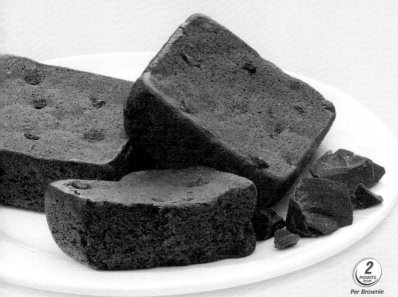

2 POINTS VALUE

Per Brownie

Chocolate Brownie

SMART

chocolateness.

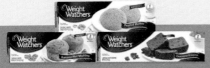

Find more information at WeightWatchers.com/brownies

WeightWatchers

Stop Dieting. Start Living.

WEIGHT WATCHERS on foods and beverages is the registered trademark of WW Foods, LLC and is used under license by Dawn Food Products, Inc. WEIGHT WATCHERS for services and *POINTS* are the registered trademarks of Weight Watchers International, Inc. and are used under license by Dawn Food Products, Inc. ©2009 Weight Watchers International, Inc. All rights reserved.

Bread & Baked Goods

POINTS VALUE

Betty Crocker Warm Delights Dessert Bowl Mixes

Cinnamon swirl cake mix, 1 package	8
Lemon swirl cake mix, 1 package	8
Minis chocolate raspberry decadence cake mix, 1	3
Minis molten caramel cake mix, 1	3
Minis molten chocolate cake mix, 1	3
Molten caramel cake mix, 1 package	7
Molten chocolate cake mix, 1 package	8

Bluebird

100 calorie iced chocolate cupcake, 1 package	1
100 calorie iced golden cupcake, 1 package	1

Cherrybrook Kitchen

Chocolate cake mix, 1 serving (1/12 of cake mix)	3
Wheat free/gluten free chocolate cake mix, 1 serving (1/8 of cake mix)	3
Yellow cake mix, 1 serving (1/12 of cake mix)	3

CHI-CHI'S

Sweet corn cake mix, 1/2 cup	2

Drake's

Coffee cakes, 2	6
Devil dogs, 1	4
Funny bones, 2	7
Ring dings, 2	8
Sunny doodles, 2	5
Yankee doodles, 2	5
Yodels, 2	7

POINTS VALUE

Entenmann's

All butter cake (single serve), 1	7
All butter French crumb cake, 1 serving (1/6 of cake)	6
All butter loaf cake, 1 serving (1/6 of loaf)	5
Banana crunch cake, 1/8	5
Black & white cake, 1/8	7
Butterscotch cake (single serve), 2	6
Carrot cake (single serve), 1/2	7
Chocolate crème cupcake, 2	7
Chocolate crumb loaf cake, 1/8	5
Chocolate fudge cake, 1/8	6
Chocolatey Swiss rolls, 2	6
Crumb cake (club size package), 1	8
Crumb cake (single serve), 1	8
Crumb coffee cake, 1 serving (1/9 cake)	6
Deluxe French cheese cake, 1 serving (1/6 of cake)	9
Enten-min's carrot cake, 1	3
Filled chocolate chip crumb cake, 1 serving (1/7 of cake)	9
Fruit cake, 1 serving (1/6 of cake)	10
Holiday cupcakes - Easter, 1	7
Holiday cupcakes - St. Patrick's Day, 1	7
Holiday cupcakes - Valentine, 1	7
Holiday devil's food cake square - Christmas, 1/8	7
Holiday devil's food cake square - Easter, 1/8	7
Holiday devil's food cake square - Halloween, 1/8	7

	POINTS VALUE
Holiday devil's food cake square - St. Patrick's Day, 1/8	7
Holiday devil's food cake square - Valentine, 1/8	7
Holiday golden chocolate cake - Christmas, 1/8	6
Holiday golden chocolate cake - Halloween, 1/8	6
Holiday golden chocolate cake - St. Patrick's Day, 1/8	6
Holiday golden chocolate cake - Valentine, 1/8	6
Holiday log cake, 1 serving (1/10 of cake)	6
Lemon coconut cake, 1/8	8
Lemon crunch cake, 1/8	9
Lemon pound cake, 1 serving (1/6 of loaf)	5
Louisiana crunch cake, 1/8	7
Marble cake (single serve), 1	6
Marble loaf cake, 1 serving (1/6 of loaf)	5
Marshmallow iced devil's food cake, 1/8	7
Mini cupcakes - Halloween, 3	7
Pound cake (club size package), 1	7
Raisin loaf cake, 1/8	4
Sour cream loaf cake, 1 serving (1/6 of loaf)	6
Sponge crème cake (single serve), 1 serving	6
Sponge crème cakes (club size package), 2	6
Swiss chocolate chip cake, 1 serving (1/7 of cake)	8
Thick fudge iced golden cake, 1/8	7

	POINTS VALUE
Ultimate chocolate truffle, 1 serving (90 g)	9
Ultimate crumb cake, 1/8	7
Ultimate Madeleine's petite butter cakes, 2	6
Entenmann's Little Bites 100 Calorie	
Carrot cake, 1	2
Golden crème cake, 1	2
Guiltless Gourmet	
Bananas foster cake with caramel sauce, 1 serving (1/3 cup mix and 1 Tbsp sauce)	4
Black velvet cake with caramel sauce, 1 serving (1/3 cup mix and 1 Tbsp sauce)	4
Hostess	
Chocolate cup cakes, 1	4
Cinnamon streusel cakes, 1	4
Devil's food zingers cake, 1	3
Ding dongs, 1	4
Ho hos, 1	3
Raspberry zingers, 1	4
Sno balls, 1	4
Suzy Q's, 1	5
Twinkies, 1	3
Vanilla zingers, 1	4
Hostess 100 Calorie	
Carrot mini cakes, 3	1
Chocolate mini cakes, 3	1
Golden mini cakes, 3	2
Lance	
Fig cake, 1 package	2

Bread & Baked Goods

	POINTS VALUE
Little Debbie	
Christmas tree cakes (chocolate), 2	4
Christmas tree cakes (vanilla), 2	5
Coffee cake (apple streusel), 1	5
Coffee cake, apple streusel, single serve, 1	5
Dessert cakes, chocolate, 1	4
Dessert cakes, spice, 1	4
Dessert cakes, yellow, 1	4
Golden crèmes, 1	3
Swiss rolls, 2	6
Little Debbie 100 Calories	
Chocolate cakes, 1	2
Yellow cakes, 1	2
Market Day	
Chocolate fudge volcano cakes, 1	11
Chocolate-chocolate chip puddin' cakes, 1 slice	6
Funnel cakes, 1	6
Mrs. Freshleys	
Swiss roll snack, 2	4
Mrs. Freshleys 100 Calorie	
Iced chocolate cupcake, 1 packet	1
Iced golden cupcake, 1 packet	1
Mrs. Freshleys Snackaway	
Chocolate cupcakes, 1	2
Lemon cupcake, 1 packet	1
Yogurt filled crème finger cakes, 1	2
Mrs. Smith's	
Carrot cake, 1 serving (1/6 cake)	6

	POINTS VALUE
Nabisco 100 Calorie Packs	
Nilla mini cakesters, 1 pouch	2
Oreo mini cakesters, 1 pouch	2
Oreo snack cakes, 1 pouch	2
Otis Spunkmeyer	
Apple crumb cake, 1 cake	9
Banana cake, 1 square	8
Blueberry crumb cake, 1 cake	9
Carrot cake, 1 square	8
Cheese crumb cake, 1 cake	10
Chocolate cake, 1 square	8
Pound cake, 1 cake	9
Otis Spunkmeyer Café Collection	
Apple cinnamon coffee cake, 1 serving (3.25 oz)	9
Cheese coffee cake, 1 serving (3.25 oz)	8
Chocolate truffle cake, 1 serving (2.65 oz)	8
Pepperidge Farm	
Chocolate coconut 3 layer cake, 1/8 cake	5
Chocolate fudge 3 layer cake, 1/8 cake	5
Chocolate fudge stripe 3 layer cake, 1/8 cake	5
Coconut 3 layer cake, 1/8 cake	5
Devil's food 3 layer cake, 1/8 cake	5
German chocolate 3 layer cake, 1/8 cake	5
Golden 3 layer cake, 1/8 cake	5
Lemon 3 layer cake, 1/8 cake	6
Peppermint 3 layer cake, 1/8 cake	5
Vanilla bean 3 layer cake, 1/8 cake	5

	POINTS VALUE

Pillsbury

Chocolate chip swirl bread coffee cake mix, prepared, 1 slice (1/14 recipe)	4
Cinnamon streusel coffee cake mix, prepared, 1 slice (1/16 recipe)	5

Pillsbury Moist Supreme

Angel food mix, baked, 1 slice (1/12 cake)	3
Banana mix, baked, 1 slice (1/12 cake)	5
Butter chocolate mix, baked, 1 slice (1/12 cake)	5
Chocolate mix, baked, 1 slice (1/12 cake)	5
Dark chocolate mix, baked, 1 slice (1/12 cake)	5
Devil's food mix, baked, 1 slice (1/12 cake)	5
French vanilla mix, baked, 1 slice (1/12 cake)	5
Funfetti mix, baked, 1 slice (1/12 cake)	5
German chocolate mix, baked, 1 slice (1/12 cake)	5
Golden butter recipe yellow mix, baked, 1 slice (1/12 cake)	5
Halloween funfetti mix, baked, 1 slice (1/12 cake)	5
Holiday funfetti mix, baked, 1 slice (1/12 cake)	5
Lemon mix, baked, 1 slice (1/12 cake)	5
Spring funfetti mix, baked, 1 slice (1/12 cake)	5
Strawberry mix, baked, 1 slice (1/12 cake)	5

	POINTS VALUE
Valentine's funfetti mix, baked, 1 slice (1/12 cake)	5
White mix, baked, 1 slice (1/12 cake)	5
Yellow mix, baked, 1 slice (1/12 cake)	5

SuperMoist

Butter pecan mix, prepared, 1 slice (1/12 cake)	6
Butter recipe yellow mix, prepared, 1 slice (1/12 cake)	6
Carrot cake mix, prepared, 1 slice (1/10 cake)	8
Cherry chip mix, prepared, 1 slice (1/10 cake)	7
Chocolate fudge mix, prepared, 1 slice (1/12 cake)	6
Confetti angel food cake mix, prepared, 1 slice (1/12 cake)	3
Dark chocolate mix, prepared, 1 slice (1/12 cake)	7
Devils food mix, prepared, 1 slice (1/12 cake)	6
French vanilla mix, prepared, 1 slice (1/12 cake)	6
German chocolate mix, prepared, 1 slice (1/12 cake)	6
Golden vanilla mix, prepared, 1 slice (1/12 cake)	6
Lemon mix, prepared, 1 slice (1/12 cake)	6
Milk chocolate mix, prepared, 1 slice (1/12 cake)	5
Rainbow chip mix, prepared, 1 slice (1/10 cake)	7
Spice mix, prepared, 1 slice (1/12 cake)	6

Bread & Baked Goods

SuperMoist (cont'd)	POINTS VALUE
Strawberry mix, prepared, 1 slice (1/12 cake)	6
Triple chocolate fudge mix, prepared, 1 slice (1/12 cake)	6
Vanilla, prepared, 1 slice (1/12 cake)	6
White angel food mix, prepared, 1 slice (1/12 cake)	3
White cake, richer recipe, 1 serving (1/12 cake)	6
White mix, prepared, 1 slice (1/12 cake)	5
Yellow mix, prepared, 1 slice (1/12 cake)	6
Weight Watchers	
Carrot cake with cream cheese icing, 1 cake	1
Chocolate cake with chocolate icing, 1 cake	1
Golden sponge cake with creamy filling, 1 cake	1
Lemon cake with lemon icing, 1 cake	1
Weight Watchers Smart Ones	
Double fudge cake, 1	4
Strawberry shortcake, 1	4

Croutons
Chatham Village

	POINTS VALUE
Caesar, 2 Tbsp	1
Fat free garlic and onion crouton, 2 Tbsp	1
Garden herb, 2 Tbsp	1
Large cut Caesar crouton, 2 Tbsp	1
Large cut cheese & garlic, 2 Tbsp	1
Large cut garlic and butter flavored crouton, 2 Tbsp	1

	POINTS VALUE
Ranch, 2 Tbsp	1
Sea salt & pepper croutons, 2 Tbsp	1
Marzetti	
Garlic & butter flavored, 2 Tbsp	1
Large cut cheese & garlic croutons, 2 Tbsp	1
Pepperidge Farm	
Classic Caesar croutons, 6	1
Four cheese and garlic croutons, 6	1
Onion and garlic croutons, 6	1
Seasoned croutons, 6	1
Whole grain seasoned croutons, 6	1
Zesty Italian croutons, 6	1

Danish/Sweet Rolls/Pastries
Amy's

	POINTS VALUE
Apple toaster pops, 1 piece (1.93 oz)	3
Cheese pizza toaster pops, 1 piece (1.93 oz)	4
Strawberry toaster pops, 1 piece (1.93 oz)	3
Betty Crocker	
Cinnamon streusel mix, prepared, 1 slice (1/14 loaf)	4
Entenmann's	
Apple danish, 1 serving (1/6 of cake)	5
Apple puffs, 1	7
Assorted honey buns - glazed (club size package), 1	8
Assorted honey buns - iced (club size package), 1	9
Cheese danish (club size package), 1	9
Cheese danish (single serve), 1	9

	POINTS VALUE
Cheese danish twist, 1/8	5
Cheese filled crumb coffee cake, 1/8	5
Cheese topped buns, 1	7
Cherry cheese danish (single serve), 1	10
Cinnamon danish, 1 serving (1/6 of cake)	5
Cinnamon danish (club size package), 1	10
Cinnamon danish (single serve), 1	10
Cinnamon hazelnut ring, 1 serving (1/6 of ring)	6
Cinnamon raisin swirl buns, 1	7
Cinnamon swirl buns, 1 (85 g)	7
Cinnamon swirl buns, 1 (90 g)	8
Crumb cake (club size package), 1	8
Fruit stollen, 1/8	5
Glazed honey bun (single serve), 1/2	8
Glazed honey buns, 1	8
Guava cheese puffs, 1	7
Hot cross buns, 1	5
Iced honey bun (single serve), 1/2	8
Old fashion apple strudel, 1/4	8
Pecan danish ring, 1 serving (1/8 danish)	6
Raspberry danish (club size package), 1	11
Raspberry danish (single serve), 1	11
Raspberry danish twist, 1 serving (1/8 danish)	5
Strawberry cheese danish, 1	10
Super cinnamon buns, 1/2	7
Walnut danish ring, 1 serving (1/8 danish)	6

	POINTS VALUE
Flavor Kist	
Toast'em pop-ups, frosted blueberry, 1	4
Toast'em pop-ups, frosted brown sugar cinnamon, 1	4
Toast'em pop-ups, frosted cherry, 1	4
Toast'em pop-ups, frosted chocolate fudge, 1	4
Toast'em pop-ups, frosted strawberry, 1	4
Toast'em pop-ups, frosted wild berry, 1	4
General Mills	
Fiber one toaster pastry, blueberry, 1	3
Fiber one toaster pastry, brown sugar cinnamon, 1	3
Fiber one toaster pastry, chocolate fudge, 1	3
Fiber one toaster pastry, strawberry, 1	3
Kellogg's	
Apple strudel, 1	4
Barbie frosted wild berry, 1	4
Splitz - chocolate vanilla, 1	4
Splitz - strawberry blueberry, 1	4
Splitz, strawberry chocolate, 1	4
Strawberry cheese danish, 1	4
Strawberry milkshake, 1	4
Kellogg's Eggo	
Bakeshop filled pastry twists, apple, 1	4
Bakeshop filled pastry twists, strawberry, 1	4
Swirlz cinnamon filled pastry, 1	3
Swirlz cinnamon mini toaster rolls, 1 (set of 4)	2
Swirlz strawberry filled pastry, 1	3
Waffles nutri-grain filled strawberry, 1	2

Bread & Baked Goods

	POINTS VALUE
Kellogg's Pop-Tarts	
Blueberry, 1	5
Brown sugar cinnamon, 1	5
Brown sugar cinnamon whole grain, 1	4
Chocolate banana split, 1	4
Chocolate chip, 1	5
Chocolate chip cookie dough, 1	4
Cinnamon roll, 1	5
Frosted blueberry, 1	4
Frosted brown sugar cinnamon, 1	5
Frosted cherry, 1	4
Frosted chocolate fudge, 1	4
Frosted chocolate fudge whole grain, 1	3
Frosted cookies and crème, 1	4
Frosted raspberry, 1	4
Frosted s'mores, 1	4
Frosted strawberry, 1	4
Frosted strawberry whole grain, 1	3
Frosted wild berry, 1	4
Hot fudge sundae, 1	4
Low fat frosted brown sugar cinnamon, 1	4
Low fat strawberry, 1	4
Strawberry, 1	5
Vanilla milkshake, 1	4
Lance	
Cinnamon roll, 1	8
Honey buns (glazed), 1	9
Honey buns (iced), 1	9
Little Debbie	
Honey buns, 1	5
Pecan spinwheels sweet rolls, 1	2

	POINTS VALUE
Market Day	
Gourmet cinnamon rolls, 1 (3 oz) (3 oz)	7
Otis Spunkmeyer	
Apple danish, 1 pastry/pastries	7
Apple demi danish, 1 pastry/pastries	3
Bear claw, 4-pack, 1 pastry/pastries	6
Breakfast claw, 8-pack, 1 pastry/pastries	6
Buttercrumb danish, 4-pack, 1 pastry/pastries	6
Cheese danish, 1 pastry/pastries	7
Cheese demi danish, 1 pastry/pastries	3
Cherry danish, 1 pastry/pastries	7
Cinnamon danish, 4-pack, 1 pastry/pastries	6
Cinnamon roll, 1 roll	8
Cinnamon roll, 4-pack, 1 roll	3
Cinnamon roll, 8-pack, 1 roll	3
Cinnamon twist, 1 pastry/pastries (1.8 oz)	5
Fruit danish, 8-pack, 1 pastry/pastries	5
Giant cinnamon roll, 1/2	6
Raisin danish, 8-pack, 1 pastry/pastries	5
Raspberry danish, 1 pastry/pastries	5
Raspberry demi danish, 1 pastry/pastries	3
Otis Spunkmeyer Café Collection	
Cinnamon chip scone, 1	8
Cinnamon swirl, 1/2 roll	4
Maple pecan scone, 1	8
Wild blueberry scone, 1	7

	POINTS VALUE
Pepperidge Farm	
Apple dumplings, 1	5
Apple turnovers, 1	6
Blueberry turnovers, 1	6
Cherry turnovers, 1	6
Peach dumplings, 1	6
Peach turnovers, 1	7
Raspberry turnovers, 1	6
Pillsbury	
Apple turnover, 1	4
Caramel rolls, 1	4
Cherry turnover, 1	4
Cinnamon bites with icing packets, 4	4
Cinnamon rolls with cream cheese icing, 1	3
Cinnamon rolls with icing, 1	3
Cinnamon rolls with icing, reduced fat, 1	3
Orange sweet rolls with icing, 1	4
Reduced fat cheese, egg, & bacon, 1	4
Pillsbury Grands!	
Cinnamon rolls with butter cream icing, 1	7
Cinnamon rolls with cream cheese icing, 1	7
Cinnamon rolls with icing, 1	9
Cinnamon rolls with icing, reduced fat, 1	6
Flaky supreme cinnamon roll, 1	9
Sugar free cinnamon roll, 1	2
Pillsbury Oven Baked	
Cinnamon, 1	6

	POINTS VALUE
Pillsbury Toaster Scrambles	
Bacon & sausage combo, 1	5
Cheese, egg & bacon, 1	5
Cheese, egg & ham, 1	5
Cheese, egg & sausage, 1	5
Reduced fat southwestern style, 1	3
Pillsbury Toaster Strudels	
Apple, 1	4
Blueberry, 1	4
Brown sugar cinnamon, 1	5
Cherry, 1	4
Chocolate fudge, 1	5
Cream cheese & raspberry, 1	5
Cream cheese & strawberry, 1	5
Danish style cream cheese, 1	5
French toast, 1	4
Raspberry, 1	4
Strawberry, 1	4
Strawberry banana, 1	4
Wildberry, 1	4
Tio Pepe's	
Cinnamon churros, 1	2
Weight Watchers Smart Ones	
Chocolate eclair, 1	3

Doughnuts
Entenmann's

	POINTS VALUE
Assorted frosted donuts softee family pack - plain, 1	4
Assorted frosted donuts softee family pack - powdered, 1	5
Assorted frosted donuts softee family pack - rich frosted, 1	8

Bread & Baked Goods

Entenmann's (cont'd)	POINTS VALUE
Chocolate donuts, 1	6
Cider donuts, 1	6
Cinnamon donuts (variety), 1	5
Cinnamon swirl buns variety pack, 1	7
Crumb topped donuts, 1	5
Crumb topped donuts (variety pack), 1	6
Eclairs, 1	5
Frosted devil's food donuts, 1	7
Frosted mini donuts, 1	4
Frosted pop'ems, 4	8
Frosted pop'ettes, 3	9
Glazed chocolate pop'ems, 4	5
Glazed donuts, 1	5
Glazed donuts (variety pack), 1	6
Glazed popems, 4 pieces	5
Holiday pop'ems - Christmas, 4	5
Holiday pop'ems - Easter, 4	5
Holiday pop'ems - Halloween, 4	5
Holiday pop'ems - Valentine, 4	5
Mini crullers, 2	5
Plain donuts (variety pack), 1	6
Plain donuts (variety), 1	4
Powdered donuts (variety), 1	5
Powdered pop'ettes, 4	6
Rainbow pop'ems, 4	5
Red, white & blue pop'ems, 4	5
Rich frosted chocolate donuts, 1	7
Rich frosted donuts (variety pack), 1	8
Softee family pack - plain donuts, 1	5
Softee frosted donuts (club size package), 1	6

	POINTS VALUE
Softee powdered donuts, 4	6
Ultimate chocolate lover's variety pack - devil's food crumb, 1	6
Ultimate chocolate lover's variety pack - frosted devil's food, 1	7
Ultimate chocolate lover's variety pack - rich frosted devil's food, 1	7
Ultimate chocolate lover's variety pack - rich frosted devil's food with drizzle, 1	7
Little Debbie	
Frosted mini donuts, 4	7
Glazed mini donuts, 1	5
Powdered mini donuts, 4	5

Flatbread/Pita/Wraps

Azumaya	
Large square wrappers, 3	3
Round wraps, 10	3
Small square wraps, 8	3
Boca	
Breakfast wraps - original, 1	4
Breakfast wraps - Southwestern flavor, 1	4
Flatout	
Mini 100% stone ground whole wheat, 1	1
Mini French toast, 1	1
Mini mediterranean herb, 1	1
Mini southwest chipotle, 1	1
Food for Life	
Organic Ezekiel 4:9 pocket bread, 1	1

	POINTS VALUE
Kangaroo	
Salad pockets, 1	2
Wheat 'n honey pita pocket bread, 1/2	1
Wheat salad pockets, 1	1
White pita pocket bread, 1/2	2
Whole grain sandwich pockets, 1	1
LaTortilla Factory Smart & Delicious	
Multigrain softwraps, 1	1
Rosemary softwraps, 1	1
Tomato basil softwraps, 1	1
Whole grain softwraps, 1	3
LaTortilla Factory Sonoma	
Organic traditional wraps, 1	4
Organic wheat wraps, 1	4
Nasoya	
Round wraps, 10	3
Wrappers, egg roll, 3	3
Wrappers, won ton, 8	3
Thomas'	
Sahara (mini) white pita bread, 1 loaf	1
Sahara 100% whole wheat (mini) pita bread, 1 loaf	1
Sahara 100% whole wheat pita bread, 1 loaf	2
Sahara white pita bread, 1 loaf	3
Tumaro's	
Chipotle chile wraps, 1	3
Garden spinach & vegetable wraps, 1	3
Honey wheat wraps, 1	3
Jalapeno & cilantro wraps, 1	3
Sun dried tomato & basil wraps, 1	3

	POINTS VALUE
Weight Watchers	
Pita pocket bread, 1	1
Western Bagel Pita Bread	
Plain pita, 1	3
Wheat pita, 1	2
Western Bagel The Alternative Pita Bread	
Plain, 1	1
Whole wheat, 1	1
## Muffins	
Betty Crocker	
Apple streusel mix (box), prepared, 1	5
Authentic corn bread mix (pouch), prepared, 1	4
Banana nut mix (box), no-cholesterol/low fat recipe, prepared, 1	3
Banana nut mix (box), prepared, 1	5
Banana nut mix (pouch), 1 serving (1/6 pouch)	2
Blueberry mix (pouch), 1 serving (1/6 pouch)	3
Chocolate chip mix (box), no cholesterol/reduced fat recipe, prepared, 1	4
Chocolate chip mix (box), prepared, 1	5
Chocolate chip mix (pouch), 1 serving (1/5 pouch)	3
Cinnabon bakery mix cinnamon streusel, prepared, 1	5
Cinnabon cinnamon streusel jumbo muffin mix (box), prepared, 1	14
Cinnamon streusel mix (box), prepared, 1	5
Cinnamon streusel mix (box), prepared, no-cholesterol/reduced fat recipe, 1	3

Bread & Baked Goods

Betty Crocker (cont'd)

Cranberry orange mix, prepared, 1 slice (1/12 loaf)	4
Double chocolate mix (box), no-cholesterol recipe, prepared, 1	4
Double chocolate mix (box), prepared, 1	5
Lemon poppyseed mix (pouch), 1 serving (1/6 pouch)	3
Sunkist lemon poppyseed mix (box), no-cholesterol/low fat recipe, prepared, 1	3
Sunkist lemon poppyseed mix (box), prepared, 1	5
Triple berry, 1 serving (1/6 pouch)	3
Twice the blueberries mix (box), no-cholesterol/low fat recipe, prepared, 1	3
Twice the blueberries mix (box), prepared, 1	3
Wild blueberry mix (box), no-cholesterol/low fat recipe, prepared, 1	3
Wild blueberry mix (box), prepared, 1	4

Betty Crocker Fiber One

Apple cinnamon muffin mix, no cholesterol recipe, prepared, 1	3
Apple cinnamon muffin mix, prepared, 1	4

Bluebird

100 calorie blueberry muffin, 1 package	1

Cherrybrook Kitchen

Chocolate chip muffin mix, 1	3

Entenmann's

Corn muffins, 1	5
Little bites - blueberry muffins, 1 pouch	4
Little bites - chocolate chip muffins, 1 pouch	4

Little bites banana chocolate chip muffins (club size package), 1 package	4
Little bites variety pack - blueberry muffins (club size package), 1 package	4
Little bites variety pack - chocolate chip muffins (club size package), 1 package	4

Entenmann's Little Bites 100 Calorie

Blueberry muffins, 1 package	2

Gladiola

Corn muffin mix, prepared, 1 (1/5 package)	4

Glory

Golden corn muffin mix, 1/2 cup	3
Homestyle cornbread mix, 1/4 cups	3

Hodgson Mill

Apple cinnamon muffin mix, 1/4 cup	2
Bran muffin mix, 1/4 cup	2
Whole wheat blueberry muffin mix, 1/4 cup	2
Whole wheat cornbread muffin mix, 1/4 cup	2
Whole wheat muffin mix, 1/4 cup	2

Hostess

Banana walnut mini muffins, 1 pouch	6
Blueberry mini muffins, 1 pouch	6
Chocolate chip mini muffins, 1 pouch	6

Jiffy Mixes

Apple cinnamon muffin mix, dry, 1 serving (1/8 package)	3
Banana muffin mix, dry, 1/4 cup	3
Blueberry muffin mix, dry, 1/4 cup	4
Bran with dates muffin mix, dry, 1/4 cup	3

	POINTS VALUE
Chocolate muffin mix, dry, 1/4 cup	4
Corn muffin mix, dry, 1/4 cup	3
Corn muffin mix, dry, 1/4 cup	3
Oatmeal muffin mix, dry, 1/4 cup	3
Raspberry muffin mix, dry, 1/4 cup	4
Kellogg's Eggo	
Muffin tops, mini blueberry, 1 set of 4	3
Muffin tops, mini chocolate-chocolate chip, 1 set of 4	3
Muffin tops, mini chocolate chip, 1 set of 4	3
Little Debbie	
Banana nut muffins, 1	5
Blueberry muffins, 1	4
Chocolate chip muffins, 1	5
Cranberry & orange muffins, 1	5
Pumpkin muffins, 1	4
Martha White	
Apple cinnamon muffin mix, prepared, 1	3
Banana chocolate chip muffin mix, prepared, 1	3
Banana nut muffin mix, prepared, 1	4
Blackberry muffin mix, prepared, 1	3
Blueberry muffin mix, prepared, 1	3
Carrot cake muffin mix, prepared, 1	3
Chocolate chip muffin mix, prepared, 1	3
Cinnamon muffin mix, prepared, 1	3
Honey bran muffin mix, prepared, 1	3
Lemon poppyseed muffin mix, prepared, 1	3
Strawberry banana muffin mix, prepared, 1	3

	POINTS VALUE
Strawberry muffin mix, prepared, 1	3
Wildberry muffin mix, prepared, 1	3
Mrs. Freshleys 100 Calorie	
Blueberry muffin, 1	1
Mrs. Freshleys Snackaway	
Blueberry muffins, 1	3
Otis Spunkmeyer	
Almond poppy seed, 1/2 (2 oz)	6
Apple, 1 (1.8 oz)	4
Apple cinnamon, 1/2 small (2 oz)	5
Apple cinnamon, 1 (2.25 oz)	6
Apple orchard, 1/2 (2 oz)	5
Banana, 1 (1.8 oz)	4
Banana, 1 (2 oz)	5
Banana, 1/2 (3.25 oz)	9
Banana caramel, 1 (2 oz)	5
Banana mini muffins, 2 (1.8 oz)	5
Banana nut, 1/2 small (2 oz)	5
Banana nut, 1 (1.9 oz)	5
Banana nut, 1 (2.25 oz)	6
Banana nut (sugar free), low carb, 1 (2 oz)	5
Banana nut, low fat, 1/2 small (2 oz)	3
Banana nut, low fat, 1 (2.25 oz)	4
Blueberry, 1/2 (3.25 oz)	8
Blueberry, 1 (1.8 oz)	4
Blueberry, 1/2 (2 oz)	5
Blueberry mini muffins, 2 (1.8 oz)	5
Blueberry streusel, 1/2 (2 oz)	5
Caramel apple, 1/2 (2 oz)	5
Cheese streusel, 1/2 small (2 oz)	5
Cheese streusel, 1 (2.25 oz)	5

Bread & Baked Goods

	POINTS VALUE
Cheese streusel, 1/2 (3.25 oz)	8
Chocolate chip, 1/2 small (2 oz)	6
Chocolate, 1 (1.8 oz)	4
Chocolate chip, 1 (2.25 oz)	6
Chocolate chocolate chip, 1/2 (3.25 oz)	8
Chocolate chocolate chip, 1 (2.25 oz)	6
Chocolate chocolate chip, 1/2 small (2 oz)	5
Chocolate chocolate chip, 1 (1.9 oz)	5
Chocolate chocolate chip mini muffins, 2 (1.8 oz)	5
Chocolate chocolate chip, low-fat, 1/2 small (2 oz)	3
Chocolate chocolate chip, low-fat, 1 (2.25 oz)	4
Chocolate raspberry, 1/2 (2 oz)	5
Cinnamon crumb coffeecake, 1 (2 oz)	5
Corn, 1/2 (3.25 oz)	9
Corn, 1 (2.25 oz)	6
Corn, 1/2 small (2 oz)	5
Cranberry orange, 1/2 (2 oz)	5
Harvest bran, 1/2 small (2 oz)	4
Harvest bran, 1 (2.25 oz)	5
Lemon, 1/2 (2 oz)	5
Orange, 1/2 (2 oz)	5
Orange, 1 small (2 oz)	5
Pumpkin walnut, 1/2 (2 oz)	5
Raspberry cheese streusel, 1/2 (2 oz)	4
Strawberry shortcake, 1 (2.25 oz)	6
Strawberry shortcake, 1 (2 oz)	5
Strawberry shortcake, 1/2 (2 oz)	5
Triple berry, 1/2 (2 oz)	5

	POINTS VALUE
Triple berry, 1/2 (3.25 oz)	8
Wild blueberry, 1 (1.9 oz)	5
Wild blueberry (no sugar added), low carb, 1 (2 oz)	4
Wild blueberry, low-fat, 1/2 small (2 oz)	3
Wild blueberry, low-fat, 1 (2.25 oz)	4
Otis Spunkmeyer Café Collection	
Banana walnut muffin, 1/2	9
Chocolate chocolate chip muffin, 1/2	8
Wild blueberry muffin, 1/2	8
Otis Spunkmeyer Delicious Essentials	
Chocolate chocolate chip muffin, 1	7
Reduced fat apple cinnamon, 1	3
Reduced fat banana, 1	4
Reduced fat chocolate chocolate chip, 1	4
Reduced fat wild blueberry, 1	4
Whole grain reduced fat apple cinnamon, 1	4
Whole grain reduced fat banana, 1	4
Whole grain reduced fat chocolate chocolate chip, 1	4
Whole grain reduced fat wild blueberry, 1	3
Otis Spunkmeyer Delicious Essentials Reduced Fat	
Apple cinnamon muffin, 1	7
Banana muffin, 1	7
Wild blueberry muffin, 1	7
Pillsbury	
Apple cinnamon mix, baked, 1 (1/6 package)	4
Banana nut mix, baked, 1 (1/6 package)	3

	POINTS VALUE
Blueberry mix, baked, 1 (1/6 package)	4
Chocolate chip mix, baked, 1 (1/6 recipe)	4
Strawberry mix, baked, 1 (1/6 recipe)	4
Wildberry mix, baked, 1 (1/6 recipe)	4
VitaMuffin	
Apple berry, 1 small	1
Blueberry bran, 1 small	1
Cranberry bran, 1 small	1
Deep chocolate, 1 small	1
Golden corn, 1 small	1
Multi bran, 1 small	1
Sugar free velvety chocolate, 1	1
Sugar-free banana nut, 1	1
VitaMuffin VitaTops	
Apple Berry, 1	1
Blueberry bran, 1	1
Cranberry bran, 1	1
Dark chocolate with pomegranate, 1	1
Deep chocolate, 1	1
Double chocolate dream, 1	1
Fudgy peanut butter, 1	1
Golden corn, 1	1
Multi bran, 1	1
Sugar free velvety chocolate, 1	1
Sugar-free banana nut, 1	1
Triple chocolate chunk, 1	1
Weight Watchers	
Banana nut muffin, 1	3
Blueberry muffin, 1	3
Double chocolate muffin, 1	3

	POINTS VALUE
Wonder	
Cinnamon raisin English muffin, 1	3
Original English muffin, 1	2
Sourdough English muffin, 1	2
Nori	
Eden	
Nori (10 sheets), 1 sheet	0
Sushi nori (7 sheets), toasted, 1 sheet	0
Rolls	
Alexia	
Ciabatta Italian Rolls, 1 roll	2
Classic French rolls, 1 roll	2
Three cheese focaccia, 1 roll	2
Whole grain rolls, 1 roll	1
Alvarado	
Sprouted wheat burger bun, 1	2
Sprouted wheat hot dog bun, 1	2
Sprouted wheat rolls, 1	1
Arnold	
Select hot dog, 1	3
Select multi-grain kaiser, 1	3
Select sandwich bun, 1	3
Select wheat hot dog roll, 1	3
Bluebird	
Pecan spins, 1	2
Cobblestone Mill	
100% whole grain wheat hot dog buns, 1	2
Honey wheat baguettes, 1/4	3
Pistolettes, 1	2
Wheat sub rolls, 1	4

Bread & Baked Goods

	POINTS VALUE
Entenmann's	
Little bites blueberry muffins (club size package), 1 package	4
Food for Life	
Organic Ezekiel 4:9 sesame sprouted grain burger bun, 1	3
Organic Ezekiel 4:9 sprouted grain burger bun, 1	3
Organic Ezekiel 4:9 sprouted grain hot dog buns, 1	3
Organic sprouted burger bun, 1	2
Organic sprouted hot dog buns, 1	2
Freihofer's	
Hamburger rolls, 1	2
Hot dog rolls, 1	2
New England hot dog rolls, 1	2
Seeded sandwich, 1	2
French Meadow Bakery	
Sprouted organic peasant rolls with Ezekiel grains, 1	3
Healthy Life Original	
Sandwich wheat buns, 1	1
Sandwich white buns, 1	1
Wheat hot dog buns, 1	1
White hot dog buns, 1	1
Healthy Life Southern Country Style	
100% whole wheat dinner rolls, 1	1
100% whole wheat hot dog buns, 1	2
100% whole wheat sandwich buns, 1	2
Maier's	
Italian club roll, 1	3
Italian steak rolls, 1	4

	POINTS VALUE
Mrs. Freshleys Snackaway	
Pecan twirls, 1	2
Nature's Own	
Butter buns, 1	2
Double fiber hamburger wheat buns, 1	1
Honey wheat buns, 1	4
Honey wheat dinner rolls, 1	1
Sugar free 100% whole grain wheat bun, 1	2
Nature's Own Whitewheat	
Hamburger buns, 1	1
Hot dog buns, 1	1
Oroweat	
100% whole wheat buns, 1	3
Cracked wheat hot dog, 1	3
Premium 100% whole wheat sandwich rolls, 1	3
Paraclete	
12" hoagie roll, 1/2	3
Dinner rolls, 1	0
Sandwich rolls, 1	1
Pepperidge Farm	
Classic 100% whole wheat hamburger buns, 1	2
Classic hamburger buns, 1	2
Classic hot dog buns, 1	3
Classic onion sandwich buns with poppy seeds, 1	3
Classic sandwich buns with sesame seeds, 1	3
Classic soft 100% whole wheat hoagie rolls with sesame seeds, 1	3

Bread & Baked Goods

	POINTS VALUE
Classic soft hoagie rolls with sesame seeds, 1	4
Classic whole grain white hamburger buns, 1	2
Classic whole grain white hot dog buns, 1	2
Farmhouse premium wheat rolls, 1	5
Hearth fired artisan French demi-baguette, 1 slice (2 3/4")	2
Hearth fired artisan hearty wheat dinner rolls, 1	2
Hot & crusty French rolls, 1	2
Hot & crusty seven grain French rolls, 1	2
Hot & crusty sourdough rolls, 1	2
Parkerhouse dinner rolls, 1	2
Party rolls, 3	3
Soft country style dinner rolls, 1	2
Pepperidge Farm Farmhouse	
Hot & crusty club pack, 1	3
Premium white rolls, 1	4
Pillsbury	
Big and buttery crescent, 1	4
Butter flake crescent, 1	3
Crusty French roll, 1	2
Garlic butter crescent, 1	3
Garlic roll, 1	3
Hot roll mix, 1/4 cup	2
Original crescent, 1	3
Place 'n bake crescent rounds, 1	3
Reduced fat crescent, 1	2
Sourdough roll, 1	2
Traditional dinner rolls, white, 1	2
Whole wheat roll, 1	1

	POINTS VALUE
Pillsbury Oven Baked	
Butterflake, 1	4
Crusty French mini loaves, 1/4 loaf	2
Soft white, 1	2
Stroehmann	
Dutch country potato hamburger, 1	3
Dutch country potato hot dog, 1	3
Dutch country wheat hamburger, 1	3
Dutch country wheat hot dog, 1	3
Hamburger, 1	2
Hot dog, 1	2
Wonder	
Stoneground wheat sandwich buns, 1	3
Wheat hamburger buns, 1	2
Wheat hot dog buns, 1	2
White hamburger buns, 1	2
White hot dog buns, 1	2
Whole grain white hamburger buns, 1	2
Whole grain white hot dog buns, 1	2
Whole grain white sandwich buns, 1	3
Wonder Light	
White hamburger buns, 1	1
White hot dog buns, 1	1

Stuffing Mix

	POINTS VALUE
Kellogg's Croutettes	
Stuffing mix, 1 cup	2
Pepperidge Farm	
Cornbread stuffing, 3/4 cup	3
Country style stuffing, 3/4 cup	2
Cubed herb seasoned stuffing, 3/4 cup	2
Herb seasoned stuffing, 3/4 cup	3

Bread & Baked Goods

Pepperidge Farm (cont'd)	POINTS VALUE
One step stuffing chicken mix, 1/2 cup	3
One step stuffing garden herb mix, 1/2 cup	3
One step stuffing turkey mix, 1/2 cup	4
Sage & onion stuffing, 3/4 cup	2
Stove Top	
Chicken flavor, as packaged, 1/2 cup	2
Chicken made with whole wheat, as packaged, 1 serving (1/5 box)	2
Chicken made with whole wheat, as prepared, 1/2 cup	3
Chicken, as prepared, 1/2 cup	4
Chicken, prepared, 1/2 cup	3
Cornbread, as packaged, 1/2 cup	2
Cornbread, as prepared, 1/2 cup	4
Cranberry flavor, as packaged, 1 serving (1/6 box)	2
Cranberry flavor, as prepared, 1/2 cup	4
Italian style roasted garlic, as packaged, 1 serving (1/6 box)	2
Italian style roasted garlic, as prepared, 1/2 cup	4
Lower sodium chicken, as packaged, 1/2 cup	2
Lower sodium chicken, as prepared, 1/2 cup	4
Monterey style mushroom & onion, as packaged, 1 serving (1/6 box)	2
Monterey style mushroom & onion, as prepared, 1/2 cup	4
Northern style long grain and wild rice, as packaged, 1 serving (1/6 box)	2

	POINTS VALUE
Northern style long grain and wild rice, as prepared, 1/2 cup	4
Pork flavor, as packaged, 1/2 cup	2
Pork flavor, as prepared, 1/2 cup	4
Savory herb, as packaged, 1 serving (1/6 box)	2
Sourdough San Francisco style, as packaged, 1 serving (1/6 box)	2
Sourdough San Francisco style, as prepared, 1/2 cup	4
Traditional sage, as packaged, 1 serving (1/6 box)	2
Turkey flavor, as packaged, 1/2 cup	2
Turkey flavor, prepared, 1/2 cup	4
Stove Top Flex Serve	
Chicken, as packaged, 1 oz	2
Homestyle herb, as packaged, 1 oz	2
Stove Top Flexible Serve	
Homestyle herb, prepared, 1/2 cup	3

Taco Shells
Bearitos
Blue taco shells, 2	3
Yellow taco shells, 2	3
Yellow tostada shells, 2	3

Garden of Eatin'
Blue taco shells, 2	3
Blue tortilla chips, salted, 15	3
Yellow taco shells, 2	3

Las Palmas
Yellow corn shells, 2	3

◈	POINTS VALUE
Old El Paso	
Hard taco shells, 3	3
Mini taco shells, 6	3
Soft taco shells (tortillas), 2	4
Stand n stuff nacho style shells, 2	3
Stand n stuff salsa shells, 2	3
Stand 'n stuff taco shells, 2	3
Super stuffer taco shells, 2	4
Taco salad shell, 1	3
Taco shells, 3	3
White corn taco shells, 3	3
Ortega	
Hard & soft taco kit, taco shells only, 2	3
Taco shells, 2	3
White corn shells, 2	3
Yellow corn shells, 2	3
Taco Bell Home Originals	
Flavored taco shells - nacho, 3	3
Flavored taco shells - ranch, 3	3
Taco shells, 3	3
Zapata	
Blue corn taco shells, 2	3
Premium taco shells, 2	2
Yellow corn taco shells, 2	3

Tortillas
Alvarado

Sprouted wheat 8" tortilla fajita, 1	3
Sprouted wheat 10" tortilla burrito, 1	3
Azteca	
Flour tortillas, 1 (9")	2
Flour tortillas, 1 (10")	3

◈	POINTS VALUE
Flour tortillas, 2 (7")	3
Low carb tortillas, 1 (6")	1
White corn tortillas, 2 (6")	1
Buena Vida	
Fat free flour tortillas, 1 (8")	2
Whole grain tortillas, 1 (8")	4
CHI-CHI'S	
Burrito tortillas (9"), 1	3
Corn tortillas (6"), 2	3
Fajita tortillas (6"), 1	1
Flour tortillas (6"), 1	2
Flour tortillas (8"), 1	3
Flour tortillas (10") 1	5
Soft taco tortillas (8"), 1	3
Don Marcos	
Healthy style fat free flour tortillas, 1	0
Food for Life	
Ezekiel 4:9 sprouted grain tortilla, 1	2
Organic Ezekiel 4:9 sprouted grain tortilla, 1	1
LaTortilla Factory	
Family pack white corn tortillas, 2	2
Tostadas, 1	1
Whole wheat low carb, high fiber garlic & herb flavor, 1	0
Whole wheat low carb, high fiber green onion flavor, 1	0
LaTortilla Factory Smart & Delicious	
Gluten free dark teff wraps, 1	3
Gluten free ivory teff wraps, 1	3
Low carb, high fiber large size, 1	1

Bread & Baked Goods

	POINTS VALUE
Low carb, high fiber original soft taco size, 1	0
Low fat low sodium burrito size, 1	2
Low fat low sodium soft taco size, 1	2
Pumpernickel softwraps, 1	1
Traditional softwraps, 1	1
Whole grain rye softwraps, 1	1
Whole grain, white whole wheat softwraps, 1	1
LaTortilla Factory Sonoma	
All natural carb cutting, 1	1
All natural gluten free dark teff, 1	3
Made with organic Mediterranean wraps, 1	3
Made with organic tomato basil wraps, 1	3
Organic multi-grain wraps, 1	3
Organic traditional wraps, 1	4
Organic yellow corn tortillas, 2	2
Manny's	
Family pack tortilla, 1	2
Fat free flour tortilla, 1	1
Mission	
96% fat free (heart healthy) tortillas - burrito size, 1	3
96% fat free (heart healthy) soft taco sized flour tortillas, 1	2
96% fat free (heart healthy) tortillas - fajita size, 1	1
96% fat free (heart healthy) whole wheat soft taco sized flour tortillas, 1	2

	POINTS VALUE
Life balance soft taco sized tortillas, 1	2
Life balance whole wheat soft taco sized tortillas, 1	2
Low carb fajita sized flour tortillas, 1	1
Low carb soft taco sized flour tortillas, 1	2
Low carb whole wheat burrito size flour tortillas, 1	4
Low carb whole wheat fajita size flour tortillas, 1	1
Multi grain fajita sized tortillas, 1	2
Multi grain soft taco sized tortillas, 1	2
White corn tortillas, 2	2
Yellow corn tortillas, 2	2
Old El Paso	
Flour tortillas for burritos, 1	3
Flour tortillas for soft tacos & fajitas, 2	3
Tostada shells, 3	4
Ortega	
Flour tortillas, 1	3
Hard & soft taco kit, tortillas only, 2	4
Tostada shells, 2	3
Taco Bell Home Originals	
Flour tortillas, 2	4
Tumaro's Healthy Flour Tortillas	
Chipotle chili & peppers, 1 small (8")	2
Chipotle chili & peppers, 1 large (10")	4
Garden spinach & vegetables, 1 small (8")	2
Garden spinach & vegetables, 1 large (10")	3

	POINTS VALUE
Honey wheat, 1 large (10")	3
Honey wheat, 1 small (8")	2
Jalapeño & cilantro, 1 small (8")	2
Jalapeño & cilantro, 1 large (10")	4
Pesto & garlic, 1 (8")	2
Premium white, 1 (8")	2
Tumaro's Low in Carb	
Garden vegetable, 8", 1	1
Garden vegetable, 10", 1	2
Green onion, 8", 1	1
Green onion, 10", 1	2

	POINTS VALUE
Multi grain, 8", 1	1
Multi grain, 10", 1	2
Salsa, 8", 1	1
Salsa, 10", 1	2
Tumaro's Soy-Full Heart	
8 grain & soy, 1	1
Apple cinnamon flatbread, 1	1
Wheat, soy & flax flatbread, 1	1
Zapata	
Premium tostada shell, 2	2

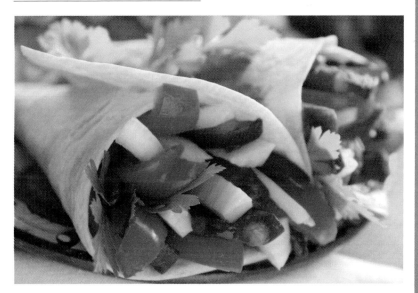

Breakfast, Cereals & Cereal Bars

	POINTS VALUE
Bran & Wheat Germ	
Hodgson Mill	
100% untoasted wheat germ, 2 Tbsp	1
Wheat germ with cinnamon & flax, 2 Tbsp	1
Kretschmer	
Honey crunch wheat germ, 1 2/3 Tbsp	1
Wheat germ - regular, 2 Tbsp	1
Tree of Life	
Wheat germ, toasted, 3 Tbsp	2
Cereal, Hot	
Amy's	
Cream of rice hot cereal bowl, 1	3
Multi-grain hot cereal bowl, 1	3
Rolled oats hot cereal bowl, 1	4
Steel-cut oats hot cereal bowl, 1	4
Arrowhead Mills	
Instant oatmeal - maple apple spice, 1 packet	2
Instant oatmeal original plain, 1 packet	2
Instant rice cereal, 1 packet	2
Cream of Wheat	
Cream of wheat, 1 minute, 3 Tbsp	2
Cream of wheat, 10 minute, 3 Tbsp	2
Cream of wheat, 2 1/2 minute, 3 Tbsp	2
Instant cream of wheat, apples 'n cinnamon, 1 packet	2
Instant cream of wheat, cinnamon swirl, 1 packet	2
Instant cream of wheat, maple brown sugar, 1 packet	2

	POINTS VALUE
Instant cream of wheat, original, 1 packet	2
Instant cream of wheat, strawberries 'n cream, 1 packet	2
Instant healthy grain, maple brown sugar, 1 packet	2
Instant Spongebob Squarepants, bikini bottom maple brown sugar, 1 packet	2
Instant Spongebob Squarepants, chocolate lagoon, 1 packet	2
Intant healthy grain, original, 1 packet	2
H-O	
Cream farina, 3 Tbsp	2
Instant oats, 1/2 cup	2
Hodgson Mill	
Bulgur wheat with soy hot cereal, 1/4 cup	2
Oat bran hot cereal, 1/4 cup	2
Steel cut oats, 1/4 cup	2
Kashi GoLean	
Creamy truly vanilla, 1 packet	2
Hearty honey and cinnamon, 1 packet	2
Kashi Heart to Heart	
Instant oatmeal raisin spice, 1 packet	2
Instant oatmeal, apple cinnamon, 1 packet	3
Instant oatmeal, maple, 1 packet	3
Kozy Shack Ready Grains	
Apple & cinnamon, 1 carton	4
Maple brown sugar, 1 carton	4
Original, 1 carton	3
Strawberry, 1 carton	4

Breakfast, Cereals & Cereal Bars

	POINTS VALUE
Martha White	
Grits, yellow, 1/4 cup	3
Nabisco	
Cream of rice, 1 serving (46 g)	3
Nature's Path	
Organic instant hot oatmeal, apple cinnamon, 1 packet	4
Organic instant hot oatmeal, flax 'n oats, 1 packet	4
Organic instant hot oatmeal, maple nut, 1 packet	4
Organic instant oatmeal, original, 1 packet	3
Quaker	
Oatmeal, lower sugar apples & cinnamon, 1 packet	2
Oatmeal, lower sugar maple & brown sugar, 1 packet	2
Quaker Oats	
Enriched hominy quick golden grits, 1/4 cup	2
Enriched white hominy grits, 1/4 cup	2
Enriched white hominy quick grits, 1/4 cup	2
Instant grits - American cheese flavor, 1 packet	2
Instant grits - butter express, 1 cup	3
Instant grits - butter flavor, 1 packet	2
Instant grits - cheddar blend, 1 packet	2
Instant grits - cheddar cheese flavor, 1 packet	2
Instant grits - country bacon, 1 packet	2
Instant grits - ham 'n cheese flavor, 1 packet	2

	POINTS VALUE
Instant grits - original flavor, 1 packet	2
Instant grits - three cheese, 1 packet	2
Instant oatmeal - apples and cinnamon, 1 packet	2
Instant oatmeal - baked apple flavor, 1 packet	3
Instant oatmeal - baked cinnamon roll, 1 packet	3
Instant oatmeal - cinnamon & spice, 1 packet	3
Instant oatmeal - crunchy apples & cinnamon, 1 packet	3
Instant oatmeal - crunchy maple brown sugar, 1 packet	3
Instant oatmeal - crunchy mixed berry, 1 packet	3
Instant oatmeal - dinosaur eggs - brown sugar cinnamon, 1 packet	3
Instant oatmeal - French toast, 1 packet	3
Instant oatmeal - honey nut, 1 packet	3
Instant oatmeal - magicolor crunch, 1 packet	3
Instant oatmeal - maple & brown sugar, 1 packet	3
Instant oatmeal - peaches & cream, 1 packet	3
Instant oatmeal - raisin-spice, 1 packet	3
Instant oatmeal - regular flavor, 1 packet	2
Instant oatmeal - strawberries & cream, 1 packet	3
Instant oatmeal express - baked apple, 1 cup	3

Breakfast, Cereals & Cereal Bars

Quaker Oats (cont'd)	POINTS VALUE
Instant oatmeal express - cinnamon roll, 1 cup	3
Instant oatmeal express - golden brown sugar, 1 cup	4
Instant oatmeal nutrition for women - apple cinnamon, 1 packet	3
Instant oatmeal nutrition for women - golden brown sugar, 1 packet	3
Instant oatmeal nutrition for women - vanilla cinnamon, 1 packet	3
Instant oatmeal weight control - banana bread, 1 packet	3
Instant oatmeal weight control - cinnamon toast, 1 packet	3
Instant oatmeal weight control - maple brown sugar, 1 packet	3
◆ Multigrain hot cereal, 1/2 cup	2
◆ Oat bran, 1/2 cup	2
◆ Old fashioned oats, 1/2 cup	2
Organic instant - maple brown sugar, 1 packet	3
◆ Organic instant - regular, 1 packet	2
◆ Quick oats, 1/2 cup	2
◆ Scotch barley, regular & quick cooking, 1/3 cup	2
◆ Whole wheat - hot natural cereal, 1/2 cup	2
Quaker Oats Simple Harvest	
Apple & cinnamon oatmeal, 1 packet	2
Maple brown sugar oatmeal, 1 packet	3
Plain oatmeal, 1 packet	2
Vanilla, almond, honey oatmeal, 1 packet	3

	POINTS VALUE
Uncle Sam	
◆ Instant oatmeal, 1 packet	2
Instant oatmeal with soymilk - cinnamon raisin, 1 packet	3
Instant oatmeal with soymilk - French vanilla, 1 packet	3
Weight Watchers	
Oatmeal – blueberry harvest, 1 cup	2
Oatmeal - maple brown sugar, 1 cup	2

Cereal, Ready to Eat
Alvarado

	POINTS VALUE
Plain granola, 1/2 cup	4
Raisin granola, 1/2 cup	4
Annie's Homegrown	
Bunny love toasted whole grain oat breakfast cereal, 3/4 cup	2
Cinna bunnies cinnamon toasted breakfast cereal, 3/4 cup	2
Honey bunnies toasted whole grain oat breakfast cereal, 3/4 cup	2
Annie's Homegrown Naturals	
Bunny crunch honey cereal, 3/4 cup	2
Fruity bunnies, 3/4 cup	2
Toasted corn & whole oat cereal with cocoa & real vanilla, 3/4 cup	2
Arrowhead Mills	
◆ Amaranth flakes, 1 cup	2
Maple buckwheat flakes, 1 cup	3
Oat bran flakes, 1 cup	2
Back To Nature	
Apple blueberry granola, 1/2 cup	3
Apple cinnamon granola, 1/2 cup	3

Breakfast, Cereals & Cereal Bars

	POINTS VALUE
Apple strawberry granola, 1/2 cup	3
Banana nut multi bran, 3/4 cup	3
Cranberry pecan granola, 1/2 cup	3
Flax & fiber crunch, 1 cup	3
French vanilla granola, 1/2 cup	4
Granola - classic, 1/2 cup	3
Granola - raisin, 1/2 cup	3
Hi protein crunch, 1/2 cup	3
Hi-fiber multibran, 1/2 cup	0
Hi-fiber multibran, 3/4 cup	2
Hi-protein crunch, 1/2 cup	2
Multigrain harvest, 1 cup	4
Oat 'n soy crisp, 3/4 cup	3
Barbara's Bakery	
Cinnamon crunch shredded oats, 1 cup	4
Organic apple cinnamon o's, 3/4 cup	2
Organic breakfast o's - fruit juice sweetened, 1 cup	2
Organic brown rice crisps - fruit juice sweetened, 1 cup	2
Organic corn flakes - fruit juice sweetened, 1 cup	2
Organic crispy wheats, 3/4 cup	2
Organic grainshop, 1/2 cup	1
Organic honey crunch'n oats, 2/3 cup	2
Organic honey nut o's, 3/4 cup	2
Organic wild puffs, cocoa graham, 3/4 cup	2
Organic wild puffs, crunchy cocoa, 3/4 cup	2
Organic wild puffs, fruit medley, 3/4 cup	2
Organic wild puffs, honey puffs, 3/4 cup	2

	POINTS VALUE
Shredded oats, 1 1/4 cups	4
Shredded spoonfuls, 3/4 cup	2
Shredded wheat, 2 biscuits	2
Ultima organic flax & granola, 1 cup	4
Ultima organic high fiber, 1/2 cup	1
Ultima organic pomegranate, 1/2 cup	1
Vanilla almond shredded oats, 1 cup	4
Weetabix minibix chocolate crisp, 1 cup	3
Weetabix minibix honey & nut, 1 cup	3
Barbara's Bakery Puffins	
Cinnamon puffins, 2/3 cup	1
Honey rice puffins, 3/4 cup	2
Original puffins, 3/4 cup	1
Peanut butter puffins, 3/4 cup	2
Benefit Nutrition	
Protein plus cereal with soy, 2/3 cup	2
Simply fiber cereal, 3/4 cup	1
Simply fiber cereal with cinnamon, 3/4 cup	1
Breadshop	
Blueberry 'n cream granola, 1/2 cup	4
Crunch oat bran, 1/2 cup	4
Gone nuts granola, 1/2 cup	5
Honey gone nuts, 1/2 cup	5
New England supernatural granola, 1/2 cup	5
Pralines 'n crème, 1/2 cup	4
Strawberry 'n cream granola, 1/2 cup	4
Super cereal, 1/2 cup	5
Supernatural granola with almond & raisin, 1/2 cup	5

Breakfast, Cereals & Cereal Bars

	POINTS VALUE
Cascadian Farm	
Cinnamon raisin granola, 2/3 cup	4
Clifford crunch, 1 cup	1
Great measure, 1 cup	3
Hearty morning, 3/4 cup	3
Honey nut o's, 1 oz	2
Multi-grain squares, 3/4 cup	2
Oats & honey granola, 2/3 cup	5
Purely o's, 1 cup	2
Raisin bran, 1 cup	3
Vanilla almond crunch, 3/4 cup	4
Wheat crunch, 3/4 cup	2
EnviroKidz	
Amazon frosted flakes, 2/3 cup	2
Gorilla munch, 1 cup	2
Koala crisp, 2/3 cup	2
Orangutan-o's, 3/4 cup	2
Peanut butter panda puffs, 1 cup	3
Erin Baker's	
Granola - ultra protein power crunch, 1/2 cup	4
Food for Life	
Organic Ezekiel 4:9 cereal, almond, 1/2 cup	3
Organic Ezekiel 4:9 cereal, cinnamon raisin, 1/2 cup	3
Organic Ezekiel 4:9 cereal, golden flax, 1/2 cup	3
◆ Organic Ezekiel 4:9 cereal, original, 1/2 cup	3

	POINTS VALUE
General Mills	
Apple cinnamon cheerios, 3/4 cup	2
Banana nut cheerios, 3/4 cup	2
Basic 4, 1 cup	4
Berry berry kix, 3/4 cup	2
Berry burst cheerios, triple berry, 3/4 cup	2
Boo berry, 1 cup	2
Cheerios, 1 cup	2
Cheerios crunch, 3/4 cup	2
Chocolate chex, 3/4 cup	3
Chocolate lucky charms, 3/4 cup	2
Cinnamon toast crunch, 3/4 cup	3
Cocoa puffs, 3/4 cup	2
Cocoa puffs combos, 3/4 cup	2
Cookie crisp, 3/4 cup	2
Corn chex, 1 cup	2
Count chocula, 3/4 cup	2
Country corn flakes, 1 cup	2
Disney's little Einstein fruity stars, 1 cup	2
Disney's Mickey Mouse clubhouse berry crunch, 1 cup	2
Disney's my friends Tigger & Pooh corn puffs, 1 cup	2
Dora the explorer, 3/4 cup	2
Double chocolate cookie crisps, 3/4 cup	2
◆ Fiber one, 1/2 cup	0
Fiber one caramel delight, 1 cup	3
Fiber one frosted shredded wheat, 1 cup	3

Breakfast, Cereals & Cereal Bars

	POINTS VALUE
Fiber one honey clusters, 1 cup	3
Fiber one raisin bran, 1 cup	3
Frankenberry, 1 cup	3
French toast crunch, 3/4 cup	3
Frosted cheerios, 3/4 cup	2
Fruity cheerios, 3/4 cup	2
Golden grahams, 3/4 cup	2
Heart healthy blend apple crunch, 1 cup	4
Heart healthy blend with fiber one, 3/4 cup	3
Honey nut cheerios, 3/4 cup	2
Honey nut chex, 3/4 cup	2
Honey nut clusters, 1 cup	4
Kaboom, 1 1/4 cups	1
Kix, 1 1/4 cups	2
Lucky charms, 3/4 cup	2
Multi-bran chex, 3/4 cup	3
Multi-grain cheerios, 1 cup	2
Nature valley crunchy oats 'n honey, 1 cup	4
Oatmeal crisp crunchy almond, 1 cup	4
Oatmeal crisp maple brown sugar, 1 cup	4
Oatmeal crisp raisin, 1 cup	4
Para su familia raisin bran, 1 1/4 cups	3
Raisin nut bran, 3/4 cup	3
Reduced sugar cinnamon toast crunch, 3/4 cup	2
Reese's puffs, 3/4 cup	2
Rice chex, 1 cup	2
Strawberry chex, 3/4 cup	3

	POINTS VALUE
Total cinnamon crunch, 1 cup	3
Total cranberry crunch, 1 1/4 cups	3
Total honey clusters, 3/4 cup	3
Total raisin bran, 1 cup	2
Total whole grain, 3/4 cup	1
Trix, 1 cup	2
Wheat chex, 3/4 cup	2
Wheaties, 3/4 cup	1
Yogurt burst cheerios berries & crème, 3/4 cup	2
Yogurt burst cheerios, strawberry, 3/4 cup	2
Yogurt burst cheerios, vanilla, 3/4 cup	2
Yogurt kix, 1 cup	2
Health Valley	
Cranberry crunch, 3/4 cup	3
Empower cereal, 1 cup	3
Heart wise cereal, 1 cup	3
Organic amaranth flakes, 3/4 cup	1
Organic fiber 7 flakes, 3/4 cup	1
Organic fiber 7 multigrain flakes, 3/4 cup	1
Organic golden flax cereal, 3/4 cup	3
Organic oat bran flakes, 3/4 cup	1
Organic oat bran flakes with raisins, 3/4 cup	1
Hodgson Mill	
Cracked wheat cereal, 1/4 cup	1
Muesli, 1/4 cup	2
Multi grain hot cereal with milled flaxseed and soy, 1/3 cup	3

Breakfast, Cereals & Cereal Bars

	POINTS VALUE
Kashi	
7 whole grain flakes, 1 cup	3
7 whole grain honey puffs, 1 cup	2
7 whole grain nuggets, 1/2 cup	4
7 whole grain puffs, 1 cup	1
Cinna-raisin crunch, 1 cup	3
Golean, 1 cup	2
Good friends caramel, 1 cup	3
Granola - cocoa beach, 1/2 cup	5
Granola - summer berry, 1/2 cup	4
Granola orchard spice, 1/2 cup	4
Honey sunshine, 3/4 cup	1
Kashi u, 1 cup (1.9 oz)	3
Mighty bites - honey crunch, 1 cup	2
Mountain medley granola, 1/2 cup	4
Organic promise island vanilla biscuit, 27 (1.9 oz)	3
Vive probiotic cereal - toasted graham & vanilla, 1 1/4 cups	3
Kashi GOLEAN	
Crunch honey almond flax, 1 cup	4
Crunch!, 1 cup	3
Kashi Heart to Heart	
Honey toasted oat, 3/4 cup	2
Wild blueberry, 1 cup	3
Kashi Organic Promise	
Autumn wheat, 1 cup	3
Cinnamon harvest, 1 cup	3
Strawberry fields, 1 cup	2

	POINTS VALUE
Kellogg's	
All-bran chocolate rolled wafers, 3	2
All-bran strawberry rolled wafers, 3	2
All-bran yogurt bites, 1 1/4 cups	3
All-bran, bran buds, 1/3 cup	1
All-bran, extra fiber, 1/2 cup ◆	0
All-bran, original, 1/2 cup	1
All-bran, strawberry medley, 1 cup	3
Apple jacks, 1 cup	2
Apple jacks cereal straws, 3	3
Barbie cereal, 1 cup	2
Caramel nut crunch, 1 cup	4
Cinnamon mini swirlz, 1 cup	2
Cocoa krispies cereal straws, 3	3
Cocoa rice krispies, 3/4 cup	2
Cocoa rice krispies coco-nilla, 3/4 cup	2
Complete wheat bran flakes, 3/4 cup	1
Corn flakes, 1 cup	2
Corn pops, 1 cup	2
Corn pops, chocolate peanut butter, 3/4 cup	2
Cracklin' oat bran, 3/4 cup	4
Crispix, 1 cup	2
Eggo crunch maple, 1 cup	2
Froot loops, 1 cup	2
Froot loops - reduced sugar, 1 1/4 cups	2
Froot loops cereal straws, 3	3
Froot loops smoothie with yogurty coated cereal pieces, 1 cup	2
Frosted flakes, 3/4 cup	2
Frosted flakes gold, 3/4 cup	2

Breakfast, Cereals & Cereal Bars

	POINTS VALUE
Frosted flakes reduced sugar, 1 cup	2
Frosted krispies, 3/4 cup	2
Fruit harvest strawberry blueberry, 3/4 cup	2
Go packs, corn pops, 1 pouch	1
Go packs, froot loops, 1 pouch	2
Go packs, frosted flakes, 1 pouch	1
Go packs, special k fruit & yogurt cereal, 1 pouch	2
Go packs, special k vanilla almond, 1 pouch	2
High school musical 3 (Disney), 1 cup	2
Honey smacks, 3/4 cup	2
Indiana jones, 1 cup	2
Keebler cookie crunch, 1 cup	2
Krispies multi-grain jumbo, 1 cup	1
Kung fu panda, 3/4 cup	2
Low fat granola with raisins, 2/3 cup	4
Low fat granola without raisins, 1/2 cup	3
Marshmallow froot loops, 1 cup	2
Mini-wheats frosted bite size, 24 pieces	3
Mini-wheats frosted bite size blueberry muffin, 24 pieces	3
Mini-wheats frosted bite size cinnamon streusel, 24 pieces	3
Mini-wheats frosted bite-size strawberry delight, 24 pieces	3
Mini-wheats frosted maple & brown sugar, 24 pieces	3
Mini-wheats frosted original, 5 pieces	3
Mini-wheats little bites honey nut, 46 pieces	3

	POINTS VALUE
Mini-wheats vanilla crème bite size, 24 pieces	3
Mini-wheats, little bites chocolate, 52 pieces	3
Mini-wheats, un-frosted bite size, 30 pieces	3
Müeslix, 2/3 cup	3
Product 19, 1 cup	2
Raisin bran, 1 cup	3
Raisin bran crunch, 1 cup	3
Raisin bran extra, 1 cup	3
Rice krispies, 1 1/4 cups	3
Rice krispies treats cereal, 3/4 cup	3
Rice Krispies with strawberries, 1 cup	2
Smart start - antioxidant, 1 cup	3
Smart start - healthy heart, 1 1/4 cups	4
Smart start, strawberry oat bites, 30 pieces	3
Smorz, 1 cup	2
Special K, 1 cup	2
Special K chocolatey delight, 3/4 cup	2
Special K cinnamon pecan, 3/4 cup	2
Special K fruit & yogurt cereal, 3/4 cup	2
Special K low carb lifestyle protein plus, 3/4 cup	1
Special K red berries, 1 cup	2
Special K vanilla almond, 3/4 cup	2
Special k, blueberry, 3/4 cup	2
Wild animal crunch, 3/4 cup	1
Kellogg's Smart Start	
Healthy heart cinnamon raisin, 1 cup	3

Breakfast, Cereals & Cereal Bars

	POINTS VALUE
Kellogg's Smart Start Healthy Heart	
Maple & brown sugar, 1 1/4 cups	4
Lifestream	
Multigrain honey puffs natural cereal, 1 cup	2
Market Day	
Apple berry breakfast bowl, 1	3
Mother's	
Cinnamon oat crunch, 1 serving (60 g)	4
Cocoa bumpers, 1 serving (33 g)	2
Graham bumpers, 1 serving (28 g)	2
Honey bumpers, 1 serving (33 g)	2
Peanut butter bumpers, 1 serving (33 g)	3
Nature's Path	
8 grain synergy flakes, 2/3 cup	1
Blueberry almond muesli organic cereal, 1/2 cup	4
Corn puffs, 1 cup	1
Flax plus granola, 1/2 cup	3
Flax plus multibran flakes, 3/4 cup	1
Fruit juice sweet cornflakes, 3/4 cup	2
Ginger zing granola, 2/3 cup	6
Hemp plus granola, 1/2 cup	2
Heritage bites, 3/4 cup	1
Heritage flakes, 3/4 cup	2
Heritage granola, 1/2 cup	2
Heritage muesli, 1/2 cup	4
Heritage o's, 3/4 cup	2
Honey'd cornflakes, 3/4 cup	2
Kamut krisp, 3/4 cup	1
Kamut puffs, 1 cup	1

	POINTS VALUE
Mesa sunrise, 3/4 cup	2
Millet puffs, 1 cup	1
Millet rice, 3/4 cup	2
Multigrain flakes, 2/3 cup	2
Multigrain with raisin, 2/3 cup	2
Oaty bites, 3/4 cup	2
Optimum power cereal, 1 cup	3
Optimum slim cereal, 1 cup	3
Optimum zen, 3/4 cup	3
Rice puffs, 1 cup	1
Soy plus granola, 1/2 cup	2
Spelt flakes cereal, 3/4 cup	2
Wheat puffs, 1 cup	1
Whole grain crispy rice cereal, 3/4 cup	2
Nutritious Living	
Dr. Sears zone cereal, 3/4 cup	3
Heartmates cereal, 3/4 cup	1
Nutritious Living Hi-Lo	
Hi-lo cereal, 1/2 cup	1
Maple pecan, 1/2 cup	1
Maple pecan cereal cup, 1 container	2
Vanilla almond, 1/2 cup	1
Vanilla almond cereal cup, 1 container	2
With strawberries, 1/2 cup	1
Post	
Bamm bamm mixed berry pebbles, 3/4 cup	2
Bran flakes, 3/4 cup	1
Cocoa pebbles, 3/4 cup	2
Fiesta fruity pebbles, 3/4 cup	2
Frosted shredded wheat spoon size, 1 cup	3

Breakfast, Cereals & Cereal Bars

	POINTS VALUE
Fruity pebbles, 3/4 cup	2
Fruity pebbles reduced sugar, 3/4 cup	2
Golden crisp, 3/4 cup	2
Grape-nut flakes, 3/4 cup	2
Grape-nut o's, 1 cup	2
Grape-nuts, 1/2 cup	3
Grape-nuts trail mix, crunch raisin almond, 1/2 cup	3
Honey bunches of oats cinnamon, 3/4 cup	2
Honey bunches of oats honey roasted, 3/4 cup	2
Honey bunches of oats with almonds, 3/4 cup	2
Honey bunches of oats with real peaches cereal, 1 serving	2
Honey bunches of oats with real strawberries cereal, 1 serving	2
Honey nut shredded wheat spoon size, 1 cup	3
Honeycomb, 1 1/2 cups	2
Oreo o's with marshmallow bits cereal, 1 serving	2
Organic grape-nuts, 1/2 cup	3
Organic honey bunches of oats honey roasted, 3/4 cup	2
Raisin bran, 1 cup	3
Shredded wheat cinnamon, 1 cup	3
◆ The original shredded wheat, 2 biscuits	2
◆ The original shredded wheat 'n bran spoon size, 1 1/4 cups	3
◆ The original shredded wheat spoon size, 1 cup	3

	POINTS VALUE
Toasties, 1 cup	2
Waffle crisp, 1 cup	2
Post Select	
Banana nut crunch, 1 cup	5
Blueberry morning, 1 1/4 cups	4
Cranberry almond crunch, 3/4 cup	4
Great grains crunchy pecan, 1/2 cup	4
Great grains raisins, dates & pecans, 1/2 cup	4
Maple pecan crunch cereal, 1 serving (52 g)	4
Organic apple cinnamon harvest, 1 cup	3
Quaker Oats	
Cap'n crunch, peanut butter, 3/4 cup	2
Cap'n crunch, peanut butter chocolate, 3/4 cup	2
Cap'n crunch, regular, 3/4 cup	2
Cap'n crunch, with crunchberries, 3/4 cup	2
Cap'n crunch's choco crunch cereal, 3/4 cup	1
Cinnamon life, 3/4 cup	2
Cinnamon oatmeal squares, 1 cup	4
Crunchy bran, 3/4 cup	1
King vitamin, 1 1/2 cups	2
Life, 3/4 cup	2
Life, chocolate oat clusters, 1 cup	4
Life, vanilla yogurt crunch, 1 1/4 cups	4
Natural granola oats, honey & raisins, 1/2 cup	4
Natural granola, low fat, 2/3 cup	4
Natural granola, oats & honey, 1/2 cup	4

Breakfast, Cereals & Cereal Bars

Quaker Oats (cont'd)	POINTS VALUE
Oat bran cereal, 1 1/4 cups	4
Oatmeal squares, 1 cup	4
Oh!s - honey graham, 3/4 cup	2
Puffed rice, 1 cup	1
Puffed wheat, 1 1/4 cups	1
Quisp, 1 cup	2
Shredded wheat, 3 biscuits	4
Toasted oatmeal cereal - honey nut, 1 cup	3
Toasted oatmeal cereal - original, 1 cup	3
Quaker Oats Simple Harvest	
Banana honey pecan cereal, 1 serving (50 g)	3
Cinnamon & honey cereal, 1 serving (52 g)	3
Sunbelt	
Berry basic cereal, 1/2 cup	5
Low fat granola cereal, 1/2 cup	4
Uncle Sam	
Cereal, 3/4 cup	3
Cereal with mixed berries, 1 cup	3
Weetabix	
Alpen - no sugar added muesli-style cereal, 2/3 cup	3
Alpen original muesli-style cereal, 2/3 cup	3
Organic crispy flakes, 3/4 cup	1
Organic crispy flakes & fiber, 1 1/4 cups	3
Organic weetabix, 2 biscuits	2

Cereal Bars
Balance

	POINTS VALUE
Almond brownie, 1 bar	4
Chocolate nutrition energy bar, 1 bar	4
Chocolate raspberry fudge, 1 bar	4
Cookie dough nutrition energy bar, 1 bar	4
Mocha chip, 1 bar	4
Peanut butter nutrition energy bar, 1 bar	4
Sweet and salty chocolate almond nutrition energy bar, 1 bar	4
Sweet and salty peanut butter nutrition energy bar, 1 bar	4
Sweet and salty yogurt nut nutrition energy bar, 1 bar	4
Trail mix chocolate chip nutrition energy bar, 1 bar	4
Trail mix cinnamon oats & honey nutrition energy bar, 1 bar	4
Trail mix fruit & nut nutrition energy bar, 1 bar	4
Yogurt honey peanut, 1 bar	4
Balance 100 Calories	
Chocolate caramel crisp nutrition energy bar, 1 bar	2
Peanut butter crisp nutrition energy bar, 1 bar	2
Vanilla caramel crisp nutrition energy bar, 1 bar	2
Balance Carbwell	
Caramel 'n chocolate nutrition energy bar, 1 bar	4

Breakfast, Cereals & Cereal Bars

	POINTS VALUE
Chocolate fudge nutrition energy bar, 1 bar	4
Chocolate peanut butter nutrition energy bar, 1 bar	4
Balance Gold	
Caramel nut blast, 1 bar	5
Chewy chocolate chip nutrition energy bar, 1 bar	5
Chocolate peanut butter, 1 bar	5
Rocky road, 1 bar	5
Triple chocolate chaos nutrition energy bar, 1 bar	5
Balance Gold Crunch	
Chocolate chocolate nutrition energy bar, 1 bar	3
Chocolate mint cookie nutrition energy bar, 1 bar	3
Cookies 'n crème nutrition energy bar, 1 bar	4
Crunchy peanut butter nutrition energy bar, 1 bar	4
S'mores nutrition energy bar, 1 bar	3
Balance Organic	
Apricot mango crisp nutrition energy bar, 1 bar	3
Cherry almond crisp nutrition energy bar, 1 bar	3
Cranberry pomegranate crisp nutrition energy bar, 1 bar	3
Barbara's Bakery	
Crunchy organic granola bar, cinnamon crisp, 2 bars	4
Crunchy organic granola bar, oats 'n' honey, 2 bars	4

	POINTS VALUE
Crunchy organic granola bar, peanut butter, 2 bars	4
Crunchy organic granola bar, toasted almond, 2 bars	4
Barbara's Bakery Fruit & Yogurt	
Apple cinnamon, 1 bar	3
Blueberry apple, 1 bar	3
Cherry apple, 1 bar	3
Strawberry apple, 1 bar	3
Cascadian Farm	
Chocolate chip, 1 bar	3
Fruit & nut: raisin, almond sunflower seed & cranberry, 1 bar	3
Granola harvest berry bars, 1 bar	3
Multi-grain bars, 1 bar	3
DrSoy	
Chocolate brownie bar, 1 bar	4
Chocolate peanut bar, 1 bar	4
Iced oatmeal cookie bar, 1 bar	4
DrSoy Healthy Snacker	
Chocolate caramel crunch, 1 bar	4
Rocky road, 1 bar	4
Entenmann's	
Apple cinnamon cereal bars, 1	2
Chocolate chip cereal bars, 1	3
Raspberry cereal bars, 1	3
Strawberry cereal bars, 1	2
Entenmann's Club Pack	
Multigrain real apple cinnamon filled cereal bars, 1 bar	3
Multi-grain real raspberry filled cereal bars, 1 bar	3

Breakfast, Cereals & Cereal Bars

Entenmann's Club Pack (cont'd)

Multi-grain real strawberry filled cereal bars, 1 bar	3

EnviroKidz

Organic crispy rice bar - berry, 1 bar	2
Organic crispy rice bar - chocolate, 1 bar	2
Organic crispy rice bar - peanut butter, 1 bar	2

Estee Smart Treats

Sugar free chocolate chip, 1	1
Sugar free chocolate crunch, 1	1
Sugar free peanut butter crunch, 1	1

Gatorade

Chocolate, 1 bar	5
Chocolate chip, 1 bar	5
Oatmeal raisin, 1 bar	5
Peanut butter, 1 bar	5

General Foods Caribou Coffee

Caramel high rise, 1 bar	3
Chocolate mocha, 1 bar	3
Mint condition, 1 bar	3
Vanilla latte, 1 bar	3

General Foods Curves

Chocolate peanut, 1 bar	1
Strawberries & cream, 1 bar	1

General Foods Fiber One

Oats & chocolate, 1 bar	2
Oats & peanut butter, 1 bar	3

General Foods Milk 'n Cereal Bar

Cinnamon toast crunch, 1 bar	4
Cocoa puffs, 1 bar	4
Honey nut cheerios, 1 bar	3

GeniSoy

Café mocha fudge, 1 bar	5
Chocolate caramel, 1 bar	3
Chocolate mint, 1 bar	5
Chunky peanut butter fudge, 1 bar	5
Cookies & cream, 1 bar	5
Honey peanut yogurt, 1 bar	5

GeniSoy Natural Choice All Natural Protein Bar

Chocolate peanut butter, 1 bar	4
Cookies & cream, 1 bar	4
Double chocolate, 1 bar	4
Lemon tart, 1 bar	4

GeniSoy Organic Protein

Apple cinnamon, 1 bar	3
Mixed berry flavor, 1 bar	3
Rich chocolate, 1 bar	3

GeniSoy Organic Protein Bars

Apple cinnamon, 1 bar	3
Mixed berry flavor, 1 bar	4
Rich chocolate, 1 bar	3

GeniSoy Ultra Bars

Chocolate caramel, 1 bar	3
Chocolate raspberry, 1 bar	3
Strawberry, 1 bar	3
Tropical, 1 bar	3

Health Valley

Apple cobbler cereal bar, 1	3
Baked apple tarts, 1 bar	3
Berry parfait yogurt bar, 1	2
Blueberry chewy granola bar, 1 bar	3

Breakfast, Cereals & Cereal Bars

	POINTS VALUE
Blueberry cobbler cereal bar, 1	3
Blueberry tarts bar, 1 bar	3
Café creations cinnamon Danish bar, 1 bar	2
Café creations vanilla crème bar, 1	3
Chocolate chip chewy granola bar, 1 bar	2
Chocolate tarts bar, 1 bar	3
Double chocolate chip chewy granola bar, 1 bar	3
Dutch apple chewy granola bar, 1 bar	2
Fig cobbler cereal bar, 1	2
French vanilla yogurt bar, 1	2
Peanut butter & chocolate bar, 1 bar	3
Peanut butter & grape bar, 1 bar	3
Peanut butter & strawberry bar, 1 bar	3
Peanut crunch chewy granola bar, 1 bar	2
Raspberry chewy granola bar, 1 bar	3
Raspberry tarts bar, 1 bar	3
Red cherry tarts bar, 1 bar	3
Strawberry cobbler cereal bar, 1	3
Strawberry tarts bar, 1 bar	3
Wild berry chewy granola bar, 1 bar	2
Healthy Snacker Bars	
Chocolate caramel crunch, 1 bar	4
Rocky road, 1 bar	4
Hostess	
Apple fruit & grain cereal bars, 1	2
Banana nut fruit & grain cereal bars, 1	3
Blueberry fruit & grain cereal bars, 1	2
Raspberry fruit & grain cereal bars, 1	2
Strawberry fruit & grain cereal bars, 1	2

	POINTS VALUE
Kashi	
Chewy granola bar, cherry dark chocolate, 1 bar	2
Chewy granola bar, chocolate raspberry, 1 bar	2
Chewy granola bar, dark chocolate coconut, 1 bar	2
Chewy granola bar, honey almond flax, 1 bar	2
Chewy granola bar, peanut butter, 1 bar	2
Chewy granola bar, pumpkin pie, 1 bar	2
Chewy granola bar, trail mix, 1 bar	2
Kashi Crunchy!	
Chocolate pretzel bar, 1 bar	3
Coffee cake bar, 1 bar	3
Kashi GOLEAN	
Original chocolate almond toffee bar, 1 bar	6
Original cookies 'n cream bar, 1 bar	6
Original malted chocolate crisp bar, 1 bar	6
Original oatmeal raisin cookie bar, 1 bar	5
Original peanut butter & chocolate bar, 1 bar	6
Kashi GOLEAN Crunchy!	
Chocolate almond bar, 1 bar	3
Chocolate caramel bar, 1 bar	2
Chocolate peanut butter bar, 1 bar	3
Kashi GOLEAN Roll!	
Caramel peanut bar, 1 bar	3
Chocolate peanut bar, 1 bar	3
Chocolate turtle bar, 1 bar	3
Fudge sundae bar, 1 bar	3
Oatmeal walnut bar, 1 bar	3

Breakfast, Cereals & Cereal Bars

	POINTS value
Kashi TLC	
Crunchy granola bar, honey toasted 7-grain, 2 bars	3
Crunchy granola bar, pumpkin spice flax, 2 bars	3
Crunchy granola bar, roasted almond crunch, 2 bars	3
Soft baked bar, baked apple spice, 1 bar	2
Soft baked bar, blackberry graham, 1 bar	2
Soft baked bar, ripe strawberry, 1 bar	2
Kellogg's	
All-bran fiber bar, apple cinnamon streusel, 1 bar	2
All-bran fiber bar, strawberry drizzle, 1 bar	2
Crunchy nut sweet & salty granola bar, chocolatey almond, 1 bar	3
Crunchy nut sweet & salty granola bar, chocolatey peanut, 1 bar	3
Crunchy nut sweet & salty granola bar, peanut butter, 1 bar	3
Fiber plus antioxidants, chocolate chip, 1 bar	2
Fiber plus antioxidants, dark chocolate almond, 1 bar	2
Kellogg's LiveBright	
Dark chocolate vanilla (DHA), 1 bar	3
Double chocolate (DHA), 1 bar	3
Kellogg's Nutri-grain	
Apple cinnamon, 1 bar	2
Blackberry, 1 bar	2

	POINTS value
Blueberry, 1 bar	2
Cherry, 1 bar	2
Fruit & nut bar, berry & almond, 1 bar	2
Fruit & nut bar, cranberry, raisin & peanut, 1 bar	2
Mixed berry, 1 bar	2
Raspberry, 1 bar	2
Strawberry, 1 bar	2
Strawberry yogurt, 1 bar	3
Vanilla yogurt, 1 bar	3
Kellogg's Special K	
Bliss bar, chocolatey dipped orange, 1 bar	2
Bliss bar, chocolatey dipped raspberry, 1 bar	2
Blueberry, 1 bar	2
Chocolatey drizzle, 1 bar	2
Cinnamon pecan, 1 bar	2
Honey nut, 1 bar	2
Peaches & berries, 1 bar	2
Protein meal replacement bar - chocolate peanut butter, 1 bar	3
Protein meal replacement bar - double chocolate, 1 bar	3
Protein meal replacement bar - honey almond, 1 bar	3
Protein meal replacement bar - strawberry, 1 bar	3
Protein meal replacement bar, chocolatey chip, 1 bar	3
Protein snack bar - chocolate delight, 1 bar	2

Breakfast, Cereals & Cereal Bars

	POINTS VALUE
Protein snack bar - chocolate peanut, 1 bar	2
Strawberry, 1 bar	2
Vanilla crisp, 1 bar	2
Kudos	
Milk chocolate granola snickers, 1 bar	2
Whole grain bars - chocolate chip, 1 bar	2
Whole grain bars - M&M's milk chocolate baking bits, 1 bar	2
Luna	
Berry almond, 1 bar	3
Caramel nut brownie, 1 bar	4
Chai tea, 1 bar	3
Chocolate raspberry, 1 bar	3
Chocolate pecan pie, 1 bar	3
Chocolate peppermint stick, 1 bar	3
Cookies 'n cream delight, 1 bar	3
Dulce de leche, 1 bar	3
Iced oatmeal raisin, 1 bar	3
Lemonzest, 1 bar	3
Nutz over chocolate, 1 bar	3
Peanut butter cookie, 1 bar	4
S'mores, 1 bar	3
Toasted nuts 'n cranberry, 1 bar	3
Luna Sunrise	
Apple cinnamon, 1 bar	3
Blueberry yogurt, 1 bar	3
Strawberries & crème, 1 bar	3
Vanilla almond, 1 bar	3
Luna Tea Cakes	
Berry pomegranate, 1 bar	3
Mint chocolate, 1 bar	2

	POINTS VALUE
Orange blossom, 1 bar	2
Vanilla macadamia, 1 bar	3
Market Day	
Quaker chewy granola bars (3 varieties), 1 bar	2
Nabisco 100 Calorie Packs	
Chips ahoy, 1 bar	2
Nutter butter, 1 bar	2
Oreo, 1 bar	2
Nabisco Honey Maid	
Oatmeal raisin bar, 1 bar	3
Soft baked blueberry bar, 1 bar	3
Nature Valley	
Granola bites, oats 'n honey, 1 pouch	1
Pecan crunch crunchy granola bar, 2 bars	4
Roasted almond crunchy granola bar, 2 bars	4
Nature Valley Chewy Granola Healthy Heart Bar	
Honey nut, 1 bar	3
Oatmeal raisin, 1 bar	3
Nature Valley Chewy Granola Trail Mix Bar	
Apple cinnamon, 1 bar	3
Fruit 'n nut, 1 bar	3
Mixed berry, 1 bar	3
Nature Valley Chewy Granola Yogurt Coated Bar	
Blueberry yogurt, 1 bar	3
Lemon yogurt, 1 bar	3
Strawberry yogurt, 1 bar	3
Vanilla yogurt, 1 bar	3

Breakfast, Cereals & Cereal Bars

	POINTS VALUE
Nature Valley Crunchy Granola Bar	
Apple crisp, 2 bars	4
Banana nut, 2 bars	4
Cinnamon, 2 bars	4
Maple brown sugar, 2 bars	4
Oats 'n honey, 2 bars	4
Peanut butter, 2 bars	4
Vanilla nut, 2 bars	4
Nature Valley Granola Sweet & Salty Bar	
Almond, 1 bar	3
Cashew, 1 bar	4
Peanut, 1 bar	4
Nature's Choice Multigrain Cereal Bars	
Apple-cinnamon, 1 bar	3
Blueberry, 1 bar	3
Cherry, 1 bar	3
Raspberry, 1 bar	3
Strawberry, 1 bar	3
Triple berry, 1 bar	3
Odwalla Bar!	
Berries gomega, 1 bar	4
Carrot, 1 bar	4
Chocolate, 1 bar	5
Chocolate chip peanut, 1 bar	5
Cranberry C monster, 1 bar	4
Peanut crunch, 1 bar	5
Super protein, 1 bar	5
Superfood, 1 bar	4
Otis Spunkmeyer Café Collection	
Double chocolate caramel bar with snickers, 2 oz	6

	POINTS VALUE
Pecan pie bar, 2 oz	6
Raspberry bar, 2 oz	5
Philadelphia Snack Bars	
Strawberry cheesecake snack bars, 1	4
Post	
Grape nuts trail mix crunch bar, fruit & nut, 1 bar	2
Honey bunches of oats, banana nut, 1 bar	2
Honey bunches of oats, cranberry almond, 1 bar	2
Honey bunches of oats, strawberry, 1 bar	2
Raisin bran, cinnamon, 1 bar	2
Raisin bran, cranberry, 1 bar	2
Quaker Fruit & Oatmeal Bar	
Oatmeal on the go, baked apple, 1 bar	3
Oatmeal on the go, cinnamon roll with raisins, 1 bar	3
Oatmeal on the go, wild berry, 1 bar	3
Quaker Oats	
Q-smart bar - cranberry almond, 1 bar	2
Q-smart bar - peanut butter chocolate, 1 bar	3
Quaker Oats Baked Fruit Crisp Bars	
Apple crisp, 1 bar	3
Mixed berry, 1 bar	3
Strawberry, 1 bar	3
Quaker Oats Baked Muffin Bars	
Banana, 1 bar	2
Blueberry, 1 bar	2
Quaker Oats Breakfast Cookie	
Chocolate chip, 1	3

Breakfast, Cereals & Cereal Bars

	POINTS VALUE
Quaker Oats Breakfast/Bites	
Apple crisp, 1 serving (37 g)	2
Raspberry with icing, 1 serving (37 g)	2
Strawberry, 1 serving (37 g)	2
Strawberry with icing, 1 serving (37 g)	2
Quaker Oats Chewy Dipps	
Chocolate chip, 1 bar	3
Peanut butter, 1 bar	3
Quaker Oats Chewy Granola Bar	
Butterfinger pieces, 1	2
Chocolate chip, 1	2
Chocolate chunk, 1	2
Cookies and cream, 1	2
Dark chocolate cherry, 1	2
Peanut butter, 1	2
Peanut butter & chocolate chip, 1	2
Peanut butter & chocolate chunk, 1	2
S'mores, 1	2
Strawberry vanilla, 1	2
Quaker Oats Chewy Granola Bar - 90 Calories	
Baked apple, 1 bar	2
Cinnamon sugar, 1 bar	2
Maple brown sugar, 1 bar	2
Oatmeal raisin, 1 bar	2
Quaker Oats Simple Harvest	
Chocolate chunk bar, 1 bar	3
Cinnamon brown sugar bar, 1 bar	3
Quaker Oats Simple Harvest Bar	
Honey roasted nuts bar, 1 bar	3

	POINTS VALUE
Quaker Oats Sweet & Salty	
Honey roasted peanut crunch bar, 2 bars	3
Oats, nuts & honey crunch bar, 2 bars	3
Toffee nut crunch bar, 2 bars	3
Real Organic Bars	
Real berry nut, 1 bar	1
Real green nut, 1 bar	1
Ruth's Foods	
Cranberry almond bar, 1	3
Cranberry trail bar, 1	4
Crannut flax bar, 1	3
Ginger almond maca bar, 1	3
Peanut butter banana bar, 1	4
Very berry flax bar, 1	4
Vote hemp bar, 1	4
Snickers	
Marathon caramel nut surge, 1 bar (singles)	6
Marathon chewy chocolate peanut, 1 bar (singles)	4
Marathon chocolate nut burst, 1 bar (singles)	6
Marathon dark chocolate crunch, 1 bar	3
Marathon honey & toasted almond, 1 bar	3
Marathon multi grain crunch, 1 bar (singles)	4
Sunbelt	
Chewy granola bars - chocolate chip, 1 bar	4
Chewy granola bars - golden almond, 1 bar	3

Breakfast, Cereals & Cereal Bars

Sunbelt (cont'd)	POINTS VALUE
Chewy granola bars - lowfat oatmeal raisin, 1 bar	3
Chewy granola bars - oats & honey, 1 bar	3
Chewy granola bars - peanut butter chip, 1 bar	4
Crunchy granola bars - oats & honey, 1 bar	3
Fruit & grain bars - apple-cinnamon, 1 bar	3
Fruit & grain bars - blueberry, 1 bar	3
Fruit & grain bars - raspberry, 1 bar	3
Fruit & grain bars - strawberry, 1 bar	3
S'mores granola treats, 1 bar	3
Uncle Sam	
Cereal bars, 1 bar	3
Weight Watchers Snack Bars	
Baked apple 'n cinnamon 1 bar	2
Banana nut bread, 1 bar	2
Chocolate chip brownie, 1 bar	2
Double chocolate delight, 1 bar	2
Fruity nutty madness, 1 bar	2
Sweet & salty, 1 bar	2
Weight Watchers Mini Bars	
Chocolate caramel mini bars, 1 bar	1
Cookies & cream mini bars, 1 bar	1
Dark chocolate raspberry mini bars, 1 bar	1
Mint cookie crisp mini bars, 1 bar	1
Peanut butter bliss mini bars, 1 bar	1
Red velvet mini bars, 1 bar	1

	POINTS VALUE
Omelets & French Toast	
Ian's	
Banana French toast stick, 1 serving (91 g)	5
Cinnamon & honey French toast sticks, 1 serving (91 g)	5
Triple berry French toast stick, 1 serving (91 g)	5
Wheat free, gluten free French toast sticks, 1 serving (91 g)	5
Kellogg's Eggo	
French toaster sticks - cinnamon, 2 sticks	5
French toaster sticks - maple, 1 piece	3
French toaster sticks - original, 2 sticks	5
Market Day	
Cinnamon crunch French toast bites, 6 pieces	7
French toast sticks, 4 pieces	6
Pillsbury	
French toast sticks - original, 6	5
Pancakes	
Aunt Jemima	
Buckwheat pancake mix, 1/4 cup	1
Buttermilk complete mix, 1/3 cup	2
Buttermilk pancake mix, 1/4 cup	2
Complete pancake mix, 1/3 cup	3
Original pancake mix, 1/3 cup	3
Reduced calorie buttermilk complete mix, 1/3 cup	2
Whole wheat mix, 1/4 cup	2

	POINTS VALUE
Batter Blaster	
Organic pancake and waffle batter, 1/4 cup (4" pancake)	2
Betty Crocker	
Complete buttermilk mix (box), 1/3 cup	4
Complete buttermilk mix (pouch), 1/2 cup	4
Complete original mix (box), 1/3 cup	4
Bisquick Shake 'N Pour	
Buttermilk, 3	4
Cherrybrook Kitchen	
Gluten free pancake and waffle mix, 1 serving (mix for 1 pancake)	2
Original pancake mix, 1 serving (mix for one 4" pancake)	2
Whole grain pancake mix, 1 serving (mix for one 4" pancake)	1
Gladiola	
Pancake & waffle mix, prepared, 1 serving (162 g)	7
Heidi's	
Cottage cheese pancake mix (original), 1/4 cup	3
Grainy day pancake mix, 1/3 cup	3
Oats n' apple pancake mix, 1/3 cup	4
Sourdough pancake mix, 1/3 cup	4
Whole wheat cottage cheese pancake mix, 1/4 cup	3
Hodgson Mill	
Buckwheat pancake mix, 1/3 cup	2
Multi grain buttermilk pancake mix with milled flaxseed, 1/3 cup	2
Whole wheat buttermilk pancake mix, 1/3 cup	2

	POINTS VALUE
Jiffy Mixes	
Buttermilk complete pancake & waffle mix, dry, 1/3 cup	4
Kellogg's Eggo	
Blueberry pancakes, 3	5
Buttermilk, 3	6
Buttermilk mini-pancakes, 11	6
Nutrigrain pancakes, 3	5
Pancakes jungle, 3	6
Pancakes, chocolate chip, 3	6
Maple Grove	
Blueberry pancake mix, dry, 1/3 cup	3
Blueberry pancake mix, prepared, 1 serving (110 g)	5
Buckwheat pancake mix, dry, 1/3 cup	2
Buttermilk & honey pancake mix, dry, 1/3 cup	3
Buttermilk & honey pancake mix, prepared, 1 serving (110 g)	5
Buttermilk pancake mix, dry, 1/3 cup	2
Buttermilk pancake mix, prepared, 1/3 cup	5
Gluten free pancake mix, dry, 1/4 cup	2
Honey buckwheat pancake mix, dry, 1/3 cup	3
Honey buckwheat pancake mix, prepared, 1 serving (110 g)	5
Multigrain pancake mix, dry, 1/3 cup	3
Sugar free pancake mix, dry, 1/3 cup	2
Wholegrain with flax seed pancake mix, dry, 1/4 cup	2
Wholegrain with flax seed pancake mix, prepared, 1 serving (110 g)	4

Breakfast, Cereals & Cereal Bars

	POINTS VALUE
Market Day	
Banana mini pancakes, 6	2
Chocolate chip mini pancakes, 6 pieces	3
Microwave pancakes, 3	4
Martha White	
Flapstax pancake mix, 1/2 cup	5
Pillsbury	
Blueberry, 3	4
Buttermilk, 3	5
Buttermilk mini's, 11	5
Chocolate burst, 3	6
Maple burst, 3	6
Mini buttermilk pancakes, 16	4
Original, 3	5
Pillsbury Mini Pancakes with Dippin' Cups	
Blueberry, 14	9
Buttermilk, 14	9
Sweet 'N Low	
Pancake mix, prepared, 1 serving (45 g)	3

Waffles

	POINTS VALUE
EnviroKidz	
Gorilla banana waffles, 2	4
Koala choco waffles, 2	4
Kashi GOLEAN	
Blueberry, 2	3
Original, 2	3
Strawberry waffles, 2	3
Kashi Heart to Heart	
Honey oat waffles, 2	3

	POINTS VALUE
Kellogg's	
Nutri-grain blueberry waffles, 2	3
Kellogg's Eggo	
Apple cinnamon, 2	4
Banana bread, 2	4
Blueberry, 2	4
Brown sugar & cinnamon flip flop waffles, 2	4
Buttermilk, 2	4
Buttery syrup mini waffles, 3	6
Chocolate chip, 2	5
Choco-nilla flip flop waffles, 2	4
Cinnamon toast mini, 1 serving (3 sets of 4 waffles)	7
French vanilla, 2	4
Homestyle, 2	4
Homestyle mini, 1 serving (3 sets of 4 waffles)	6
Lego waffles, 2	4
Nutri-grain, 2	3
Nutri-grain cinnamon, 2	3
Nutri-grain low fat, 2	2
Shrek homestyle, 2	4
Special K - low fat waffles, 2	3
Strawberry, 2	4
Waffles - French toast, 1	3
Waffles - special k red berries low fat, 2	3

	POINTS VALUE
Lifestream	
8 grain sesame, 2	5
Buckwheat wildberry, 2	5
Flax plus, 2	5
Hemp plus, 2	4
Mesa sunrise, 2	4
Soy plus, 2	4
Maple Grove	
Belgian waffle mix, dry, 1/4 cup	3

	POINTS VALUE
Nature's Path	
Optimum power waffles, 2	3
Pillsbury	
Blueberry, 2	4
Buttermilk, 2	4
Homestyle, 2	4
Waffle sticks - homestyle, 6	5

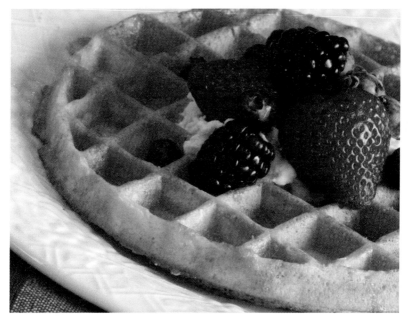

Candy, Cookies & Desserts

Breath Mints
Tic Tac

Cinnamon, 1 piece	0
Fresh mints, 1 piece	0
Orange mints, 1 piece	0
Spearmints, 1 piece	0
Wintergreen, 1 piece	0

Candy
3 Musketeers

3 musketeers bar, 1 small bar (fun size)	1
3 musketeers bar, 1 large bar	6
3 musketeers bar, 7 pieces (miniatures)	4
3 musketeers bar - mint, 1 bar (fun size)	2
3 musketeers bar - mint, 2 pieces (35 g)	4

Andes

Cherry jubilee thins, 8 pieces	5
Creme de menthe changemaker, 3 pieces	5
Creme de menthe thins, 8 pieces	5
Mint parfait thins, 8 pieces	5
Mocha mint, 4 pieces	5
Peppermint crunch, 4 pieces	5
Sugar free crème de menthe, 6 pieces	4
Toffee crunch thins, 8 pieces	5

Annabelle Candy Company

Abba-zabba bar, 1 bar	5
Abba-zabba sour apple, 1 bar	5
Big hunk candy bar, 1 bar	5
Look bar, 1 bar	4
Skinny hunk, 1 bar	2
U-no bar, 1 bar	6

Annie's Homegrown

Organic bunny fruit snacks, berry patch, 1 pouch	1
Organic bunny fruit snacks, tropical treat, 1 pouch	1

Be Happy & Healthy

Yummy gummy in my tummy, 18 pieces	3

Brookside

Cocoa clodhoppers, 1 package	3
Dark chocolate almonds, 8 pieces	5
Macaroons, 11 pieces	4
Starbuds, 11 pieces	4
Vanilla clodhoppers, 1 package	3
X-treme fruit bites, atomic apple, 1 package	1
X-treme fruit bites, charg-n cherry, 1 package	1
X-treme fruit bites, chili lime fusion, 1 package	1
X-treme fruit bites, citrus cyclone, 1 package	1

Cadbury's

Caramello, 1 bar	5
Crème egg, 1 piece	3
Dairy milk chocolate bar, 7 blocks	5
Fruit & nut chocolate bar, 7 blocks	4
Mini-eggs, 12 pieces	4
Roast almond chocolate bar, 7 blocks	5
Royal dark chocolate bar, 7 blocks	4

Cambridge Brands

Caramel apple sugar babies, 22 pieces	3
Charleston chew vanilla, 1 (53 g)	5

Candy, Cookies & Desserts

	POINTS VALUE
Charleston chew, chocolate, 1 (53 g)	5
Charleston chew, strawberry, 1 (53 g)	5
Charleston chew, vanilla, 13 pieces (39 g)	4
Charleston mini chews, 1 serving (24 g)	4
Chocolate sugar babies, 19 pieces	4
Easter sugar babies, 22 pieces	3
Holiday sugar babies, 22 pieces	3
Junior caramels, 2 boxes (24 g)	2
Junior caramels, 13 pieces	4
Junior mints, 16 pieces	3
Junior mints, 1 box (18 g)	2
Junior mints deluxe, 3 pieces	4
Junior mints inside-out, 15 pieces	4
Sugar babies, 2 boxes (35 g)	3
Sugar babies, 27 pieces	3
Sugar daddy, junior pop, 3	3
Sugar daddy, large pop, 1	4
Sugar mama, 7 pieces	3
Cella's	
Dark chocolate covered cherries, 3 pieces	3
Milk chocolate covered cherries, 3 pieces	4
Charm's	
Blow pop mini's, 8 pieces	1
Blow pop, junior, 1	1
Blow pop, regular, 1	1
Blow pop, super, 1	3
Blue razzberry blow pops, 1	1
Charm's way -2- sour blow pop, junior, 1	1

	POINTS VALUE
Charm's way -2- sour blow pop, regular, 1	1
Charm's way -2- sour blow pop, super, 1	3
Fluffy stuff, 1 bag	2
Fluffy stuff, 1 small bag	1
Maxxed energy pop, 1	2
Sour balls, 1	0
Sour pop, regular flat pop, 1	1
Squares, 2 pieces	0
Sweet pop, junior flat pop, 1	1
Sweet pop, regular flat pop, 1	1
Sweet/sour pop, regular flat pop, 1	1
Tear jerkers cotton candy, 1 bag	2
Tropical stormz, 1	1
Zip-a-dee-doo-da pop, 3	1
Dove	
Dark chocolate, 1 bar (36.9 g)	5
Dark chocolate, 1 bar (3 bar pack)	4
Dark chocolate, 5 pieces	5
Dark chocolate - 63% cacao, 1 bar	4
Dark chocolate - 71% cacao, 1 bar	5
Dark chocolate - cranberry almond, 1 bar	4
Dark chocolate - roasted almond, 1 bar	4
Dark chocolate with mint caramel, 5 pieces (miniatures)	5
Dark chocolate with raspberry caramel, 5 pieces (miniatures)	5
Milk chocolate, 1 bar (36.9 g)	5
Milk chocolate, 1 bar (3 bar pack)	4
Milk chocolate, 5 pieces	5

Candy, Cookies & Desserts

Dove (cont'd)	POINTS VALUE
Milk chocolate - blueberry almond, 1 bar	4
Milk chocolate - extra creamy, 1 bar	4
Milk chocolate - peanut toffee crunch, 1 bar	4
Milk chocolate - roasted almond, 1 bar	4
Milk chocolate - roasted hazelnut, 1 bar	5
Sugar free dark chocolates - double chocolate crème, 5 pieces (miniatures)	4
Sugar free dark chocolates - mint crème, 5 pieces (miniatures)	5
Sugar free dark chocolates - raspberry crème, 5 pieces (miniatures)	5

Dove Miniatures

	POINTS VALUE
Caramel, 5 pieces	5
Dark chocolate - roasted almond, 5 pieces	5
Dark chocolate - tiramisu caramel, 5 pieces	5
Milk chocolate - roasted almond, 5 pieces	5
Milk chocolate caramel, 5 pieces	5

Estee

	POINTS VALUE
Dark chocolate bars, 7 squares	5
Milk chocolate bars, 7 squares	6
Milk chocolate with almonds bar, 7 squares	6
Milk chocolate with crisp rice bar, 1 bar	10
No sugar added caramels, 5 pieces	3
Peanut brittle - no sugar added, 1 1/2 oz	5
Peanut butter cups, 5	5

	POINTS VALUE
Sugar free assorted fruit gum drops, 11 pieces	2
Sugar free assorted fruit hard, 3 pieces	0
Sugar free hard butterscotch, 3 pieces	0
Sugar free hard peppermint, 3 pieces	0
Sugar free hard tropical fruit, 3 pieces	0
Sugar free toffee hard, 3 pieces	0

Estee Smart Treats

	POINTS VALUE
Sugar free chocolate fudge candy bar, 1	2
Sugar free cookie dough candy bar, 1	1
Sugar free gourmet jelly beans, 26 pieces	2
Sugar free gummy bears, 17 pieces	1
Sugar free raspberry candy bar, 1	2
Sugar free sour citrus slices, 15 pieces	2

Fastbreak

	POINTS VALUE
Fastbreak, 1 bar	6

Ferrero Rondnoir

	POINTS VALUE
Fine dark chocolates, 1 package	4

Fling

	POINTS VALUE
Dark chocolate bar, 1	2
Milk chocolate bar, 1	2
Milk chocolate hazelnut bar, 1	2

Fling Singles

	POINTS VALUE
Milk chocolate bar, 2	4

Guylian

	POINTS VALUE
Belgian dark chocolate orange, no sugar added, 8 squares	3
Belgian dark chocolate, no sugar added, 8 squares	3

	POINTS VALUE
Belgian milk chocolate, no sugar added, 8 squares	3
Extra dark 70% cocoa, no sugar added, 8 squares	4
La trufflina, 3 pieces	5
Opus (assorted Belgian chocolates), 3 pieces	6
Seashells, 4 pieces	6
Guylian Solitaire	
Assorted dark chocolates, 6 pieces	3
Guylian Solitaire Extra Dark	
Extra dark 70% cocoa, 6 pieces	3
Guylian Twists	
Assorted dark, 5 pieces	6
Dark chocolate orange cream, 5 pieces	6
Milk chocolate truffle, 5 pieces	6
Original praline, 4 pieces	5
Hershey's	
100 calorie pretzel bar, 1 bar	2
100 calorie wafer bar, 1 bar	2
5th avenue, 1 bar (56 g)	6
Almond joy bar, 1 bar (45 g)	5
Baking bits Heath - English toffee, 1 Tbsp	2
Chips, mini milk chocolate bars, 1 Tbsp	2
Chips, peanut butter, 1 Tbsp	2
Chips, semi-sweet, 1 Tbsp	2
Chips, special dark, 1 Tbsp	2
Chips, white, 1 Tbsp	2
Chocolate covered marshmallow eggs, 1	2
Cookies n crème, 1 bar (43 g)	5

	POINTS VALUE
Dark chocolate (100 calorie bar), 1 bar	2
Dark chocolate nuggets with almonds, 4 pieces	4
Extra dark chocolate bar, 3 blocks	3
Good & plenty, 1 box (51 g)	4
Heath milk chocolate English toffee bar, 1 bar (39 g)	5
Hershey-ets (pastel), 42 pieces	4
Hugs, 9 pieces	5
Kissables, 1 package	4
Kisses milk chocolate with almonds, 9 pieces	5
Kisses milk chocolates, 9 pieces	5
Kisses milk chocolates filled with caramel, 9 pieces	5
Kisses milk chocolates filled with peanut butter, 9 pieces	5
Kisses, dark chocolate, 9 pieces	4
Kisses, milk chocolates filled with cherry cordial crème, 9 pieces	4
Kit kat wafer bar, 1 (4-piece bar)	5
Kit Kat wafer bar, white chocolate, 1 (4-piece bar)	5
Milk chocolate bar, 1 bar (43 g)	5
Milk chocolate bar with almonds, 1 bar (41 g)	5
Milk duds, 1 box (52 g)	5
Mini robin eggs, 1 box (52 g)	5
Miniatures, 5 pieces	5
Mr. Goodbar, 1 bar (49 g)	6
Nuggets, chocolate, 4 pieces	5
Nuggets, chocolates with raisins and almonds, 4 pieces	5

Candy, Cookies & Desserts

Hershey's (cont'd)

	POINTS VALUE
Nuggets, chocolates with toffee and almonds, 4 pieces	5
Nuggets, chocolate with almond, 4 pieces	5
Payday, 1 bar (52 g)	5
Rolo, 1 package	5
Special dark, 1 bar (41 g)	4
Symphony almond and toffee, 1 bar (42 g)	5
Symphony milk chocolate, 5 blocks	5
Take 5 candy bar, 1 package	5
Whatchamacallit, 1 bar (45 g)	5
Zagnut, 1 bar (49 g)	5

Hershey's Bliss

Dark chocolate, 6 pieces	5
Milk chocolate, 6 pieces	5
Milk chocolate, chocolate crème filled, 6 pieces	5

Hershey's Sugar Free

Sugar-free dark chocolate, 5 pieces	3
York peppermint patties, 3 pieces	2

Hershey's Sugar Free Bars

Chocolate, 5 pieces	4
Dark chocolate, 5 pieces	3

Jelly Belly

Jelly beans, 1 package (1 oz)	2

Jolly Rancher

Fruit chews, 1 package (58 g)	4
Gummis, 9 pieces	2
Hard candy twists assortment, 3 pieces	1
Jelly beans, 30 pieces	2

	POINTS VALUE
Lollipops, 1 piece	1

Kellogg's Yogos

Yogurty covered fruit bits, berry berry banana, 1 pouch	2
Yogurty covered fruit snack, watermelon splash, 1 pouch	2

Kraft

Caramels, 5 pieces	3

Kraft Jet-Puffed

Bunnymallows marshmallows, 15 pieces	2
Funmallows miniature marshmallows, 1 serving (30 g)	2
Holidaymallows marshmallows, 28 pieces	2
Marshmallow crème, 1 serving (13 g)	1
Marshmallow, mini, 2/3 cup	2
Marshmallow, regular, 4 pieces	2
Miniature marshmallows, 1 packet	2

Lance

Cinnamon chewz, 11 pieces	2
Fruit chewz, 11 pieces	2
Peanut bar, 1	6
Peanut bar, 1 small	6
Peppermint chewz, 11 pieces	2
Strawberry chewz, 11 pieces	2

M&M's

Almond chocolate candies, 1 1/2 oz	5
Almond chocolate candies, 1 bag (34 g)	4
Dark chocolate candies, 1 bag (42.5 g)	5
Dark chocolate candies, 1/3 cup	5
Milk chocolate, 1 1/2 oz	5

	POINTS VALUE
Milk chocolate, 1 bag (47.9 g)	5
Milk chocolate, 1 small bag (fun size)	2
Peanut butter chocolate candies, 1 1/2 oz	6
Peanut butter chocolate candies, 1 bag (39.7 g)	6
Peanut chocolate candies, 1 1/2 oz	5
Peanut chocolate candies, 1 bag (49.3 g)	6
Peanut chocolate candies, 1 small bag (fun size)	2
M&M's Minis	
Milk chocolate candies, 1 pack	3
Milk chocolate candies, 1 tube	4
Mamba	
Fruit chews, 6 pieces	2
Sour fruit chews, 6 pieces	2
Merci	
Assortment of European chocolates, 4 pieces	7
Milka	
Milk chocolate, 1 serving (33 g)	4
Truffle bar cookies & crème, 1 serving (33 g)	4
Milky Way	
Midnight bar, 5 pieces (miniatures)	4
Midnight bar, 1 bar (singles)	5
Milky way bar, 1 bar (fun size)	2
Milky way bar, 5 small bars (miniatures)	4
Milky way bar, 1 large bar	6
Munch	
Nut bar, 1	5

	POINTS VALUE
Nabisco 100 Calorie Packs	
Chips ahoy candy bites, 1 pouch	2
Oreo candy bites, 1 pouch	2
Nestle	
100 Grand, 1 bar (43 g)	4
Baby Ruth, 1 (59.5 g)	7
Baby Ruth - fun size, 2	3
Baby Ruth sugar free, 1 bar (36.8 g)	3
Bit-o-honey, 1 (48.1 g)	4
Buncha crunch, 1 bag	4
Butterfinger, 1 (59.5 g)	6
Butterfinger - fun size, 1	2
Butterfinger BB's, 1 bag	5
Butterfinger bunny, 1 serving (1.5 oz)	5
Butterfinger crisp mini, 4 bars (44 g)	5
Butterfinger crisp single, 1 bar (50 g)	6
Butterfinger heart bag, 5 pieces	4
Butterfinger heart singles, 1 piece	4
Butterfinger pieces in milk chocolate, 1 serving (1/5 bar)	4
Butterfinger pumpkins, 5 pieces	5
Chunky bar, 1 (39.6 g)	5
Creme eggs - baby ruth, 1	4
Crunch, 1 (43.9 g)	5
Crunch - fun size, 4	5
Crunch assorted minis, 4 pieces	5
Crunch bunny, 1 serving (1.5 oz)	5
Crunch dark, 1 bar (1.4 oz)	4
Crunch dark heart, 1 piece	3
Crunch dark stixx, 1 stick	2
Crunch dark with caramel, 1 bar (1.52 oz)	5

Candy, Cookies & Desserts

Nestle (cont'd)	POINTS VALUE
Crunch disk (Easter/Xmas), 1	4
Crunch harvest pumpkins, 5 pieces	4
Crunch heart bag, 5 pieces	4
Crunch heart singles, 1 piece	3
Crunch stixx, 1 stick	2
Crunch sugar free, 4 bars	4
Crunch sugar free, 1 bar (1.1 oz)	4
Crunch with caramel, 1 bar (1.52 oz)	5
Crunch with caramel, 2 bars (fun size)	4
Fun dips (3 cells), 1 serving (2/3 of a stick and 1 packet powder)	1
Goobers, 1 bag (39.1 g)	5
Jingles crunch, 5 pieces	4
Jingles dark chocolate, 5 pieces	5
Jingles milk chocolate, 5 pieces	5
Jingles milk chocolate with butterfingers, 5 pieces	4
Milk chocolate, 1 (41.1 g)	5
Mini shock tarts, 20 pieces	1
Nerds rope, 1	2
Nesteggs caramel, 5 pieces	5
Nesteggs crunch, 5 pieces	4
Nesteggs dark chocolate, 6 pieces	5
Nesteggs milk chocolate, 5 pieces	5
Nesteggs milk chocolate with butterfingers, 5 pieces	5
Nesteggs peanut butter, 5 pieces	5
Nips, butter rum, 2 pieces	1
Nips, caramel, 2 pieces	1
Nips, chocolate parfait, 2 pieces	1
Nips, coffee, 2 pieces	1

	POINTS VALUE
Nips, peanut butter parfait, 2 pieces	1
Oh Henry!, 1 (26 g)	3
Pixy stix (3 pack), 3	1
Raisinets, 1 bag (44.7 g)	4
Sno caps, 1/4 cup	4
Spree - mini chewy, 16 pieces	1
Spree - regular, 8 pieces	1
SweeTarts - mini chewy, 23 pieces	1
SweeTarts - regular, 8 pieces	1
Treasures - chocolate crème, 3 pieces	4
Treasures - peanut butter, 3 pieces	4
Treasures - w/caramel, 3 pieces	4
Turtles, 2 pieces	4
White crunch, 1 (39.6 g)	5
Wonderball, 1	3
Odense	
Marzipan, 2 Tbsp	4
Pangburn's	
Millionaires, 2 pieces	6
Peter Paul	
Mounds, 1 package (49 g)	5
Planters	
Original peanut bar, 1 package (45 g)	5
Reed's	
Rootbeer, 1 piece	1
Reese's	
100 calorie wafer bar, 1 bar	3
Clusters, pecan caramel, 3 pieces	5
Crispy crunchy bar, 1 bar	6
Miniature peanut butter cups, 5 pieces	5
Nutrageous, 1 bar	6

	POINTS VALUE
Peanut butter cup, 1 package (2 cups)	5
Peanut butter cup miniatures, 5 pieces	5
Pieces, 1 package	5
Reesesticks, 1 package	5
Whipps, 1 bar	5
Reese's Sugar Free	
Peanut butter cups, miniature, 5 pieces	4
Riesen	
Chewy chocolate caramel, with 45% cacao, 4 pieces	4
Russell Stover	
Assorted chocolates, 2 pieces	3
Cherry cordials, 3 pieces	3
Chocolate covered nuts, 3 pieces	5
Double pecan delight, 2 pieces	6
French chocolate mint miniatures, 5 pieces	5
Milk chocolate toffee sticks, 4	6
Mint patties, 3 pieces	4
Pecan delight, 2 pieces	7
Pecan delight bars, 2 pieces	4
Truffle assortment, 3 pieces	5
Russell Stover Elegant	
Assorted chocolates, 3 pieces	5
Russell Stover Internationale	
French café vanilla crème, 2 pieces	4
German black forest truffle, 2 pieces	4
Swiss lodge mocha cream, 2 pieces	4
Russell Stover Private Reserve	
70% cacao toasted south seas coconut, 3 pieces	5
Assorted box, 3 pieces	5

	POINTS VALUE
Milk chocolate mocha ganache, 2 pieces	4
Triple chocolate mousse, 2 pieces	5
Vanilla bean brulee, 2 pieces	4
Russell Stover Private Reserve Origin Select	
Assorted box, 3 pieces	5
Belgian, 3 pieces	6
Ecuador dark, 3 pieces	4
Ghana dark, 3 pieces	4
Venezuela dark, 3 pieces	5
Russell Stover Urban	
Assorted chocolates, 3 pieces	5
Skittles	
Original bite size candies, 1 bag (fun size)	2
Original bite size candies, 1 1/2 oz (about 1/4 cup)	4
Original bite size candies, 1 single bag (singles)	5
Skittles sour, 1 bag (51 g)	4
Skittles sour, 1 small bag (fun size)	2
Skittles sour, 1 1/2 oz	3
Tropical bite size candies, 1 single bag (singles)	5
Tropical bite size candies, 1 bag (fun size)	2
Tropical bite size candies, 1 1/2 oz (about 1/4 cup)	4
Wild berry bite size candies, 1 single bag (singles)	5
Wild berry bite size candies, 1 1/2 oz (about 1/4 cup)	4
Wild berry bite size candies, 1 bag (fun size)	2

Candy, Cookies & Desserts

	POINTS VALUE
Snickers	
Snickers almond, 1 bar (49.9 g)	5
Snickers almond bar, 4 pieces (miniatures)	4
Snickers almond bar, 1 (fun size)	2
Snickers bar, 1 large bar	7
Snickers bar, 4 miniatures	4
Snickers bar, 1 bar (fun size)	2
Starburst	
Fruit chews, California fruits, 8 pieces	4
Fruit chews, California fruits, 1 package (58.7 g)	5
Fruit chews, fruit & crème, 8	3
Fruit chews, fruit & crème, 8 small (fun size)	3
Fruit chews, fruit & crème, 1 package (58.7 g)	5
Fruit chews, original fruits, 8 pieces	4
Fruit chews, original fruits, 1 package (58.7 g)	5
Fruit chews, tropical fruits, 8 pieces	4
Fruit chews, tropical fruits, 1 package (58.7 g)	5
Gummibursts, 1 bag (42.5 g)	3
Jelly beans original fruits, 1/4 cup	3
Sour gummibursts, 1 bag (42.5 g)	3
Sunbelt	
Fruit jammers gummy bears, 1 pouch	2
Terry's	
Milk chocolate orange, 1 serving (44 g)	5
Pure milk chocolate, 1 serving (44 g)	6

	POINTS VALUE
Tic Tac	
Cherry passion, 1 piece	0
Citrus twist, 1 piece	0
Toblerone	
Swiss bittersweet with honey & almond nougat, 1 serving (33 g)	4
Swiss milk chocolate with honey & almond nougat, 1 (50 g)	6
Swiss milk chocolate with honey & almond nougat, 1 serving (40 g)	5
Swiss milk chocolate with honey & almond nougat, 1 small (35 g)	4
Swiss milk chocolate with honey & almond nougat, 1 small serving (33 g)	4
Swiss minis milk chocolate with honey & almond nougat, 1 serving (38 g)	5
Swiss white confection with honey & almond nougat, 1 serving (33 g)	4
Toffifay	
Caramel/hazelnut/chocolate candy, 5 pieces	5
Tootsie Roll	
Candy cane pops, 1	1
Caramel apple pops, 1	1
Caramel tootsie pops, 1	1
Chocolate tootsie pops, 1	1
Crows, 12 pieces	3
Mason dots, 12 pieces	3
Mini chews, 2 boxes	2
Mini chews, 30 pieces	4
Mini chews, 1 large serving (36 g)	3
Tootsie frooties, 13 pieces	3

	POINTS VALUE
Tootsie fruit rolls, 6 pieces	3
Tootsie miniature pops, 1	1
Tootsie miniature pops sugar free, 1	1
Tootsie pops, 1 small	1
Tootsie pops, 1 regular	1
Tootsie roll, 1/2 large	3
Tootsie roll, 1/2 regular	2
Tootsie roll, 1 serving (40 g)	3
Tootsie roll, 3 snack bars	3
Tootsie roll, 6 regular (midgees)	3
Tootsie roll, 13 small (midgees)	3
Tootsie roll, 4 pieces	3
Tropical dots, 12 pieces	3
Wild berry dots, 12	3
Wild berry pops, 1	1
Tree of Life	
Carob malt balls, 1 serving (40 g)	5
Trolli Gummy Candy	
Classic bears, 1 serving (40 g)	3
Melon-o's, 1 serving (39 g)	3
Peachie-o's, 1 bag (35 g)	2
Peachie-o's, 1 serving (39 g)	3
Road kill, 1 serving (39 g)	3
Rocket racers, 1 serving (38 g)	2
Small brite crawlers, 1 serving (39 g)	2
Sour apple-o's, 1 serving (39 g)	3
Sour brite crawler eggs, 1 serving (40 g)	3
Sour brite crawlers, 1 serving (36 g)	2
Sour brite crawlers, 1 bag (43 g)	3
Sour brite octopus, 1 serving (36 g)	2
Squiggles, 1 serving (38 g)	3

	POINTS VALUE
Stingin' red ants hot cinnamon, 1 bag (35 g)	2
Stingin' red ants hot cinnamon, 1 serving (39 g)	3
Strawberry puffs, 1 serving (39 g)	3
Tropical Nut & Fruit	
Chocolate pops, Halloween, 1 serving (40 g)	5
Lindor truffles, 3 balls	6
Triple treat almonds, 9 pieces	4
Triple treat cashews, 9 pieces	5
Triple treat pecans, 9 pieces	4
Twix	
Caramel cookie bar, 1 large bar (family pack)	3
Caramel cookie bar, 3 pieces	3
Caramel cookie bar, 1 small bar (fun size)	2
Caramel cookie bar, 2 bars	7
Peanut butter cookie bar, 1 small bar (family pack)	3
Peanut butter cookie bar, 2 large bars	7
Peanut butter cookie bar, 1 bar (fun size)	2
Twizzlers	
100 calorie rainbow, 1 package	2
Cherry bites, 17 pieces	3
Pull-n-peel cherry, 2 pieces	3
Sourz assortment, 1 package	4
Strawberry, 1 package	5
Twerpz, 1 package	4
Young & smylie, black licorice, 11 pieces	3

Candy, Cookies & Desserts

Twizzlers (cont'd)	POINTS VALUE
Young & smylie, peach mango, 11 pieces	3
Young & smylie, strawberry, 11 pieces	3
Weight Watchers	
Cappuccino cream melts, 2 pieces	0
Weight Watchers by Whitman's	
Almond nougat, 3 pieces	3
Caramel medallions, 3 pieces	3
Coconut, 3 pieces	3
Crispy butter cream caramel, 3 pieces	3
Double chocolate mousse, 3 pieces	3
English toffee squares, 3 pieces	3
Mint patties, 3 pieces	3
Nougie nutty chew, 3 pieces	3
Peanut butter crunch, 4 pieces	3
Peanut butter cups, 2 pieces	4
Pecan crowns, 3 pieces	3
Weight Watchers Fruities	
Blackberry, 3 pieces	0
Cherry, 3 pieces	0
Strawberry, 3 pieces	0
Welch's Fruit 'n Yogurt Snacks	
Blueberry, 1 pouch	2
Strawberry, 1 pouch	2
Werther's Original	
Caramel chocolate, dark with 42% cacao, 6 pieces	6
Caramel chocolate, milk, 6 pieces	6
Caramel coffee, 4 pieces	1
Caramel mint, 4 pieces	1

	POINTS VALUE
Chewy caramels, 6 pieces	4
Creamy caramel filled hard candies, 2 pieces	1
Hard candies, 3 pieces	2
Sugar free caramel coffee, 5 pieces	1
Sugar free caramel mint, 5 pieces	1
Sugar free hard candies, 5 pieces	1
Whitman's	
Assorted sampler, 4 pieces	5
Whitman's Soho	
Assorted chocolates, 3 pieces	6
Whoppers	
Malted milk balls, 1 package (49 g)	5
Mini Eggs, 31 pieces	4
Whoppers, peanut butter, 17 pieces	4
Wonka	
Bottle caps, 8 pieces	1
Chewy gobs, 9 pieces	1
Chewy runts, 13 pieces	1
Chewy tart n tinys, 1 Tbsp	1
Egg breakers, 6 pieces	1
Freckled eggs, 9 pieces	1
Fruit runts, 12 pieces	1
Gobstopper, 9 pieces	1
Heartbreaker, 8 pieces	1
Laffy taffy, 5 bars	3
Merry mix, 11 pieces	1
Nerds, 1 Tbsp	1
Nerds gum ball, 1	1
Oompas, 1 serving (52 g)	4
Runts, hearts, 1 serving (15 g)	1

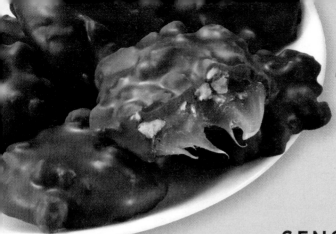

Pecan
Crowns®

1
POINTS
VALUE

Per Piece

SENSIBLE

tastiness.

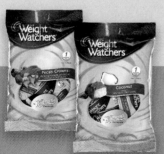

WeightWatchers®

Stop Dieting. Start Living.

Whitman's
CANDIES

Find more information at WeightWatchers.com/chocolate

IGHT WATCHERS on foods and beverages is the registered trademark of WW Foods, LLC and is used under license by Whitman's Candies, Inc. WEIGHT WATCHERS for services and *POINTS*
are the registered trademarks of Weight Watchers International, Inc. and are used under license by Whitman's Candies, Inc. © 2009 Weight Watchers International, Inc. All rights reserved.

Candy, Cookies & Desserts

Wonka (cont'd)	POINTS VALUE
Shock tarts, 8 pieces	1
Shock tarts gum ball, 1	1
Snowball gobs, 6 pieces	1
Tangy taffy, 1 bar	4
Tart n tinys, 1 Tbsp	1
Wonka bar, 1 bar	6
Wrigley's Eclipse	
Cinnamon sugarfree mints, 3 pieces	0
Peppermint sugarfree mints, 3 pieces	0
Winterfrost sugarfree mints, 3 pieces	0
York	
100 calorie wafer bar, 1 bar	2
Mints, candy coated, 3	0
Peppermint pattie, 1 pattie	3
Peppermint pattie, bite size, 3 pieces	3

Cookies
Annie's Homegrown

	POINTS VALUE
Bunny graham friends, chocolate, 30	3
Bunny graham friends, chocolate chip, 30	3
Bunny graham friends, honey, 30	3
Austin	
Animal crackers - sea-licious, 1 package (28 g)	3
Zoo animal crackers, 1 package (28 g)	2
Bakehouse Foods	
Café mocha cookies, 11	1
Chocolate chip cookies, 9	2
Chocolate peanut butter chip, 10	2
Cinnamon chocolate, 10	1
Dutch chocolate cookies, 10	1
English toffee, 10	2

	POINTS VALUE
French vanilla cookies, 11	1
Halloween, 11	1
Key lime cookies, 11	1
Orange cream, 11	1
Peanut butter chocolate chip, 10	2
Spring time/Easter, 11	1
Valentine's day, 11	1
Vanilla bouquet cookies, 11	1
Winter holidays, 11	1
Barbara Dee	
Winter mint cookies, 4	4
Barbara's Bakery	
Fat free wheat free fig bars, 1	1
Fat free wheat free raspberry fig bars, 1	1
Fat free whole wheat apple cinnamon fig bars, 1	1
Fat free whole wheat fig bars, 1	1
Low fat blueberry fig bars, 1	1
Low fat traditional fig bars, 1	1
Organic 100 calorie mini cookies, chocolate, 1 package	2
Organic 100 calorie mini cookies, ginger, 1 package	2
Organic 100 calorie mini cookies, oatmeal, 1 package	2
Snackimals animal cookies, chocolate chip, 10	3
Snackimals animal cookies, oatmeal - wheat free, 10	3
Snackimals animal cookies, snickerdoodle, 10	3
Snackimals animal cookies, vanilla, 10	3

	POINTS VALUE
Snackimals, vanilla (made with organic grains), 10	3
Barry's Bakery	
French twist no trans fat American apple pie, 1	1
French twist no trans fat café mocha, 1	1
French twist no trans fat California almond, 1	1
French twist no trans fat chocolate, 1	1
French twist no trans fat chocolate chip, 1	1
French twist no trans fat key lime, 1	1
French twist no trans fat maple French toast, 1	1
French twist no trans fat original, 1	1
French twist no trans fat vanilla, 1	1
French twist no trans fat wild raspberry, 1	1
Merangos, banana, 11	2
Merangos, café mocha, 12	2
Merangos, chocolate, 11	2
Merangos, chocolate chip, 10	2
Merangos, cinnamon, 11	2
Merangos, coconut, 11	2
Merangos, French vanilla, 12	2
Merangos, mint, 11	2
Merangos, mint chocolate chip, 11	2
Merangos, rainbow, 11	2
Merangos, tropical, 11	2
Merangos, very berry, 11	2
Mini peaks banana, 100 pieces	2

	POINTS VALUE
Mini peaks cappuccino, 100 pieces	2
Mini peaks chocolate, 100 pieces	2
Mini peaks chocolate mint, 100 pieces	2
Mini peaks cinnamon, 100 pieces	2
Mini peaks coconut, 100 pieces	2
Mini peaks mint, 100 pieces	2
Mini peaks mint chocolate chip, 100 pieces	2
Mini peaks mocha, 100 pieces	2
Mini peaks rainbow, 100 pieces	2
Mini peaks tropical, 100 pieces	2
Mini peaks vanilla, 100 pieces	2
Mini peaks verry berry, 100 pieces	2
Parisan sweets grande meringues, café mocha, 4	2
Parisan sweets grande meringues, chocolate, 4	2
Parisan sweets grande meringues, key lime, 4	2
Parisan sweets grande meringues, rainbow, 4	2
Parisan sweets grande meringues, vanilla, 4	2
Parisan sweets mini meringues, café mocha, 100	2
Parisan sweets mini meringues, chocolate, 100	2
Parisan sweets mini meringues, key lime, 100	2
Parisan sweets mini meringues, rainbow, 100	2
Parisan sweets mini meringues, vanilla, 100 pieces	2

Candy, Cookies & Desserts

Barry's Bakery (cont'd)

Parisan sweets petite meringues, café mocha, 12	2
Parisan sweets petite meringues, chocolate, 12	2
Parisan sweets petite meringues, key lime, 12	2
Parisan sweets petite meringues, rainbow, 12	2
Parisan sweets petite meringues, vanilla, 12	2
Betty Crocker	
Gingerbread cookie, prepared, 2	4
Holiday sugar cookie, prepared, 2	4
Rainbow chocolate candy cookie mix, prepared, 2	4
Walnut chocolate chip cookie mix, prepared, 2	4
Betty Crocker Cookie Mixes (Box)	
Hershey's kisses peanut butter, prepared, 1	3
Betty Crocker Cookie Mixes (Pouch)	
Chocolate chip cookie mix, prepared, 2	4
Chocolate chip snack size, prepared, 2	3
Chocolate peanut butter chip cookie mix, prepared, 2	3
Double chocolate chunk cookie mix, prepared, 2	3
Oatmeal chocolate chip cookie mix, prepared, 2	4
Oatmeal cookie mix, prepared, 2	3
Peanut butter cookie mix, prepared, 2	3
Peanut butter snack size, prepared, 2	3
Betty Crocker Pouch Dessert Mixes	
Sugar cookie mix, prepared, 2	4

Betty Crocker Supreme Dessert Bar Mixes	
Cookie brownie bar, prepared, 1	5
Breadshop	
Low fat animal cookies, 15	2
Cherrybrook Kitchen	
Chocolate chip mini cookies, 6	3
Chocolate chip mini cookies - gluten free, 6	3
Fudge brownie mini cookies, 6	3
Snickerdoodle mini cookies, 6	3
Vanilla graham mini cookies, 6	3
Chippery	
Chocolate chip cookie dough, 1 small	4
Chocolate chip cookie dough, 1 medium	5
Chocolate chip cookie dough, 1 large	7
Chocolate chunk cookie dough, 1 small	4
Chocolate chunk cookie dough, 1 regular	6
Chocolate chunk cookie dough, 1 medium	8
Chocolate chunk cookie dough, 1 large	13
Chocolate chunk triple nut cookie dough, 1	5
Cranberry walnut cookie dough, 1	4
Cranberry walnut cookie dough, 1 large	8
Heath English toffee cookie dough, 1 small	4
Heath English toffee cookie dough, 1 medium	9
Heath English toffee cookie dough, 1 large	13
M&M cookie dough, 1 small	4

	POINTS VALUE
M&M cookie dough, 1 medium	6
M&M cookie dough, 1 large	8
Oatmeal raisin cookie dough, 1 small	4
Oatmeal raisin cookie dough, 1 medium	5
Oatmeal raisin cookie dough, 1 regular	8
Oatmeal raisin cookie dough, 1 large	12
Peanut butter cookie dough, 1 small	5
Peanut butter cookie dough, 1 regular	6
Peanut butter cookie dough, 1 medium	10
Peanut butter cookie dough, 1 large	14
Peanut butter milk chocolate with reese's peanut butter cups, 1	5
Snickerdoodle cookie dough, 1 small	4
Snickerdoodle cookie dough, 1 medium	6
Snickerdoodle cookie dough, 1 large	9
Sugar cookie dough, 1 small	4
Sugar cookie dough, 1 medium	6
Sugar cookie dough, 1 large	9
Triple chocolate cookie dough, 1 small	4
Triple chocolate cookie dough, 1 regular	6
Triple chocolate cookie dough, 1 medium	9
Triple chocolate cookie dough, 1 large	13
White chunk macadamia nut, 1 small	5
White chunk macadamia nut, 1 regular	6
White chunk macadamia nut, 1 medium	9
White chunk macadamia nut, 1 large	14

	POINTS VALUE
Dunkaroos	
Cinnamon graham w/vanilla frosting, 1 tray	3
Honey graham cookie with chocolate chips & chocolate frosting, 1 tray	3
Eagle Brand Premium Dessert Kits	
Magic cookie bar, 1 piece (1 1/2" x 1 1/2")	3
Entenmann's	
Black & white cookie, 1	8
Chocolate chip cookie - single, 1	8
Chocolate chip cookies, 2	3
Easter sprinkled cookies, 3	3
Gourmet raspberry cookies, 2	3
Holiday collection butter cookie - Christmas, 2	3
Holiday collection butter cookie - St. Patrick's day, 2	3
Holiday collection butter cookie - Valentine, 2	3
Little bites brownie (club size package), 1 package	5
Little bites variety pack - fudge brownie (club size package), 1 package	5
Milk chocolate chip cookies, 3	4
Original chocolate chip cookies, 3	3
Original recipe chocolate chip cookies, 3	3
Soft baked chocolate chunk cookie, 1	5
St. Patrick's sprinkled cookies, 3	3
Ultimate brownies, 1	3
Valentine's sprinkled cookies, 3	3

Candy, Cookies & Desserts

	POINTS value
Erin Baker's	
Organic brownie bites - classic walnut, 1	2
Erin Baker's Breakfast Cookie	
Banana toasted flax, 1	6
Banana walnut, 1	6
Caramel apple, 1	5
Chocolate chunk raisin, 1	6
Double chocolate chunk, 1	6
Double chocolate chunk cherry, 1	6
Fruit & nut, 1	6
Gingerbread, 1	6
Mocha cappuccino, 1	6
Morning glory, 1	6
Organic breakfast cookie mini, double chocolate chunk, 1	2
Organic breakfast cookie mini, fruit & nut, 1	2
Organic breakfast cookie mini, oatmeal raisin, 1	2
Organic breakfast cookie mini, peanut butter, 1	2
Peanut butter, 1	7
Peanut butter & jelly, 1	6
Pumpkin spice, 1 cookie	5
Vegan chocolate chunk, 1	6
Vegan peanut butter chocolate chunk, 1	7
Estee	
Banana split crème wafer, 5	4
Chocolate chip cookie, 4	3
Chocolate crème wafers, 5	4
Chocolate sandwich cookies, 3	4

	POINTS value
Fudge cookies, 4	3
Lemon creme wafers, 5	4
Lemon thins, 4	3
Oatmeal raisin cookies, 4	3
Original sandwich cookies, 3	4
Peanut butter creme wafers, 5	3
Peanut butter sandwich cookie, 3	4
Shortbread cookies, 4	3
Vanilla and strawberry crème wafer, 5	4
Vanilla crème wafer, 5	4
Vanilla sandwich cookie, 3	4
Vanilla thins, 4	3
Estee Smart Treats	
Sugar free old fashioned vanilla, 1	1
Sugar free, reduced fat chocolate chip, 4	3
Sugar free, reduced fat coconut, 4	3
Famous Amos	
Chocolate chip, 4	3
Chocolate chip & pecan, 4	3
Chocolate sandwich crème, 3	4
Coconut bar cookies, 4	3
Crème oatmeal macaroon sandwich, 3	4
Crème vanilla sandwich, 3	4
Lemon, 5	3
Oatmeal raisin, 4	3
Sandwich crème peanut butter, 3	4
Vanilla animal cookies, 10	3
Gamesa	
Emperador vanilla crème sandwich cookies, 2	3

	POINTS VALUE
Girl Scouts	
Caramel dulce de leche, 3	5
Chalet, 3	4
Do-si-dos, 2	3
Samoas, 2	3
Sugar free chocolate chip, 3	4
Tagalongs, 2	3
Thin mints, 4	4
Trefoils, 5	4
Grandma's	
Limited edition holiday cinnamon sugar flavored big cookies, 1	4
Limited edition holiday gingerbread flavored big cookies, 1	3
Peanut butter sandwich crème, 5	5
Rich n' chewy chocolate chip, soft, 1 package	6
Vanilla mini sandwich cookies, 9	3
Vanilla sandwich crème, 5	5
Grandma's Homestyle Big Cookies	
Chocolate chip, 1	5
Fudge chocolate chip, 1	4
Lemon iced big cookies, 1	4
Oatmeal raisin, 1	4
Peanut butter, 1	4
Sugar big cookies, 1	4
Hain Pure Foods	
Low fat vanilla animal cookies, 10	3
Health Valley	
Biscotti cookies, chocolate, 2	2
Chocolate mint sandwich cookies, 2	3

	POINTS VALUE
Chocolate sandwich cookies, 2	3
Double chocolate chunk cookies, 1	3
Double chocolate sandwich cookies, 2	3
Low fat healthy chips double chocolate, 3	2
Low fat raisin oatmeal, 3	2
Mini chocolate chip cookies, 4	3
Mini chocolate chocolate chip cookies, 4	3
Mini peanut butter cookies, 4	3
Oatmeal cookies, chocolate chip, 1	2
Oatmeal cookies, peanut, 1	2
Vanilla flavored sandwich cookies, 2	3
Hershey's	
Cookie, mini kiss, chocolate chip, 1 package	2
Cookie, soft baked, 1/2	4
Peanut butter snack barz, 1 bar	6
Ian's	
Organic chocolate chip cookie buttons, 1 serving (23 g)	2
Organic double chocolate chip cookie buttons, 1 serving (23 g)	2
Organic mini vanilla wafers, 1 pouch	2
Wheat free/gluten free chocolate chip cookie buttons, 1 serving (30 g)	3
Irene's Bakery	
Fat free assorted biscotti, 1	0
Fat free chocolate almond biscotti, 1	1
Fat free cranberry biscotti, 1	0

Candy, Cookies & Desserts

Jacks	POINTS VALUE
Butter thins, 8	3
Chocolatey chip thins, 8	3
Wafers vanilla, 9	3
Jackson's	
Lemon jumbles, 3	4
Wafers vanilla, 8	3
Joseph's Sugar Free Cookies	
Almond, 4	2
Chocolate chip, 4	2
Chocolate peanut butter, 4	2
Chocolate raspberry bite size cake, 4	2
Chocolate walnut, 4	2
Coconut, 4	2
Lemon, 4	2
Oatmeal, 4	2
Oatmeal chocolate chip with pecans, 4	2
Peanut butter, 4	2
Pecan chocolate chip, 4	2
Pecan shortbread, 4	2
Strawberry coconut, 4	2
Kashi	
Happy trail mix, 1	2
Oatmeal dark chocolate, 1	2
Oatmeal raisin flax, 1	2
Keebler	
Animal cookies - frosted, 8	4
Animal cookies frosted, 1 package (40 g)	5
Animal cookies iced, 6	3
Animal cookies iced, 1 package (40 g)	4
Bug bites cinnamon grahams, 13	3

	POINTS VALUE
Chips deluxe chocolate lovers, 1	2
Chips deluxe coconut, 2	4
Chips deluxe fudge striped caramel chip, 1	3
Chips deluxe fudge striped original, 1	3
Chips deluxe original, 2	4
Chips deluxe peanut butter chocolate, 1	2
Chips deluxe peanut butter cups, 1	2
Chips deluxe rainbow, 1	2
Chips deluxe rainbow, bite size, 1 package (40 g)	5
Chips deluxe soft n' chewy, 1	2
Chips deluxe, chocolate malt chunk, 2	4
Chips deluxe, oatmeal chocolate chip, 2	3
Chips deluxe, rainbow-gripz, 1 pouch	3
Country style oatmeal with raisins, 2	3
Danish wedding, 4	3
El fudge butter flavored, 1	2
EL fudge, double stuffed, 2	4
Fig bars, 2	2
Fudge shoppe caramel filled, 2	4
Fudge shoppe deluxe grahams, 3 pieces	3
Fudge shoppe fudge sticks, 3	4
Fudge shoppe fudge stripes, 3	3
Fudge shoppe fudge stripes, mini, 1 package	5
Fudge shoppe grasshopper fudge mint, 4	3
Fudge shoppe merry mint patties holiday, 2	3

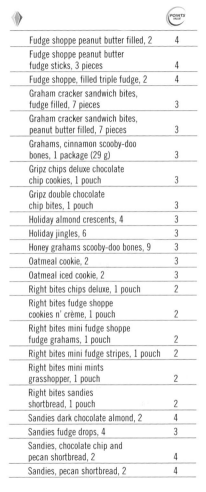

	POINTS VALUE
Fudge shoppe peanut butter filled, 2	4
Fudge shoppe peanut butter fudge sticks, 3 pieces	4
Fudge shoppe, filled triple fudge, 2	4
Graham cracker sandwich bites, fudge filled, 7 pieces	3
Graham cracker sandwich bites, peanut butter filled, 7 pieces	3
Grahams, cinnamon scooby-doo bones, 1 package (29 g)	3
Gripz chips deluxe chocolate chip cookies, 1 pouch	3
Gripz double chocolate chip bites, 1 pouch	3
Holiday almond crescents, 4	3
Holiday jingles, 6	3
Honey grahams scooby-doo bones, 9	3
Oatmeal cookie, 2	3
Oatmeal iced cookie, 2	3
Right bites chips deluxe, 1 pouch	2
Right bites fudge shoppe cookies n' crème, 1 pouch	2
Right bites mini fudge shoppe fudge grahams, 1 pouch	2
Right bites mini fudge stripes, 1 pouch	2
Right bites mini mints grasshopper, 1 pouch	2
Right bites sandies shortbread, 1 pouch	2
Sandies dark chocolate almond, 2	4
Sandies fudge drops, 4	3
Sandies, chocolate chip and pecan shortbread, 2	4
Sandies, pecan shortbread, 2	4

	POINTS VALUE
Sandies, reduced fat pecan shortbread, 2	4
Sandies, simply shortbread, 2	4
Soft batch chocolate chunk, 1	7
Soft batch oatmeal raisin, 1	2
Soft batch peanut butter, 1	2
Soft batch, chocolate chip, 1	2
Vanilla wafers, 8	3
Vanilla wafers mini, 18	3
Vienna fingers, 2	3
Vienna fingers, reduced fat, 2	3
Kellogg's Rice Krispies Treats	
Crispy marshmallow squares, 1 bar	2
Original (shrek), 1 bar	2
Original holiday, 1 bar	2
Strawberry, 1 bar	2
Kraft	
Cameo crème sandwich cookies, 1 serving (31 g)	4
Cameo crème sandwich cookies, 1 package (4-count)	6
Cameo crème sandwich cookies - mini, 9	3
Cameo crème sandwich cookies - mini, 1 package	4
South beach diet cookies - oatmeal chocolate chip, 2	2
South beach diet cookies - oatmeal chocolate chip, 1 package	2
South beach diet cookies - peanut butter, 2	2
South beach diet cookies - peanut butter, 1 package	2

Candy, Cookies & Desserts

	POINTS VALUE
Kraft Handi-Snacks	
Teddy grahams bearwiches - honey, 1 serving (26 g)	3
Lance	
Bite size chocolate chip cookies, 4	3
Choc-o-lunch, 5 small	4
Choc-o-lunch, 6	4
Lem-o-lunch, 5	5
Malt, 6	4
Nut-o-lunch, 5	4
Oatmeal crèmes, 1 small	5
Oatmeal crèmes, 1	7
Peanut butter crème filled wafer, 1 package	7
Peanut butter crème filled wafer, 1 bar	5
Peanut butter nekot, 6	6
Strawberry creme filled vanilla cookies, 5	5
Strawberry crème filled wafers, 4	4
Vanilla crème filled wafers, 4	4
Van-o-lunch, 6	5
Van-o-lunch, 5 small	5
Little Debbie	
Apple flips cookies, 1	3
Caramel cookie bars, 1	4
Cherry cordials (Christmas & Valentine), 1	4
Chocolate chip creme pies, 1	4
Chocolate cremes, 1	3
Christmas gingerbread cookies, 1	2
Cookie wreaths cookies, 1	2
Easter marshmallow treats, 1 bar	2

	POINTS VALUE
Easter puffs cookies, 1	3
Fall marshmallow treats, 1 bar	2
Fig bars, 1	3
Fudge rounds, 1	3
German chocolate cookie rings with caramel & coconut, 1	3
Gingerbread cookies, 1	2
Holiday marshmallow treats, 1 bar	2
Jelly crème pies, 1	4
Marshmallow pie, banana, single serve, 1	4
Marshmallow pie, chocolate, single serve, 1	4
Marshmallow pies (banana), 1	4
Marshmallow pies chocolate flavored, 1	4
Marshmallow supremes, 1	3
Marshmallow treat, single serve, 1 bar	4
Marshmallow treats, 1 bar	2
Nutty bar singles, 1	3
Nutty bar thins, 2	5
Nutty bars wafer bars, 2	8
Oatmeal creme pies, 1	4
P.b. & j. oatmeal pies, 1	3
Pumpkin delights filled cookies, 1	3
Raisin crème pies, 1	4
Smores cookie, 1	4
Snow puffs, 1	2
Spirit of America marshmallow treats, 1 bar	2
Star crunch cosmic snacks, 1	3
Stars & stripes marshmallow puffs, 1	4

Candy, Cookies & Desserts

	POINTS VALUE
Little Debbie 100 Calories	
Be my valentine marshmallow treats, 1 bar	2
Little Debbie Less than 100 Calories	
Nutty bar peanut butter stix, 1	2
Manischewitz	
Almond biscotti - sugar free, 2	2
Coconut macaroons - reduced sugar, 2	2
Market Day	
Chocolate chip cookie dough, 2	3
Chocolate chip cookie meltdown, 1	12
Trail mix breakfast cookies, 1	4
Mi-Del	
Chocolate snaps, 5	3
Cinnamon graham bite size cookies, 12	2
Ginger snaps, 5	3
Gluten free arrowroot animal cookies, 10	3
Gluten free chocolate caramel bite size cookies, 23	2
Gluten free chocolate chip cookies, 5	3
Gluten free cinnamon snaps, 5	3
Gluten free ginger snaps, 5	3
Gluten free pecan cookies, 5	3
Gluten free royal vanilla sandwich cookies, 3	4
Lemon snaps, 5	3
Oatmeal chocolate chip bite size cookies, 23	3
Oatmeal snaps, 5	3
Organic ginger snaps, 5	3
Organic snickerdoodle bite size cookies, 23	3

	POINTS VALUE
Organic vanilla snaps, 5	3
Vanilla snaps, 5	3
Miss Meringue	
Fat free cappuccino, 4	2
Fat free vanilla, 4	2
Fat free vanilla rainbow, 4	2
Low fat chocolate chip, 4	2
Low fat mint chocolate chip, 4	2
Low fat triple chocolate chip, 4	2
Miss Meringue Chocolettes	
Chocolaty crunch, 8	3
Mint, 10	3
Strawberry vanilla, 10	3
Vanilla, 10	3
Miss Meringue Minis	
Apple spice, 13	2
Chocolate chip, 12	3
Creamsicle, 13	2
Fat free chocolate mini cookies, 13	2
Fat free vanilla, 13	2
Low fat mint chocolate chip, 12	2
Peppermint crush, 9	2
Rainbow vanilla, 13	2
Watermelon, 13	2
Miss Meringue Sugar Free	
Chocolate meringue cookies, 13	0
Vanilla meringue cookies, 13	0
Mrs. Denson's	
Organic chocolate chip cookies, 1	2
Organic oatmeal raisin cookies, 1	2
Wheat free chocolate chip macaroon, 1	3

Candy, Cookies & Desserts

Mrs. Denson's (cont'd)

	POINTS VALUE
Wheat free oatmeal raisin cookies, 1	2
Wheat free quinoa macaroon, 1	2
Mrs. Freshleys Snackaway	
Peanut butter wafers, 1	1
Yogurt filled oatmeal crème cookies, 1	1
Murray	
Animal cookies, 12	3
Animal cookies - iced, 12	3
Big 'uns, 2	3
Chocolatey chip thins, 8	3
Cinnamon graham, 8	3
Cookie jar classics butter, 8	3
Cookie jar classics coconut, 6	3
Cookie jar classics ginger, 6	3
Cookie jar classics lemon, 6	3
Crème sandwich assorted, 3	3
Crème sandwich banana, 3	3
Crème sandwich chocolate, 3	3
Crème sandwich lemon, 3	3
Crème sandwich peanut butter, 3	3
Crème sandwich strawberry, 3	3
Crème sandwich vanilla, 3	3
Duplex crème sandwich cookies, 3	3
Dutch windmill, 3	4
Honey graham, 8	3
Iced lemon - low fat, 7	2
Low fat iced oatmeal, 7	2
Old fashioned ginger snaps, 5	3
Old fashioned holiday gingerbread men, 5	3
Old fashioned holiday shortbread classics, 7	3

	POINTS VALUE
Old fashioned iced ginger snaps, 5	3
Old fashioned iced oatmeal, 5	3
Southern kitchen - chocolate chip, 2	3
Southern kitchen - coconut, 2	3
Southern kitchen - oatmeal, 2	3
Southern kitchen - oatmeal iced, 2	3
Southern kitchen - peanut butter, 2	3
Strawberry thins, 8	3
Sugar free chocolate bites, 1 pouch	1
Sugar free chocolate chip, 3	4
Sugar free chocolate chip with pecans, 3	4
Sugar free double fudge, 3	4
Sugar free fudge dipped grahams, 4	3
Sugar free fudge dipped mint, 4	3
Sugar free fudge dipped shortbread, 5	3
Sugar free fudge dipped wafers, 4	3
Sugar free gingersnaps, 7	3
Sugar free oatmeal, 3	3
Sugar free peanut butter, 3	4
Sugar free pecan shortbread, 3	4
Sugar free sandwich crème chocolate, 3	3
Sugar free sandwich crème lemon, 3	3
Sugar free sandwich crème vanilla, 3	3
Sugar free shortbread, 8	3
Sugar free shortbread bites, 1 pouch	1
Sugar free vanilla wafer, 9	3
Sugar free wafer duplex, 5	3
Sugar free wafers - lemon, 4	2
Sugar free wafers - vanilla, 4	2
Sugar wafers - peanut butter, 5	4

	POINTS VALUE
Sugar wafers - strawberry, 5	3
Sugar wafers - vanilla, 5	3
Vanilla wafer, 8	3
Nabisco	
Biscos sugar wafers, 1 serving (28 g)	3
Biscos waffle cremes, 4	4
Chips ahoy, 3	4
Chips ahoy cookie barz, 1	4
Chips ahoy, candy blasts, 1 serving (15 g)	2
Chips ahoy, chewy real chocolate chip, 1 serving (27 g)	3
Chips ahoy, mini chocolate chip bite-size go-pak, 1 package (35 g)	4
Chips ahoy, mini chocolate chip bite-size go-pak, 1 serving (31 g)	3
Chips ahoy, reduced-fat, 3	3
Chips ahoy, soft baked chunky chocolate chip, 1 serving (28 g)	3
Famous chocolate wafers, 1 serving (32 g)	3
Fig newtons, 2	2
Fig newtons fat free fruit chewy cookies, 2	2
Ginger snaps, 1 serving (28 g)	3
Golden oreo crème sandwich cookies - original crème, 1 package (51 g)	6
Honey maid cookies - oatmeal, 3	3
Honey maid cookies - oatmeal raisin, 3	3
Honey maid cookies - oatmeal raisin mini, 1 package (56 g)	5
Honey maid graham bars - banana flavored, 1	3

	POINTS VALUE
Lorna doone shortbread cookies, 1 serving (29 g)	3
Lorne doone shortbread cookies, 1 (28 g)	3
Lorne doone shortbread cookies, 1 package (42 g)	5
Mallomars pure chocolate cookies, 1 serving (27 g)	3
Newtons fruit chewy cookies - fig, 1 package (28 g)	2
Newtons fruit chewy cookies - fig fat free, 1	2
Newtons fruit chewy cookies - fig, 100% whole grain, 2	2
Newtons snackable dessert cookies - strawberry shortcake, 2	3
Nutter butter bites sandwich cookies - peanut butter, 1 package (42 g)	5
Nutter butter patties - peanut crème, 5 (32 g)	4
Nutter butter sandwich bites, 1 serving (35 g)	4
Nutter butter sandwich bites go-pak, 1 serving (30 g)	3
Nutter butter sandwich bites snak saks, 1 serving (49 g)	5
Nutter butter sandwich cookies, 1 package (53 g)	6
Nutter butter sandwich cookies, 1 serving (28 g)	3
Oreo, 3 (34 g)	4
Oreo chocolate crème mini, 1 serving (43 g)	5

Candy, Cookies & Desserts

Nabisco (cont'd)

	POINTS VALUE
Oreo chocolate crème mini sandwich cookies, 1 serving (35 g)	4
Oreo chocolate crème mini snak saks, 1 serving (29 g)	3
Oreo chocolate fudge covered sandwich cookies, 1 serving (19 g)	2
Oreo chocolate mini bite size, 1 serving (35 g)	4
Oreo chocolate mini bite size go-pak, 1 serving (29 g)	3
Oreo chocolate mini bite size packs 2 go, 1 serving (42 g)	4
Oreo chocolate sandwich cookies, 1 serving (57 g)	6
Oreo chocolate sandwich cookies, 1 package (2 count)	2
Oreo chocolate sandwich cookies - double delight peanut butter 'n, 2	3
Oreo chocolate sandwich cookies - double stuff smilin', 2	3
Oreo chocolate sandwich cookies - mini chocolate crème, 1 package (50 g)	5
Oreo chocolate sandwich cookies - mini white crème, 1 package (49 g)	5
Oreo chocolate sandwich cookies - sugar free, 2	2
Oreo cookie barz, 1	4
Oreo double delight mint'n crème sandwich cookies, 1 serving (29 g)	3
Oreo double stuf packs 2 go, 1 serving (42 g)	5
Oreo double stuf sandwich cookies, 1 serving (29 g)	3
Oreo double stuff sandwich cookies- chocolate crème, 2	3

	POINTS VALUE
Oreo double stuff sandwich cookies- chocolate crème, 1 package (15 g)	2
Oreo golden original sandwich cookies, 1 serving (35 g)	4
Oreo golden with chocolate creme sandwich cookies, 1 serving (35 g)	4
Oreo Halloween orange creme sandwich cookies, 1 serving (29 g)	3
Oreo mini bite size snak saks, 1 serving (28 g)	3
Oreo spring purple creme sandwich cookies, 1 serving (29 g)	3
Raspberry newtons, 2	2
Social tea biscuits, 1 serving (31 g)	3
Soft cookies - chips ahoy, 1	4
Strawberry newtons, 2	2
Twirls, marshmallow fudge, 1 serving (30 g)	3

Nabisco 100 Calorie Packs

	POINTS VALUE
Alpha bits mini cookies, 1 pouch	2
Barnum's animals choco crackers, 1 pouch	2
Chips ahoy thin crisps, 1 pouch	2
Lorna doone shortbread cookie crisps, 1 pouch	2
Mini teddy grahams cinnamon cubs, 1 pouch	2
Oreo thin crisps, 1 pouch	2
Planters peanut butter cookie crisps, 1 pouch	2

Nabisco SnackWell's

	POINTS VALUE
Chocolate chip, 3	3
Crème sandwich, 1 package (48 g)	5

Candy, Cookies & Desserts

	POINTS VALUE
Crème sandwich, 2	2
Sandwich cookies - crème, 1 package (24 g)	2
Sugar free lemon creme, 3	3
Sugar free shortbread, 3	3
Nabisco Teddy Grahams	
Graham snacks - chocolate, 1 package (21 g)	2
Natural Nectar	
Chocolate whole grain wafers, 5	3
Cinnamon sticks, 5	4
Lady fingers, 5	3
Pretzel cookies, 2	4
Strawberry whole grain wafers, 5	3
Vanilla whole grain wafers, 5	3
O'coco's	
Cinnamon organic chocolate crisps, 1 container	2
Mocha organic chocolate crisps, 1 container	2
Original organic chocolate crisps, 1 container	2
Otis Spunkmeyer	
Café au lait brownie, 1 serving (3.3 oz)	9
Otis Spunkmeyer Café Collection	
Chocolate chunk cookie, 2 oz (2.5 servings per cookie)	6
Oatmeal raisin cookie, 2 oz (2.5 servings per cookie)	5
White chocolate macadamia nut cookie, 2 oz (2.5 servings per cookie)	6

	POINTS VALUE
Otis Spunkmeyer Chippery Thaw and Serve	
Sugar, 1 small (1.3 oz)	4
Sugar, 1 (2 oz)	6
Triple chocolate, 1 (2 oz)	6
Triple chocolate, 1 small (1.3 oz)	4
Otis Spunkmeyer Delicious Essentials	
Butter sugar cookie, 1 (1 oz)	2
Carnival, 1 (1 oz)	2
Chocolate chip, 1 (2 oz)	5
Chocolate chip, 1 (1 oz)	2
Oatmeal raisin, 1 (1 oz)	2
Otis Spunkmeyer Express	
Chocolate chunk, 1 (2 oz cookie) (57 g)	6
Chocolate chunk, 1/2 small (4 oz cookie) (57 g)	6
Chocolate chunk, 1 serving (2/5 of 5 oz cookie) (57 g)	6
Double chocolate chip, 1 (2 oz cookie) (57 g)	6
Double chocolate chip, 1/2 small (4 oz cookie) (57 g)	6
Oatmeal raisin, 1 (2 oz cookie) (57 g)	5
Oatmeal raisin, 1/2 small (4 oz cookie) (57 g)	5
Oatmeal raisin, 1 serving (2/5 of 5 oz cookie) (57 g)	5
Peanut butter, 1 (2 oz cookie) (57 g)	6
Peanut butter, 1/2 small (4 oz cookie) (57 g)	6
White chunk macadamia nut, 1 cookie (2 oz cookie) (21 g)	6

Candy, Cookies & Desserts

Otis Spunkmeyer Express (cont'd)	POINTS VALUE
White chunk macadamia nut, 1/2 (4 oz cookie) (10.5 g)	3
White chunk macadamia nut, 1 serving (2/5 of 5 oz cookie) (21 g)	6
Otis Spunkmeyer Otis Express	
Chocolate chunk, 1 (2 oz)	6
Double chocolate chip, 1 (2 oz)	6
Oatmeal raisin, 1 (2 oz)	5
Peanut butter, 1 (2 oz)	6
Otis Spunkmeyer Spunkies Sweet Discovery	
Chocolate chip, 4 (30 g)	3
Peanut butter, 4 (1.1 oz)	3
Otis Spunkmeyer Sugar Free	
Chocolate chip cookie, 1 (1.1 oz)	3
Double chocolate cookie, 1 (1.1 oz)	2
Lemon cookie, 1 (1.1 oz)	3
Otis Spunkmeyer Supreme Indulgence	
Buttery pecan decadence, 1/2 (1.5 oz)	4
Buttery pecan decadence, 1/2 (2 oz)	6
Chocolate peanut butter flutter, 1/2 (1.5 oz)	4
Chocolate peanut butter flutter, 1 (2 oz)	6
Chunky chocolate supreme, 1/2 (2 oz)	6
Chunky chocolate supreme, 1 (2 oz)	6
Chunky chocolate supreme, 1/2 (1.5 oz)	4
Cranberry white chocolate duo, 1/2 (1.5 oz)	4
Double chunky chocolate dream, 1/2 (1.5 oz)	4
Honey nut chocolate buzz, 1/2 (1.5 oz)	4
Lemon white chunk, 1/2 (2 oz)	6
Lemon white chunk, 1/2 (1.5 oz)	4

	POINTS VALUE
Nutty white chocolate delight, 1/2 (1.5 oz)	5
Nutty white chocolate delight, 1 (2 oz)	6
Oatmeal cinnaraisin cravin', 1/2 (2 oz)	5
Oatmeal cinnaraisin cravin', 1 (2 oz)	5
Oatmeal cinnaraisin cravin', 1/2 (1.5 oz)	4
Shortbread, 1/2 (1.5 oz)	10
Otis Spunkmeyer Sweet Discovery	
All American, 1 (1.3 oz)	4
Apple cinnamon raisin breakfast cookie, 1 (1.33 oz)	3
Apple cinnamount, 1 (1.3 oz)	4
Boo-licious, 1 (1.3 oz)	3
Butter sugar, 1 (2 oz)	6
Butter sugar, 1 bite size (0.75 oz)	2
Butter sugar, 1 (1.3 oz)	4
Butter sugar, 1/2 (2 oz)	6
Buttercrunch toffee, 1 (2 oz)	6
Buttercrunch toffee, 1/2 small (2 oz)	6
Buttercrunch toffee, 1 (1.3 oz)	4
Café vienna, 1 (1.3 oz)	4
Carnival, 1/2 (2 oz)	6
Carnival, 1 (1.3 oz)	4
Carnival, 1 (2 oz)	6
Chocolate chip, 1 (2 oz)	6
Chocolate chip, 1 (1.3 oz)	4
Chocolate chip, 1/2 (2 oz)	6
Chocolate chip, 1 (3 oz)	8
Chocolate chip, 1 bite size (0.75 oz)	2
Chocolate chip pecan, 1 (1.3 oz)	4
Chocolate chip walnut, 1 (2 oz)	6

Candy, Cookies & Desserts

	POINTS VALUE
Chocolate chip walnut, 1 (1.3 oz)	4
Chocolate obsession, 1 (1.3 oz)	4
Chocolate with reese's pieces, 1 (1.3 oz)	4
Cranberry oatmeal, 1 (37 g)	3
Double chocolate brownie cookie, 1 (1.3 oz)	4
Double chocolate chip, 1/2 (2 oz)	6
Double chocolate chip, 1 (2 oz)	6
Double chocolate chip, 1 bite size (0.75 oz)	2
Double chocolate chip, 1 (1.3 oz)	4
Holiday carnival, 1 (1.3 oz)	4
Milk chocolate chunk, 1 (1.3 oz)	4
Milk chocolate chunk, 1 (2 oz)	6
Oatmeal raisin, 1 (85 g)	7
Oatmeal raisin, 1 bite size (0.75 oz)	2
Oatmeal raisin, 1/2 (2 oz)	5
Oatmeal raisin, 1 (2 oz)	5
Oatmeal raisin, 1 (1.3 oz)	3
Peanut butter, 1 (85 g)	9
Peanut butter, 1/2 (2 oz)	6
Peanut butter, 1 bite size (0.75 oz)	2
Peanut butter, 1 (2 oz)	6
Peanut butter, 1 (1.3 oz)	4
Peanut butter chocolate chunk, 1/2 (2 oz)	5
Peanut butter chocolate chunk, 1 (2 oz)	5
Peanut butter chocolate chunk, 1 (1.3 oz)	4
Red, white and blue, 1 (1.3 oz)	4
Rocky road, 1 (2 oz)	5
Rocky road, 1 (1.3 oz)	4

	POINTS VALUE
S'mores, 1 (1.3 oz)	4
Spring carnival, 1 (1.3 oz)	4
Strawberry shortcake, 1 (1.3 oz)	4
Triple chocolate, 1 (1.3 oz)	4
Triple chocolate, 1 (2 oz)	6
Turtle, 1/2 (2 oz)	6
Turtle, 1 (2 oz)	6
Turtle, 1 (1.3 oz)	4
White chocolate macadamia nut, 1 (85 g)	9
White chocolate macadamia nut, 1 (2 oz)	6
White chocolate macadamia nut, 1 (0.75 oz)	4
White chocolate macadamia nut, 1 bite size (0.75 oz)	2
White chocolate macadamia nut, 1/2 (2 oz)	6
Yogurt raisin sensation, 1 (0.75 oz)	4
Otis Spunkmeyer Sweet Discovery Reduced Fat	
100% whole grain butter sugar cookie, 1 (1.33 oz)	3
100% whole grain carnival cookie, 1 (1.33 oz)	3
100% whole grain chocolate chip cookie, 1 (1.33 oz)	3
100% whole grain chocolate chip cookie, 1 (1.33 oz)	3
100% whole grain oatmeal raisin cookie, 1 (1.33 oz)	3
Butter sugar cookie, 1 (1.33 oz)	3
Carnival cookie, 1 (1.33 oz)	3

Candy, Cookies & Desserts

Otis Spunkmeyer Sweet Discovery Reduced Fat (cont'd)	POINTS VALUE
Chocolate chip cookie, 1 (1.33 oz)	3
Chocolate chip cookie, 1 (2 oz)	5
Oatmeal raisin, 1 (1.33 oz)	3
Otis Spunkmeyer Traditional Recipe	
Carnival, 1 (2.5 oz)	7
Carnival, 1 (1.5 oz)	4
Chocolate chip, 1 (1.5 oz)	4
Chocolate chip, 1 (2.5 oz)	7
Double chocolate chip, 1 (1.5 oz)	4
Double chocolate chip, 1 (2.5 oz)	7
Oatmeal raisin, 1 (1.5 oz)	4
Oatmeal raisin, 1 (2.5 oz)	7
Peanut butter, 1 (1.5 oz)	5
Peanut butter, 1 (2.5 oz)	8
Ranger, 1 (1.5 oz)	4
Ranger, 1 (2.5 oz)	7
Sugar, 1 (2.5 oz)	7
Sugar, 1 (1.5 oz)	4
White chocolate macadamia nut, 1 (2.5 oz)	8
White chocolate macadamia nut, 1 (1.5 oz)	4
Otis Spunkmeyer Value Zone	
Double chocolate chip, 1 (2.5 oz)	7
Double chocolate chip, 1 small (1 oz)	3
Oatmeal raisin, 1 (1 oz)	3
Oatmeal raisin, 1 small (0.67 oz)	2
Ranger, 1 (1 oz)	3
Reduced fat carnival, 1 (1 oz)	2
Reduced fat chocolate chip, 1 (1 oz)	2
Reduced fat oatmeal raisin, 1 (1 oz)	2
Reduced fat sugar, 1 (1 oz)	2

	POINTS VALUE
Otis Spunkmeyer Value Zone Reduced Fat	
100% whole grain chocolate brownie cookie, 1 (1 oz)	2
100% whole grain chocolate brownie cookie, 1 (2 oz)	4
100% whole grain chocolate chip cookie, 1 (1 oz)	2
100% whole grain oatmeal raisin cookie, 1 (1 oz)	2
Otis Spunkmeyer Value Zone Reduced Fat 100% Whole Grain	
Chocolate brownie cookie dough, 1 serving (1.5 oz)	3
Chocolate chip cookie dough, 1 serving (1.5 oz)	3
Oatmeal raisin cookie dough, 1 serving (1.5 oz)	3
Payaso	
Animal cookies, 15	2
Maria cookies, 8	3
Peek Freans	
Cinnamon crisp, 3	4
Crème biscuits - bourbon, 2	3
Digestive, 3	4
Digestive family, 2	4
Family shortcake (fudge covered shortcake), 2	3
Garden, 2	4
Orange blossom, 3	3
Pecan passion, 2	4
Toffee crisp, 3	4

	POINTS VALUE
Pepperidge Farm	
100 calorie pack chessmen cookies, 1 packet	2
100 calorie pack chocolate chessmen cookies, 1 packet	2
100 calorie pack chocolate chunk cookies, 1 packet	2
Amaretto Milano cookies, 2	3
Black & white Milano cookies, 3	4
Bordeaux cookies, 4	3
Brussels cookies, 3	3
Butter chessmen cookies, 3	3
Chesapeake dark chocolate chunk pecan cookies, 1	3
Chocolate chessmen cookies, 3	3
Chocolate cookie collection, 2	3
Chocolate fudge pirouettes, 2	3
Chocolate hazelnut creme-filled pirouettes, 2	3
Chocolate mint Milano cookies, 2	3
Chocolate petite truffle cookies, 5	4
Chocolate raspberry Milano cookies, 2	3
Dark chocolate chunk soft baked Nantucket cookies, 1	4
Dark chocolate crispy crepes, 6	3
Dark chocolate drenched Milano cookies, 1	2
Dark chocolate drenched mint Milano cookies, 1	2
Distinctive entertaining cookie collection, 3	3
Double chocolate Milano cookies, 2	3
French vanilla pirouettes, 2	3

	POINTS VALUE
Geneva cookies, 3	4
Ginger family cookie collection, 4	3
Gingerman homestyle cookies, 4	3
Golden orchard assortment, 3	3
Milano cookies, 3	4
Milk chocolate caramel medallion, 4	4
Milk chocolate crispy crepes, 6	3
Milk chocolate drenched Milano cookies, 1	2
Milk chocolate medallion, 5	4
Milk chocolate Milano cookies, 3	4
Mini butter cookie canister, 9	3
Mini gingerman cookie canister, 12	3
Mini Milano cookies, 6	4
Mini mint Milano cookies, 6	4
Mini Sausalito cookies, 4	4
Mint Brussels cookies, 3	4
Mint chocolate pirouette, 2	3
Mint milano cookies, 2	3
Montieri apple tart cookies, 2	2
Montieri peach tart cookies, 2	2
Montieri raspberry tart cookies, 2	2
Nantucket dark chocolate chunk cookies, 1	3
Nantucket double chocolate chunk cookies, 1	3
Orange Milano cookies, 2	3
Raspberry Milano cookies, 2	3
Sausalito milk chocolate chunk macademia nut cookies, 1	3
Sausalito milk chocolate chunk macademia nut soft baked cookies, 1	4

Candy, Cookies & Desserts

Pepperidge Farm (cont'd)	POINTS VALUE
Shortbread homestyle cookies, 2	3
Soft baked Captiva dark chocolate brownie cookies, 1	3
Soft baked carmel milk chocolate chunk caramel cookies, 1	3
Soft baked milk chocolate cookies, 1	3
Soft baked molasses cookies, 1	3
Soft baked oatmeal cookies, 1	3
Soft baked oatmeal cranberry cookies, 1	3
Soft baked Santa Cruz oatmeal raisin cookies, 1	3
Soft baked snickerdoodle cookies, 1	3
Soft baked sugar cookies, 1	3
Specialty cookie collection gift box, 3	3
Sugar free Milano cookies, 3	4
Sugar free mint Milano cookies, 3	4
Sugar homestyle cookies, 3	3
Tahiti cookies, 2	4
Tahoe white chocolate chunk macadamia nut cookies, 1	3
Toasted coconut petite truffle cookies, 5	4
Verona apple caramel cookies, 3	3
Verona apricot raspberry cookies, 3	3
Verona blueberry cookies, 3	3
Verona strawberry cookies, 3	3
Perfect Bite Cookies	
Sugar free chocolate chip, 3	2
Sugar free lemon, 3	2
Sugar free oatmeal, 3	2
Sugar free peanut butter, 3	2

	POINTS VALUE
Pillsbury	
Holiday shapes (sugar), 2	3
Sugar cookie dough sheets, 1 serving (1/12 package)	4
Pillsbury Create 'N Bake	
Chocolate chip cookies, 1 ball	3
Chocolate chip walnut cookies, 1 ball	3
Double chocolate chip & chip cookies, 1 ball	3
Oatmeal chocolate chip cookies, 1 ball	3
Peanut butter cookies, 1 ball	3
Sugar cookies, 1 slice	3
Pillsbury Ready To Bake!	
Chocolate candy cookies, 1	2
Chocolate chip, 1	2
Chocolate chip mini bites, 4	3
Chocolate chip with walnuts, 1	2
Chocolate chunk & chip, 1	2
Oatmeal chocolate chip cookies, 1	2
Peanut butter blossom cookies, 1	3
Reeses pieces, 1	2
S'mores, 1	2
Sugar, 1	2
Sugar free chocolate chip, 1	2
Pillsbury Ready To Bake! Big Deluxe Classics	
Chocolate chip, 1	5
Oatmeal raisin, 1	4
Peanut butter cup, 1	4
Triple chocolate indulgence cookies, 1	5
Turtle, 1	5
White chunk macadamia nut, 1	5

	POINTS VALUE
Pillsbury Simply Bake Bars	
Peanut butter chocolate chunk bars, 1 serving (1/9 package)	4
Turtle supreme bars, 1 serving (1/9 package)	4
Pillsbury Tub Cookie Dough	
Chocolate chip, 1 oz	3
Quaker Oats Breakfast Cookie	
Apple cinnamon, 1	3
Oatmeal raisin, 1	3
Reese's	
Cookie, soft baked, 1/2	3
Roberts	
Assorted, 7	4
Butter artificially flavored, 4	3
Chocolate chip, 4	3
Chocolate cremes, 3	4
Coconut bars, 4	3
Coconut chocolate chip, 4	3
Fudge grahams, 4	3
Fudge striped, 5	4
Gingersnaps, 4	3
Lemon cremes, 3	4
Oatmeal raisin, 4	3
Peanut butter cremes, 3	4
Pecan shortee, 4	3
Sprinkled butter (holiday), 5	3
Striped chocolate chip, 4	4
Vanilla cremes, 3	4

	POINTS VALUE
Rocks n' Rolls	
Almond French munching cookies, 1 serving (30 g)	2
Almond/orange gluten-free madeleines cookies, 1	3
Almond/orange with dark chocolate, 1	3
Chocolate French munching cookies, 1 serving (30 g)	2
Cinnamon French munching cookies, 1 serving (30 g)	2
Lemon & vanilla French munching cookies, 1 serving (30 g)	2
Lemon/vanilla gluten-free madeleines cookies, 1	3
Lemon/vanilla with white chocolate, 1	3
Orange chocolate chip French munching cookies, 1 serving (30 g)	2
Praline French munching cookies, 1 serving (30 g)	2
Raspberry chocolate chip French munching cookies, 1 serving (30 g)	2
Santa Fe Farms Fat Free Cookies	
Chocolate chocolate chip, 4	1
Chocolate mint chip, 4	1
Ginger, 4	1
Sathers	
Chocolate chip, 4	4
Regal grahams, 4	3
Shortbread, 5	4
Stella D'oro	
Almond delight cookies, 1 serving (30 g)	4
Almond toast cookies, 1 serving (27 g)	2
Angel wings cookies, 1 serving (30 g)	4

Candy, Cookies & Desserts

Stella D'oro (cont'd)	POINTS VALUE
Anginetti cookies, 1 serving (30 g)	3
Anisette sponge cookies, 1 serving (25 g)	2
Anisette toast, 1 serving (34 g)	3
Banana walnut toast cookies, 1 serving (26 g)	2
Biscotti, almond, 1 serving (20 g)	2
Biscotti, chocolate almond, 1 serving (20 g)	2
Biscotti, chocolate chunk, 1 serving (20 g)	2
Biscotti, French vanilla, 1 serving (20 g)	2
Blueberry toast cookies, 1 serving (26 g)	2
Breakfast treats, chocolate, 1 serving (23 g)	2
Breakfast treats, mini, original, 1 serving (28 g)	3
Breakfast treats, original, 1 serving (22 g)	2
Cinnamon raisin toast cookies, 1 serving (26 g)	2
Egg jumbo cookies, 1 serving (33 g)	3
Holiday fruit slices, 2	3
Lady stella cookie assortment, 3 (28 g)	3
Margherite, 2	3
Margherite cookies, mini, 1 serving (34 g)	3
Mini anisette toast cookies, 1 serving (34 g)	3
Roman egg biscuits, 1 serving (32 g)	3
Swiss fudge, 3 (34 g)	4
Viennese cinnamon breakfast treats, 1 serving (22 g)	2

	POINTS VALUE
Stella D'oro Holiday	
Pfeffernusse spice drops, 1 serving (25 g)	2
Sunbelt	
Hearty grain cookies, oatmeal blueberry, 1	3
Hearty grain cookies, oatmeal raisin, 1	3
Sunshine	
Hydrox chocolate sandwich, 3	4
Tree of Life	
Coconut macaroon, unsulphured, 1 oz	4
Walkers	
Pure butter chocolate chip shortbread, 2 pieces	3
Pure butter shortbread, 1 piece	3
Pure butter shortbread rounds, 1 piece	2
Pure butter shortbread triangles, 2 pieces	3
Weight Watchers	
Chocolate chip soft cookie, 1 cookie	1
Oatmeal raisin soft cookie, 1 cookie	1
Peanut butter soft cookie, 1 cookie	1
World of Grains	
Apple cinnamon cookies, 1 package	2
Blueberry cookies, 1 package	2
Cranberry cookies, 1 package	2
Multigrain cookies, 1 packet	2
Oatmeal raisin cookies, 1 package	2

Frozen Yogurt
Blue Bell	
Banana split nonfat, 1/2 cup	2
Country vanilla, lowfat, 1/2 cup	2

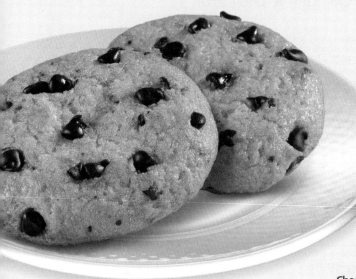

1 POINTS VALUE

Per Cookie

**Chocolate Chip
Soft Cookie**

SMART

sweetness.

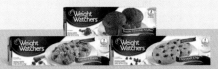

Find more information at WeightWatchers.com/cookies

)WeightWatchers®

Stop Dieting. Start Living.

WEIGHT WATCHERS on foods and beverages is the registered trademark of WW Foods, LLC and is used under license by Dawn Food Products, Inc. WEIGHT WATCHERS for services and *POINTS* are the registered trademarks of Weight Watchers International, Inc. and are used under license by Dawn Food Products, Inc. ©2009 Weight Watchers International, Inc. All rights reserved.

Candy, Cookies & Desserts

Blue Bell (cont'd)	POINTS VALUE
Strawberry nonfat, 1/2 cup	2
The great divide lowfat frozen yogurt, 1/2 cup	2
Blue Bunny	
Brownie fudge fantasy fat free frozen yogurt, 1/2 cup	2
Double strawberry frozen yogurt bar, 1	3
Fat free homemade chocolate frozen yogurt, 1/2 cup	2
Fat free homemade vanilla frozen yogurt, 1/2 cup	2
Fat free strawberry cheesecake frozen yogurt, 1/2 cup	2
Raspberry frozen yogurt bar, 1	3
Fruitfull	
Blueberry, 1 bar	2
Chocolate yogurt bar, 1 bar	3
Vanilla, 1 bar	3
Stonyfield Farm Organic	
Low fat cookies'n dream, 1/2 cup	3
Low fat crème - caramel, 1/2 cup	3
Low fat minty chocolate chip, 1/2 cup	3
Low fat raspberry white chocolate chunk, 1/2 cup	3
Nonfat after dark chocolate, 1/2 cup	2
Nonfat gotta have java, 1/2 cup	2
Nonfat gotta have vanilla, 1/2 cup	2
Nonfat vanilla fudge swirl, 1/2 cup	2
Turkey Hill	
Banana split, 1/2 cup	2
Chocolate cherry cordial, fat free, 1/2 cup	2

	POINTS VALUE
Chocolate chip cookie dough, low fat, 1/2 cup	2
Chocolate marshmallow, fat free, 1/2 cup	2
Fudge ripple, fat free, 1/2 cup	2
Green tea mango, 1/2 cup	2
Mint cookies 'n cream, low fat, 1/2 cup	2
Neapolitan, fat free, 1/2 cup	2
Nutty caramel caribou (limited edition), 1/2 cup	2
Orange cream swirl, 1/2 cup	2
Peach mango, 1/2 cup	2
Pomegranate blueberry & cream with acai, 1/2 cup	2
Raspberry lemonade, 1/2 cup	2
Southern lemon pie, 1/2 cup	2
Strawberry kiwi passion fruit, 1/2 cup	2
Vanilla bean, fat free, 1/2 cup	2

Fruit Cobblers/Crisps

Marzetti

	POINTS VALUE
Apple crisp mix, 1 serving (1/8 package)	2

Mrs. Smith's

	POINTS VALUE
Apple cobbler, 1 serving (1/8 cobbler)	5
Blackberry cobbler, 1 serving (1/8 cobbler)	5
Cherry cobbler, 1 serving (1/8 cobbler)	5
Peach cobbler, 1 serving (1/8 cobbler)	5

Gelatins

Certo

	POINTS VALUE
Fruit pectin, 2 pouches	0

Candy, Cookies & Desserts

	POINTS VALUE
Del Monte	
Mango chiller, 1 cup	3
Peaches in peach flavored gel, 1 cup	2
Peaches in strawberry banana flavored gel-lite, 1 cup	1
Raspberry chiller, 1 cup	3
Strawberry chiller, 1 cup	3
Jell-O	
Apple, 1/4 package	2
Apricot, prepared, 1/2 cup	2
Berry blue, prepared, 1/2 cup	2
Black cherry, prepared, 1/2 cup	2
Cherry, prepared, 1/2 cup	2
Color changing grape flavor extreme, 1/4 package	2
Cranberry raspberry, prepared, 1/2 cup	2
Cranberry, prepared, 1/2 cup	2
Grape, prepared, 1/2 cup	2
Lemon, prepared, 1/2 cup	2
Lime, prepared, 1/2 cup	2
Mexican gelatina lime, 1/8 package	1
Mexican gelatina orange, 1/8 package	1
Mexican gelatina pineapple, 1/8 package	1
Mexican gelatina strawberry, 1/8 package	1
Mixed fruit, prepared, 1/2 cup	2
Orange, prepared, 1/2 cup	2
Peach, prepared, 1/2 cup	2
Pineapple, prepared, 1/2 cup	2
Raspberry, prepared, 1/2 cup	2

	POINTS VALUE
Strawberry banana, prepared, 1/2 cup	2
Strawberry, prepared, 1/2 cup	2
Sugar free gelatin strawberry, 1/8 package	0
Sugar-free black cherry, 1/4 package	0
Sugar-free cherry, prepared, 1/2 cup	0
Sugar-free cranberry, prepared, 1/2 cup	0
Sugar-free lemon, prepared, 1/2 cup	0
Sugar-free lime, prepared, 1/2 cup	0
Sugar-free mixed fruit, prepared, 1/2 cup	0
Sugar-free orange, prepared, 1/2 cup	0
Sugar-free raspberry, prepared, 1/2 cup	0
Sugar-free strawberry banana, prepared, 1/2 cup	0
Sugar-free strawberry kiwi, prepared, 1/2 cup	0
Sugar-free strawberry, prepared, 1/2 cup	0
Summer breezes pina colada, 1/4 package	2
Summer breezes strawberry daquiri, 1/4 package	2
Watermelon, prepared, 1/2 cup	2
Wild strawberry, prepared, 1/2 cup	2
Jell-O Fruit Passions	
Peaches & pineapple 'n orange, 1 serving	1
Peaches 'n strawberry, 1 serving	1
Pineapple & peaches 'n lemon-lime, 1 serving	1
Pineapple 'n raspberry, 1 serving	1
Tropical fruit 'n peach, 1 serving	1

Candy, Cookies & Desserts

	POINTS VALUE
Jell-O Gel Cups X-Treme	
Cherry & blue raspberry, 1	1
Jell-O Gelatin Snacks	
Orange, 1	1
Raspberry, 1	1
Strawberry, 1	1
Strawberry/orange, 1	1
Strawberry/raspberry, 1	1
Sugar free lemon lime, 1	0
Jell-O Sugar Free Low Calorie Gelatin Snacks	
Cherry/black-cherry, 1	0
Orange, 1	0
Orange lemon-lime, 1	0
Peach, 1	0
Peach & watermelon, 1	0
Raspberry, 1	0
Raspberry/orange, 1	0
Strawberry, 1	0
Strawberry-kiwi, 1	0
Strawberry-kiwi & tropical berry, 1	0
Tropical berry, 1	0
Jell-O Sugar-Based Gelatin Snacks	
Watermelon & green apple, 1	1
Knox	
Unflavored gelatin, 1/4 envelope	0
Kool-Aid Gels	
Cherry tropical punch, 1 container	1
Grape, 1 container	1
Ice blue raspberry, 1 container	1
Oh yea orange, 1 container	1

	POINTS VALUE
Orange, 1 container	1
Soarin' strawberry, 1 container	1
Payaso	
Strawberry gelatin dessert, 1/8 package	2
Sure Jell	
Fruit pectin for homemade jams & jellies, 1 serving (0.5 g)	0
Fruit pectin for lower sugar recipes, 1 serving (0.5 g)	0
Jam pectin no cook, 1 serving (0.5 g)	0
## Gum, Chewing	
Big League Chew	
Grape, 8 pieces	0
Original, 8 pieces	0
Sour apple, 8 pieces	0
Strawberry, 8 pieces	0
Watermelon, 8 pieces	0
Extra	
Cool green apple, 1 stick	0
Hubba Bubba Bubble Jug	
Tropical fruit, 1 tsp	1
Watermelon, 1 tsp	1
Hubba Bubba Bubble Tape	
Awesome original, 1 piece	0
Cotton candy, 1 piece	0
Gushing grape, 1 piece	0
Sour apple, 1 piece	0
Sour blue raspberry, 1 piece	0
Sour watermelon, 1 piece	0
Triple treat, 1 piece	0

Candy, Cookies & Desserts

	POINTS VALUE
Hubba Bubba Max	
Cherry-lemonade, 1 piece	1
Grape-berry, 1 piece	1
Sour double berry, 1 piece	1
Strawberry-watermelon, 1 piece	1
Hubba Bubba Ouch Multiflavor	
Grape, 1 stick	0
Sour watermelon, 1 stick	0
Strawberry, 1 stick	0
Juicy Fruit	
Tropikiwi kick, 2 pellets	0
Orbit	
Bubblemint, 1 piece	0
Cinnamint, 1 piece	0
Citrusmint, 1 piece	0
Peppermint, 1 piece	0
Spearmint, 1 piece	0
Sweet mint, 1 piece	0
Wintermint, 1 piece	0
Orbit White	
Bubblemint, 2 pieces	0
Peppermint, 2 pieces	0
Spearmint, 2 pieces	0
Trident Splash	
Apple with raspberry, 1 piece	0
Citrus with blackberry, 1 piece	0
Orange swirl, 1 piece	0
Peppermint swirl, 1 piece	0
Strawberry with lime, 1 piece	0
Summer spearmint, 1 piece	0

	POINTS VALUE
Wrigley's	
Big red, 1 stick	0
Doublemint, 1 stick	0
Juicy fruit, 1 stick	0
Juicy fruit grapemelon, 2 pieces	0
Juicy fruit strappleberry, 2 pieces	0
Spearmint, 1 stick	0
Winterfresh, 1 stick	0
Wrigley's Eclipse	
Cherry chill, 2 pieces	0
Lemon burst, 2 pieces	0
Peppermint, 2 pieces	0
Polar ice, 2 pieces	0
Spearmint, 2 pieces	0
Winterfresh, 2 pieces	0
Wrigley's Extra Sugarfree	
Cinnamon, 1 stick	0
Classic bubble gum, 1 stick	0
Peppermint, 1 stick	0
Polar ice, 1 piece	0
Spearmint, 1 stick	0
Wildberry frost, 1 stick	0
Winterfresh, 1 stick	0
Wrigley's Freedent	
Peppermint, 1 stick	0
Spearmint, 1 stick	0
Winterfresh, 1 stick	0

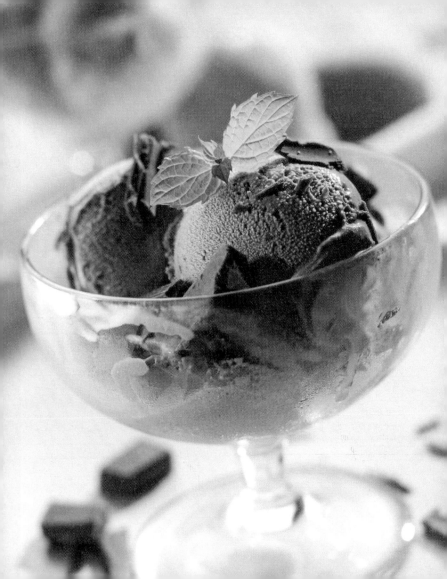

POINTS VALUE

Ice Cream

Blue Bell

Almond bar, 1 bar	5
Banana pudding, 1/2 cup	4
Banana split, 1/2 cup	4
Banana split no sugar added lowfat, 1/2 cup	1
Belle bar, 1 bar	5
Birthday cake cups, 1 container (72 g)	4
Buttered pecan, 1/2 cup	5
Buttered pecan bars, 1 bar	5
Buttered pecan no sugar added lowfat, 1/2 cup	1
Caramel turtle fudge ice cream, 1/2 cup	5
Chocolate chip, 1/2 cup	4
Chocolate chip cookie dough, 1/2 cup	5
Chocolate covered cherries bars, 1 bar	5
Chocolate extreme, 1/2 cup	5
Chocolate French silk, 1/2 cup	3
Chocolate fudge bar, 1 bar	2
Cookies n cream, 1/2 cup	4
Cookies n cream light, 1/2 cup	4
Cookies 'n cream sandwich, 1	4
Country cone, cookies 'n cream, 1	6
Country cone, vanilla, 1	7
Country vanilla no sugar added lowfat, 1/2 cup	1
Créme pops, 1 bar	1
Double vanilla ice cream sandwich, 1	4
Dream bar, 1 bar	2
Dutch chocolate, 1/2 cup	4
Dutch chocolate cups, 1 container (81 g)	4

Dutch chocolate, no sugar added lowfat, 1/2 cup	1
French vanilla, 1/2 cup	4
Fudge blast, 1 bar	4
Fudge bombstik, 1 bar	5
Great divide bars, 1 bar	5
Homemade vanilla, 1 container (81 g)	4
Homemade vanilla, 1/2 cup	4
Homemade vanilla bars, 1 bar	5
Homemade vanilla cup, 1 container (81 g)	4
Homemade vanilla light, 1/2 cup	3
Ice cream sandwich, 1	4
Krunch bar, 1 bar	5
Milk chocolate, 1/2 cup	4
Mini sandwiches, 2	4
Mini vanilla country cones, 1 cone	2
Mint chocolate chip, 1/2 cup	4
Moo-llennium crunch, 1/2 cup	5
Mooo bars, 1 bar	4
Natural vanilla bean, 1/2 cup	4
Neapolitan ice cream sandwich, 1	4
No sugar added fudge bars, 1 bar	1
No sugar added krunch bars, 1 bar	2
No sugar added mooo bars, 1 bar	2
Orange swirl country cooler, 1/2 cup	3
Peaches & homemade vanilla, 1/2 cup	4
Pecan pralines 'n cream, 1/2 cup	5
Pop 'n fudge, banana fudge bar, 1 bar	2
Pop 'n fudge, chocolate fudge bar, 1 bar	3
Pop 'n fudge, orange and cherry pop, 1 bar	1
Rainbow sherbet pop up, 1 bar	2
Rocky road, 1/2 cup	4

Candy, Cookies & Desserts

Blue Bell (cont'd)	POINTS VALUE
Southern blackberry cobbler, 1/2 cup	4
Southern hospitality, 1/2 cup	4
Strawberries & homemade vanilla, 1/2 cup	4
Strawberries & homemade vanilla bars, 1 bar	5
Strawberry, 1/2 cup	3
The great divide, 1/2 cup	4
The great divide ice cream, light, 1/2 cup	3
The great divide ice cream, no sugar added lowfat, 1/2 cup	1
Ultimate neapolitan, 1/2 cup	4
Ultimate neapolitan - light, 1/2 cup	3
Blue Bunny	
Banana split ice cream, 1/2 cup	4
Big star bar double chocolate, 1	3
Birthday cake flavored light ice cream sandwich, 1	3
Butter pecan 100 calorie bar, 1	2
Champ caramel ice cream cone, 1 cone	8
Champ ice cream cone variety pack, caramel nut, 1 cone	8
Champ ice cream cone variety pack, fudge nut, 1 cone	8
Champ ice cream cone variety pack, homemade vanilla, 1 cone	8
Chocolate chip cookie dough ice cream, 1/2 cup	4
Chocolate chip ice cream, 1/2 cup	3
Chocolate fudge bars, 2 bars	3
Chocolate ice cream, 1/2 cup	3
Chocolate lovers' champ ice cream cones, 1 cone	7

	POINTS VALUE
Chocolate malt cups, 1 cup	5
Chocolate raspberry cheesecake light ice cream, 1/2 cup	2
Chocolate sundae crunch bar, 1 bar	4
Chocolate sundae cups, 1 cup	3
Chocolate/vanilla flavored ice cream, 1/2 cup	3
Classic vanilla sundae cones, 1 cone	6
Cookies & cream ice cream, 1/2 cup	3
Crunch bar, 1 bar	4
Double chocolate yogurt granola sandwich, 1	4
Double fudge bars, 2 bars	3
Double strawberry light ice cream, 1/2 cup	2
Double strawberry yogurt granola sandwich, 1	3
English toffee bars, 1 bar	3
French vanilla flavored ice cream, 1/2 cup	3
Fudge bar, 1 bar	2
Fudge ice cream bar, 1 bar	1
Fudge twirl ice cream, 1/2 cup	3
Goin' bananas bar, 2 bars	3
Homemade vanilla ice cream bars, 1 bar	4
Homemade vanilla ice cream sandwiches, 1	4
Ice cream sandwich, 1	4
Jolly rancher pops - watermelon, lemon, and green apple, 1 bar	1
Mint bon bon ice cream, 1/2 cup	3
Mississippi mud ice cream sandwich, 1	4
Neapolitan ice cream, 1/2 cup	3
Neapolitan ice cream sandwich, 1	4
New York vanilla flavored ice cream, 1/2 cup	3

Candy, Cookies & Desserts

	POINTS VALUE
Orange and vanilla low fat ice cream bar, 1 bar	2
Orange dream bar, 1 bar	2
Original banana split ice cream, 1/2 cup	3
Original bunny tracks ice cream, 1/2 cup	4
Original butter pecan ice cream, 1/2 cup	4
Original chocolate caramel commotion ice cream, 1/2 cup	4
Original chocolate chip cookie dough ice cream, 1/2 cup	4
Original chocolate chip ice cream, 1/2 cup	3
Original chocolate ice cream, 1/2 cup	3
Original cookies & cream ice cream, 1/2 cup	4
Original French vanilla flavored ice cream, 1/2 cup	3
Original homemade vanilla flavored ice cream, 1/2 cup	3
Original hot fudge sundae ice cream, 1/2 cup	4
Original mint chip ice cream, 1/2 cup	3
Original neapolitan ice cream, 1/2 cup	3
Original orange dream, 1/2 cup	3
Original Ozark black walnut ice cream, 1/2 cup	4
Original peanut butter brownie sensation ice cream, 1/2 cup	4
Original strawberry cheesecake ice cream, 1/2 cup	3
Original strawberry ice cream, 1/2 cup	3
Original tin roof sundae ice cream, 1/2 cup	4
Original vanilla flavored ice cream, 1/2 cup	3
Peanut butter fudge light ice cream, 1/2 cup	2
Rainbow sherbet cups, 1 cup	2

	POINTS VALUE
Raspberry and vanilla low fat ice cream bars, 1 bar	2
Rocky road ice cream sandwich, 1	4
Root beer float bars, 1 small bar	2
Root beer float bars, 1 bar	2
Star bar, 1 bar	3
Strawberry marble ice cream, 1/2 cup	3
Strawberry sundae crunch bar, 1 bar	4
Strawberry sundae cups, 1 cup	3
Super chunky cookie dough ice cream, 1/2 cup	4
Super fudge brownie light ice cream, 1/2 cup	2
Toffee 100 calorie bar, 1	2
Triple chocolate light ice cream sandwich, 1	3
Vanilla flavored ice cream, 1/2 cup	3
Vanilla flavored ice cream cups, 1 cup	3
Vanilla fudge ice cream bar, 1	1
Vanilla light ice cream, 1/2 cup	2
Vanilla nutty sundae cones, 1 bar	5
Vanilla orange crème bar, 1	2
Vanilla raspberry crème bar, 1	2
Yogurt smoothie fat free frozen yogurt bar, peach, 1 bar	1
Yogurt smoothie fat free frozen yogurt bar, strawberry, 1 bar	1
Blue Bunny Carb Freedom	
Chocolate almond fudge dairy dessert, 1/2 cup	2
Blue Bunny Champ	
Banana split super cone, 1	5
Hot fudge brownie super cone, 1	5
Malt shoppe sundae super cone, 1	5

Candy, Cookies & Desserts

	POINTS VALUE
Blue Bunny Champ (cont'd)	
Strawberry cone, 1 cone	5
Blue Bunny Doubles	
Banana split ice cream bar, 1	4
Peanut butter cup ice cream bar, 1	5
S'mores ice cream bar, 1	4
Blue Bunny Fat Free No Sugar Added	
Caramel toffee crunch ice cream, 1/2 cup	1
Vanilla flavored ice cream, 1/2 cup	1
Vanilla flavored ice cream, 1/2 cup	1
Blue Bunny FrozFruit	
Coconut cream bar, 1 bar	4
Blue Bunny Hi Lite	
Chocolate lite ice cream, 1/2 cup	2
Cookies & cream lite ice cream, 1/2 cup	3
Fudge nut sundae lite ice cream, 1/2 cup	3
Homemade vanilla lite ice cream, 1/2 cup	3
Mint chip lite ice cream, 1/2 cup	3
Vanilla flavored lite ice cream, 1/2 cup	2
Vanilla light ice cream, 1/2 cup	2
Blue Bunny No Sugar Added	
Banana split reduced fat ice cream, 1/2 cup	2
Blue Bunny Personals	
Banana split ice cream, 1/2 cup	4
Bunny tracks light ice cream, 1/2 cup	2
Double strawberry light ice cream, 1/2 cup	2
Peanut butter fudge light, 1/2 cup	2
Peanut butter panic ice cream, 1/2 cup	5
Premium bunny tracks light ice cream, 1/2 cup	2
Premium chocolate raspberry cheesecake light ice cream, 1/2 cup	2

	POINTS VALUE
Premium double strawberry ice cream, 1/2 cup	3
Premium turtle sundae, 1/2 cup	4
Super chunky cookie dough ice cream, 1/2 cup	4
Super fudge brownie ice cream, 1/2 cup	4
Super fudge brownie light ice cream, 1/2 cup	2
Blue Bunny Premium	
All natural vanilla bean ice cream, 1/2 cup	4
Bordeaux cherry chocolate ice cream, 1/2 cup	4
Bunny tracks ice cream, 1/2 cup	5
Bunny tracks ice cream (pint), 1/2 cup	5
Bunny tracks light ice cream, 1/2 cup	2
Butter pecan ice cream, 1/2 cup	4
Butter Pecan ice cream (pint), 1/2 cup	4
Butter pecan light ice cream, 1/2 cup	2
Chocolate chip cookie ice cream, 1/2 cup	4
Chocolate chunk ice cream, 1/2 cup	4
Coffee break ice cream, 1/2 cup	3
Cookies & cream ice cream (pint), 1/2 cup	4
Cookies and cream ice cream, 1/2 cup	4
Double strawberry ice cream, 1/2 cup	3
Double strawberry ice cream (pint), 1/2 cup	3
Fat free no sugar added brownie sundae ice cream, 1/2 cup	1
French vanilla flavored ice cream, 1/2 cup	4
Homemade chocolate ice cream, 1/2 cup	4
Homemade chocolate ice cream (pint), 1/2 cup	4
Homemade turtle sundae ice cream, 1/2 cup	4

Candy, Cookies & Desserts

	POINTS VALUE
Homemade turtle sundae ice cream (pint), 1/2 cup	6
Homemade vanilla flavored ice cream, 1/2 cup	4
Homemade vanilla flavored ice cream (pint), 1/2 cup	4
Mint chocolate chunk ice cream, 1/2 cup	4
Monster cookie ice cream, 1/2 cup	4
No sugar added bunny tracks ice cream, 1/2 cup	3
No sugar added butter pecan ice cream, 1/2 cup	3
No sugar added cherry vanilla flavored ice cream, 1/2 cup	2
No sugar added chocolate chip cookie reduced fat ice cream, 1/2 cup	3
No sugar added chocolate chunk cookie reduced fat ice cream, 1/2 cup	3
No sugar added double strawberry ice cream, 1/2 cup	2
No sugar added rocky road ice cream, 1/2 cup	3
No sugar added turtle sundae ice cream, 1/2 cup	3
No sugar added vanilla flavored ice cream, 1/2 cup	2
Peanut butter cookie ice cream, 1/2 cup	5
Peanut butter panic ice cream, 1/2 cup	6
Pistachio almond ice cream, 1/2 cup	3
Rocky road ice cream, 1/2 cup	4
Super fudge brownie ice cream, 1/2 cup	4
Toasted almond fudge ice cream, 1/2 cup	4
Vanilla flavored ice cream, 1/2 cup	3
Vanilla flavored ice cream (pint), 1/2 cup	4

	POINTS VALUE
Blue Bunny Sweet Carb Freedom	
Black raspberry bar, 1 bar	2
Blue Bunny Sweet Freedom	
Black raspberry bar, 1 bar	2
Candy bar, 1 bar	6
Chocolate almond fudge dairy dessert, 1/2 cup	2
Chocolate ice cream lites - no sugar added, 1 bar	2
Chocolate peanut butter dairy dessert, 1/2 cup	3
Fudge lites, no sugar added, 2 bars	1
Ice cream lites, no sugar added, 1 bar	2
Ice cream sandwiches, 1	2
Krunch lites, no sugar added, 1 bar	2
Dove	
Beyond vanilla ice cream, 1/2 cup	6
Caramel pecan perfection ice cream, 1/2 cup	9
Chocolate & brownie affair ice cream, 1/2 cup	7
Chocolate & cherry courtship ice cream, 1/2 cup	7
Chocolate with almonds ice cream bar, 1 bar	7
Dark chocolate with vanilla ice cream bar, 1 bar	6
Give into mint ice cream, 1/2 cup	7
Ice cream miniatures chocolate with French vanilla, 1 piece	2
Ice cream miniatures chocolate with vanilla ice cream, 1 piece	2
Ice cream miniatures flavor collection, 1 piece	2

Candy, Cookies & Desserts

Dove (cont'd)

POINTS VALUE

Irresistibly raspberry ice cream, 1/2 cup	6
Milk chocolate ice cream bar, 1 bar	6
Toffee and caramel moment ice cream, 1/2 cup	7
Unconditional chocolate ice cream, 1/2 cup	7
Vanilla with chocolate soul ice cream, 1/2 cup	7

Fruitfull

Banana bar, 1 bar	2
Coconut bar, 1 bar	3
Horchata, 1 bar	6
Mango cream bar, 1 bar	4
Peaches 'n cream bar, 1 bar	3
Pina colada bar, 1 bar	2
Raspberry cream, 1 bar	2
Strawberry cream bar, 1 bar	2

Greek Gods

Baklava ice cream, 1/2 cup	6
Chocolate fig ice cream, 1/2 cup	6
Honey pomegranate ice cream, 1/2 cup	6

Happy Indulgence Decadent Dips

Banana cream bar (chocolate-dipped), 1 bar	6
Banana split bar (chocolate-dipped), 1 bar	7
Cherry cream bar (chocolate-dipped), 1 bar	7
Coconut cream bar (chocolate-dipped), 1 bar	7
Mud pie bar (chocolate-dipped), 1 bar 1 bar	10
Strawberry cream bar (chocolate-dipped), 1 bar	7

POINTS VALUE

Klondike

Original Vanilla ice cream bars, 1 piece	7

Market Day

Apple blossoms, 1	8
Root beer float cups, 1	6

Nestle

Classic vanilla drumsticks, 1	9

Stonyfield Farm Organic Super Premium

After dark chocolate, 1/2 cup	6
Chocolate raspberry swirl, 1/2 cup	6
Cookies'n Dream, 1/2 cup	7
Crème caramel, 1/2 cup	6
Gotta have java, 1/2 cup	6
Gotta have vanilla, 1/2 cup	6
Vanilla chai, 1/2 cup	6

Turkey Hill

Double decker ice cream sandwich, 1	4
Ice cream sandwich, strawberry cheesecake (limited edition), 1	4
Ice cream sandwich, vanilla bean, 1	4
Vanilla fudge sundae cones, 1	8

Turkey Hill All Natural Recipe

Chocolate, 1/2 cup	4
Coffee, 1/2 cup	3
Mint chocolate chip, 1/2 cup	4
Neapolitan, 1/2 cup	3
Nutty neapolitan, 1/2 cup	4
Vanilla bean, 1/2 cup	3

Turkey Hill Creamy Commotions

Chocolate malt chip, 1/2 cup	4
Lana's strawberry cheesecake, 1/2 cup	4

Candy, Cookies & Desserts

	POINTS VALUE
Moose tracks, 1/2 cup	4
Snyder's chocolate pretzel, 1/2 cup	4
Tastykake chocolate cupcake, 1/2 cup	4
Tastykake peanut butter kandy kake, 1/2 cup	5
Turkey Hill Duetto	
Cherry, 1/2 cup	3
Chocolate & coconut, 1/2 cup	3
Chocolate coconut, 1/2 cup	3
Lemon, 1/2 cup	3
Mango, 1/2 cup	2
Pombluberry, 1/2 cup	3
Raspberry, 1/2 cup	3
Rootbeer, 1/2 cup	3
Strawberry banana, 1/2 cup	2

	POINTS VALUE
Turkey Hill Light Recipe	
Banana split, 1/2 cup	2
Chocolate chip cookie dough, 1/2 cup	2
Chocolate nutty moose tracks, 1/2 cup	3
Cookies 'n cream, 1/2 cup	2
Dulce de chocolate, 1/2 cup	3
Extreme cookies n' cream, 1/2 cup	3
Ice cream sandwich, 1	3
Raspberry chocolate chunk, 1/2 cup	3
Skinny minty, 1/2 cup	3
Vanilla bean, 1/2 cup	2
Turkey Hill Light Recipe Ice Cream	
Choco malt chip, 1/2 cup	2
Chocolate chip, 1/2 cup	3
Moose tracks, 1/2 cup	3

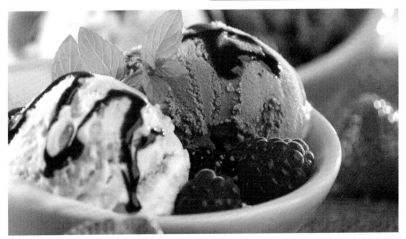

Candy, Cookies & Desserts

Turkey Hill Light Recipe Ice Cream (cont'd)	*POINTS VALUE*
Peanut butter mania, 1/2 cup	3
Snyder's chocolate pretzel, 1/2 cup	3
Strawberry cheesecake, 1/2 cup	3
Turkey Hill No Sugar Added	
Cherry fudge ripple, 1/2 cup	1
Dutch chocolate, 1/2 cup	1
Peanut brittle, low fat, 1/2 cup	2
Vanilla bean, 1/2 cup	1
Turkey Hill Premium	
Baked apple dumpling, 1/2 cup	4
Black cherry, 1/2 cup	3
Black raspberry, 1/2 cup	3
Butter pecan, 1/2 cup	4
Choco mint chip, 1/2 cup	4
Chocolate chip cookie dough, 1/2 cup	4
Chocolate marshmallow, 1/2 cup	4
Chocolate peanut butter cup, 1/2 cup	4
Coconut cream pie, 1/2 cup	4
Colombian coffee, 1/2 cup	3
Cookies n' cream, 1/2 cup	4
Dutch chocolate, 1/2 cup	3
Egg nog, 1/2 cup	3
French vanilla, 1/2 cup	3
Fried ice cream, 1/2 cup	4
Fudge ripple, 1/2 cup	3
Gertrude Hawk box of chocolate (limited edition), 1/2 cup	4
Junior mint, 1/2 cup	4
Neapolitan, 1/2 cup	3
Orange cream swirl, 1/2 cup	3
Original vanilla, 1/2 cup	3

	POINTS VALUE
Peaches n' cream, 1/2 cup	3
Peanut Butter Ripple, 1/2 cup	4
Peppermint stick (limited edition), 1/2 cup	4
Pineapple upside down cake (limited edition), 1/2 cup	4
Rocky road, 1/2 cup	4
Rum raisin, 1/2 cup	3
Southern lemon pie, 1/2 cup	4
Strawberries and cream, 1/2 cup	3
Tin roof sundae, 1/2 cup	4
Vanilla and chocolate, 1/2 cup	3
Vanilla bean, 1/2 cup	3
Vanilla Swiss almond, 1/2 cup	4
Turkey Hill Premium Ice Cream	
Banana split, 1/2 cup	3
Eagles touchdown sundae, 1/2 cup	4
Party cake, 1/2 cup	4
Phillies graham slam, 1/2 cup	5
Turkey Hill Stuff'd	
Chocolate mint moose tracks, 1/2 cup	3
Chocolate nutty moose tracks, 1/2 cup	3
Praline pecan paradise, 1/2 cup	2
Weight Watchers	
Candy bar ice cream bar, 1 bar	3
Chocolate chip cookie dough cup, 1 cup	2
Chocolate fudge brownie cup, 1 cup	2
Chocolate round ice cream sandwich, 1 sandwich	2
Cookies and cream cup, 1 cup	2
Chocolate mousse bars, 2 bars	2
English toffee crunch bar, 2 bars	2

2 POINTS VALUE

Per Sandwich
**Chocolate
Ice Cream
Sandwich**

INDULGENT

tastiness.

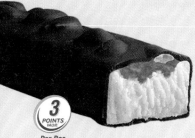

3 POINTS VALUE

Per Bar
**Candy Bar
Ice Cream Bar**

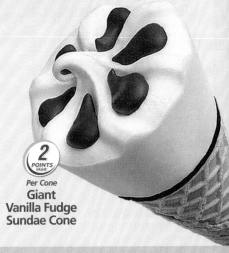

2 POINTS VALUE

Per Cone
**Giant
Vanilla Fudge
Sundae Cone**

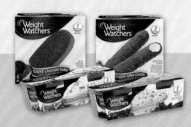

WeightWatchers®

Stop Dieting. Start Living.

Find more information at WeightWatchers.com/icecream

WEIGHT WATCHERS on foods and beverages is the registered trademark of WW Foods, LLC and is used under license by Wells' Dairy, Inc. WEIGHT WATCHERS for services and **POINTS** are the registered trademarks of Weight Watchers International, Inc. and are used under license by Wells' Dairy, Inc. ©2009 Weight Watchers International, Inc. All rights reserved.

Candy, Cookies & Desserts

Weight Watchers (cont'd)	POINTS VALUE
Giant chocolate cookies 'n cream bar, 1 bar	2
Giant chocolate fudge sundae cone, 1 cone	2
Giant cookies 'n chocolate cream bar, 1 bar	2
Giant fudge bar, 1 bar	1
Giant latte bar, 1 bar	1
Giant mint fudge cone, 1 cone	2
Giant orange sorbet & ice cream bar, 1 bar	2
Giant vanilla fudge sundae cone, 1 cone	2
Giant wildberry sorbet & ice cream bar, 1 bar	2
Key lime sherbet & ice cream bar, 2 bars	2
Mint ice cream sandwich, 1 sandwich	2
Mint chocolate chip cup, 1 cup	2
Passion fruit sherbet & ice cream bar, 2 bars	2
Peanut butter delight cup, 1 cup	3
Strawberry sherbet & ice cream bar, 2 bars	2
Turtle sundae cup, 1 cup	3
Vanilla ice cream sandwich, 1 sandwich	2
Vanilla round ice cream sandwich, 1 sandwich	2

Weight Watchers Smart Ones

Brownie a la mode, 1	4
Chocolate chip cookie dough sundae, 1	3
Mint chocolate chip sundae, 1	3
Mocha fudge sundae, 1	3
Peanut butter cup sundae, 1	3

Ice Cream Cones & Toppings

Blue Bunny

Chocolate ice cream cups, 1	2

	POINTS VALUE
Cool Whip	
Chocolate, 2 Tbsp	1
Extra creamy whipped topping, 2 Tbsp	1
Free whipped topping, 2 Tbsp	0
French vanilla, 2 Tbsp	1
Lite whipped topping, 2 Tbsp	0
Strawberry, 2 Tbsp	1
Sugar free whipped topping, 2 Tbsp	0
Whipped topping, 2 Tbsp	1
Dream Whip	
Whipped topping mix, 1 serving (1/16 envelope)	0
Whipped topping mix, prepared as directed, 2 Tbsp	0
Fisher Chef's Naturals	
Nut topping, 2 Tbsp	2
Hershey's Shell Topping	
Chocolate, 2 Tbsp	6
Heath, 2 Tbsp	5
Reese, 2 Tbsp	5
Hershey's Sugar Free	
Syrup, 2 Tbsp	0
Keebler	
Ice cream cup fudge-dipped fudge shoppe, 1 cup	1
Ice cream waffle bowl, 1 bowl	1
Ice cream waffle cone, 1 cone	1
Sugar cones, 1	1
Nabisco	
Oreo chocolate ice cream cones, 1	1
Oreo crunchies, 1 serving	1

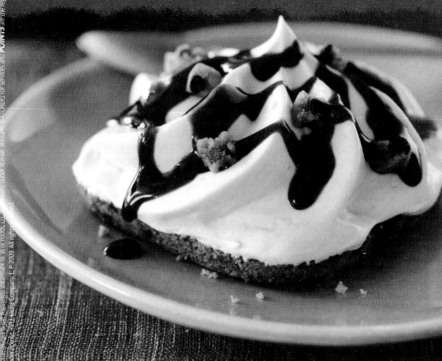

Guess who?

Satisfy your cravings with Weight Watchers® Smart Ones® Chocolate Chip Cookie Dough Sundae. Creamy ice cream, topped with cookie dough pieces and rich fudge sauce. And, with a *POINTS*® value of 3, it's deliciously smart, too.

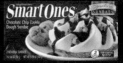

SAVE $4.00 at www.eatyourbest.com/food

WEIGHT WATCHERS is the registered trademark of WEIGHT WATCHERS International, Inc. and are used under license. *POINTS* are the registered trademarks of Weight Watchers International, Inc. and are used under license. SMART ONES and the SMART ONES logo are registered trademarks of H.J. Heinz Company, L.P. © 2009 All rights reserved.

Candy, Cookies & Desserts

	POINTS VALUE
Nabisco Comet	
Ice cream cups, 1	0
Ice cream cups rainbow, 1	0
Sugar cones, 1	1
Planters	
Nut topping, 2 Tbsp	3
Reddi-wip	
Chocolate, 2 Tbsp	0
Extra creamy, 2 Tbsp	1
Fat free, 2 Tbsp	0
Original, 2 Tbsp	0
Smucker's	
Light hot fudge topping, 2 Tbsp	1
Sugar free hot fudge topping, 2 Tbsp	2

Ices, Sherbets, Sorbets, Frozen Fruit Bars

	POINTS VALUE
Blue Bell	
Bullets, 1 bar	1
Lime sherbet, 1/2 cup	3
Megabite, 1 bar	3
Mini rainbows, 1 bar	1
Orange sherbet, 1/2 cup	3
Pineapple sherbet, 1/2 cup	3
Rainbow, 1/2 cup	3
Rainbow freeze, 1 bar	2
Sugar free bullets, 1 bar	0
Blue Bunny	
Lemonade bomb pop, 1 bar	1
Lime fat free sherbet, 1/2 cup	2
Lucas chamoy bar, 1 bar	1

	POINTS VALUE
Lucas pelucas bar, 1 bar	1
Orange fat free sherbet, 1/2 cup	2
Pineapple fat free sherbet, 1/2 cup	2
Polar pops, all flavors, 1 bar	1
Rainbow fat free sherbet, 1/2 cup	2
Raspberry fat free sherbet, 1/2 cup	2
Slush pops (grape, cherry, orange), 1 bar	1
Sour bomb pops (watermelon, orange blast, green apple), 1 bar	1
Sugar free bomb pops, 1 bar	0
The original bomb pop (cherry, lime, blue raspberry), 1 bar	1
Twin pops, all flavors, 1 bar	1
Blue Bunny FrozFruit	
Pomegranate cherry fruit bar, 1 bar	2
Raspberry acai fruit bar, 1 bar	1
Strawberry fruit bar, 1 bar	1
Fruit A Freeze	
All natural chocolate covered creamy banana bar, 1	5
All natural chocolate covered creamy strawberry bar, 1	5
All natural creamy coconut bar, 1	4
All natural creamy strawberry milk bar, 1	2
Banana milk bar, 1 bar	3
Creamy cappuccino milk bar, 1	3
Lime bar, 1	1
Mango pineapple bar, 1	1
Fruit Goodness	
Banana, 1 bar	2
Coconut, 1 bar	2

Candy, Cookies & Desserts

	POINTS VALUE
Lime, 1 bar	1
Mango cream, 1 bar	3
Strawberry, 1 bar	1
Strawberry cream, 1 bar	2
Fruitfull	
Fuzzynavel bar, 1 bar	1
Green tea melon, 1 bar	2
Guava bar, 1 bar	1
Lemon, 1 bar	2
Lemon bar, 1 bar	2
Lime bar, 1 bar	2
Passionate cherry bar, 1 bar	2
Pineapple bar, 1 bar	2
Raspberry bar, 1 bar	1
Strawberry bar, 1 bar	1
Tamarind, 1 bar	2
Tropical splash bar, 1 bar	2
Watermelon bar, 1 bar	1
Kool-Aid	
Kool pops freezer bars, 1	1
Luigi's	
No sugar added cherry, with splenda, 1 cup	1
No sugar added lemon with splenda, 1 cup	1
Luigi's Real Italian Ice	
Cherry, 1 cup	2
Lemon, 1 cup	2
Variety pack (lemon/strawberry), 1 cup	2
Variety pack, mango, 1 cup	3
Variety pack, pina colada, 1 cup	3

	POINTS VALUE
Luigi's Swirl Real Italian Ice	
Blue razzin' lemonade, 1 cup	3
Strawberry banana blast, 1 cup	3
Minute Maid	
Cherry juice bar, 1 bar	1
Grape juice bar, 1 bar	1
Juice bar, grape, 1 bar	1
Orange juice bar, 1 bar	1
Soft frozen cherry limeade, 1 tube	1
Soft frozen lemonade, 1 tube	1
Soft frozen limeade, 1 tube	1
Soft frozen raspberry lemonade, 1 tube	1
Popsicle	
Sugar free popsicle, orange, cherry, grape, 1	0
Sharon's	
Coconut, 1/2 cup	3
Dutch chocolate, 1/2 cup	3
Lemon, 1/2 cup	2
Mango, 1/2 cup	2
Mixed berry, 1/2 cup	2
Passion fruit, 1/2 cup	2
Raspberry, 1/2 cup	2
Strawberry sorbet, 1/2 cup	2
Turkey Hill	
Cherry orchard, 1/2 cup	2
Fruit rainbow sherbet, 1/2 cup	2
Orange grove sherbet, 1/2 cup	2
Turkey Hill Venice Ice	
Lemon & cherry, 1/2 cup	2
Mango, 1/2 cup	2

Candy, Cookies & Desserts

Turkey Hill Venice Ice (cont'd)	POINTS VALUE
Pomegranate blueberry with acai, 1/2 cup	2
Raspberry, 1/2 cup	2
Whole Fruit	
Coconut sorbet, 1/2 cup	4
Lemon sorbet, 1/2 cup	3
Mango sorbet, 1/2 cup	3
Peach sorbet, 1/2 cup	3
Pomberry sorbet, 1/2 cup	2
Raspberry sorbet, 1/2 cup	2
Strawberry sorbet, 1/2 cup	2

Mousses
Sans Sucre Sugar Free

	POINTS VALUE
Mousse mix, cheesecake, 1/2 cup	2
Mousse mix, chocolate, 1/2 cup	1
Mousse mix, chocolate cheesecake, 1/2 cup	2
Mousse mix, French vanilla, 1/2 cup	2
Mousse mix, key lime, 1/2 cup	2
Mousse mix, lemon, 1/2 cup	2
Mousse mix, mocha cappuccino, 1/2 cup	1
Mousse mix, strawberry, 1/2 cup	2

Weight Watchers Smart Ones
Chocolate mousse, 1	3

Pies
Amy's
Apple pie, 1/2	5

Entenmann's
Apple pie (single serve), 1 (99 g)	10
Apple snack pie (club size package), 1	10

	POINTS VALUE
Apple snack pie (single serve), 1	10
Cherry pie (single serve), 1 (135 g)	10
Cherry snack pie (single serve), 1 (99 g)	10
Coconut custard pie, 1 serving (1/5 of pie)	8
Homestyle apple pie, 1 serving (1/6 of pie)	8
Lemon snack pie (single serve), 1	11
Peach pie (single serve), 1	9
Pineapple pie (single serve), 1	10
Pumpkin pie, 1 serving (1/5 of pie)	7
Sweet Potato Pie, 1 slice (1/6 of pie)	7
Lance	
Pecan pie, 1	8
Market Day	
Apple deep dish pie, 1 serving (1/12 pie)	8
No sugar added apple pie, 1 slice	7
Mrs. Smith's	
Apple pie, 1 serving (1/8 pie)	8
Apple pie, no sugar added, 1 serving (1/6 pie)	4
Blueberry pie, 1 serving (1/8 pie)	7
Boston cream pie, 1 serving (1/8 pie)	4
Cherry pie, 1 serving (1/8 pie)	8
Chocolate cream pie, 1 serving (1/4 pie)	8
Coconut cream pie, 1 serving (1/4 pie)	8
Coconut custard pie, 1 serving (1/8 pie)	6
Dutch apple crumb pie, 1 serving (1/8 pie)	7

	POINTS VALUE
Hearty pumpkin pie, 1 serving (1/8 pie)	5
Key lime pie, 1 serving (1/9 pie)	10
Lemon meringue pie, 1 serving (1/8 pie)	7
Mince pie, 1 serving (1/8 pie)	9
Peach pie, 1 serving (1/8 pie)	7
Pecan pie, 1 serving (1/5 pie)	12
Pumpkin custard pie, 1 serving (1/8 pie)	5
Red raspberry pie, 1 serving (1/8 pie)	8
Sweet potato pie, 1 serving (1/8 pie)	7
Mrs. Smith's Restaurant Classics	
French silk chocolate pie, 1 serving (1/9 pie)	14
Mrs. Smith's Special Recipe	
Deep dish apple pie, 1 serving (1/12 pie)	7
Deep dish cherry pie, 1 serving (1/12 pie)	8
Deep dish peach pie, 1 serving (1/12 pie)	7
Homemade pumpkin pie, 1 serving (1/10 pie)	6
Mrs. Smith's Traditional Recipe Slices	
Apple pie slices sweetened with splenda, 1 slice	6
Mixed berry pie slices sweetened with splenda, 1 slice	5
Weight Watchers Smart Ones	
Key lime pie, 1	4

	POINTS VALUE
## Puddings	
Jell-O	
Flan mix, 1/4 package	2
Lemon, prepared, 1/2 cup	3
Milk chocolate, prepared, 1/2 cup	3
Sugar free chocolate mint fudge sundae, 1	1
Sugar free dulce de leche vanilla caramel sundae, 1	1
Sugar free mochaccino chocolate coffee sundae, 1	1
Vanilla, prepared, 1/2 cup	3
Jell-O 100 Calorie Packs	
Smoothies, 1	2
Jell-O Americana	
Custard dessert, prepared, 1/2 cup	3
Jell-O Cook & Serve	
Americana custard mix, 1 serving (1/6 package)	2
Banana cream mix, 1 serving (22 g)	2
Banana cream, prepared, 1/2 cup	3
Butterscotch mix, 1/4 package	2
Butterscotch, prepared, 1/2 cup	3
Chocolate fudge mix, 1/4 package	2
Chocolate fudge, prepared, 1/2 cup	3
Chocolate mix, 1/4 package	2
Chocolate, prepared, 1/2 cup	3
Coconut cream mix, 1/4 package	2
Coconut cream, prepared, 1/2 cup	3
Flan, prepared, 1/2 cup	3

Candy, Cookies & Desserts

Jell-O Cook & Serve (cont'd)	POINTS VALUE
Lemon mix, 1 serving (1/6 package)	1
Milk chocolate mix, 1/4 package	2
Vanilla mix, 1/4 package	2
Jell-O Fat Free 100 Calorie Packs Pudding Snacks	
Caramel vanilla, 1	2
Chocolate, 1	2
Chocolate/vanilla swirls, 1	2
Devil's food & chocolate, 1	2
Tapioca, 1	2
Vanilla, 1	2
Jell-O Fat Free Cook & Serve	
Rice mix, 1/4 package	2
Rice, prepared, 1/2 cup	3
Tapioca mix, 1/4 package	2
Tapioca, prepared, 1/2 cup	3
Jell-O Fat Free Sugar Free Instant	
Banana cream mix, 1/4 package	1
Butterscotch mix, 1/4 package	1
Butterscotch, prepared, 1/2 cup	1
Cheesecake mix, 1/4 package	1
Cheesecake, prepared, 1/2 cup	1
Chocolate fudge mix, 1/4 package	1
Chocolate fudge, prepared, 1/2 cup	1
Chocolate mix, 1/4 package	1
Chocolate, prepared, 1/2 cup	1
Lemon mix, 1/4 package	1
Lemon, prepared, 1/2 cup	1
Pistachio mix, 1/4 package	1
Pistachio, prepared, 1/2 cup	1
Vanilla mix, 1/4 package	1

	POINTS VALUE
Vanilla, prepared, 1/2 cup	1
White chocolate, 1/2 cup	1
White chocolate mix, 1/4 package	1
Jell-O Fat Free, Sugar Free Cook & Serve	
Banana cream, prepared, 1/2 cup	1
Chocolate mix, 1 serving (1/6 package)	0
Chocolate mix, 1/4 package	0
Chocolate, prepared, 1/2 cup	1
Chocolate, prepared, 1/2 cup	1
Vanilla mix, 1/4 package	0
Vanilla, prepared with skim milk, 1/2 cup	1
Jell-O Instant	
Banana cream mix, 1/4 package	2
Banana cream, prepared, 1/2 cup	3
Butterscotch mix, 1/4 package	2
Butterscotch, prepared, 1/2 cup	3
Cheesecake mix, 1/4 package	2
Cheesecake, prepared, 1/2 cup	3
Chocolate cherry mix, 1/4 package	2
Chocolate fudge mix, 1/4 package	2
Chocolate fudge, prepared, 1/2 cup	3
Chocolate mix, 1/4 package	2
Chocolate, prepared, 1/2 cup	3
Coconut cream mix, 1/4 package	2
Coconut cream, prepared, 1/2 cup	3
Devil's food mix, 1/4 package	2
Devil's food, prepared, 1/2 cup	3
French vanilla mix, 1/4 package	2
French vanilla, prepared, 1/2 cup	3
Lemon mix, 1/4 package	2

	POINTS VALUE
Lemon, prepared, 1/2 cup	3
Oreo cookies 'n cream with cookie pieces mix, 1 serving (31 g)	2
Pistachio mix, 1/4 package	2
Pistachio, prepared, 1/2 cup	3
Pumpkin spice mix, 1/4 package	2
Pumpkin spice, prepared, 1/2 cup	3
Vanilla mix, 1/4 package	2
Vanilla, prepared, 1/2 cup	3
White chocolate mix, 1/4 package	2
White chocolate, prepared, 1/2 cup	3
Jell-O Pudding Snacks	
Chocolate, 1	2
Chocolate/vanilla oreo parfait, 1	2
Chocolate/vanilla swirls, 1	2
Tapioca, 1	2
Vanilla, 1	2
Jell-O Sugar Free Pudding	
Chocolate, 1	1
Chocolate vanilla swirls, 1	1
Creamy caramel, 1	1
Double chocolate, 1	1
Vanilla, 1	1
Jell-O Sugar Free Pudding Snacks	
Banana fudge sundae, 1	1
Chocolate mint fudge sundae, 1	1
Dulce de leche sundae, 1	1
Mochaccino sundae, 1	1
Jell-O X-Treme Pudding Sticks	
Variety pak, 1	1

	POINTS VALUE
Kozy Shack	
Banana pudding, 1/2 cup	3
Banana pudding, prepared with 1% milk, 4 oz	1
Chocolate-covered strawberries (limited edition), 1/2 cup	3
Chocolate pudding, 1/2 cup	3
Chocolate pudding, prepared with 1% milk, 4 oz	1
Chocolate soy pudding, 1 serving	2
Cinnamon raisin rice pudding, 1/2 cup	3
Country peach (limited edition), 1/2 cup	3
Crème caramel flan, 4 oz	3
European style rice pudding, 1/2 cup	3
Key lime (limited edition), 1/2 cup	3
No sugar added apple pie a la mode, 3 1/2 oz	1
No sugar added chocolate pudding, 4 oz	0
No sugar added rice pudding, 4 oz	1
No sugar added tapioca pudding, 4 oz	1
Original rice pudding, 1/2 cup	3
Pumpkin (limited edition), 1/2 cup	3
Tapioca pudding, 1/2 cup	3
Vanilla soy pudding, 1 serving	2
Kozy Shack Ready Grains	
Rice with fruit, no sugar added - acai mango, 1 serving	1
Rice with fruit, no sugar added - blueberry pomegranate, 1 serving	1
Rice with fruit, no sugar added - strawberry guava, 1 serving	1

Candy, Cookies & Desserts

	POINTS VALUE
Kraft Handi-Snacks	
Banana, 1	2
Butterscotch, 1	2
Chocolate, 1	2
Chocolate (fat free), 1	1
Chocolate fudge, 1	2
Doubles banana split, 1	2
Doubles chocolate chip cookie, 1	2
Doubles fudge rocky road, 1	2
Pudding doubles, chocolate vanilla, 1 cup	2
Rice pudding, 1 cup	2
Sugar free chocolate, 1	1
Sugar free creamy caramel, 1	1

	POINTS VALUE
Sugar free vanilla, 1	1
Tapioca, 1	2
Vanilla, 1	2
Vanilla (fat free), 1	2
Minute	
Rice pudding, as packaged, 1 serving (25 g)	2
Tapioca, 1 Tbsp	0
Uncle Ben's	
Rice pudding mix, smooth and creamy cinnamon & raisins, 1/2 cup (cooked)	3
Rice pudding mix, smooth and creamy French vanilla, 1/3 cup	2

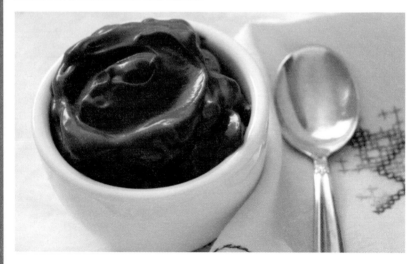

Condiments, Sauces & Gravies

	POINTS VALUE

Asian Sauces

A Taste of Thai

Fish sauce, 1 Tbsp	0
Garlic chili pepper sauce, 1 tsp	0
Pad Thai sauce, 2 Tbsp	2
Panang curry base, 1 tsp	1
Peanut satay sauce, 2 Tbsp	2
Peanut sauce mix, 1/4 envelope	1
Red curry base, 1 tsp	0
Sweet red chili sauce, 1 tsp	0

Cherchies

Asian grilling & stir fry sauce with sherry, 2 Tbsp	2

Contadina

Sweet & sour sauce, 2 Tbsp	1

Eden

Wasabi powder, 1 tsp	0

Eden Organic

Genmai miso, organic, 1 Tbsp	0
Hacho miso, organic, 1 Tbsp	1
Mugi miso, organic, 1 Tbsp	0
Shiro miso, organic, 1 Tbsp	0
Shoyu, 1 Tbsp	0
Shoyu, reduced sodium, 1 Tbsp	0
Tamari, organic, imported, 1 Tbsp	0

Eden Selected

Shoyu - imported, 1 Tbsp	0

House of Tsang

Bangkok padang sauce, 1 Tbsp	1
Classic stir fry sauce, 1 Tbsp	1
General Tsao sauce, 1 tsp	1

	POINTS VALUE
Ginger flavored soy sauce, 1 Tbsp	0
Hoisin sauce, 1 tsp	0
Hunan smokehut hibachi grill sauce, 1 Tbsp	1
Imperial citrus stir fry, 1 Tbsp	1
Kobe steak hibachi grill sauce, 1 Tbsp	1
Korean teriyaki sauce, 1 Tbsp	1
Low sodium ginger flavored soy sauce, 1 Tbsp	0
Low sodium soy sauce, 1 Tbsp	0
Oyster flavored stir fry, 1 Tbsp	1
Saigon sizzle sauce, 1 Tbsp	1
Spicy brown bean sauce, 1 tsp	0
Sweet & sour stir fry sauce, 1 Tbsp	1
Sweet ginger sesame hibachi grill sauce, 1 Tbsp	1
Szechuan spicy stir fry sauce, 1 Tbsp	1
Teriyaki hibachi grill sauce, 1 Tbsp	1
Thai peanut hibachi grill sauce, 1 Tbsp	1

Kahiki

Tempura chicken nuggets, sauce only, 1 Tbsp	1

Kraft

Sweet 'n sour sauce, 1 dipping cup	1

Litehouse

Classic stir fry, 2 Tbsp	1
Teriyaki stir fry, 2 Tbsp	1

San-J

Asian bbq sauce, 2 Tbsp	1
Organic shoyu, 1 Tbsp	0

Condiments, Sauces & Gravies

San-J (cont'd)	POINTS VALUE
Organic wheat free tamari reduced sodium, 1 Tbsp	0
Organic wheat free tamari, 1 Tbsp	0
Reduced sodium tamari, 1 Tbsp	0
Sweet & tangy sauce, 2 Tbsp	1
Szechuan, 1 tsp	0
Tamari, 1 Tbsp	0
Teriyaki sauce, 1 Tbsp	0
Thai peanut, 2 Tbsp	1
Seeds of Change	
Jalfrezi simmer sauce, 1/3 cup	2
Korma simmer sauce, 1/3 cup	3
Madras simmer sauce, 1/3 cup	1
Tikka masala simmer sauce, 1/3 cup	2
Simply Asia	
General Tsao stir-fry sauce, 2 Tbsp	2
Ginger teriyaki stir-fry sauce, 2 Tbsp	1
Kung Pao stir-fry sauce, 2 Tbsp	1
Mandarin orange stir-fry sauce, 2 Tbsp	1
Szechwan stir-fry sauce, 2 Tbsp	2
Thai Kitchen	
10-minute simmer sauce, green curry, 1/2 cup	2
10-minute simmer sauce, Panang curry, 1/2 cup	2
10-minute simmer sauce, red curry, 1/2 cup	2
10-minute simmer sauce, yellow curry, 1/2 cup	2
Peanut satay sauce dipping & all-purpose sauce, 2 Tbsp	2
Premium fish sauce, 1 Tbsp	0

	POINTS VALUE
Premium fish sauce, less sodium, 1 Tbsp	0
Spicy Thai chili all-purpose sauce & marinade, 1 Tbsp	0
Tree of Life	
Organic shoyu soy sauce, 1 Tbsp	0
Organic wheat free tamari soy sauce, 1 Tbsp	0

Barbecue/Grilling Sauces

A1	
Original, 2 Tbsp	1
Annie's Naturals	
Organic hot chipotle bbq sauce, 2 Tbsp	1
Organic original bbq sauce, 2 Tbsp	1
Organic smokey maple bbq sauce, 2 Tbsp	1
Boar's Head	
Gourmet barbecue sauce - hot & spicy, 2 Tbsp	1
Gourmet barbecue sauce - sweet & mild, 2 Tbsp	1
Bull's Eye	
Brewers best with guinness, 2 Tbsp	1
Honey garlic bonanza, 2 Tbsp	1
Honey smoke, 2 Tbsp	1
Honey teriyaki, 2 Tbsp	1
Original, 2 Tbsp	1
Premium select, 2 Tbsp	1
Ragin' buffalo bbq sauce, 2 Tbsp	1
Smokehouse hickory, 2 Tbsp	1
Smokin' chipotle barbecue sauce, 2 Tbsp	1
Spicy honey, 2 Tbsp	1

Condiments, Sauces & Gravies

	POINTS VALUE
Spicy hot, 2 Tbsp	1
Steakhouse with A1 barbecue sauce, 2 Tbsp	1
Sweet & sticky barbecue sauce, 2 Tbsp	1
Sweet hickory, 1 Tbsp	0
Sweet hickory smoke, 2 Tbsp	1
Sweet homestyle blend, 2 Tbsp	1
Texas style mesquite, 2 Tbsp	1
Consorzio	
BBQ sauce, original, 2 Tbsp	1
Emeril's	
Kicked up bbq sauce, 2 Tbsp	1
Sweet & easy molasses bbq sauce, 2 Tbsp	1
Sweet original bbq sauce, 2 Tbsp	1
Tropical bbq sauce, 2 Tbsp	1
Goldwater's	
Bisbee barbeque sauce, 2 Tbsp	1
Heinz Thick & Rich	
Cajun style barbecue sauce, 2 Tbsp	1
Chunky barbecue sauce, 2 Tbsp	1
Hawaiian barbecue sauce, 2 Tbsp	1
Honey mustard barbeque sauce, 2 Tbsp	1
Jack Daniel's	
Hickory brown sugar, 2 Tbsp	1
Honey smokehouse, 2 Tbsp	1
Spicy original recipe, 2 Tbsp	1
Jack Daniel's No. 7	
Original recipe, 2 Tbsp	1
K.C. Masterpiece	
Classic blend bbq sauce, 2 Tbsp	0
Hickory barbecue sauce, 2 Tbsp	1

	POINTS VALUE
Hickory brown sugar barbecue sauce, 2 Tbsp	1
Honey barbecue sauce, 2 Tbsp	1
Hot'n spicy original barbecue sauce, 2 Tbsp	1
Mesquite barbecue sauce, 2 Tbsp	1
Original barbecue sauce, 2 Tbsp	1
Kraft	
30 calorie light original, 2 Tbsp	0
Brown sugar, 2 Tbsp	1
Char-grill, 2 Tbsp	1
Classic recipe, 2 Tbsp	1
Hickory smoke, 2 Tbsp	1
Hickory smoke molasses, 2 Tbsp	1
Hickory smoke onion bits, 2 Tbsp	1
Honey, 2 Tbsp	1
Honey hickory smoke, 2 Tbsp	1
Honey mustard, 2 Tbsp	1
Honey roasted garlic, 2 Tbsp	1
Hot, 2 Tbsp	1
Kansas City style, 2 Tbsp	1
Mesquite smoke, 2 Tbsp	1
Onion bits, 2 Tbsp	1
Original, 2 Tbsp	1
Roasted garlic, 2 Tbsp	1
Spicy honey, 2 Tbsp	1
Steakhouse style, 2 Tbsp	1
Sweet smokehouse hickory, 2 Tbsp	1
Teriyaki, 2 Tbsp	1
Teriyaki sesame ginger, 2 Tbsp	1
Thick 'n spicy Cajun, 2 Tbsp	1

Condiments, Sauces & Gravies

	POINTS VALUE
Kraft Carb Well	
Barbeque sauce original, 2 Tbsp	0
Kraft Thick 'N Spicy	
Hickory bacon, 2 Tbsp	1
Hickory smoke, 2 Tbsp	1
Honey, 2 Tbsp	1
Mesquite smoke, 2 Tbsp	1
Original, 2 Tbsp	1
Muirhead	
Barbeque sauce, 1 Tbsp	1
Naturally Fresh	
BBQ sauce, 2 Tbsp	1
Open Pit	
Hot bbq sauce, 2 Tbsp	1
Original bbq sauce, 2 Tbsp	1
Original onion bbq sauce, 2 Tbsp	1
Thick & tangy chile lime bbq sauce, 2 Tbsp	1
Thick & tangy original bbq sauce, 2 Tbsp	1
Walden Farms	
BBQ hickory smoked sauce, 2 Tbsp	0
BBQ honey sauce, 2 Tbsp	0
BBQ original sauce, 2 Tbsp	0

Gravies

	POINTS VALUE
Boston Market Gravies	
Poultry gravy, 2 oz	1
Campbell's	
Au jus gravy, 1/4 cup	0
Beef gravy, 1/4 cup	1
Brown gravy with onions, 1/4 cup	1
Chicken gravy, 1/4 cup	1
Country style cream gravy, 1/4 cup	1
Country style sausage gravy, 1/4 cup	2
Fat free beef gravy, 1/4 cup	0
Fat free chicken gravy, 1/4 cup	0
Fat free turkey gravy, 1/4 cup	0
Golden pork gravy, 1/4 cup	1
Mushroom gravy, 1/4 cup	0
Turkey gravy, 1/4 cup	1
Campbell's Microwavable Gravies	
Beef gravy, 1/4 cup	1
Chicken gravy, 1/4 cup	1
Turkey gravy, 1/4 cup	1
Durkee	
Au jus branded mix, 1 tsp	0
Brown gravy mix, 2 tsp	0
Chicken gravy mix, 1 Tbsp	1
Country gravy mix, 1 1/3 Tbsp	1
Mushroom in brown gravy mix, 2 tsp	0
Onion in brown gravy mix, 2 tsp	0
Pork gravy mix, 2 tsp	0
Turkey gravy mix, 2 tsp	0
Franco-American	
Slow roast beef gravy, 1/4 cup	1
Slow roast chicken gravy, 1/4 cup	0
Slow roast fat free beef gravy, 1/4 cup	0
Slow roast fat free chicken gravy, 1/4 cup	0
Slow roast fat free turkey gravy, 1/4 cup	0
Slow roast turkey gravy, 1/4 cup	1

Condiments, Sauces & Gravies

	POINTS VALUE		POINTS VALUE
French's		**Tofurky**	
Au jus branded mix, 1 tsp	0	Mushroom & giblet gravy, 2 Tbsp	1
Brown gravy mix, 2 tsp	0	**Tony Chachere's**	
Chicken gravy mix, 1 Tbsp	0	Creole instant roux mix, 1 tsp	0
Pork gravy mix, 2 tsp	0	Southern pantry brown gravy mix, 1 1/2 tsp	0
Sausage flavored country gravy mix, 1 1/3 Tbsp	1	Southern pantry white gravy mix, 2 tsp	0
Turkey gravy mix, 2 tsp	1	**Horseradish/Horseradish Sauce**	
Heinz		**Boar's Head**	
Fat free beef gravy, 1/4 cup	0	Horseradish and beets grated in vinegar, 1 tsp	0
Fat free chicken gravy, 1/4 cup	0	Pub style horseradish sauce, 1 tsp	0
Fat free turkey gravy, 1/4 cup	0	**Heinz**	
Heinz HomeStyle		Horseradish sauce, 1 tsp	1
Beef gravy, 1/4 cup	1	**Kraft**	
Bistro style au jus, 1/4 cup	0	Cream style horseradish, 1 tsp	0
Chicken gravy, 1/4 cup	1	Horseradish sauce, 1 tsp	0
Country sausage, 1/4 cup	1	Prepared horseradish, 1 tsp	0
Cream of chicken gravy, 1/4 cup	1	**Manischewitz**	
Mushroom gravy, 1/4 cup	0	Creamy horseradish sauce - original, 1 tsp	1
Onion gravy, 1/4 cup	1	Creamy horseradish sauce - wasabi, 1 tsp	0
Pork gravy, 1/4 cup	0	Creamy horseradish sauce with dill, 1 tsp	0
Turkey gravy, 1/4 cup	1	Creamy horseradish sauce with lemon, 1 tsp	0
McCormick		**Marzetti**	
Brown gravy dry seasoning mix, 1 Tbsp	0	Horseradish sauce, 1 Tbsp	1
Chicken gravy dry seasoning mix, 2 tsp	0		
Turkey gravy dry seasoning mix, 2 tsp	0		
Pillsbury			
Brown, mix, 2 tsp	0		
Chicken style, mix, 2 tsp	0		
Homestyle, mix, 2 tsp	0		

Condiments, Sauces & Gravies

Hot & Latin Sauces

Bufalo

	POINTS VALUE
Chipotle hot sauce, 1 tsp	0
Especial hot sauce, 1 tsp	0
Jalapeno hot sauce, 1 tsp	0
Picante clasica hot sauce, 1 tsp	0

CHI-CHI'S

Fiesta squeezable taco sauce, 1 Tbsp	0
Picante medium, 2 Tbsp	0
Picante mild, 2 Tbsp	0

Emeril's

Kicked up green pepper sauce, 1 tsp	0
Kicked up red sauce, 1 tsp	0
Wing sauce, 1 tsp	0

Glory

Hickory smoked hot sauce, 1 tsp	0
Louisiana style hot sauce, 1 tsp	0
Spicy vidalia hot sauce, 1 tsp	0

La Estrellita

Enchilada sauce, mild, 1/2 cup	1

Las Palmas

Enchilada sauce - hot, 1/4 cup	0
Enchilada sauce - medium, 1/4 cup	0
Enchilada sauce - mild, 1/4 cup	0
Green enchilada sauce, 1/4 cup	1
Red chile sauce, 1/4 cup	0
Tomato enchilada sauce, 1/4 cup	0

Old El Paso

Enchilada sauce, hot, 1/4 cup	1
Enchilada sauce, medium, 1/4 cup	1
Enchilada sauce, mild, 1/4 cup	1

	POINTS VALUE
Green chilli enchilada sauce, 1/4 cup	1
Picante - hot, 2 Tbsp	0
Picante - medium, 2 Tbsp	0
Picante - mild, 2 Tbsp	0
Taco sauce, hot, 1 Tbsp	0
Taco sauce, medium, 1 Tbsp	0
Taco sauce, mild, 1 Tbsp	0
Taco toppers - mild taco sauce, 2 Tbsp	0
Thick 'n chunky picante - hot, 2 Tbsp	0
Thick 'n chunky picante - medium, 2 Tbsp	0
Thick 'n chunky picante - mild, 2 Tbsp	0

Ortega

Enchilada sauce, 1/4 cup	0
Green taco sauce, mild, 1 Tbsp	0
Picante sauce - hot, 2 Tbsp	0
Picante sauce, medium, 2 Tbsp	0
Picante sauce, mild, 2 Tbsp	0
Taco sauce, 1 Tbsp	0

Pace

Enchilada sauce, 1/4 cup	0
Green taco sauce, 1 Tbsp	0
Organic picante sauce, 2 Tbsp	0
Picante, 2 Tbsp	0
Taco sauce, 2 Tbsp	0

Sunsun

Louisiana hot sauce, 1 tsp	1

Taco Bell Home Originals

Hot restaurant sauce, 1 tsp	0
Medium taco sauce, 2 Tbsp	0
Mild taco sauce, 2 Tbsp	0

	POINTS VALUE
Tostitos	
All natural medium picante sauce, 2 Tbsp	0
Trappey's	
Red devil cayenne pepper sauce, 1 tsp	0
Zapata	
Hot sauce, 1 tsp	0

Ketchup

	POINTS VALUE
Annie's Naturals	
Organic ketchup, 1 Tbsp	0
Del Monte	
Ketchup, 1 Tbsp	0
Sauce, chili, 1 Tbsp	0
Estee	
No salt added ketchup, 1 Tbsp	0
Heinz	
Chili sauce, 1 Tbsp	0
Hot ketchup made with Tabasco, 1 Tbsp	0
Kid's EZ squirt blastin' green, 1 Tbsp	0
Kid's ketchup with vitamin c, 1 Tbsp	0
Light harvest ketchup, 1 Tbsp	0
Organic tomato ketchup, 1 Tbsp	0
Reduced sugar tomato ketchup, 1 Tbsp	0
Tomato ketchup, 1 Tbsp	0
Tomato ketchup, no salt added, 1 Tbsp	0
Heinz Ketchup Kick'rs	
Hot and spicy flavored tomato ketchup, 1 Tbsp	0
La Estrellita	
Green vegetarian chile, medium, 1/2 cup	1
Green vegetarian chile, mild, 1/2 cup	1
Hot green vegetarian chile, 1/2 cup	1

	POINTS VALUE
Muir Glen Organic	
Tomato ketchup, 1 Tbsp	0
Tree of Life	
Organic ketchup, 1 Tbsp	0
Walden Farms	
Ketchup, 1 Tbsp	0

Marinades

	POINTS VALUE
A1	
Seafood marinade, ginger teriyaki with orange, 1 Tbsp	1
Seafood marinade, mango chipotle, 1 Tbsp	1
Seafood marinade, roasted garlic with lemon, 1 Tbsp	0

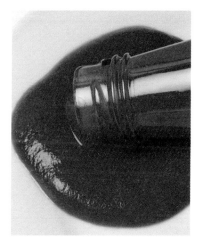

Condiments, Sauces & Gravies

	POINTS VALUE
Annie's Naturals	
Organic mango cilantro, 1 Tbsp	0
Organic smokey tomato marinade, 1 Tbsp	1
Organic spicy ginger marinade, 1 Tbsp	1
Organic steak marinade, 1 Tbsp	1
Organic teriyaki marinade, 1 Tbsp	1
Annie's Naturals All Natural	
Baja lime, 1 Tbsp	1
Consorzio	
Roasted garlic marinade, 1 Tbsp	1
Sesame orange, 1 Tbsp	1
Consorzio All Natural	
California teriyaki, 1 Tbsp	1
Roasted garlic and balsamic, 1 Tbsp	1
Durkee Grill Creations	
Chipotle marinade, dry mix, 1 tsp	0
Emeril's	
Ginger teriyaki, 1 Tbsp	1
Herbed lemon pepper, 1 Tbsp	2
Hickory maple chipotle, 1 Tbsp	1
Lemon rosemary gaaahlic, 1 Tbsp	2
Orange herb poppyseed, 1 Tbsp	4
Roasted vegetable, 1 Tbsp	4
Sesame Asian, 1 Tbsp	4
Grill Mates	
Mesquite marinade, 2 tsp	0
Zesty herb marinade, 1 tsp	0
House of Tsang	
Mandarin marinade soy sauce, 1 Tbsp	1

	POINTS VALUE
House of Tsang Simply Tsang	
Ginger sesame marinade, 1 Tbsp	0
Jamaican jerk marinade, 1 Tbsp	1
Japanese steakhouse marinade, 1 Tbsp	1
Sweet & sour marinade, 1 Tbsp	1
Teriyaki marinade, 1 Tbsp	1
K.C. Masterpiece	
Chipotle & lime marinade, 1 Tbsp	0
Garlic herb marinade, 1 Tbsp	1
Ginger teriyaki marinade, 1 Tbsp	1
Honey teriyaki with sesame marinade, 1 Tbsp	1
Mesquite marinade, 1 Tbsp	1
Roasted garlic balsamic marinade, 1 Tbsp	0
Spiced Caribbean jerk marinade, 1 Tbsp	1
Steakhouse marinade, 1 Tbsp	0
Zesty lemon pepper marinade, 1 Tbsp	1
Mrs. Dash	
Garlic lime 10-minute marinade, 1 Tbsp	1
Lemon herb peppercorn 10-minute marinade, 1 Tbsp	1
Mesquite grille 10-minute marinade, 1 Tbsp	1
Southwestern chipotle 10-minute marinade, 1 Tbsp	1
Spicy teriyaki 10-minute marinade, 1 Tbsp	1
Zesty garlic herb 10-minute marinade, 1 Tbsp	1
Naturally Fresh	
Lemon pepper marinade, 2 Tbsp	3
Marinade, all natural, 2 Tbsp	0
Southwestern marinade, 2 Tbsp	2

Condiments, Sauces & Gravies

	POINTS VALUE
San-J	
Japanese steak marinade, 1 Tbsp	0

Mayonnaise
Best Foods

Canola mayonnaise, 1 Tbsp	3
Light mayonnaise, 1 Tbsp	1
Mayonnaise with olive oil, 1 Tbsp	1
Real mayonnaise, 1 Tbsp	3
Reduced fat mayonnaise, 1 Tbsp	1

Boar's Head

Real mayonnaise, 1 Tbsp	3
Savory remoulade Cajun style mayonnaise, 1 Tbsp	3
Sun dried tomato pesto mayonnaise, 1 Tbsp	1

Hain Pure Foods

Canola mayonnaise dressing, 1 Tbsp	3
Lite safflower mayonnaise, 1 Tbsp	1
Safflower mayonnaise, 1 Tbsp	3

Hellmann's

Canola mayonnaise, 1 Tbsp	3
Light mayonnaise, 1 Tbsp	1
Mayonnaise with olive oil, 1 Tbsp	1
Real mayonnaise, 1 Tbsp	3
Reduced fat mayonnaise, 1 Tbsp	1

Kraft

Fat free mayonnaise dressing, 1 Tbsp	0
Light mayonnaise, 1 Tbsp	1
Real mayonnaise, 1 Tbsp	3
Real mayonnaise hot 'n spicy super easy squeeze, 1 Tbsp	3

Kraft Mayonesa

Real mayonnaise with lime juice, 1 Tbsp	3

	POINTS VALUE
Smart Balance	
Omega plus light mayo, 1 Tbsp	1
Smart Beat	
Fat free mayonnaise, 1 Tbsp	0
Spectrum Naturals	
Canola mayonnaise, 1 Tbsp	3
Dijon mayonnaise, organic, 1 Tbsp	3
Eggless vegan mayonnaise, organic, 1 Tbsp	1
Light canola mayonnaise, eggless, vegan, 1 Tbsp	1
Mayonnaise, organic, 1 Tbsp	3
Naturals spread, 1 Tbsp	3
Olive oil mayonnaise, organic, 1 Tbsp	3
Roasted garlic mayonnaise, organic, 1 Tbsp	3
Soy mayonnaise, organic, omega 3 with flax oil, 1 Tbsp	3
Wasabi mayonnaise, organic, 1 Tbsp	3

Mustard
Annie's Naturals

Organic Dijon mustard, 1 tsp	1
Organic honey mustard, 1 tsp	0
Organic horseradish mustard, 1 tsp	0
Organic yellow mustard, 1 tsp	1

Boar's Head

Delicatessen style mustard, 1 tsp	0
Honey mustard, 1 tsp	0

Cherchies

Champagne mustard, 1 tsp	0
Cranberry mustard, 1 tsp	0
Hot banana pepper mustard, 1 Tbsp	0
Key lime mustard, 1 Tbsp	1

Condiments, Sauces & Gravies

	POINTS VALUE
Eden Organic	
Organic brown mustard, 1 tsp	0
Organic yellow mustard, 1 tsp	0
Emeril's	
Dijon mustard, 1 Tbsp	0
Horseradish mustard, 1 Tbsp	0
NY Deli style mustard, 1 Tbsp	0
Smoooth honey mustard, 1 Tbsp	0
French's	
Classic yellow mustard, 1 tsp	0
Honey dijon mustard, 1 tsp	0
Honey mustard, 1 tsp	0
Horseradish mustard, 1 tsp	0
Spicy brown mustard, 1 tsp	0
Grey Poupon	
Country dijon mustard, 1 tsp	0
Deli mustard, 1 tsp	0
Harvest course ground, 1 tsp	0
Hearty spicy brown mustard, 1 tsp	0
Mild & creamy, 1 tsp	0
Savory honey mustard, 1 tsp	0
Heinz	
Spicy brown mustard, 1 tsp	0
Yellow mustard, 1 tsp	0
Kraft	
Horseradish mustard, 1 tsp	0
Yellow mustard, 1 tsp	0
Muirhead	
Dijon mustard, 1 Tbsp	1
Honey mustard, 1 Tbsp	2
Horseradish mustard, 1 Tbsp	2

	POINTS VALUE
Tree of Life	
Organic dijon mustard, 1 tsp	0
Organic stone ground mustard, 1 tsp	0
Organic yellow mustard, 1 tsp	0
Organic yellow squeeze mustard, 1 tsp	0
Westbrae Natural	
Dijon style mustard, 1 tsp	0
Olives	
Faraon	
Spanish olives, 7	1
Spanish pimiento stuffed olives, 5 olives	1
Sardo	
Cocktail olives, 6	1
Kalamata olives, 4	1
Manzanilla olives, 5	1
Plain green olives, 2	1
Sliced green olives, 1 Tbsp	1
Stuffed queen olives, 2	0
Other Sauces	
Annie's Naturals	
Organic Worcestershire sauce, 1 Tbsp	0
Austex American Originals	
Hot dog chili sauce with onion, 1 Tbsp	0
Hot dog chili sauce, classic, 1 Tbsp	0
Boar's Head	
Brown sugar & spice ham glaze cooking sauce, 2 Tbsp	2
Jalapeño pepper sauce, 1 tsp	0
Boboli	
Pizza sauce, 1/2 pouch	1

Condiments, Sauces & Gravies

	POINTS VALUE
Castleberry's American Originals	
Hot dog chili sauce with onion, 1 Tbsp	0
Hot dog chili sauce, classic, 1 Tbsp	0
Cherchies	
Apple butter cooking & dipping sauce, 2 Tbsp	1
Raspberry chipotle cooking & dipping sauce, 2 Tbsp	1
Chincoteague	
Red clam sauce, 1/2 cup	2
White clam sauce, 1/2 cup	3
Contadina	
Deluxe pizza sauce, 1/4 cup	0
Fully prepared pizza sauce, 1/4 cup	0
Pizza sauce, flavored with pepperoni, 1/4 cup	1
Pizza sauce, four cheese, 1/4 cup	0
Pizza sauce, original, 1/4 cup	0
Pizza squeeze, 1/4 cup	0
Del Monte	
Homestyle original, 1/4 cup	1
Sloppy Joe sauce, bbq, 1/4 cup	1
Dona Maria	
Mole, 2 Tbsp	4
Mole verde, 2 Tbsp	6
Nopalitos, 2 Tbsp	0
Pipian, 2 Tbsp	6
Durkee	
Famous sandwich & salad sauce, 1 Tbsp	2
Eden	
Ponzu sauce, 1 Tbsp	0

	POINTS VALUE
Faraon	
Casera Mexican sauce - red, 2 Tbsp	0
Goldwater's	
Grand Canyon cranberry grill sauce, 2 Tbsp	1
Heinz	
Worcestershire sauce, 1 tsp	0
Hormel	
Not-so-sloppy-Joe sauce, 1/4 cup	1
Jackaroo	
Meat sauce, 2 Tbsp (individual 4-oz portion cup)	1
Lucky Leaf	
Lite strawberry fruit 'n sauce, no sugar added, 4 oz	1
Manischewitz	
Tomato & mushroom sauce, 1/4 cup	1
Muir Glen Organic	
Premium pizza sauce, 1/4 cup	1
Muirhead	
Apple cranberry chutney, 1 Tbsp	0
Apple pineapple chutney, 1 Tbsp	0
Apple pomegranate chutney, 1 Tbsp	0
Chocolate raspberry sauce, 1 Tbsp	1
Tangy cherry chutney, 1 Tbsp	1
Naturally Fresh	
Buffalo wing sauce, 2 Tbsp	2
Ocean Spray	
Jellied cranberry sauce, 1/4 cup	2
Whole berry cranberry sauce, 1/4 cup	2

Condiments, Sauces & Gravies

	POINTS VALUE
Old El Paso	
Taco toppers zesty ranch, 2 Tbsp	2
Progresso	
Lobster, 1/2 cup	2
Red clam with tomato & basil, 1/2 cup	1
White clam (authentic), 1/2 cup	3
White clam with garlic & herbs, 1/2 cup	3
Ragu Old World Style	
Pizza sauce, 1/4 cup	0
Ragu Pizza Quick	
Traditional, 1/4 cup	1
Spice Islands	
Chipotle sauce, 1 Tbsp	0
Sweet red chili dipping & all-purpose sauce, 2 Tbsp	1
Tree of Life	
Lime & chili chutney, 1 Tbsp	1
Major grey chutney, 1 Tbsp	1
Mango pomegranate chutney, 1 Tbsp	1
Mango raisin chutney, 1 Tbsp	1
Organic cranberry sauce, jellied, 1/4 cup	2
Organic sesame tahini, 2 Tbsp	4
Pineapple chutney, 1 Tbsp	1
Walden Farms	
Scampi sauce, 2 Tbsp	0
Yoshida	
Cracked pepper & garlic, 1 Tbsp	1
Gourmet sauce, 1 Tbsp	1
Hawaiian sweet & sour, 2 Tbsp	1
Spicy wing and rib sauce, 2 Tbsp	1
Traditional teriyaki, 1 Tbsp	0

	POINTS VALUE
Zapata	
Cheese sauce, mild, 1/4 cup	1
Cheese sauce, spicy, 1/4 cup	1

Pasta Sauces

Amy's	
Family marinara pasta sauce, 1/2 cup	1
Garlic mushroom pasta sauce, 1/2 cup	2
Low sodium marinara sauce, 1/2 cup	1
Puttanesca sauce, 1/2 cup	1
Roasted garlic pasta sauce, 1/2 cup	3
Tomato basil pasta sauce, 1/2 cup	2
Tomato basil pasta sauce, light in sodium, 1/2 cup	2
Aunt Millie's	
Italian sausage sauce, 1/2 cup	1
Marinara, 1/2 cup	1
Meat sauce, 1/2 cup	2
Traditional sauce, 1/2 cup	1
Barilla	
Marinara Sauce, 1/2 cup	1
Tomato & basil sauce, 1/2 cup	1
Bertolli	
Alfredo with mushrooms, 1/4 cup	2
Creamy alfredo, 1/4 cup	3
Fire roasted tomato with cabernet, 1/2 cup	2
Five cheese, 1/2 cup	2
Italian sausage, romano & garlic, 1/2 cup	1
Marinara, 1/2 cup	1
Marinara with burgundy wine, 1/2 cup	2
Mediterranean olive, 1/2 cup	2

Condiments, Sauces & Gravies

	POINTS VALUE
Mushroom and garlic, 1/2 cup	1
Olive oil & garlic, 1/2 cup	1
Organic olive oil garlic, 1/2 cup	1
Organic tomato & basil, 1/2 cup	2
Portobello mushroom with merlot, 1/2 cup	2
Tomato & basil, 1/2 cup	1
Vidalia onion & roasted garlic, 1/2 cup	1
Vodka sauce, 1/2 cup	3
CIBO Naturals	
Artichoke lemon pesto, 1/4 cup	6
Cilantro lime pesto, 1/4 cup	8
Classic basil pesto, 1/4 cup	9
Roasted red pepper pesto, 1/4 cup	2
Sun dried tomato pesto (vegan), 1/4 cup	7
Classico	
Cabernet marinara, 1/2 cup	1
Caramelized onion and garlic, 1/2 cup	1
Creamy alfredo, 1/4 cup	3
Fire roasted tomato and garlic, 1/2 cup	1
Florentine spinach & cheese, 1/2 cup	2
Four cheese, 1/2 cup	1
Four cheese alfredo, 1/4 cup	2
Garden vegetable primavera, 1/2 cup	1
Italian sausage with green peppers & onions, 1/2 cup	2
Mushroom & ripe olives, 1/2 cup	1
Organic spinach & garlic, 1/2 cup	1
Organic tomato, herbs and spices, 1/2 cup	1
Roasted garlic, 1/2 cup	1

	POINTS VALUE
Roasted garlic alfredo, 1/4 cup	2
Roasted red pepper alfredo, 1/4 cup	2
Spicy red pepper, 1/2 cup	1
Spicy tomato & basil, 1/2 cup	1
Spicy tomato & pesto, 1/2 cup	2
Sun dried tomato pesto, 1/4 cup	2
Sun-dried tomato, 1/2 cup	1
Sun-dried tomato alfredo, 1/4 cup	2
Tomato & basil, 1/2 cup	1
Traditional sweet basil, 1/2 cup	1
Triple mushroom, 1/2 cup	1
Contadina	
Deluxe marinara sauce, 1/2 cup	1
Deluxe spaghetti sauce, 1/2 cup	1
Italian paste - tomato paste product with roasted garlic, 2 Tbsp	1
Italian paste - tomato paste product with tomato pesto, 2 Tbsp	1
Italian style tomato sauce, 1/4 cup	0
Spaghetti sauce, 1/2 cup	1
Tomato paste - 100% tomatoes, 2 Tbsp	0
Tomato puree, 1/4 cup	0
Tomato sauce, 1/4 cup	0
Tomato sauce - extra thick & zesty, 1/4 cup	0
Tomato sauce - garlic and onion, 1/4 cup	0
Del Monte	
Four cheese, 1/2 cup	1
Organic tomato sauce, 1/4 cup	0
Sauce, tomato no salt added, 1/4 cup	0

Condiments, Sauces & Gravies

Del Monte (cont'd)	POINTS VALUE
Tomato & basil, 1/2 cup	1
Traditional, 1/2 cup	1
With garlic and onion, 1/2 cup	1
With green peppers and mushrooms, 1/2 cup	1
With meat, 1/2 cup	1
With mushrooms, 1/2 cup	1
Del Monte Chunky	
Garlic & herb, 1/2 cup	1
Italian herb, 1/2 cup	1
Eden Organic	
Pizza pasta sauce, 1/2 cup	1
Spaghetti sauce, 1/2 cup	1
Spaghetti sauce - no salt, 1/2 cup	1
Ellen Rose	
Artichoke & olive pesto, 2 Tbsp	2
Pesto sauce, 2 Tbsp	3
Sun dried tomato pesto, 2 Tbsp	5
Emeril's	
Homestyle marinara, 1/2 cup	2
Kicked up tomato, 1/2 cup	1
Mushroom & onion, 1/2 cup	2
Puttanesca, 1/2 cup	2
Roasted gaaahlic, 1/2 cup	1
Roasted red pepper, 1/2 cup	1
Vodka, 1/2 cup	3
Faraon	
◆ Tomato sauce, 1/4 cup	0
Lucini	
Rustic tomato basil sauce, 1/2 cup	2
Spicy Tuscan tomato sauce, 1/2 cup	2

	POINTS VALUE
Monterey Pasta Company	
Mediterranean sauce, 1/2 cup	2
Pesto cream sauce, 1/4 cup	3
Pesto sauce with garlic and basil, 1/4 cup	8
Roasted garlic alfredo sauce, 1/2 cup	6
Sweet tomato basil sauce, 1/2 cup	1
Tomato cream sauce with gorgonzola, 1/2 cup	5
Muir Glen Organic	
Cabernet marinara pasta sauce, 1/2 cup	1
Chunky tomato & herb pasta sauce, 1/2 cup	1
Fire roasted tomato pasta sauce, 1/2 cup	1
Four cheese pasta sauce, 1/2 cup	1
Garden vegetable pasta sauce, 1/2 cup	1
Garlic roasted garlic sauce, 1/2 cup	1
Italian herb pasta sauce, 1/2 cup	1
Portabello mushroom pasta sauce, 1/2 cup	1
◆ Premium chunky tomato sauce, 1/4 cup	0
◆ Premium tomato sauce, 1/4 cup	0
Spicy tomato pasta sauce, 1/2 cup	1
Sun dried tomato pasta sauce, 1/2 cup	1
Muirhead	
Tomato sauce, 1 Tbsp	0
Naturally Fresh	
Marinara, 2 Tbsp (individual 4-oz portion cup)	0

Prego

	POINTS VALUE
Flavored with meat, 1/2 cup	2
Fresh mushroom, 1/2 cup	1
Fresh mushroom - plastic container, 1/2 cup	1
Heart smart fresh mushroom Italian sauce, 1/2 cup	2
Heart smart traditional Italian sauce, 1/2 cup	1
Italian sausage & garlic, 1/2 cup	2
Marinara, 1/2 cup	2
Mini meatball, 1/2 cup	2
Mushroom & garlic, 1/2 cup	1
Onion & garlic, 1/2 cup	2
Organic mushroom, 1/2 cup	1
Organic tomato & basil, 1/2 cup	1
Ricotta parmesan, 1/2 cup	1
Roasted garlic & herb, 1/2 cup	1
Roasted garlic parmesan, 1/2 cup	1
Roasted red pepper & garlic, 1/2 cup	1
Three cheese, 1/2 cup	1
Tomato basil & garlic, 1/2 cup	1
Traditional, 1/2 cup	1
Traditional - plastic container, 1/2 cup	1

Prego Chunky Garden

Garden combination, 1/2 cup	1
Mushroom & green peppers, 1/2 cup	1
Mushroom supreme, 1/2 cup	1
Tomato onion & garlic, 1/2 cup	1

Progresso

	POINTS VALUE
Tomato puree, 1/4 cup	0

Ragu Cheese Creations

Classic alfredo, 1/4 cup	3
Double cheddar, 1/4 cup	3
Lite parmesan alfredo, 1/4 cup	2
Roasted garlic parmesan, 1/4 cup	3

Ragu Chunky Gardenstyle

Garden combination, 1/2 cup	2
Mama's special garden sauce, 1/2 cup	2
Mushroom & green pepper, 1/2 cup	2
Mushrooms & green pepper, 1/2 cup	2
Roasted red pepper & onion, 1/2 cup	2
Sundried tomato & sweet basil, 1/2 cup	2
Super chunky mushroom, 1/2 cup	2
Super chunky mushroom, 1/2 cup	2
Super vegetable primavera, 1/2 cup	2
Tomato, basil & Italian cheese, 1/2 cup	2
Tomato, garlic & onion, 1/2 cup	2

Ragu Light

No sugar added tomato & basil, 1/2 cup	1
Tomato & basil, fat free, 1/2 cup	1

Ragu Old World Style

Flavored with meat, 1/2 cup	1
Marinara, 1/2 cup	2
Mushroom, 1/2 cup	1
Traditional, 1/2 cup	1

Condiments, Sauces & Gravies

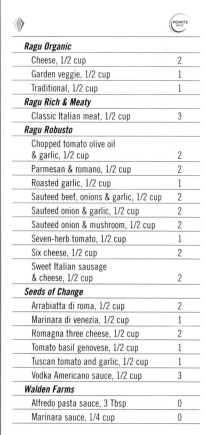

	POINTS VALUE
Ragu Organic	
Cheese, 1/2 cup	2
Garden veggie, 1/2 cup	1
Traditional, 1/2 cup	1
Ragu Rich & Meaty	
Classic Italian meat, 1/2 cup	3
Ragu Robusto	
Chopped tomato olive oil & garlic, 1/2 cup	2
Parmesan & romano, 1/2 cup	2
Roasted garlic, 1/2 cup	1
Sauteed beef, onions & garlic, 1/2 cup	2
Sauteed onion & garlic, 1/2 cup	2
Sauteed onion & mushroom, 1/2 cup	2
Seven-herb tomato, 1/2 cup	1
Six cheese, 1/2 cup	2
Sweet Italian sausage & cheese, 1/2 cup	2
Seeds of Change	
Arrabiatta di roma, 1/2 cup	2
Marinara di venezia, 1/2 cup	1
Romagna three cheese, 1/2 cup	2
Tomato basil genovese, 1/2 cup	1
Tuscan tomato and garlic, 1/2 cup	1
Vodka Americano sauce, 1/2 cup	3
Walden Farms	
Alfredo pasta sauce, 3 Tbsp	0
Marinara sauce, 1/4 cup	0

	POINTS VALUE
## Pickles	
B&G	
Bread & butter chips, unsalted, 6 pieces	1
Bread & butter pickles, 1 oz	1
Deli style zesty spear, 2/3	0
Dill pickles, 1/2	0
Hamburger dill chips, 1 oz	0
Hamburger dill toppers, 1 1/2 pieces	0
Kosher baby dills, 2	0
Kosher dill gherkins, 1 oz	0
Kosher dill sandwich toppers, 1 1/2 pieces	0
Kosher dills, 1 oz	0
New York deli pickles, 1 1/2	0
New York deli toppers, 1 1/2 pieces	0
No salt kosher dills, 1/2	0
Pickle in a pouch, 1 pouch	0
Polish dill toppers, 1 1/2 pieces	0
Sour pickles, 1/2	0
Sweet gherkins, 1 oz	1
Sweet midget gherkins, 3	1
Sweet mixed pickles, 6 1/2	1
Sweet pickles, 1/2	1
Tiny treats, 1 serving (1 oz)	1
B&G Sandwich Toppers	
Bread & butter, 1 1/2 pieces	1
Boar's Head	
Sweet pickle chips with horseradish, 3	1

	POINTS VALUE
Cascadian Farm	
Baby dills, 1	0
Bread & butter chips, 5 slices	1
Kosher dills, 1	0
Kosher dills - reduced sodium, 1	0
Claussen	
Bread 'n butter chips, 4 slices	0
Burger slices, kosher dill, 1 slice	0
Deli style hearty garlic wholes, 1/2	0
Deli style kosher dill halves, 1/2	0
Deli style kosher dill spears, 1	0
Kosher dill halves, 1/2	0
Kosher dill mini, 1	0
Kosher dill spears, 1	0
Kosher dill wholes, 1/2	0
New York deli style half sour wholes, 1/2	0
Sandwich slices deli style hearty garlic, 2 slices	0
Sandwich slices kosher dill, 2 slices	0
Sandwich slices, bread 'n butter, 2 slices	1
Heinz	
Baby kosher dills, 1 oz	0
Bread & butter sandwich slices, 1 oz	1
Dill pickles, 1 oz	0
Genuine dill pickles, 1 oz	0
Hamburger dill chips, 1 oz	0
Kosher dill sandwich slices, 1 oz	0

	POINTS VALUE
Kosher dill spears, 1 oz	0
Kosher dills, 1 oz	0
Old fashioned bread and butter pickles, 1 oz	0
Polish dills, 1 oz	0
Sweet gherkins, 1 oz	1
Sweet pickles, 1 oz	1
Mrs. Fanning's	
Bread 'n butter pickles, 1 oz	1
Vlasic	
Bread & butter chips no sugar added, 3	0
Bread & butter sandwich stackers, 2	1
Bread & butter spears, 3/4	1
Bread & butter spears no sugar added, 1 serving (3/4 spear)	0
Kosher baby dills, 1	0
Kosher crunchy dills, 1 serving (1/2 pickle)	0
Kosher dill sandwich stackers, 2	0
Kosher dill snack'mms, 2 pickles	0
Kosher dill spears, 1 serving (3/4 spear)	0
Kosher midget dills, 3	0
Sweet bread & butter chips, 3	1
Sweet gherkins no sugar added, 3	0
Sweet relish no sugar added, 1 Tbsp	0
Zesty dill sandwich stackers, 2	0
Zesty garlic whole pickles, 1 serving (1/2 pickle)	0

Condiments, Sauces & Gravies

POINTS VALUE

POINTS VALUE

Relish

B&G

Dill relish, 1 Tbsp	0
Emerald relish, 1 Tbsp	0
Hamburger relish, 1 Tbsp	0
Hot dog relish, 1 Tbsp	0
India relish, 1 Tbsp	0
Piccalilli relish, 1 Tbsp	0
Sweet relish, 1 Tbsp	0
Unsalted sweet relish, 1 Tbsp	0

Cascadian Farm

Sweet relish, 1 Tbsp	1

Claussen

Premium sweet pickle relish, 1 Tbsp	0
Sweet pickle relish, 1 Tbsp	0

Del Monte

Sweet pickle relish, 1 Tbsp	0

Heinz

Hamburger relish, 1 Tbsp	0
Hot dog relish, 1 Tbsp	0
India relish, 1 Tbsp	0
Sweet relish, 1 Tbsp	0
Zesty relish, 1 Tbsp	0

Vlasic

Dill relish, 1 Tbsp	0
Dill Tabasco relish, 1 Tbsp	0

Seafood Sauces

Cherchies

Seafood seasoning sauce, 1 Tbsp	0

Del Monte

Sauce, seafood cocktail, 1/4 cup	2

Heinz

Seafood cocktail sauce, 1/4 cup	1
Tartar sauce, 2 Tbsp	3
Zesty cocktail sauce, 1/4 cup	1

Kraft

Cocktail sauce, 1/4 cup	1
Lemon & herb flavor tartar sauce, 2 Tbsp	4
Nonfat tartar sauce, 2 Tbsp	1
Tartar sauce, 2 Tbsp	2

Marzetti

Cocktail sauce, 1/4 cup	3
Tartar sauce, 2 Tbsp	3

McCormick

Cocktail sauce, 1/4 cup	2
Tartar sauce, 2 Tbsp	4

Naturally Fresh

Seafood cocktail, 2 Tbsp (individual 4-oz portion cup)	0
Seafood cocktail sauce, 2 Tbsp	1
Tartar sauce, 2 Tbsp (individual 4-oz portion cup)	4
Tartar sauce, 2 Tbsp	4

Walden Farms

Seafood sauce, 2 Tbsp	0

Steak & Meat Sauces

A1

	POINTS VALUE
Bold & spicy, 1 Tbsp	0
Bold & spicy with Tabasco, 1 Tbsp	0
Carb well steak sauce, 1 Tbsp	0
Chicago steak house, 1 Tbsp	0
Cracked peppercorn, 1 Tbsp	0
Kobe sesame teriyaki, 1 Tbsp	1
New York steakhouse, 1 Tbsp	0
Roasted garlic, 1 Tbsp	0
Smokey mesquite, 1 Tbsp	1
Steak house New Orleans Cajun, 1 Tbsp	1
Steak house teriyaki, 1 Tbsp	1
Steak sauce, 1 Tbsp	0
Steakhouse classic, 1 Tbsp	0
Steakhouse garlic & herb, 1 Tbsp	0
Steakhouse Jamaican jerk, 1 Tbsp	1
Steakhouse Texas mesquite, 1 Tbsp	0
Supreme garlic, 1 Tbsp	1
Teriyaki, 1 Tbsp	1
Thick & hearty, 1 Tbsp	1

Emeril's

	POINTS VALUE
Steak sauce, 1 Tbsp	0

Heinz

57 sauce, 1 Tbsp	0
Traditional steak sauce, 1 Tbsp	0

Jack Daniel's

Ez marinader honey teriyaki, 1 Tbsp	1
ez marinader mesquite, 1 Tbsp	1
Ez marinader slow roasted garlic and herb, 1 Tbsp	0
Original steak sauce, 1 Tbsp	0
Smokey steak sauce, 1 Tbsp	0

Weber Grill Creations

Black peppercorn marinade, dry mix, 1 tsp	0
Italian herb, dry mix, 1 1/2 tsp	0
Mesquite, dry mix, 1 tsp	0
Tomato garlic pesto marinade, dry mix, 1 tsp	0
White wine & herb, dry mix, 1 tsp	0

Wright's

Hickory liquid smoke, 1 tsp	0
Mesquite liquid smoke, 1 tsp	0

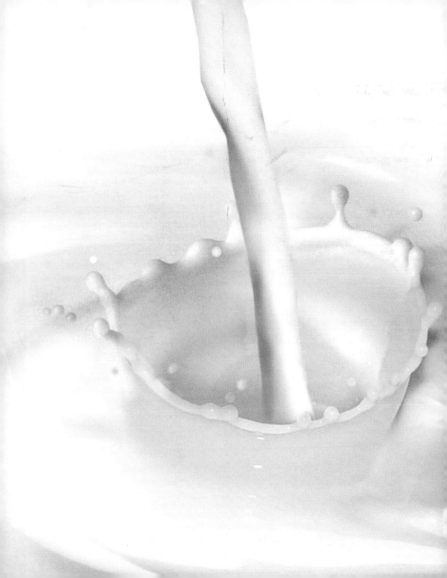

Butter & Butter Substitutes

Butter Buds

	POINTS VALUE
Powdered mix, 1 tsp	0
Sprinkles, 1 tsp	0

Land O Lakes

Butter, salted stick, 1 Tbsp	3
Butter, unsalted stick, 1 Tbsp	3
Country morning blend, soft, 1 Tbsp	3
Country morning blend, stick, 1 Tbsp	3
Garlic flavored butter, 1 Tbsp	3
Honey butter, 1 Tbsp	2
Light butter, salted stick, 1 Tbsp	2
Light butter, whipped salted, 1 Tbsp	1
Spreadable butter with canola oil, 1 Tbsp	3
Whipped butter, salted, 1 Tbsp	2
Whipped butter, unsalted, 1 Tbsp	2

Molly McButter

Natural butter, 1 tsp	0
Natural cheese, 1 tsp	0

Smart Balance

Butter blend stick, regular, 1 serving (14 g)	3
Butter blend stick, unsalted, 1 serving (14 g)	3
Butter blended stick, omega, 1 serving (14 g)	3

Cheese

4C

Grated Italian pecorino Romano sharp cheese, 1 serving (5 g)	1

	POINTS VALUE
Grated Parmesan & Romano cheese, 1 serving (5 g)	1
Grated Parmesan cheese, 1 serving (5 g)	1
Homestyle grated Parmesan cheese, 1 serving (5 g)	1
Homestyle grated Parmesan/Romano cheese, 1 serving (5 g)	1
Homestyle grated pecorino Romano cheese, 1 serving (5 g)	1

Alpine Lace

Reduced fat American cheese, 1 oz	2
Reduced fat American cheese yellow shingle pack slices, 1 slice	2
Reduced fat Cheddar cheese, 1 oz	2
Reduced fat co-jack cheese, 1 slice	2
Reduced fat mozzarella cheese, single pack, 1 slice	2
Reduced fat provolone shingle pack slices, 1 slice	2
Reduced fat provolone with smoke, 1 oz (about a 1" cube)	2
Reduced fat Swiss cheese, 1 slice	2
Reduced fat Swiss cuts, 1 oz (about a 1" cube)	2
Reduced fat Swiss shingle pack slices, 1 slice	2
Reduced salt muenster, 1 oz (about a 1" cube)	3
Reduced salt muenster cheese, 1 slice	2

Athenos

Blue cheese crumbles, 3 Tbsp	3
Blue cheese crumbles, 1/4 cup	3
Feta cheese garlic & herb, 1 oz	2

Dairy & Eggs

Athenos (cont'd)	POINTS VALUE
Feta cheese traditional, 1 oz	2
Feta cheese traditional crumbles, 1/4 cup	2
Feta cheese with garlic & herb, 1/4 cup	2
Feta cheese with tomato & basil, 1 oz	2
Feta cheese with tomato basil crumbles, 1/4 cup	2
Gorgonzola cheese crumbles, 3 Tbsp	3
Reduced fat feta cheese slab, 1 oz	2
Boar's Head	
25% lower sodium - 25% lower fat American cheese - yellow & white, 1 oz	2
28% lower sodium - blue cheese crumbled, 1/4 cup	2
American cheese (loaf) - yellow or white, 1 oz	3
American cheese 120 sliced - yellow or white, 1 slice	2
American cheese 160, sliced - yellow or white, 2 slices	3
Baby Swiss cheese, 1 oz	3
Canadian Cheddar cheese 3 yr. old, 1 oz	3
Cream cheese, 2 Tbsp	3
Cream havarti cheese plain with dill, 1 oz	3
Cream havarti cheese plain with jalapeño, 1 oz	3
Creamy blue cheese crumbled, 1/4 cup	2
Creamy gorgonzola cheese crumbled, 1/4 cup	3
Double gloucester Cheddar cheese, 1 oz	3
Edam cheese, 1 oz	2

	POINTS VALUE
Feta cheese, 1 oz	2
Fontina cheese, 1 oz	3
Gold label prem. imported Swiss cheese, 1 oz	3
Gouda cheese, 1 oz	3
Grana padano cheese - pre-cut, 1 oz	3
Gruyere cheese pre-cut, 1 oz	3
Horseradish Cheddar cheese, 1 oz	3
Imported Italian grated pecorino Romano cheese, 1 Tbsp	1
Imported Italian pecorino Romano cheese - wedge, 1 Tbsp	1
Insalata panino, 1 oz	2
Lacey Swiss cheese, 1 oz	2
Low sodium muenster cheese, 1 oz	3
Lower sodium provolone cheese, 1 oz	3
Mild & creamy asiago cheese, 1 oz	3
Monterey Jack cheese with jalapeño, 1 oz	3
Monterey Jack cheese, plain, 1 oz	3
Muenster cheese, 1 oz	3
Natural Swiss cheese, 1 oz	3
Neufchatel cheese, 2 Tbsp	2
No salt added natural Swiss cheese, 1 oz	3
Picante/sharp provolone cheese, 1 oz	3
Pre-cut asiago cheese, 1 oz	4
Pre-cut creamy gorgonzola cheese, 1 oz	3
Premium imported grated Parmesan cheese, 1 Tbsp	0
Queso para freir cheese, 1 oz	2
Sharp American cheese - white, 1 oz	3

	POINTS VALUE
Sharp Cheddar cheese (white & yellow), 1 oz	3
Vermont Cheddar cheese (white or yellow), 1 oz	3

Borden 2% Blocks

Reduced fat sharp Cheddar cheese, 1 oz	2

Borden 2% Milk Singles

American reduced fat pasteurized prepared cheese product, 1 slice	1

Borden 2% Shreds

Finely shredded reduced fat mild Cheddar cheese, 1/4 cup	2
Shredded reduced fat Cheddar & Monterey Jack cheese, 1/4 cup	2

Borden Big! Singles

American pasteurized prepared cheese product, 1 slice	2

Borden Blocks

Colby and Monterey Jack cheese (chunks), 1 oz	3
Medium Cheddar cheese, 1 oz	3
Mild Cheddar cheese, 1 oz	3
Sharp Cheddar cheese, 1 oz	3

Borden Essentials

American reduced fat pasteurized prepared cheese product, 1 slice	1

Borden Essentials String Cheese

Low-moisture part-skim mozzarella cheese, 1 stick	2

Borden Fat Free Singles

American nonfat process cheese product with added calcium, 1 slice	1

	POINTS VALUE
Sharp nonfat process cheese product with added calcium, 1 slice	1
Swiss nonfat process cheese product with added calcium, 1 slice	1

Borden Kid Builder Singles

American pasteurized prepared cheese product, 1 slice	2

Borden Kid Builder String Cheese

Low-moisture part-skim mozzarella cheese with added vitamins, 1 stick	2

Borden Shreds

2% shredded reduced fat Mexican cheese blend, 1/4 cup	2
Finally shredded Cheddar melt cheese, 1/4 cup	3
Finely shredded Cheddar & Monterey Jack cheese, 1/4 cup	3
Finely shredded colby & Monterey Jack cheese, 1/4 cup	3
Finely shredded Italian cheese blend, 1/4 cup	2
Finely shredded low moisture, post skim Mozzarella cheese, 1/4 cup	2
Finely shredded mild Cheddar cheese, 1/4 cup	3
Finely shredded sharp Cheddar cheese, 1/4 cup	3
Mexican cheese blend (Cheddar, Monterey Jack, asadero, quesadilla), 1/4 cup	3
Shredded Cheddar & Monterey Jack cheese, 1/4 cup	3
Shredded Cheddar and Monterey Jack cheeses with taco seasonings, 1/4 cup	3

Dairy & Eggs

Borden Shreds (cont'd) POINTS VALUE

Shredded low-moisture part-skim mozzarella cheese, 1/4 cup	2
Shredded mild Cheddar cheese, 1/4 cup	3
Shredded sharp Cheddar cheese, 1/4 cup	3
Borden Singles	
American (white) pasteurized prepared cheese product, 1 slice (21 g)	2
American pasteurized prepared cheese product, 1 small slice (19 g)	2
American pasteurized prepared cheese product, 1 large slice (21 g)	2
Grilled cheese melts - pasteurized prepared cheese product, 1 slice (21 g)	2
Borden String Cheese	
Low-moisture, part-skim string cheese, mozzarella, 1 serving (23 g)	2
Boursin Light	
Garlic & fine herbs Gournay cheese, 1 2/3 Tbsp	1
Breakstone's	
Lowfat cottage cheese - 2% milkfat with added calcium & vitamin D, small curd, 1/2 cup	2
Ricotta cheese, 1/4 cup	3
Breakstone's 4-Pack	
2% milkfat, small curd (snack size), 4 oz	2
Breakstone's TempTee	
Whipped cream cheese, 2 Tbsp	2

POINTS VALUE

Cabot	
50% reduced fat jalapeno Cheddar cheese, 1 oz (1" cube)	2
50% reduced fat sharp Cheddar cheese, 1 oz	2
50% reduced fat single serve Cheddar, 3/4 oz (1 bar)	1
50% reduced fat sliced Cheddar cheese, 1 slice	2
75% reduced fat sharp Cheddar cheese, 1 oz (1" cube)	1
Cheddar cheese, 1 oz (1" cube)	3
Fancy blend shredded cheese, 1/4 cup	3
Habanero Cheddar, 1 oz (1" cube)	3
Monterey Jack, 1 oz	3
Pepper Jack, 1 oz (1" cube)	3
Shredded - 50% reduced fat, Cheddar cheese, 1/4 cup	2
Swiss slices, 1 slice	3
Cache Valley	
Colby & Monterey Jack cheese, 1 oz	3
Colby and Monterey Jack cheese, 1 oz	3
Low-moisture part-skim mozzarella cheese, 1 oz	2
Medium Cheddar cheese, 1 oz	3
Mild Cheddar cheese, 1 oz	3
Monterey Jack cheese, 1 oz	3
Sharp Cheddar cheese, 1 oz	3
Swiss cheese, 1 oz	3
Cache Valley Shreds	
Shredded colby and Monterey Jack cheese, 1/4 cup	3

	POINTS VALUE
Shredded medium Cheddar cheese, 1/4 cup	3
Shredded mild Cheddar cheese, 1/4 cup	3
Cache Valley String Cheese	
Low-moisture part-skim mozzarella cheese, 1 stick	2
Daisy Brand	
Low fat cottage cheese, 1/2 cup	2
DiGiorno	
Asiago cheese wedge, grated, 2 tsp	1
Asiago cheese, wedge & cubes, 1 oz	3
Fior di latte fresh mozzarella cheese, 3 balls	2
Fresh twist Parmesan cheese, grated, 2 Tbsp	1
Full moisture asiago cheese, shredded, 1/4 cup	3
Full moisture Parmesan, shredded, 1/4 cup	3
Full moisture pecorino Romano cheese, shredded, 1/4 cup	3
Full moisture Romano cheese, shredded, 1/4 cup	3
Full moisture shaved Parmesan cheese, shredded, 1/4 cup	3
Gourmet mozzarella cheese, 1 oz	2
Romano cheese wheels, grated, 2 tsp	1
Three cheese blend, shredded, 1/4 cup	3
DiGiorno Full-moisture Grated	
Parmesan cheese, 2 tsp	1
Romano cheese, 2 tsp	1

	POINTS VALUE
Finlandia	
Imported double Gloucester deli slices, 1 slice	2
Imported gouda deli slices, 1 slice	2
Imported havarti deli slices, 1 slice	2
Imported light Swiss deli slices, 1 slice	1
Imported muenster deli slices, 1 slice	2
Imported Swiss deli slices, 1 slice	2
Imported thin sliced Swiss deli slices, 1 slice	1
Follow Your Heart	
♦ Vegan gourmet Monterey Jack cheese alternative, 1 oz	2
♦ Vegan gourmet Cheddar cheese alternative, 1 oz	1
Vegan gourmet cream cheese alternative, 2 Tbsp	2
♦ Vegan gourmet mozzarella cheese alternative, 1 oz	1
♦ Vegan gourmet nacho cheese alternative, 1 oz	1
Friendship	
1% lowfat cottage cheese - no salt added, 1/2 cup	2
1% lowfat cottage cheese with pineapple, 1/2 cup	2
1% lowfat cottage cheese, regular, 1/2 cup	2
1% lowfat cottage cheese, whipped, 1/2 cup	2
2% digestive health cottage cheese, 1/2 cup	1
2% pot style cottage cheese, 1/2 cup	2

Dairy & Eggs

Friendship (cont'd)	POINTS VALUE
4% California style cottage cheese, 1/2 cup	3
4% cottage cheese with pineapple, 1/2 cup	3
Farmer cheese, 2 Tbsp	1
Farmer cheese no salt added, 2 Tbsp	1
◆ Nonfat cottage cheese, 1/2 cup	2
Nonfat cottage cheese with pineapple, 1/2 cup	2
Galaxy Foods	
Rice Cheddar flavor shreds, 1/3 cup	2
Rice Cheddar flavored block, 1 oz	2
Rice mozzarella flavor shreds, 1/3 cup	2
Rice mozzarella flavored block, 1 oz	2
Rice Parmesan flavored grated topping, 2 tsp	0
Rice slices - American flavor, 1 slice	1
Rice slices Cheddar flavor, 1 slice	1
Rice slices mozzarella flavor, 1 slice	1
Rice slices pepper Jack flavor, 1 slice	1
Rice slices Swiss flavor, 1 slice	1
◆ Vegan Cheddar flavor alternative slices, 1 slice	1
◆ Vegan Cheddar flavor block, 1 oz	1
◆ Vegan mozzarella flavor, 1 slice	1
◆ Vegan mozzarella flavor block, 1 oz	1
◆ Vegan Parmesan flavored grated topping, 2 tsp	0
◆ Veggie American flavor alternative, 1 slice	1
◆ Veggie Cheddar & pepper Jack cheese flavor alternative - shreds, 1/4 cup	2

	POINTS VALUE
◆ Veggie Cheddar flavor alternative, 1 slice	1
◆ Veggie Cheddar flavor alternative - shreds, 1/4 cup	2
◆ Veggie Cheddar flavor alternative - block, 1 oz	2
◆ Veggie Cheddar with jalapeño flavor, 1 slice	1
◆ Veggie Monterey Jack & Cheddar alternative - shreds, 1/4 cup	2
◆ Veggie mozzarella flavor alternative, 1 slice	1
◆ Veggie mozzarella flavor alternative - shreds, 1/4 cup	2
◆ Veggie mozzarella flavor alternative - block, 1 oz	2
◆ Veggie Parmesan flavor topping - grated, 2 tsp	0
◆ Veggie Parmesan/mozzarella/Romano flavor alternative - shreds (low fat), 1/4 oz	2
◆ Veggie pepper Jack flavor alternative slices, 1 slice	1
◆ Veggie Swiss flavor alternative, 1 slice	1
◆ Veggie Smoked provolone flavor alternative slices, 1 slice	1
GG Golden Guernsey Dairy	
4% cottage cheese, 1/2 cup	3
◆ Fat free cottage cheese, 1/2 cup	2
Low fat cottage cheese, 1/2 cup	2
Gourmet Goat	
Goat cream cheese log, 1 slice	2

Dairy & Eggs

POINTS VALUE

Greek Gods

Mediterranean yogurt cheese spread, 2 Tbsp	2

Horizon Organic

Lowfat cottage cheese, 1/2 cup	2
Reduced fat cream cheese, 2 Tbsp	2
Regular cottage cheese, 1/2 cup	3
Spreadable cream cheese, 2 Tbsp	3

Jarlsberg

Lite sliced, 1 slice	1
Sliced, 1 slice	2

Knudsen

Cottage cheese - 4% milkfat, small curd, 1/2 cup	3
Cottage cheese - 4% milkfat, large curd, 1/2 cup	3
Lowfat cottage cheese - 2% milkfat with added calcium & vitamin D, small curd, 1/2 cup	2

Knudsen Cottage Doubles

Lowfat cottage cheese and blueberry topping, 1 container	3
Lowfat cottage cheese and peach topping with added calcium and vitamin D, 1 container	3
Lowfat cottage cheese and pineapple topping, 1 container	3
Lowfat cottage cheese and raspberry topping, 1 container	3
Lowfat cottage cheese and strawberry topping, 1 container	3

Knudsen Free

Free fat free cottage cheese, 1/2 cup	2

Knudsen LiveActive

2% milkfat cottage cheese, small curd, 1 container	1

Kraft

1% milk reduced-fat singles, 1 slice	2
2% milk reduced fat colby & 2% milk reduced-fat Monterey Jack crumbles, 1/4 cup	2
2% milk reduced fat sharp Cheddar, 4 slices	2
2% milk reduced fat sharp Cheddar stick, 1	2
2% milk reduced-fat shredded mozzarella, 1 cup	2
3-cheese blend crumbles (Monterey Jack, colby and Cheddar), 1/4 cup	3
American pasteurized prepared cheese product, 1 slice	2
Blue cheese crumbles, 3 Tbsp	3
Cheddar & Monterey Jack (shredded), 1/4 cup	3
Cheddar, medium (shredded), 1/4 cup	3
Cheddar, mild (shredded), 1/4 cup	3
Cheddar, sharp (shredded), 1/4 cup	3
Classic melts shredded American, mild Cheddar & Monterey Jack, 1/4 cup	3
Colby & Monterey Jack (shredded), 1/4 cup	3
Colby & Monterey Jack cubes, 4 pieces	3
Cracker cuts baby Swiss slices, 3 slices	3
Cracker cuts extra sharp Cheddar, 4 slices	3
Cracker cuts marbled colby & Monterey Jack slices, 3 slices	3

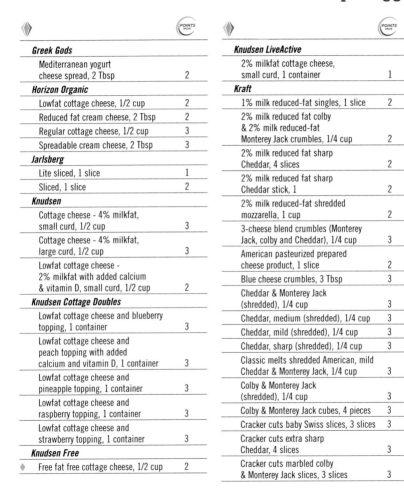

Dairy & Eggs

Kraft (cont'd)	POINTS value
Cracker cuts mild Cheddar slices, 3 slices	3
Cracker cuts sharp Cheddar and marbled colby & high-moisture Monterey Jack, 4 slices	3
Cracker cuts sharp Cheddar slices, 3 slices	3
Easy cheese American, 1 serving (32 g)	2
Easy cheese Cheddar, 1 serving (32 g)	2
Easy cheese Cheddar 'n bacon, 1 serving (32 g)	2
Easy cheese pasteurized cheese snack, original cream cheese, 2 Tbsp	3
Easy cheese sharp Cheddar, 1 serving (32 g)	2
Extra sharp Cheddar sticks, 1	3
Feta crumbles, 1/4 cup	2
Grate it fresh Parmesan, 2 Tbsp	1
Grated Parmesan & Romano blend, 2 tsp	1
Italian style five cheese - cheese shreds, 1 oz	2
Italian-style crumbles (low-moisture part-skim mozzarella, provolone, asiago and Romano), 1/4 cup	2
Low-moisture part-skim mozzarella (shredded), 1/4 cup	2
Low-moisture part-skim mozzarella, 1 oz	2
Low-moisture part-skim mozzarella crumbles, 1/4 cup	2
Macaroni & cheese topping, 2 tsp	1
Mediterranean-style crumbles (provolone, feta & Parmesan), 1/4 cup	2

	POINTS value
Mexican blend shredded cheese, 1/4 cup	3
Mexican style crumbles (sharp Cheddar, asadero, and queso quesadilla), 1/4 cup	3
Mexican style natural shredded four cheese blend, 1/4 cup	3
Mexican style pasteurized prepared cheese product, 1 slice	2
Mexican style shredded queso quesadilla/asadero cheeses, 1/4 cup	2
Mild Cheddar & Monterey Jack cubes, 7 pieces	3
Mild Cheddar sticks, 1	3
Mild Cheddar, wax dipped, 1 oz	3
Mild marbled Cheddar, 1 oz	3
♦ Nonfat grated topping, 2 tsp	0
Organic pasteurized prepared cheese product, 1 slice	2
Organic shredded Cheddar, 1/4 cup	3
Organic shredded low-moisture part-skim mozzarella, 1/4 cup	2
Organic string cheese, 1 stick	2
Parmesan, grated, 2 tsp	1
Parmesan style topping, 2 tsp	1
Parmesan, shredded, 1/4 cup	3
Pasteurized process American slices, 1 slice	2
Pasteurized process cheese food cheese n' onion, 1 oz	2
Pasteurized process cheese food with bacon & smoke flavor, 1 oz	2
Pasteurized process cheese food with garlic & natural flavor, 1 oz	3

	POINTS VALUE
Pasteurized process cheese food, garlic, 1 oz	2
Pimento, spread, 2 Tbsp	2
Pineapple, spread, 2 Tbsp	2
Reduced fat Cheddar & Monterey Jack cubes, 7 pieces	2
Reduced fat Italian style shredded cheese blend, 1/4 cup	2
Reduced fat Mexican style crumbles, 1/4 cup	2
Reduced fat Parmesan style grated topping, 2 tsp	0
Reduced-fat Monterey Jack pasteurized prepared cheese product with jalapeno pepper, 1 slice	1
Roka brand blue, spread, 2 Tbsp	2
Sharp Cheddar cubes, 7 pieces	3
Sharp cheese crumbles, 1/4 cup	3
Shredded 2% milk reduced fat sharp Cheddar with added calcium, 1/4 cup	2
Shredded queso asadero low-moisture part-skim cheese, 1/4 cup	2
Shredded queso quesadilla low-moisture whole milk cheese, 1/4 cup	2
Shredded sharp white Cheddar, 1/4 cup	3
Singles American pasteurized prepared cheese, 1 slice	2
Smoky Swiss & Cheddar hickory smoked pasteurized process cheese food, 1 oz	2
String cheese reduced fat mozzarella made with 2% milk, 1 stick	2
Swiss (shredded), 1/4 cup	3
Three cheese, shredded, 1/4 cup	3
Traditional feta crumbles, 1/4 cup	2

	POINTS VALUE
Whole milk low-moisture mozzarella (shredded), 1/4 cup	2
Kraft 2%	
Colby & Monterey Jack (shredded), 1/4 cup	2
Kraft 2% Milk Natural Cheese	
Cheddar, mild, 1 oz	2
Cheddar, sharp, 1 oz	2
Colby, 1 oz	2
Mexican four cheese - cheese shreds, 1 oz	2
Monterey Jack, 1 oz	2
Kraft 2% Milk Reduced Fat Natural Shredded Cheese	
Cheddar, mild (with calcium), 1/4 cup	2
Cheddar, sharp (with calcium), 1/4 cup	2
Mozzarella (with calcium), 1/4 cup	2
Kraft 2% Milk Singles	
American, 1 slice	1
American, 2/3 oz	1
Mozzarella, 1 slice	1
Sharp Cheddar, 3/4 oz	1
Swiss, 3/4 oz	1
Kraft Breakstone's Temp-Tee	
Pasteurized whipped cream cheese, 2 Tbsp	2
Kraft Classic Melts	
Cheddar & American, 1 serving (28 g)	3
Four cheese, 1 serving (28 g)	3
Kraft Cracker Barrel	
2% milk reduced fat extra sharp Cheddar sticks, 1	2

Dairy & Eggs

Kraft Cracker Barrel (cont'd)	POINTS VALUE
Baby Swiss, 1 oz	3
Cheddar, aged reserve extra sharp, 1 oz	3
Cheddar, extra sharp, 1 oz	3
Cheddar, marbled sharp, 1 oz	3
Cheddar, sharp, 1 oz	3
Cheddar, Vermont sharp white, 1 oz	3
Cracker cuts 2% milk reduced fat extra sharp Cheddar slices, 3 slices	2
Cracker cuts extra sharp, 1 oz	3
Cracker cuts Vermont sharp white, 1 oz	3
Emmentaler slices, 1 slice	2
Extra sharp Cheddar sticks, 1	3
Extra sharp Cheddar, colored, 1 oz	3
Extra sharp Cheddar, uncolored, 1 oz	3
Extra sharp Cheddar spread, 2 Tbsp	3
Extra sharp white Cheddar sticks, 1	3
Fontina slices, 1 slice	2
Havarti slices, 1 slice	2
Natural sharp Cheddar slices, 1 slice	2
Sharp Cheddar cheese sticks, 1	3
Sharp Cheddar spread, 2 Tbsp	3
Shredded 2% milk reduced fat extra sharp Cheddar, 1/4 cup	2
Shredded 2% milk reduced fat sharp Cheddar, 1/4 cup	2
Shredded extra sharp Cheddar, 1/4 cup	3
Vermont sharp Cheddar slices, 1 slice	2
Vermont sharp Cheddar sticks, 1	3
White colby slices, 1 slice	2

	POINTS VALUE
Kraft Cracker Barrel 2%	
Cheddar, extra sharp, 1 oz	2
Cheddar, sharp, 1 oz	2
Cheddar, Vermont sharp, 1 oz	2
Kraft Deli Deluxe	
American slices, 1 slice (19 g)	2
American slices, 1 medium slice (21 g)	2
American slices, 1 large slice (28 g)	3
Colby Jack slices, 1 slice	2
Grated Romano, 2 Tbsp	1
Low-moisture part-skim mozzarella slices, 1 slice	2
Mild Cheddar slices, 1 slice	2
Monterey Jack slices with jalapeno peppers, 1 slice	2
Muenster slices, 1 slice	2
Pasteurized process American, 1 oz	3
Pasteurized process Cheddar, 1 slice	2
Pasteurized process Swiss slices, 1 slice	2
Provolone with smoked flavor added, 1 slice	3
Reduced fat 2% milk Cheddar slices, 1 slice	2
Reduced fat 2% milk pasteurized process American with added calcium & vitamin D, 1 slice	2
Reduced fat 2% milk Swiss, 1 slice	2
Sharp Cheddar slices, 1 slice	2
Sharp pasteurized process Cheddar slices, 1 slice	3
Swiss slices, 1 small slice (21 g)	2

	POINTS VALUE
Swiss slices, 1 medium slice (23 g)	2
Swiss slices, 1 large slice (28 g)	3
Thin Swiss slices, 2 slices (28 g)	3
Kraft Deluxe Singles Pasteurized Process Cheese	
American, 1 oz	2
Pimento, 1 slice	2
Swiss, 1 slice	2
Kraft Free	
♦ Cheddar (shredded), 1/4 cup	1
♦ Mozzarella (shredded), 1/4 cup	1
Kraft Free Singles	
♦ American, 3/4 oz	1
♦ Mozzarella, 1 slice	1
♦ Sharp Cheddar, 1 slice	1
♦ Swiss, 1 slice	1
Kraft Italian Style	
Mozzarella & Parmesan (shredded), 1/4 cup	2
Kraft Mexican Style	
Cheddar and Monterey Jack (shredded), 1/4 cup	3
Four cheese (shredded), 1/4 cup	3
Taco cheese (shredded), 1/4 cup	3
Kraft Natural Cheese	
Cheddar, mild, 1 oz	3
Cheddar, mild, 7 cubes	3
Cheddar, medium, 1 oz	3
Cheddar, sharp, 1 oz	3
Cheddar, extra sharp, 1 oz	3
Cheddar & Monterey Jack marbled, 1 oz	3
Colby, 1 oz	3

	POINTS VALUE
Colby & Monterey Jack, 1 oz	3
Colby & Monterey Jack, marbled, 1 oz	3
Colby & Monterey Jack, marbled, 7 cubes	3
Low-moisture part-skim mozzarella, 1 oz	2
Monterey Jack, 1 oz	3
Monterey Jack with jalapeño peppers, 1 oz	3
Kraft Parm Plus!	
Garlic & herb, 2 tsp	0
Seasoning blend zesty red pepper, 2 tsp	0
Kraft Philadelphia	
Chive & onion (tub), 2 Tbsp	3
Chive, whipped, 2 Tbsp	2
Garden vegetable, 2 Tbsp	2
Honey nut flavor, 2 Tbsp	2
Neufchatel cheese (brick), 1 oz	2
Original (brick), 1 oz	3
Original (tub), 2 Tbsp	3
Original, whipped, 2 Tbsp	2
Pineapple, 2 Tbsp	2
Salmon (tub), 2 Tbsp	2
Strawberry, 2 Tbsp	2
Whipped cinnamon 'n brown sugar cream cheese, 2 Tbsp	2
Whipped garlic 'n herb cream cheese, 2 Tbsp	2
Whipped mixed berry cream cheese, 2 Tbsp	2
Whipped ranch cream cheese, 2 Tbsp	2

Dairy & Eggs

	POINTS VALUE
Kraft Philadelphia Free	
Fat free cream cheese, 1 oz	1
Strawberry, 2 Tbsp	1
Kraft Philadelphia Light	
Chive and onion, 2 Tbsp	2
Garden vegetable, 2 Tbsp	2
Garlic, 2 Tbsp	2
Jalapeño, 2 Tbsp	2
Original, 2 Tbsp	2
Strawberry, 2 Tbsp	2
Kraft Philly Flavors	
Cheesecake, 2 Tbsp	3
Kraft Pizza	
Four cheese (shredded), 1/4 cup	2
Low-moisture mozzarella and Cheddar (shredded), 1/4 cup	2
Low-moisture mozzarella and provolone (shredded), 1/4 cup	2
Kraft Polly-O	
Mozzarella reduced fat string cheese, 1 serving	2
Kraft Rip-Ums	
Pasteurized processed cheese food with added calcium American, pizza, 1	2
Kraft Singles	
American slices, 1 slice	2
Kraft Singles Pasteurized Process Cheese Food	
American, 1 slice	2
Sharp, 1 slice	2
Swiss, 1 slice	2
Kraft String-Ums	
String cheese, 1 stick	2

	POINTS VALUE
Kraft To Go!	
Cheddar cheese cubes & mini ritz crackers, 1 tray	5
Marble colby & Monterey Jack cheese cubes & triscuit crackers, 1 tray	4
Monterey Jack cheese with jalapeno peppers & mini wheat thins, 1 tray	4
Kraft Twist-Ums	
Low-moisture part-skim mozzarella string cheese, 1 stick	2
Low moisture part-skim mozzarella and Cheddar string cheese, 1 stick	2
Kraft Velveeta	
Extra thick slices, 1 serving (34 g)	2
Mild Mexican, 1 oz	2
Pasteurized prepared cheese product, 1 oz	2
Pasteurized prepared cheese product slices, 1 slice	1
Pepper Jack pasteurized prepared cheese product with jalapeno pepper, 1 oz	2
Plain, 1 oz	2
Shredded pasteurized process mild Cheddar, 1/4 cup	3
Shreds, 1/4 cup	2
Kraft Velveeta Light	
Reduced fat pasteurized process cheese product, 1 oz	1
Kraft Velveeta Singles	
American, 1 slice	2
Land O Lakes	
American cheese product white, 1 slice	2
American cheese product white vertical slices, 2 slices	3

	POINTS VALUE
American cheese product yellow slices, 1 slice	2
American cheese product yellow vertical slice, 2 slices	3
American cheese white shingle slices, 1 slice	2
American cheese white stack slices, 1 slice	2
American cheese white vertical slices, 1 slice	2
American cheese yellow shingle slices, 1 slice	2
American cheese yellow stack slices, 1 slice	2
American cheese yellow, vertical slices, 1 slice	2
American Swiss loaf, 1 oz (about a 1" cube)	3
Baby Swiss loaf, 1 oz	3
Baby Swiss shingle slices, 1 slice	2
Chedarella cheese, 1 oz	3
Chedarella print, 1 oz	3
Cheddar cheese, mild, medium, sharp, extra sharp - yellow & white, 1 oz	3
Cheddar longhorn style mild yellow, 1 oz (about a 1" cube)	3
Cheddar medium yellow shingle slices, 1 slice	2
Cheddar mild yellow horn, 1 oz (about a 1" cube)	3
Cheddar sharp white loaf, 1 oz (about a 1" cube)	3
Cheddar sharp yellow loaf, 1 oz (about a 1" cube)	3

	POINTS VALUE
Chedarella shingle slices, 1 slice	3
Co-Jack cheese, 1 oz	3
Co-Jack horn, 1 oz (about a 1" cube)	3
Colby cheese, 1 oz	3
Colby horn, 1 oz	3
Colby shingle slices, 1 slice	2
Havarti shingle slices, 1 slice	2
Hot pepper cheese product, 1 oz	3
Hot pepper monterey jack cheese, 1 oz	3
Jalapeno cheese food shingle slices, 1 slice	2
Light 50% reduced fat American cheese white loaf, 1 oz (about a 1" cube)	2
Light 50% reduced fat American cheese yellow loaf, 1 oz (about a 1" cube)	2
Monterey Jack cheese, 1 oz	3
Mozzarella cheese, 1 oz	2
Mozzarella low-moisture part-skim, 1 oz (about a 1" cube)	2
Mozzarella shingle slices, 1 slice	2
Muenster, 1 oz	3
Muenster shingle slices, 1 slice	2
Onion cheese food loaf, 1 oz (about a 1" cube)	2
Pepper Jack horn, 1 oz (about a 1" cube)	3
Pepper Jack shingle slices, 1 slice	2
Process American loaf, yellow, 1 oz (about a 1" cube)	3
Process extra sharp Cheddar yellow loaf, 1 oz (about a 1" cube)	3
Process Monterey Jack cheese with jalapeno peppers loaf, 1 oz (about a 1" cube)	3

Dairy & Eggs

Land O Lakes (cont'd)	POINTS VALUE
Provolone no-smoke, 1 oz (about a 1" cube)	3
Provolone no-smoke shingle slices, 1 slice	2
Provolone stack slices, 1 slice	2
Provolone with smoke, 1 oz (about a 1" cube)	3
Provolone with smoke shingle slices, 1 slice	2
Reduced fat provolone with smoke slices, 1 slice	2
Sharp American cheese, yellow shingle slices, 1 slice	2
Sharp Cheddar shingle slices, 1 slice	2
Swiss cheese, 1 oz	3
Swiss loaf, 1 oz	3
Variety pack, 25% reduced fat muenster, 1 slice	2
Variety pack, 25% reduced fat provolone, 1 slice	2
Variety pack, 25% reduced fat Swiss, 1 slice	2
Variety pack, American, 1 slice	2
Variety pack, co-Jack, 1 slice	2
Variety pack, colby, 1 slice	2
Variety pack, mild Cheddar, 1 slice	2
Variety pack, provolone, 1 slice	2
Variety pack, Swiss, 1 slice	2
Land O Lakes Deli	
American cheese loaf, sharp, white, 1 oz	3
American cheese white loaf, less sodium, 1 oz	3

	POINTS VALUE
Brick cheese, 1 oz	3
Co-Jack cheese, single pack, 1 slice	2
Land O Lakes Hillview	
American cheese product, white loaf, 1 large slice	2
American cheese product, white loaf, 2 slices	3
American cheese product, white loaf, 1 oz (about a 1" cube)	3
American cheese product, yellow loaf, 2 slices	3
American cheese product, yellow loaf, 1 large slice	2
American cheese product, yellow loaf, 1 oz (about a 1" cube)	3
Land O Lakes Naturally Slender	
American cheese product, white single slices, 1 slice	2
Cheese product, white loaf, 1 oz (about a 1" cube)	2
Cheese product, white with red bell & green jalapeno peppers loaf, 1 oz (about a 1" cube)	2
Cheese product, yellow loaf, 1 oz (about a 1" cube)	2
Land O Lakes New Yorker	
American cheese product, white, 2 slices	3
American cheese product, white, 1 oz (about a 1" cube)	3
American cheese product, yellow, 1 slice	3
American cheese product, yellow, 1 oz (about a 1" cube)	3

	POINTS VALUE
Hot pepper American cheese food, 1 oz (about a 1" cube)	2
Muenster, 1 oz (about a 1" cube)	3
Provolone with smoke, 1 oz (about a 1" cube)	3
Swiss loaf, 1 oz (about a 1" cube)	3
Land O Lakes Reduced Fat Snack'N Cheese To-Go	
Co-Jack cheese portions, 1 piece	2
Mild Cheddar cheese, 1 piece	2
Land O Lakes Snack'N Cheese To-Go	
Chedarella, 1 portion (21 g)	2
Co-Jack, 1 portion (21 g)	2
Mild cheddar, 1 portion (21 g)	2
Land O Lakes Starfield	
American cheese product, yellow loaf, 1 oz (about a 1" cube)	3
Laughing Cow, The	
Gourmet cheese & baguettes, 1 serving (21 g)	1
Light creamy French onion cheese wedges, 1 wedge	1
Light creamy garlic & herb cheese wedges, 1 wedge	1
Light creamy Swiss original flavor cheese wedges, 1 wedge	1
Light gourmet cheese bites, 5 pieces	1
Mini babybel, bonbel, 1 piece	2
Mini babybel, gouda, 1 piece	2
Mini babybel, light original, 1 cheese	1
Mini babybel, mild Cheddar, 1 piece	2
Mini babybel, original, 1 piece	2

	POINTS VALUE
Lifetime	
Low fat jalapeno Jack, 1 oz	1
Low fat sharp Cheddar, 1 oz	1
Low fat Swiss, 1 oz	1
Light N' Lively	
Lowfat cottage cheese with added calcium, 1/2 cup	2
Light N' Lively 4-Pack	
Lowfat cottage cheese with added calcium, 4 oz	2
Light N' Lively Free	
◆ Fat free cottage cheese with calcium, 1/2 cup	2
Litehouse	
Bleu cheese crumbles, 1 oz	2
Madame Chevre Elite	
Cranberry with port in a cup, 2 Tbsp	1
Goat cream cheese log, 1 slice	2
Roasted red pepper in a cup, 2 Tbsp	1
Market Day	
American cheese, 1 slice	2
String cheese, 1 oz (about 1" cube)	2
Morning Glory	
4% cottage cheese, 1/2 cup	3
◆ Fat free cottage cheese, 1/2 cup	2
Low fat cottage cheese, 1/2 cup	2
Mozzarella Fresca	
Bocconcini, 1 serving (1 oz)	2
Ciliegine, 1 serving (1 oz)	2
Fresh mozzarella - snack cheese, 1 serving (1 oz)	2

Dairy & Eggs

Mozzarella Fresca (cont'd)	POINTS VALUE
Fresh mozzarella ball (packed in water), 1 serving (1 oz)	2
Fresh mozzarella ball (vacuum packed), 1 serving (1 oz)	2
Fresh mozzarella log (vacuum packed), 1 serving (1 oz)	2
Low fat ricotta, 1 serving (1 oz)	1
Marinated fresh mozzarella, 1 serving (1 oz)	4
Mascarpone, 1 serving (1 oz)	4
Medallions, 1 serving (1 oz)	2
Ovoline, 1 serving (1 oz)	2
Perlini, 1 serving (1 oz)	2
Whole milk ricotta, 1 serving (1 oz)	1
Philadelphia	
Blueberry, 2 Tbsp	2
Cream cheese spread, 1 pouch	2
Fat free cream cheese, 1 oz	1
Raspberry, 2 Tbsp	2
Swirls - brown sugar'n cinnamon, 2 Tbsp	2
Swirls - garlic 'n herb, 2 Tbsp	2
Swirls - triple berry, 2 Tbsp	2
Philadelphia Jammin' Swirls	
Blueberry, 2 Tbsp	2
Strawberry, 2 Tbsp	2
Polly-O	
Asiago cheese, 1 oz	3
Caruso low-moisture mozzarella cheese, 1 oz	2
Caruso low-moisture part-skim mozzarella cheese, 1 oz	2

	POINTS VALUE
Fat free mozzarella cheese loaf, 1 oz	1
Fat free ricotta, 1/4 cup	1
Fior di latte fresh mozzarella cheese, 1 1/2 oz	3
Fresh mozzarella cheese, 1 oz	2
Fresh, fancy shredded Parmesan cheese, 1/4 cup	3
Full moisture shredded Parmesan cheese, 1/4 cup	3
Gourmet mozzarella cheese, 1 oz	2
Low-moisture part-skim mozzarella cheese, 1/4 cup	2
Low-moisture part-skim mozzarella cheese, 1 oz	2
Low-moisture whole-milk mozzarella cheese, 1 oz	2
Part skim ricotta cheese, 1/4 cup	2
Provolone cheese (not smoked), 1 oz	3
Reduced fat mozzarella cheese loaf, 1 oz	1
Ricotta, 1/4 cup	3
Ricotta cheese alphabet, 1/4 cup	3
Shredded, whole milk mozzarella, 1 oz	2
Smoked low-moisture whole milk mozzarella loaf, 1 oz	2
Smoked low-moisture whole milk mozzarella loaf, 1 slice	2
String cheese reduced fat mozzarella cheese made with 2% milk, 1	2
Whole milk mozzarella, 1 serving	2
Polly-O String-Ums	
Low moisture part-skim mozzarella, 1 stick	2

Dairy & Eggs

	POINTS VALUE
Président	
Brie light, 1 oz	2
◆ Crumbled feta, fat free California tomato, 1 oz	1
◆ Crumbled feta, fat free Mediterranean herbs, 1 oz	1
◆ Crumbled feta, fat free plain, 1 oz	1
◆ Fat free feta, 1 cube (1")	1
◆ Fat free feta, California tomato & basil, 1 cube (approx. 1")	1
◆ Fat free feta, Mediterranean herbs, 1 cube (approx. 1")	1
Sandwich-Mate	
Swiss imitation pasteurized process cheese food, 1 slice	1
Sandwich-Mate Singles	
American imitation pasteurized process cheese food, 1 slice	1
ShredMate	
Shredded imitation Cheddar cheese, 1/4 cup	2
Smart Balance	
Cream cheese, 1 serving (30 g)	2
Creamy cheddar slices, 1 slice	1
Light cream cheese, 1 serving (30 g)	2
Part skim Cheddar-style product, 1 oz	2
Part-skim mozzarella style product, 1 oz	2
Regular cream cheese, 1 serving (30 g)	2
Smart Beat	
◆ Fat free American, mellow Cheddar, lactose free slices, 1 slice	1
◆ Fat free American, sharp Cheddar slices, 1 slice	1

	POINTS VALUE
Sonoma Cheese Company	
Blue Jack, 1 serving (1 oz)	3
Garlic Jack, 1 serving (1 oz)	3
Habanero Jack, 1 serving (1 oz)	3
Hot pepper Jack, 1 serving (1 oz)	3
Mediterranean Jack, 1 serving (1 oz)	3
Pesto Jack, 1 serving (1 oz)	3
Traditional Jack, 1 serving (1 oz)	3
SoyaKaas	
Cream cheese - garden vegetable, 1 oz	2
Cream cheese - garlic & herb, 1 oz	2
Cream cheese original - plain, 1 oz	2
◆ Fat free jalapeño, 1 oz	1
◆ Fat free mild Cheddar style, 1 oz	1
◆ Fat free mozzarella style, 1 oz	1
◆ Garlic & herb, 1 oz	2
◆ Gouda (block), 1 slice	2
◆ Grated Parmesan style, 1 oz	1
◆ Jalapeño Mexi-kaas, 1 oz	2
◆ Mild Cheddar style, 1 oz	2
◆ Monterey Jack style, 1 oz	2
◆ Mozzarella style, 1 oz	2
◆ Sliced American Cheddar style, 1 slice	1
◆ Sliced white Cheddar style, 1 slice	1
◆ Smoked Cheddar style, 1 oz	2
◆ White Cheddar horseradish (block), 1 oz	2
Temptee	
Cream cheese, 2 Tbsp	2
Tofu Rella	
◆ Cheddar (chunk), 1 oz	2
◆ Garlic-herb (chunk), 1 oz	2

Dairy & Eggs

Tofu Rella (cont'd)

	POINTS VALUE
Jalapeño jack (chunk), 1 oz	2
Monterey jack (chunk), 1 oz	2
Mozzarella (chunk), 1 oz	2

Tree of Life

Natural cheese, mild Cheddar, 1 serving (1 oz)	3
Natural cheese, mozzarella, 1 serving (1 oz)	2
Natural cheese, razor sharp Cheddar, 1 serving (1 oz)	3
Natural cheese, sharp Cheddar, 1 serving (1 oz)	3
Natural cheese, Swiss, 1 serving (1 oz)	3
Organic cheese, 33% reduced fat Cheddar, 1 serving (1 oz)	2
Organic cheese, jalapeno Jack, 1 serving (1 oz)	3
Organic cheese, mild Cheddar, 1 serving (1 oz)	3
Organic cheese, Monterey Jack style, 1 serving (1 oz)	3
Organic cheese, mozzarella, 1 serving (1 oz)	2

Vegie Kaas

Cheddar style, 1 oz	1
Mozzarella style, 1 oz	1

Weight Watchers

Light string cheese, 1 piece	1
Natural reduced fat Cheddar cheese snacks, 2 pieces	2
Natural reduced fat medium Cheddar, 2 slices	2
Natural reduced fat pepper Jack, 2 slices	2

	POINTS VALUE
Natural reduced fat shredded Cheddar cheese, 1 pouch	2
Natural reduced fat shredded Mexican style blend, 1/3 cup	2
Natural reduced fat shredded mozzarella cheese, 1/3 cup	2
Natural reduced fat Swiss cheese, 2 slices	2
Pepper Jack singles, 1 slice	1
Reduced fat cream cheese spread, 1 oz	1
Reduced fat singles, 1 slice	1
Reduced fat whipped cream cheese, 2 Tbsp	1

Wholesome Valley Organic

American flavor slice, 1 slice	1
Cheddar flavor slice, 1 slice	1
Mozzarella flavor slice, 1 slice	1

Woolwich Dairy

Goat feta slice, 1 slice	3
Goat mozzarella, 1 slice	3
White goat Cheddar, 1 slice	3

Cream/Creamers
Breakstone's

Fat free sour cream, 2 Tbsp	1
Reduced fat sour cream, 2 Tbsp	1
Sour cream, 2 Tbsp	2

Carnation Coffee-Mate

Amaretto, liquid, 1 Tbsp	1
Chocolate raspberry, liquid, 1 Tbsp	1
Cinnamon vanilla creme, liquid, 1 Tbsp	1
Cinnamon vanilla crème, powder, 4 tsp	1

1 POINTS VALUE

Per Stick
**Natural
Light String
Cheese**

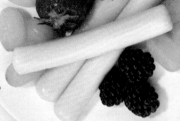

SMART
cheesiness.

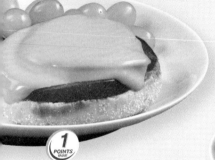

1 POINTS VALUE

Per Slice
**Reduced Fat
Singles**

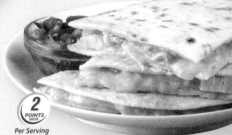

2 POINTS VALUE

Per Serving
**Reduced Fat
Mexican-Style
Shredded Cheese**

WeightWatchers

Stop Dieting. Start Living.

WEIGHT WATCHERS on foods and beverages is the registered trademark of WW Foods, LLC and is used under license by Schreiber Foods, Inc. WEIGHT WATCHERS for services and **POINTS** are the registered trademarks of Weight Watchers International, Inc. and are used under license by Schreiber Foods, Inc. © 2009 Weight Watchers International, Inc. All rights reserved.

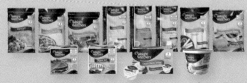

Visit WeightWatchers.com/cheese for more information.

Dairy & Eggs

Carnation Coffee-Mate (cont'd)	POINTS VALUE
Coconut crème, liquid, 1 Tbsp	1
Coconut crème, powder, 4 tsp	1
Creamy chocolate, powder, 4 tsp	1
Crème brulee, liquid, 1 Tbsp	1
Crème brulee, powder, 4 tsp	1
Fat free, liquid, 1 Tbsp	0
Fat free, powder, 1 tsp	0
Fat free cinnamon vanilla crème, liquid, 1 Tbsp	1
Fat free French vanilla, liquid, 1 Tbsp	1
Fat free French vanilla, powder, 4 tsp	1
Fat free hazelnut, liquid, 1 Tbsp	1
French vanilla, liquid, 1 Tbsp	1
French vanilla, powder, 4 tsp	1
Hazelnut, liquid, 1 Tbsp	1
Hazelnut, powder, 4 tsp	1
Irish creme, liquid, 1 Tbsp	1
Lite, powder, 1 tsp	0
Low fat, liquid, 1 Tbsp	0
Regular, liquid, 1 Tbsp	0
Regular, powder, 1 tsp	0
Sugar free French vanilla, liquid, 1 Tbsp	0
Sugar free French vanilla, powder, 1 Tbsp	1
Sugar free hazelnut, liquid, 1 Tbsp	0
Sugar free hazelnut, powder, 1 Tbsp	1
Sugar free vanilla caramel, powder, 1 Tbsp	1
Toasted almond, liquid, 1 Tbsp	1
Toffee nut, liquid, 1 Tbsp	1
Toffee nut, powder, 4 tsp	1
Vanilla caramel, liquid, 1 Tbsp	1

	POINTS VALUE
Vanilla caramel, powder, 4 tsp	1
Vanilla chai spice, liquid, 1 Tbsp	1
Vanilla chai spice, powder, 4 tsp	1
Vanilla nut, liquid, 1 Tbsp	1
Follow Your Heart	
Vegan gourmet sour cream alternative, 2 Tbsp	1
Friendship	
All-natural sour cream, 2 Tbsp	2
Fresh salsa sour cream, 2 Tbsp	1
Light sour cream, 2 Tbsp	1
Nonfat sour cream, 2 Tbsp	1
Toasted onion sour cream, 2 Tbsp	2
GG Golden Guernsey Dairy	
Half & half, 1 fl oz	1
Reduced fat sour cream, 2 Tbsp	1
Sour cream, 2 Tbsp	2
International Delight	
Amaretto, 1 Tbsp	1
Belgian white chocolate macadamia, 1 Tbsp	1
Caribbean cinnamon crème, 1 Tbsp	1
Chocolate cream, 1 Tbsp	1
Dulce de leche, 1 Tbsp	1
English almond toffee, 1 Tbsp	1
French vanilla, 1 Tbsp	1
French vanilla, fat free, 1 Tbsp	1
Hazelnut, 1 Tbsp	1
Irish crème, 1 Tbsp	1
Southern butter pecan, 1 Tbsp	1
Sugar free French vanilla, 1 Tbsp	1
Sugar free hazelnut, 1 Tbsp	1

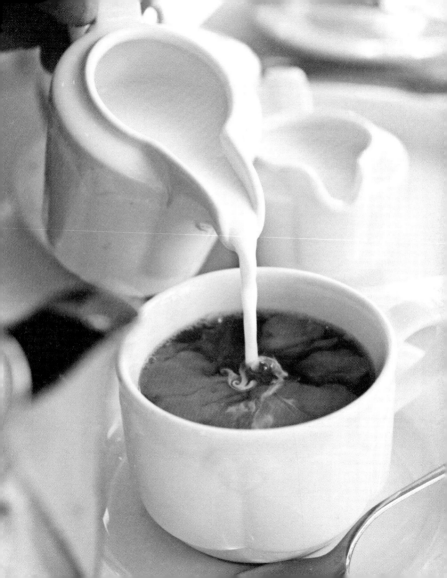

Dairy & Eggs

Knudsen

		POINTS VALUE
Fat free sour cream, 2 Tbsp	1	
Hampshire sour cream, 2 Tbsp	2	
Light sour cream, 2 Tbsp	1	

Land O Lakes

Fat free half & half, 2 Tbsp	0	

Morning Glory

Fat free sour cream, 2 Tbsp	1	
Half & half, 1 fl oz	1	
Reduced fat sour cream, 2 Tbsp	1	
Sour cream, 2 Tbsp	2	

Silk

French vanilla, 1 Tbsp	0	
Hazelnut, 1 Tbsp	0	
Original, 1 Tbsp	0	

Egg & Egg Substitutes

Better'N Eggs

All Whites, 1/4 cup	1	(5)
Better'N Eggs, 1/4 cup	1	(5)

Egg Beaters

Cheese & chive, 1/4 cup	1	
Egg white, refrigerated, 3 Tbsp	1	(5)
Frozen, 1/4 cup	1	(5)
Garden vegetable, refrigerated, 1/4 cup	1	(5)
Refrigerated, 1/4 cup	1	(5)
Southwestern, refrigerated, 1/4 cup	1	(5)

Eggland's Best

Brown egg, 1 large	2	(5)
Cage free egg, 1 extra large	2	(5)

		POINTS VALUE
Cage free egg, 1 large	2	(5)
Egg, 1 large	2	(5)
Egg, 1 extra large	2	(5)
Egg, 1 jumbo	2	(5)
Hard cooked and peeled eggs, 1 medium	2	(5)
Organic egg, 1 large	2	(5)
Organic egg, 1 extra large	2	(5)

Gold Circle Farms

Cage free dha omega 3 eggs, 1	2	(5)
Cage free dha omega 3 liquid egg product, 1/4 cup	1	(5)
DHA omega-3, grade A extra large egg, 1	2	(5)
DHA Omega-3, grade A large egg, 1	2	(5)

Horizon Organic

Extra large organic eggs, 1	2	(5)
Jumbo organic eggs, 1	2	(5)
Large organic eggs, 1	2	(5)
Medium organic eggs, 1	2	(5)
Omega 3 organic eggs, 1	2	(5)
Organic hard boiled eggs, 1	2	(5)
Organic liquid egg product, 1/4 cup	1	(5)

Market Day

Mini cheese omelets, 1 (2 oz)	1	

Nature's Harmony

Grade A large eggs, 1 large	2	(5)

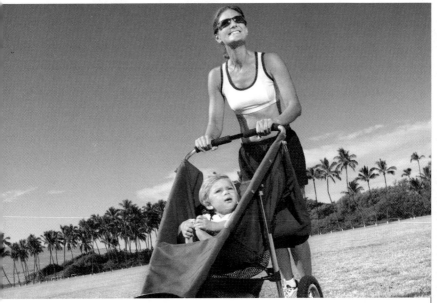

"FOR MY LIFESTYLE,
NOTHING BUT THE BEST."

What you eat matters to you. You want foods that offer the very best in taste and nutrition. That's why there are Eggland's Best eggs.

Eggland's Best delivers more of the farm-fresh flavor you love. They're 100% natural. Plus, compared with ordinary eggs, they provide:

- 10 times more vitamin E
- 3 times more Omega 3 (100 mg)
- 25% less saturated fat
- 19% less cholesterol; 175 mg (58% DV) vs. 215 mg (71% DV)

So why settle for ordinary when you can have the best? Eggland's Best.

www.eggland.com

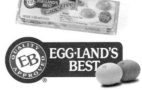

Better taste. Better nutrition. Better eggs.

THE BETTER EGG

Dairy & Eggs

◆ (POINTS VALUE)

Luncheon/Deli Lunches
Oscar Mayer Lunchables

Cheese & salsa nacho lunch, 1 package	9

Margarine
Blue Bonnet

Light soft spread, 1 Tbsp	1
Light stick, 1 Tbsp	2
Original soft spread, 1 Tbsp	2
Stick, 1 Tbsp	3

Country Crock

Light margarine plus omega, 1 Tbsp	1
Margarine with calcium, 1 Tbsp	1
Regular margarine plus omega, 1 Tbsp	2

Country Crock Shedd's Spread

Light margarine, 1 Tbsp	1

Earth Balance

All natural buttery spread, 1 Tbsp	3
Buttery stick, 1 serving	3
Organic whipped buttery spread, 1 serving	2

Fleischmann's

Light soft spread, 1 Tbsp	1
Made with olive oil soft spread, 1 Tbsp	2
Original soft spread, 1 Tbsp	2
Original stick, 1 Tbsp	3
Unsalted soft spread, 1 Tbsp	2
Unsalted stick, 1 Tbsp	3

I Can't Believe It's Yogurt!

Fat free margarine, 1 Tbsp	0
Light stick, 1 Tbsp	2
Light tub, 1 Tbsp	1

◆ (POINTS VALUE)

Original stick, 1 Tbsp	3
Original tub, 1 Tbsp	2
Sweet cream and calcium, 1 Tbsp	2

I Can't Believe It's Not Butter!

Mediterranean blend, 1 Tbsp	2
Mediterranean blend light, 1 Tbsp	1

Land O Lakes

Margarine, soft, 1 Tbsp	3
Margarine, stick, 1 Tbsp	3

Molly McButter

Lite sodium, 1 tsp	0
Roasted garlic, 1 tsp	0

Nucoa

No burn margarine, soft, 1 Tbsp	3
No-burn margarine, stick, 1 Tbsp	3

Parkay

Light soft, 1 Tbsp	1
Light stick, 1 Tbsp	1
Original soft spread, 1 Tbsp	2
Original squeeze, 1 Tbsp	2
Original stick, 1 Tbsp	2

Promise

Buttery spread, 1 Tbsp	2
Free, 1 Tbsp	0
Light, 1 Tbsp	1

Smart Balance

37% light spread, 1 Tbsp	1
64% with flax oil margarine, 1 Tbsp	2
67% buttery spread, 1 Tbsp	2
Extra virgin olive oil spread, light, 1 serving (11 g)	1

	POINTS VALUE
Extra virgin olive oil spread, regular, 1 serving (11 g)	2
Light buttery spread with flax, 1 Tbsp	1
Low sodium buttery spread, 1 serving (11 g)	2
Omega spread, light, 1 serving (13 g)	1
Omega spread, regular, 1 serving (13 g)	2
Organic whipped buttery spread (margarine), 1 Tbsp	2
Smart Balance Omega Plus	
Buttery spread with phytosterols, 1 Tbsp	2
Smart Beat	
Fat free squeeze margarine, 1 Tbsp	0
Trans fat free super light margarine, 1 Tbsp	1
Soy Garden	
Natural buttery spread, 1 Tbsp	3

Milk & Milk Based Drinks/ Flavorings for Milk

	POINTS VALUE
Carnation	
Malted milk chocolate, 3 Tbsp	2
Malted milk original, 3 Tbsp	2
◆ Nonfat dry milk, 1 serving (1/3 cup dry)	2
Friendship	
Lowfat buttermilk, 1 cup	3
GG Golden Guernsey Dairy	
Chocolate malt milk, 1 cup	6
Chocolate milk, 1 cup	5
Cultured reduced fat buttermilk, 1 cup	3
◆ Fat free milk, 1 cup	2
Low fat chocolate milk, 1 cup	3
Low fat milk, 1%, 1 cup	2

	POINTS VALUE
Reduced fat milk, 2%, 1 cup	3
Strawberry flavored low fat milk, 1 cup	4
Vitamin D milk, 1 cup	4
Grip It. Sip It.	
Chocolate malt milk, 1 cup	6
Chocolate milk, 1 cup	5
◆ Fat free milk, 1 cup	2
Low fat chocolate milk, 1 cup	3
Milk and coffee, 1 cup	3
Reduced fat milk, 2%, 1 cup	3
Strawberry flavored low fat milk, 1 cup	4
Vitamin D milk, 1 cup	4
Horizon Organic	
Lowfat eggnog, 1/2 cup	3
Market Day	
Nesquik low fat chocolate milk, 1 serving (8 oz)	3
Morning Glory	
Chocolate malt milk, 1 cup	6
Chocolate milk, 1 cup	5
Cultured reduced fat buttermilk, 1 cup	3
◆ Fat free milk, 1 cup	2
Low fat chocolate milk, 1 cup	3
Low fat milk, 1%, 1 cup	2
Reduced fat milk, 2%, 1 cup	3
Strawberry flavored low fat milk, 1 cup	4
Strawberry flavored reduced fat milk, 1 cup	4
Vitamin D milk, 1 cup	4
Nesquik	
Buncha reduced fat banana, 1 cup	4
Chocolate powder, 2 Tbsp	2

Dairy & Eggs

Nesquick (cont'd)

Double chocolate powder, 2 Tbsp	2
Fat free chocolate milk, 1 cup	3
Lowfat chocolate, 1 cup	4
Lowfat double chocolate, 1 cup	3
Lowfat strawberry, 1 cup	4
Lowfat vanilla, 1 cup	3
Lowfat very vanilla, 1 cup	3
No sugar added chocolate powder, 2 Tbsp	1
Reduced fat chocolate, 1 cup	4
Reduced fat double chocolate, 1 cup	4
Reduced fat strawberry, 1 cup	4
Reduced fat very vanilla, 1 cup	4
Strawberry powder, 2 Tbsp	2

Odwalla

Super protein chocolate, 8 fl oz	4
Super protein vanilla al'mondo, 8 fl oz	4

Over the Moon

1% low fat milk, 1 cup	3
Fat free chocolate milk, 1 cup	3
Fat free milk, 1 cup	2

Quaker

Milk chiller - chocolate, 8 fl oz	3
Milk chiller - strawberry, 8 fl oz	3

Silk

Cultured soy - banana, 1 container	3

Smart Balance

1% milk, 1 serving (8.75 oz)	3
Chocolate milk, 1 serving (8.75 oz)	3
Lactose free milk, 1 serving (8.75 oz)	2
Skim milk, 1 serving (8.75 oz)	2

Stonyfield Farm

Fat free milk, 1 cup	2
Lowfat (1%) milk, 1 cup	2
Reduced fat (2%) milk, 1 cup	3
Whole milk, 1 cup	4

Thai Kitchen

Coconut milk, 2 fl oz	3
Coconut milk, unsweetened, premium, 2 fl oz	3
Lite coconut milk, 2 fl oz	1
Organic coconut milk, 2 fl oz	3
Organic lite coconut milk, 2 fl oz	1

Tofu Town

Eggnog, 1/2 cup	4

Yogurt & Yogurt Drinks

Chobani

Blueberry nonfat, 6 oz	3
Honey nonfat, 6 oz	3
Peach nonfat, 6 oz	3
Plain lowfat, 6 oz	3
Plain lowfat, 8 oz	4
Plain nonfat, 6 oz	2
Plain nonfat, 8 oz	3
Plain original, 6 oz	6
Plain original, 8 oz	8
Strawberry nonfat, 6 oz	3
Vanilla nonfat, 6 oz	2
Vanilla nonfat, 8 oz	3

Colombo

Plain (low fat), 8 oz	3
Vanilla (low fat), 8 oz	5

Colombo Classic

	POINTS VALUE
Banana/strawberry, 8 oz	5
Black cherry parfait, 8 oz	5
Blackberry burst, 8 oz	5
Blueberry, 8 oz	5
Cherry, 8 oz	5
Fruit burst, 8 oz	5
Peach, 8 oz	5
Raspberry, 8 oz	5
Strawberry, 8 oz	5
Vanilla, 8 oz	5
White chocolate raspberry, 8 oz	5

Colombo Fat Free

Plain, 8 oz	2
Vanilla, 8 oz	3

Colombo Light

Blueberry, 8 oz	2
Boston cream pie, 8 oz	2
Cherry vanilla, 8 oz	2
Juicy peach, 8 oz	2
Key lime pie, 8 oz	2
Lemon meringue, 8 oz	2
Mixed berries, 8 oz	2
Orange crème, 8 oz	2
Raspberry, 8 oz	2
Strawberry, 8 oz	2
Strawberry/banana, 8 oz	2
White chocolate raspberry, 8 oz	2

Colombo Low Fat

French vanilla, 8 oz	4

FAGE

Total 0%, 8 oz	2
Total 2%, 8 oz	3
Total 5%, 5 1/2 oz	4
Total cherry, 5 1/2 oz	5
Total classic, 8 oz	8
Total honey, 5 1/2 oz	6
Total peach, 5 1/2 oz	5
Total strawberry, 5 1/2 oz	5
Total cherry 2%, 5 1/2 oz	3
Total honey 2%, 5 1/2 oz	4
Total peach 2%, 5 1/2 oz	3
Total strawberry 2%, 5 1/2 oz	3

Friendship

Plain yogurt, 1 cup	3

Greek Gods

Fig, 6 oz	6
Non fat, plain, 6 oz	1
Pomegranate, 6 oz	6
Reduced fat vanilla cinnamon & orange, 6 oz	4
Traditional, 4 oz	4
Traditional Greek yogurt, honey flavored, 6 oz	6

Horizon Organic

Lemon blended lowfat yogurt, 1 container (6 oz)	3
Mixed berry fat free yogurt, 1 container (6 oz)	3
Organic blueberry fat free yogurt, 1 container (6 oz)	3

Dairy & Eggs

Horizon Organic (cont'd)	POINTS VALUE
Organic blueberry low fat yogurt, 1 container (6 oz)	3
Organic cherry fat free yogurt, 1 container (6 oz)	2
Organic lemon low fat yogurt, 1 container (6 oz)	3
Organic mixed berry fat free yogurt, 1 container (6 oz)	3
Organic peach fat free yogurt, 1 container (6 oz)	3
Organic peach low fat yogurt, 1 container (6 oz)	3
Organic raspberry fat free yogurt, 1 container (6 oz)	2
Organic raspberry low fat yogurt, 1 container (6 oz)	3
Organic strawberry banana low fat yogurt, 1 container (6 oz)	3
Organic strawberry fat free yogurt, 1 container (6 oz)	3
Organic strawberry fat free yogurt, 1 container (6 oz)	2
Organic strawberry low fat yogurt, 1 container (6 oz)	3
Organic vanilla fat free yogurt, 1 container (6 oz)	3
Peach blended lowfat yogurt, 1 container (6 oz)	3
Stonyfield Farm Fat Free Yogurt	
Black cherry, 1 container (6 oz)	2
Blackberry, 1 container (6 oz)	3
Blueberry, 1 container (6 oz)	2
Chocolate underground, 1 container (6 oz)	3

	POINTS VALUE
French vanilla, 1 container (6 oz)	3
Key lime, 1 container (6 oz)	3
Lotsa lemon, 1 container (6 oz)	3
Peach, 1 container (6 oz)	2
Plain, 1 container (6 oz)	2
Raspberry, 1 container (6 oz)	2
Strawberry, 1 container (4 oz)	1
Stonyfield Farm Oikos	
Blueberry, 1 container (5.3 oz)	2
Honey, 1 container (5.3 oz)	2
Plain, 1 cup (8 oz)	3
Plain, 1 container (5.3 oz)	2
Vanilla, 1 container (5.3 oz)	2
Stonyfield Farm Organic Fat Free Yogurt	
French vanilla, 1 cup	4
Plain, 1 cup	2
Stonyfield Farm Organic Lowfat Yogurt	
Banilla, 8 oz	4
Blueberry, fruit on the bottom, 1 container (6 oz)	3
Caramel, 1 container (6 oz)	4
Just peachy, fruit on the bottom, 1 container (6 oz)	3
Luscious lemon, fruit on the bottom, 1 container (6 oz)	3
Maple vanilla, 1 container (6 oz)	3
Mocha latte, 1 container (6 oz)	3
Plain, 1 container (6 oz)	2
Plain, 8 oz	3
Raspberry, fruit on the bottom, 1 container (6 oz)	3
Strawberry, 8 oz	4

	POINTS VALUE
Strawberry, fruit on the bottom, 1 container (6 oz)	2
Vanilla, 1 container (6 oz)	3
Vanilla, 8 oz	4
Stonyfield Farm Organic Lowfat YoKids Squeezers	
Berry blitz, 1 tube	1
Chillin' cherry, 1 tube	1
Screamin' strawberry, 1 tube	1
Stonyfield Farm Organic Probiotic Fat Free Yogurt	
Yocalcium, apricot mango, 1 container (6 oz)	2
Yocalcium, strawberry raspberry, 1 container (6 oz)	2
Yocalcium, wild berry, 1 container (6 oz)	2
Stonyfield Farm Organic Whole Milk Yogurt	
Chocolate underground, 1 container (6 oz)	5
French vanilla, 1 container (6 oz)	4
French vanilla, 1 cup (8 oz)	5
Plain, 1 cup (8 oz)	4
Strawberries & cream, 1 container (6 oz)	4
Wild blueberry, 1 container (6 oz)	4
Stonyfield Farm O'Soy Multipack	
Strawberry & peach, 1 container (4 oz)	2
Stonyfield Farm O'Soy Organic Cultured Soy	
Blueberry, fruit on the bottom, 1 container (6 oz)	3

	POINTS VALUE
Chocolate, 1 container (6 oz)	3
Peach, fruit on the bottom, 1 container (6 oz)	3
Raspberry, fruit on the bottom, 1 container (6 oz)	3
Strawberry, fruit on the bottom, 1 container (6 oz)	3
Vanilla, 1 container (6 oz)	3
Stonyfield Farm Yo Baby	
Apple, 1 container (4 oz)	3
Banana, 1 container (4 oz)	3
Peach, 1 container (4 oz)	2
Pear, 1 container (4 oz)	2
Simply plain, 1 container (4 oz)	2
Vanilla, 1 container (4 oz)	2
Stonyfield Farm Yo Baby Drinkable Yogurt	
Banana, 1 bottle (6 oz)	4
Peach, 1 bottle (6 oz)	4
Stonyfield Farm Yo Baby Plus Cereal	
Raspberry pear with DHA, 1 container (4 oz)	2
Strawberry banana with DHA, 1 container (4 oz)	2
Stonyfield Farm Yo Baby Plus Cereal Plus Iron	
Apple, 1 container (4 oz)	2
Mixed berry, 1 container (4 oz)	2
Stonyfield Farm YoKids Organic Yogurt	
Banilla, 1 container (4 oz)	2
Raspberry, 1 container (4 oz)	2
Strawberry, 1 container (4 oz)	2
Strawberry vanilla, 1 container (4 oz)	2

Dairy & Eggs

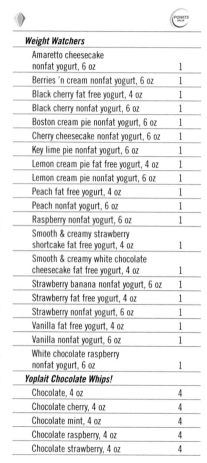

POINTS VALUE

Weight Watchers

Amaretto cheesecake nonfat yogurt, 6 oz	1
Berries 'n cream nonfat yogurt, 6 oz	1
Black cherry fat free yogurt, 4 oz	1
Black cherry nonfat yogurt, 6 oz	1
Boston cream pie nonfat yogurt, 6 oz	1
Cherry cheesecake nonfat yogurt, 6 oz	1
Key lime pie nonfat yogurt, 6 oz	1
Lemon cream pie fat free yogurt, 4 oz	1
Lemon cream pie nonfat yogurt, 6 oz	1
Peach fat free yogurt, 4 oz	1
Peach nonfat yogurt, 6 oz	1
Raspberry nonfat yogurt, 6 oz	1
Smooth & creamy strawberry shortcake fat free yogurt, 4 oz	1
Smooth & creamy white chocolate cheesecake fat free yogurt, 4 oz	1
Strawberry banana nonfat yogurt, 6 oz	1
Strawberry fat free yogurt, 4 oz	1
Strawberry nonfat yogurt, 6 oz	1
Vanilla fat free yogurt, 4 oz	1
Vanilla nonfat yogurt, 6 oz	1
White chocolate raspberry nonfat yogurt, 6 oz	1

Yoplait Chocolate Whips!

Chocolate, 4 oz	4
Chocolate cherry, 4 oz	4
Chocolate mint, 4 oz	4
Chocolate raspberry, 4 oz	4
Chocolate strawberry, 4 oz	4

Yoplait Go-Gurt

Banana split, 1 tube	2
Berry blue, 1 tube	2
Berry bubblegum, 1 tube	2
Blue razzberry, 1 tube	2
Chill out cherry, 1 tube	2
Cool cotton candy, 1 tube	2
Crazy berry bolt, 1 tube	2
Melon berry, 1 tube	2
Paradise punch, 1 tube	2
Rad raspberry, 1 tube	2
Red rush, 1 tube	2
Shrek's donkeyberry blast, 1 tube	2
Shrek's ogreberry, 1 tube	2
Strawberry banana burst, 1 tube	2
Strawberry kiwi, 1 tube	2
Strawberry kiwi kick, 1 tube	2
Strawberry milkshake, 1 tube	2
Strawberry milkshake, 1 tube	2
Strawberry splash, 1 tube	2
Watermelon melt down, 1 tube	2

Yoplait Kids Yogurt

Banana, 4 oz	2
Peach, 4 oz	2
Strawberry, 4 oz	2
Strawberry banana, 4 oz	2
Strawberry vanilla, 4 oz	2
Vanilla, 4 oz	2

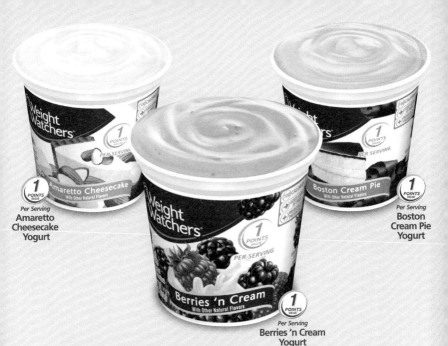

SMART *snackiness.*

Indulge yourself by checking out these and other great-tasting yogurt flavors with a **POINTS**® value of 1 at **WeightWatchers.com/yogurt**

WeightWatchers®

Stop Dieting. Start Living.

WEIGHT WATCHERS on foods and beverages is the registered trademark of WW Foods, LLC and is used under license by Gilsa Products and Services, Co. WEIGHT WATCHERS for services and **POINTS** are the registered trademarks of Weight Watchers International, Inc. and are used under license by Gilsa Products and Services, Co. ©2009 Weight Watchers International, Inc. All rights reserved.

Dairy & Eggs

Yoplait Kids Yogurt Drink

Banana, 1 container	2
Mixed berry, 1 container	2
Strawberry, 1 container	2
Strawberry banana, 1 container	2

Yoplait Light

Apple turnover, 6 oz	2
Apricot mango, 6 oz	2
Banana cream pie, 6 oz	2
Berries 'n cream, 6 oz	2
Blackberry, 6 oz	2
Blueberry, 4 oz	1
Blueberry, 6 oz	2
Boston cream pie, 6 oz	2
Cherry, 4 oz	1
Cherry, 6 oz	2
Key lime pie, 6 oz	2
Lemon cream pie, 6 oz	2
Orange créme, 6 oz	2
Peach, 4 oz	1
Peach, 6 oz	2
Raspberry, 6 oz	2
Strawberry, 4 oz	1
Strawberry, 6 oz	2
Strawberry banana, 6 oz	2
Strawberry orange sunrise, 6 oz	2
Very vanilla, 6 oz	2
White chocolate strawberry, 6 oz	2

Yoplait Light Thick & Creamy

French vanilla, 6 oz	2
Key lime, 6 oz	2
Lemon meringue pie, 6 oz	2
Mixed berry, 6 oz	2
Orange crème, 6 oz	2
Peaches 'n cream, 6 oz	2
Strawberry cream, 6 oz	2

Yoplait Original

Mango, 4 oz	2
Pina colada, 4 oz	2
Raspberry, 4 oz	2
Strawberry banana, 4 oz	2

Yoplait Original 99% Fat Free

Banana crème, 6 oz	4
Berry banana, 6 oz	4
Blackberry harvest, 6 oz	4
Blueberry, 6 oz	4
Blueberry crumble, 6 oz	4
Boysenberry, 6 oz	4
Cherry, 6 oz	4
French vanilla, 6 oz	4
Guava, 6 oz	4
Harvest peach, 6 oz	4
Key lime pie, 6 oz	4
Lemon burst, 6 oz	4
Mandarin orange, 6 oz	4
Mango, 6 oz	4
Mixed berry, 6 oz	4

	POINTS VALUE
Orange créme, 6 oz	4
Original coconut cream pie, 6 oz	4
Passion fruit, 6 oz	4
Peach, 4 oz	2
Peach, 8 oz	5
Peach cobbler, 6 oz	4
Pina colada, 6 oz	4
Pineapple, 6 oz	4
Plain fat free, 6 oz	2
Plain fat free, 1 cup	3
Raspberry, 6 oz	4
Strawberry, 4 oz	2
Strawberry, 6 oz	4
Strawberry, 8 oz	5
Strawberry banana, 6 oz	4
Strawberry banana, 8 oz	5
Strawberry cheesecake, 6 oz	4
Strawberry kiwi, 6 oz	4
Strawberry mango, 6 oz	4
Tropical peach, 6 oz	4
Vanilla, 8 oz	5
White chocolate raspberry, 6 oz	4
Yoplait Thick & Creamy	
Banana, 6 oz	4
Blackberry harvest, 6 oz	4
Blueberries & cream, 6 oz	4
Crème caramel, 6 oz	4
Key lime pie, 6 oz	4
Lemon supreme, 6 oz	4
Orange crème, 6 oz	4

	POINTS VALUE
Peaches 'n cream, 6 oz	4
Raspberry cheesecake, 6 oz	4
Royal raspberry, 6 oz	4
Strawberries & cream, 6 oz	4
Strawberry, 6 oz	4
Strawberry banana, 6 oz	4
Vanilla, 6 oz	4
Yoplait Trix	
Berry bolt, 4 oz	2
Bubble gum, 4 oz	2
Cotton candy, 4 oz	2
Rainbow sherbet, 4 oz	2
Raspberry rainbow, 4 oz	2
Strawberry banana bash, 4 oz	2
Strawberry kiwi, 4 oz	2
Strawberry punch, 4 oz	2
Triple cherry, 4 oz	2
Very berry melon, 4 oz	2
Watermelon burst, 4 oz	2
Wild berry blue, 4 oz	2
Yoplait Whips!	
Creamy latte, 1 container (4 oz)	3
Dulce de leche, 1 container (4 oz)	3
Key lime pie, 1 container (4 oz)	3
Lemon meringue, 1 container (4 oz)	3
Orange crème, 1 container (4 oz)	3
Peaches n' cream, 1 container (4 oz)	3
Raspberry mousse, 1 container (4 oz)	3
Strawberry mist, 1 container (4 oz)	3

Fish & Seafood

Anchovies
Yankee Clipper
	POINTS VALUE	
Anchovies flat fillets, 6	1	
Anchovies rolled fillets, 5 pieces	1	

Clams
Bumble Bee
Chopped clams, 1/4 cup	1	(5)
Fancy whole baby clams, 2 oz	1	(5)

Cape Cod
Premium hand shucked breaded fried clams, 4 oz	8	

Chincoteague
Breaded fried clams, 3 oz	6	
Chopped arctic clams, 1/4 cup	0	(5)
Chopped ocean clams, 1/4 cup	1	(5)
Chopped sea clams, 1/4 cup	1	(5)
Minced ocean clams, 1/4 cup	1	(5)
Ocean clam juice, 1/2 cup	0	
Sea clam juice, 1/2 cup	0	

Snow's
All natural clam juice, 1 Tbsp	0	
Chopped clams in clam juice, 1/4 cup	1	(5)
Minced clams in clam juice, 1/4 cup	1	(5)

Sol-Mex
Baby clams, 1/2 cup	1	(5)

Yankee Clipper
Baby clams, boiled in water, 1 serving (2 oz)	1	(5)
Minced clams, 1/4 cup	1	(5)
Smoked baby clams, 1 can	3	

Crab
Bumble Bee
	POINTS VALUE	
Lump crabmeat, 2 oz (drained)	1	(5)
White crabmeat, 2 oz (drained)	1	(5)

Market Day
Crab cakes, 1 (2 oz)	2	
Pre-split king crab legs, 3 pieces	2	(5)

Sol-Mex
Crab meat, 1/2 cup	2	(5)

Trans-Ocean
Crab classic surimi seafood, 1 serving (85 g)	2	

Yankee Clipper
Fancy crabmeat, 1 serving (2 oz)	1	(5)
Fancy crabmeat with leg meat, 1 serving (2 oz)	1	(5)
Fancy crabmeat, lump, 1 serving (2 oz)	1	(5)

Flounder
Gorton's
Premium fillets, flounder, 1	6	

Market Day
Flounder del ray, 1 serving (6 oz)	4	

Gefilte Fish
Manischewitz
Sweet gefilte fish, 1 piece	1	

Haddock
Gorton's
Premium fillets, haddock, 1	6	

Fish & Seafood

Herring

Acme

Pickled herring in cream sauce, 1/4 cup	2
Pickled herring in cream sauce, 5 pieces	2
Pickled herring in wine, 5 pieces	2

Oysters

Bumble Bee

◆ Whole oysters, 2 oz	2	(5)

Yankee Clipper

Smoked oysters, 1 can	3	
◆ Whole boiled oysters, 1/4 cup	1	(5)

Salmon

Acme

Baked salmon salad, 4 Tbsp	5	
Kippered salmon (vacuum-packed), 2 oz	3	
◆ Pre-sliced all natural smoked salmon, 2 oz	2	(5)
◆ Pre-sliced cold smoked salmon, 5 slices	3	(5)

Bumble Bee

◆ Pink salmon, 1 serving (2.2 oz)	2	(5)
◆ Red salmon, 1 serving (2.2 oz)	3	(5)
◆ Skinless and boneless pink salmon, 2 oz (drained)	1	(5)

Deming's

◆ Pink salmon, 1/4 cup	2	(5)
◆ Red sockeye Alaska salmon, 1/4 cup	3	(5)

Double "Q"

◆ Pink Alaska salmon, 1/4 cup	2	(5)
◆ Red sockeye salmon, 1/4 cup	3	(5)

Market Day

Classic salmon, 1 serving (2" wide piece)	7
Mediterranean salmon, 1 serving (12 oz)	10
Seasoned salmon, 4 oz (raw, about 2" wide piece)	7
Wild Alaskan grilled salmon, 1 fl oz	2

Phillips

Salmon cakes, 1 cake	6

Season Brand

◆ Salmon medium red salted, 1/4 cup	2	(5)
◆ Salmon pink - no salt, 1/4 cup	2	(5)
◆ Salmon pink - salt, 1/4 cup	2	(5)

SnackMasters Natural Gourmet Jerky

Salmon - original, 1 oz	2

Sardines

Bumble Bee

◆ Sardines in hot sauce, 1 can	4	
Sardines in mustard, 1 can	3	
Sardines in oil, 1 cup (drained)	3	
◆ Sardines in water, 1 can (drained)	3	(5)

Season Brand

Sardine fillet lemon pepper, 1 can	9
Sardine fillets lemon garlic, 1 serving (106 g)	9
Sardine fillets sweet tangy, 1 serving (106 g)	10

Fish & Seafood

Season Brand (cont'd) | POINTS VALUE

Sardines skin bone water, 1 serving (85 g)	4 (5)
Sardines in water, 1 can	3 (5)
Sardines in water, salted, 1 can	5 (5)
Sardines in water, unsalted, 1 can	4 (5)

Sol-Mex

Sardines in tomato sauce - hot, 1/4 cup	2

Yankee Clipper

Sardines in mustard sauce, 1/4 cup	2
Sardines in soybean oil, 1/4 cup	3
Sardines in tomato sauce, 1/4 cup	2

Scallops
Market Day

Seasoned scallops, 1 serving (4 oz)	4

Shrimp
Bumble Bee

Deveined small shrimp, 1/4 cup (drained)	1 (5)
Deveined medium shrimp, 1/4 cup (drained)	1 (5)
Deveined large shrimp, 1/4 cup (drained)	1 (5)
Regular broken shrimp, 1/4 cup (drained)	1 (5)
Regular jumbo shrimp, 1/4 cup (drained)	1 (5)
Regular large shrimp, 1/4 cup (drained)	1 (5)
Regular medium shrimp, 1/4 cup (drained)	1 (5)

POINTS VALUE

Regular small shrimp, 1/4 cup (drained)	1 (5)
Tiny shrimp, 2 oz (drained)	1 (5)

Gorton's

Popcorn shrimp, 22 (3.5 oz)	6

Gorton's Popcorn Shrimp

Beer batter popcorn shrimp, 1 serving (about 18 shrimp)	7
Garlic & herb popcorn shrimp, 1 serving (about 22 shrimp)	6
Original popcorn shrimp, 1 serving (about 20 shrimp)	6

Gorton's Shrimp Temptations

Beer batter, 5	6
Jumbo butterfly, 5	5
Lemon butter, 4 oz	3
Scampi, 4 oz	3

Market Day

Garlic & herb shrimp, 15	3
Jumbo party shrimp with sauce, 3 oz	1
Large shrimp, 4 oz	1 (5)
Oven-ready butterfly shrimp, 4 (3 oz)	5
Parmesan seasoned shrimp, 1 serving (42) (4 oz)	3
Popcorn shrimp, 21	5

Phillips

Breaded shrimp, 5	3
Buffalo shrimp, 5 pieces (with 3/4 oz sauce)	3
Coconut shrimp, 5	6

	POINTS VALUE
Phillips Steamer Creations	
Garlic & herb shrimp, 8	4
Honey chipotle shrimp, 8	4
Steamed spiced shrimp, 8	3

Tilapia
Gorton's
Premium fillets, tilapia, 1	6

Market Day
Tilapia fillets, 1 serving (4 oz)	2	(5)
Tortilla crusted tilapia, 1 piece (5.3 oz)	6	

Tuna
Bumble Bee
Chunk light tuna in water, 1/4 cup (drained)	1	(5)
Chunk light tuna in water (3 oz can), 1 can	1	(5)
Chunk light tuna with a touch of lemon in water, 1/4 cup (drained)	1	(5)
Chunk white albacore in water, 1/4 cup	1	(5)
Chunk white albacore in water, 1/4 cup (drained)	1	(5)
Chunk white albacore in water (3 oz can), 1 can (drained)	1	(5)
Fat free tuna salad with crackers (salad only), 1 cup	1	
Premium albacore tuna in water, 1 pouch	2	(5)
Premium albacore tuna in water (pouch), 2 oz	1	(5)
Prime fillet albacore steak entrees, lemon and cracked pepper, 4 oz	2	

Prime fillet albacore steak entrees, mesquite grilled, 4 oz	2	
Prime fillet solid white albacore in water, 2 oz (drained)	1	(5)
Solid light tuna - tonno in olive oil, 2 oz (drained)	3	
Solid white albacore in water, 1 can (3 oz)	1	(5)
Solid white albacore in water, 2 oz (drained)	1	(5)
Solid white albacore in water, 1 can (drained)	1	(5)

Bumble Bee Lunch on the Run
Tuna salad - complete lunch kit, cookie only, 1	3
Tuna salad - complete lunch kit, crackers only, 6	2
Tuna salad - complete lunch kit, diced peaches only, 4 oz	2
Tuna salad - complete lunch kit, entire kit, 1	12
Tuna salad - complete lunch kit, tuna only, 1 serving (2.9 oz)	6

Bumble Bee Sensations
Seasoned tuna medleys with crackers, crackers only, 6	2
Seasoned tuna medleys with crackers, lemon & pepper, tuna only, 3 oz	2
Seasoned tuna medleys with crackers, spicy Thai chili, tuna only, 3 oz	4
Seasoned tuna medleys with crackers, sundried tomato & basil, tuna only, 3 oz	2

Fish & Seafood

	POINTS VALUE
Coral	
Chunk light tuna in oil, 1/4 cup (2 oz)	2
◆ Chunk light tuna in water, 1/4 cup (drained)	1 (5)
Progresso	
Light solid tuna in olive oil, 1/4 cup	3
Light solid tuna in olive oil, 1 can	4
Solid white albacore tuna in olive oil, 1/4 cup	2
Season Brand	
◆ Tuna, pouch, albacore, in water, 1 pouch	2 (5)
◆ Tuna, pouch, light, in water, 1 pouch	2 (5)
SnackMasters Natural Gourmet Jerky	
Ahi tuna - original, 1 oz	2
Tree of Life	
◆ Wild chunk light Tongol tuna in spring water, 1/4 cup	1 (5)

Whitefish
Acme
◆ Whitefish (vacuum packed), 2 oz	3 (5)

Other Fish Products
Acme
Whitefish chunk, 2 oz	3

Eden
Bonito flakes - cured, steamed & dried, 2 Tbsp	0

Fanci Food
Snails, very large, 6 pieces	1

	POINTS VALUE
Gorton's Grilled Fillets	
Cajun blackened, 1 fillet	2
Classic char-grilled, 1 fillet	2
Garlic butter, 1 fillet	2
Italian herb, 1 fillet	2
Lemon butter, 1 fillet	2
Lemon pepper, 1 fillet	2
Phillips	
Coconut mahi mahi, 3 pieces	7
Tree of Life	
◆ Wild chunk light Tongol tuna in spring water, no salt added, 1/4 cup	1 (5)
Yankee Clipper	
◆ Clam juice, 1 Tbsp	0

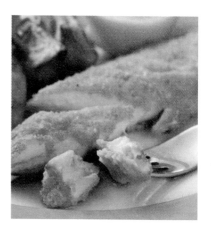

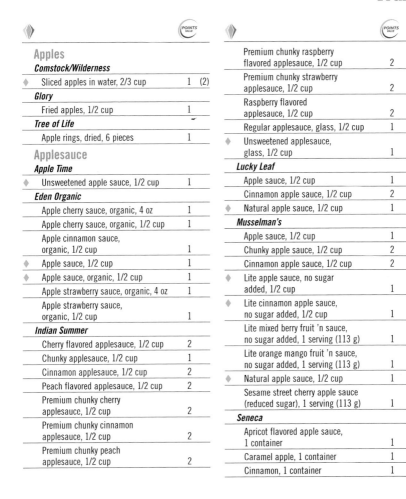

Apples

Comstock/Wilderness

Sliced apples in water, 2/3 cup	1	(2)

Glory

Fried apples, 1/2 cup	1

Tree of Life

Apple rings, dried, 6 pieces	1

Applesauce

Apple Time

Unsweetened apple sauce, 1/2 cup	1

Eden Organic

Apple cherry sauce, organic, 4 oz	1
Apple cherry sauce, organic, 1/2 cup	1
Apple cinnamon sauce, organic, 1/2 cup	1
Apple sauce, 1/2 cup	1
Apple sauce, organic, 1/2 cup	1
Apple strawberry sauce, organic, 4 oz	1
Apple strawberry sauce, organic, 1/2 cup	1

Indian Summer

Cherry flavored applesauce, 1/2 cup	2
Chunky applesauce, 1/2 cup	1
Cinnamon applesauce, 1/2 cup	2
Peach flavored applesauce, 1/2 cup	2
Premium chunky cherry applesauce, 1/2 cup	2
Premium chunky cinnamon applesauce, 1/2 cup	2
Premium chunky peach applesauce, 1/2 cup	2

Premium chunky raspberry flavored applesauce, 1/2 cup	2
Premium chunky strawberry applesauce, 1/2 cup	2
Raspberry flavored applesauce, 1/2 cup	2
Regular applesauce, glass, 1/2 cup	1
Unsweetened applesauce, glass, 1/2 cup	1

Lucky Leaf

Apple sauce, 1/2 cup	1
Cinnamon apple sauce, 1/2 cup	2
Natural apple sauce, 1/2 cup	1

Musselman's

Apple sauce, 1/2 cup	1
Chunky apple sauce, 1/2 cup	2
Cinnamon apple sauce, 1/2 cup	2
Lite apple sauce, no sugar added, 1/2 cup	1
Lite cinnamon apple sauce, no sugar added, 1/2 cup	1
Lite mixed berry fruit 'n sauce, no sugar added, 1 serving (113 g)	1
Lite orange mango fruit 'n sauce, no sugar added, 1 serving (113 g)	1
Natural apple sauce, 1/2 cup	1
Sesame street cherry apple sauce (reduced sugar), 1 serving (113 g)	1

Seneca

Apricot flavored apple sauce, 1 container	1
Caramel apple, 1 container	1
Cinnamon, 1 container	1

Fruit

Seneca (cont'd)

	POINTS VALUE
Golden delicious, 1 container	1
♦ Natural, 1 container	1
Peach mango, 1 container	1
Regular, 1 container	1
Wild berry, 1 container	1

Tree of Life

Organic apple sauce, cinnamon, 1/2 cup	2
♦ Organic apple sauce, unsweetened, 1/2 cup	1
Organic cinnamon apple sauce, 1/2 cup	2
Organic cinnamon apple sauce, 1/2 cup	2

Tree Top

Blue raspberry flavored apple sauce, 1 container	1
Cinnamon apple sauce, 1 container	1
♦ Natural apple sauce, no sugar added, 1 container	1
Original apple sauce, 1 container	1
Strawberry flavored apple sauce, 1 container	1

Wilderness

♦ Applesauce, unsweetened, 1/2 cup	1
Cherry flavored applesauce, 1/2 cup	2
Chunky applesauce, 1/2 cup	1
Cinnamon applesauce, 1/2 cup	2
Peach flavored applesauce, 1/2 cup	2
Premium chunky cherry applesauce, 1/2 cup	2

	POINTS VALUE
Premium chunky cinnamon applesauce, 1/2 cup	2
Premium chunky peach applesauce, 1/2 cup	2
Premium chunky raspberry flavored applesauce, 1/2 cup	2
Premium chunky strawberry applesauce, 1/2 cup	2
Raspberry flavored applesauce, 1/2 cup	2
Regular applesauce, glass, 1/2 cup	1

Apricots

Del Monte

Lite unpeeled apricot halves in extra lite syrup, 1/2 cup	1
Unpeeled apricot halves in heavy syrup, 1/2 cup	2

Del Monte Orchard Select

Unpeeled apricot halves in light syrup, 1/2 cup	1

Dole

♦ Apricots, 3 pieces	1 (2)

Sun-Maid

California apricots, 1 oz	1
Mediterranean apricots, 1 oz	1

Tropical Nut & Fruit

Turkish apricots, 5 pieces	1
Turkish apricots, 5 pieces	1

Avocado

Brooks

♦ Slimcado, 1/2	3

POINTS VALUE

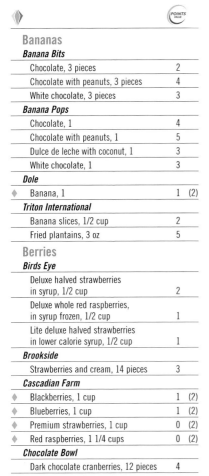

Bananas

Banana Bits

Chocolate, 3 pieces	2
Chocolate with peanuts, 3 pieces	4
White chocolate, 3 pieces	3

Banana Pops

Chocolate, 1	4
Chocolate with peanuts, 1	5
Dulce de leche with coconut, 1	3
White chocolate, 1	3

Dole

Banana, 1	1	(2)

Triton International

Banana slices, 1/2 cup	2
Fried plantains, 3 oz	5

Berries

Birds Eye

Deluxe halved strawberries in syrup, 1/2 cup	2
Deluxe whole red raspberries, in syrup frozen, 1/2 cup	1
Lite deluxe halved strawberries in lower calorie syrup, 1/2 cup	1

Brookside

Strawberries and cream, 14 pieces	3

Cascadian Farm

Blackberries, 1 cup	1	(2)
Blueberries, 1 cup	1	(2)
Premium strawberries, 1 cup	0	(2)
Red raspberries, 1 1/4 cups	0	(2)

Chocolate Bowl

Dark chocolate cranberries, 12 pieces	4

Dole

Cranberries, 1/2 cup	0	(2)
Fresh frozen blackberries, 1 cup	1	(2)
Fresh frozen blueberries, 1 cup	1	(2)
Fresh frozen burst o berry, 1 cup	1	
Fresh frozen red raspberries, 1 cup	1	(2)
Fresh frozen sliced strawberries with sugar, 1/2 cup	3	
Fresh frozen whole strawberries, 1 cup	0	(2)
Fresh frozen wild blueberries, 1 cup	1	(2)
Raspberries 1 cup	0	(2)
Strawberries, 8	0	(2)

Ocean Spray

Fresh cranberries, 1/2 cup	0	(2)

Ocean Spray Craisins

Sweetened dried cranberries, cherry flavor, 1/3 cup	2
Sweetened dried cranberries, orange flavor, 1/3 cup	2
Sweetened dried cranberry, original flavor, 1/3 cup	2

Sun-Maid

Cape Cod cranberries, 1 oz	2

Tree of Life

Blueberries, dried, 1/4 cup	2	
Cranberries, dried, 1 serving (40 g)	2	
Organic blueberries, frozen, 1 cup	1	(2)
Organic red raspberries, frozen, 2/3 cup	1	(2)
Organic whole strawberries, frozen, 3/4 cup	1	(2)

Tropical Nut & Fruit

Dried blueberries, 1/4 cup	2

Fruit

Cherries

Cascadian Farm

◆ Sweet cherries, 1 cup	1	

Del Monte

Dark, pitted cherries in heavy syrup, 1/2 cup	2	

Dole

◆ Cherries, 1 cup	1	(2)
◆ Fresh frozen dark sweet cherries, 1 cup	1	

Eden

Dried Montmorency cherries, 1/4 cup	2	

Futuro

◆ Yellow cherries, 1 oz	0	(2)

Great Expectations

Maraschino cherries with stems, 1	0	

Tree of Life

Dried cherries, 1 serving	2	
◆ Organic dark sweet cherries, frozen, 1/2 cup	2	(2)

Tropical Nut & Fruit

Bing cherries, 1/4 cup	2	
Dried cherries, 1/4 cup	2	

Dried Fruit

Bare Fruit

100% organic bake dried bananas & cherries, 1 serving (18 g)	1	
100% organic bake dried cherries, 1 serving (18 g)	1	
100% organic bake dried cinnamon apple chips, 1 serving (12 g)	0	
100% organic bake dried cinnamon apple chips, 1 large serving (18 g)	1	
100% organic bake dried fuji apple chips, 1 serving (12 g)	0	
100% organic bake dried granny smith apple chips, 1 serving (12 g)	0	
100% organic bake dried mangos, 1 serving (18 g)	1	
100% organic bake dried pears, 1 serving (12 g)	0	
100% organic bake dried pears, 1 large serving (18 g)	1	
100% organic baked dried pineapple & mangos, 1 serving (18 g)	1	

Be Happy & Healthy

Sour wiggle giggle, 6 pieces	3	

Betty Crocker Fruit Smoothie Blitz

All flavors and shapes, big pouch, 1 big pouch	3	

Crispy Green

Crispy apples, 1 bag	1	
Crispy apricots, 1 bag	1	
Crispy peaches, 1 bag	1	
Crispy pears, 1 bag	1	
Crispy pineapple, 1 bag	1	

Dole

California seedless raisins, 1/4 cup	2	
Chopped raisins, 1 oz	2	
Cinnaraisins, 1/4 cup	3	
Golden raisins, 1/4 cup	2	
Pitted, 1/4 cup	2	

	POINTS VALUE
Estee	
Chocolatey covered raisins, 1/4 cup	4
Fruit by the Foot	
All flavors, 1 roll	2
Fruit by the Foot Mini Feet	
All flavors, 1 roll	1
Fruit Gushers	
All flavors, 1 pouch	2
Fruit Roll-Ups	
All flavors, 1 roll	1
Fruit Roll-Ups Mini Rolls	
All flavors, 1 roll	1
Fruit Shapes	
All flavors, 1 pouch	2
Kashi	
Fruitabu organic smooshed apple twirl, 1	2
Fruitabu organic smooshed flat - organic apple, 1 pouch	1
Fruitabu organic smooshed flat - organic grape, 1 pouch	1
Fruitabu organic smooshed flat, organic raspberry, 1 pouch	1
Fruitabu organic smooshed flat, organic strawberry, 1 pouch	1
Fruitabu organic smooshed fruit, organic apricot, 1 pouch	1
Fruitabu organic smooshed grape flavored twirl, 1	2
Fruitabu organic smooshed strawberry flavored twirl, 1	2
Fruitabu sploooshers - organic grape flavored tube, 1 tube	1
Fruitabu sploooshers - organic raspberry flavored tube, 1 tube	1

	POINTS VALUE
Fruitabu sploooshers - organic strawberry flavored tube, 1 tube	1
Kashi Stretch Island	
Fruit leather - autumn apple, 1 pouch	1
Fruit leather, abundant apricot, 1 pouch	1
Fruit leather, cranberry raspberry, 1 pouch	1
Fruit leather, harvest grape, 1 pouch	1
Fruit leather, mango sunrise, 1 pouch	1
Fruit leather, orchard cherry, 1 pouch	1
Fruit leather, pineapple coconut, 1 pouch	1
Fruit leather, ripened raspberry, 1 pouch	1
Fruit leather, strawberry pomegranate, 1 pouch	1
Fruit leather, summer strawberry, 1 pouch	1
Kellogg's	
Fruit leather - ripened raspberry, 1 pouch	1
Yogos rollers - yogurty striped- chacha cherry, 1 roll	2
Yogos rollers - yogurty striped- punch-a-licious, 1 roll	2
Yogos rollers - yogurty striped- strawberry splits, 1 roll	2
Kellogg's Kashi	
Fruit leather - harvest grape, 1 pouch	1
Fruit leather - mango sunrise, 1 pouch	1
Fruit leather - orchard cherry, 1 pouch	1
Fruit leather - summer strawberry, 1 pouch	1

Fruit

Kellogg's Yogos

Bits crashers, berry melon mania, 1 pouch	2
Bits crashers, tangy rainbow splash, 1 pouch	2
Rollers - yogurty striped fruit roll, orange cream, 1	2
Yogurty covered fruit bits, crazy berries, 1 pouch	2
Yogurty covered fruit bits, island explosion, 1 pouch	2
Yogurty covered fruit bits, strawberry slam, 1 pouch	2
Yogurty fruit flavored sour bits, big bitin' apple, 1 pouch	2
Yogurty fruit flavored sour bits, bitin' berry blast, 1 pouch	2

Market Day

Fruit snacks variety pack, 1 serving (22.7 g)	2

Nature Valley Fruit Crisps

Cinnamon apple fruit ripples, 1 pouch	1
Strawberry apple fruit ripples, 1 pouch	1

Sunbelt

Fruit jammers snacks, 1 pouch	2

Sun-Maid

Calimyrna figs, 1 oz	1
Fruit bits, 1 oz	2
Golden raisins, 1 oz	2
Golden raisins and cherries, 1 oz	2
Mission figs, 1 oz	1
Mixed fruit, 1 oz	1
Pitted dates, 1 oz	1

Raisins, 1 oz	2
Tart cherries, 1 oz	2
Tropical pineapple, 1 oz	2
Tropical trio, 1 oz	2
Vanilla yogurt raisins, 1 oz	3
Washington apples, 1 oz	2
Zante currants, 1 oz	2

Sunsweet

Antioxidant blend, 1/4 cup	1
Berry blend, 1/4 cup	2
Blueberries, 1/4 cup	2
Cherries, 1/4 cup	2
Chopped dates, 1/4 cup	2
Cranberries, 1 bag	2
Cranberries, 1 1/2 oz	2
Dried apricots, 1 1/2 oz	1
Jumbo red raisins, 1/4 cup	2
Lemon essence prunes, 1 1/2 oz	1
Orange essence prunes, 1 1/2 oz	1
Orchard mix, 1/4 cup	1
Pitted dates, 1 1/2 oz	2
Pitted prunes, 1 1/2 oz	1
Tropical mix, 1/3 cup	3

Sunsweet Ones

Super select California prunes, 4	1

Sunsweet Smart 60 Calorie Packs

Cherry essence prunes, 1 bag	1
Prunes, 1 bag	1

Sunsweet Smart 70 Calorie Packs

Mediterranean apricots, 1 bag	1
Premium Thailand mango, 1 bag	1

Fruit

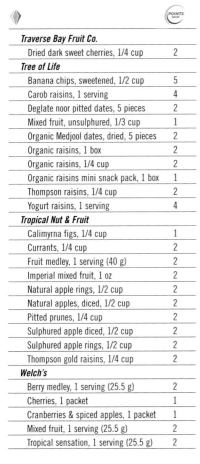

Traverse Bay Fruit Co.

Dried dark sweet cherries, 1/4 cup	2

Tree of Life

Banana chips, sweetened, 1/2 cup	5
Carob raisins, 1 serving	4
Deglate noor pitted dates, 5 pieces	2
Mixed fruit, unsulphured, 1/3 cup	1
Organic Medjool dates, dried, 5 pieces	2
Organic raisins, 1 box	2
Organic raisins, 1/4 cup	2
Organic raisins mini snack pack, 1 box	1
Thompson raisins, 1/4 cup	2
Yogurt raisins, 1 serving	4

Tropical Nut & Fruit

Calimyrna figs, 1/4 cup	1
Currants, 1/4 cup	2
Fruit medley, 1 serving (40 g)	2
Imperial mixed fruit, 1 oz	2
Natural apple rings, 1/2 cup	2
Natural apples, diced, 1/2 cup	2
Pitted prunes, 1/4 cup	2
Sulphured apple diced, 1/2 cup	2
Sulphured apple rings, 1/2 cup	2
Thompson gold raisins, 1/4 cup	2

Welch's

Berry medley, 1 serving (25.5 g)	2
Cherries, 1 packet	1
Cranberries & spiced apples, 1 packet	1
Mixed fruit, 1 serving (25.5 g)	2
Tropical sensation, 1 serving (25.5 g)	2

X-Treme Fruit Bites

Grape blast, 1 bag	1
Lemon xplosion, 1 bag	1
Mega mango, 1 bag	1
Strawberry blast, 1 bag	1

Fruit Cocktail/Salad

Cascadian Farm

Harvest berries, 1 cup	0

Del Monte

Cherry mixed fruit (plastic cup), 1/2 cup	1
Chunky mixed fruits in heavy syrup, 1/2 cup	2
Citrus salad in extra light syrup, 1/2 cup	2
Fruit cocktail in heavy syrup, 1/2 cup	2
Fruit cocktail in water, artificially sweetened, 1/2 cup	1
Fruit naturals chunky mixed fruits in fruit juice, 1/2 cup	1
Fruit naturals fruit cocktail in fruit juices, 1/2 cup	1
Lite chunky mixed fruits in extra light syrup, 1/2 cup	1
Lite fruit cocktail in extra light syrup, 1/2 cup	1
Mixed fruit - artificially sweetened, 1 container	0
Mixed fruit in cherry flavored gel, 1 cup	2
Tropical fruit in extra light syrup, 1/2 cup	1
Tropical fruit salad in pineapple & passion fruit juices, 1/2 cup	1
Very cherry mixed fruit, 1/2 cup	2

Fruit

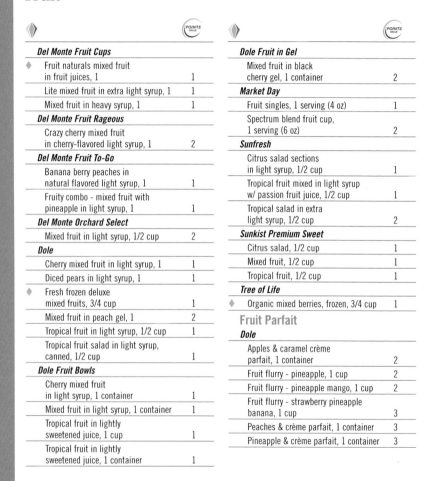

Del Monte Fruit Cups

Fruit naturals mixed fruit in fruit juices, 1	1
Lite mixed fruit in extra light syrup, 1	1
Mixed fruit in heavy syrup, 1	1

Del Monte Fruit Rageous

Crazy cherry mixed fruit in cherry-flavored light syrup, 1	2

Del Monte Fruit To-Go

Banana berry peaches in natural flavored light syrup, 1	1
Fruity combo - mixed fruit with pineapple in light syrup, 1	1

Del Monte Orchard Select

Mixed fruit in light syrup, 1/2 cup	2

Dole

Cherry mixed fruit in light syrup, 1	1
Diced pears in light syrup, 1	1
Fresh frozen deluxe mixed fruits, 3/4 cup	1
Mixed fruit in peach gel, 1	2
Tropical fruit in light syrup, 1/2 cup	1
Tropical fruit salad in light syrup, canned, 1/2 cup	1

Dole Fruit Bowls

Cherry mixed fruit in light syrup, 1 container	1
Mixed fruit in light syrup, 1 container	1
Tropical fruit in lightly sweetened juice, 1 cup	1
Tropical fruit in lightly sweetened juice, 1 container	1

Dole Fruit in Gel

Mixed fruit in black cherry gel, 1 container	2

Market Day

Fruit singles, 1 serving (4 oz)	1
Spectrum blend fruit cup, 1 serving (6 oz)	2

Sunfresh

Citrus salad sections in light syrup, 1/2 cup	1
Tropical fruit mixed in light syrup w/ passion fruit juice, 1/2 cup	1
Tropical salad in extra light syrup, 1/2 cup	2

Sunkist Premium Sweet

Citrus salad, 1/2 cup	1
Mixed fruit, 1/2 cup	1
Tropical fruit, 1/2 cup	1

Tree of Life

Organic mixed berries, frozen, 3/4 cup	1

Fruit Parfait

Dole

Apples & caramel crème parfait, 1 container	2
Fruit flurry - pineapple, 1 cup	2
Fruit flurry - pineapple mango, 1 cup	2
Fruit flurry - strawberry pineapple banana, 1 cup	3
Peaches & crème parfait, 1 container	3
Pineapple & crème parfait, 1 container	3

Grapefruit

Del Monte

	POINTS VALUE
Red grapefruit in extra light syrup, 1/2 cup	1
Red grapefruit in extra light syrup (color added), 1/2 cup	1

Sunfresh

Red grapefruit in slightly sweetened grapefruit juice, 1/2 cup	1
Red grapefruit sections in light syrup, 1/2 cup	2
White grapefruit sections in light syrup, 1/2 cup	2

Sunkist Premium Sweet

Red grapefruit, 1/2 cup	1

Grapes

Dole

Grapes, 1 1/2 cups	2 (2)

Kiwifruit

Dole

Kiwi, 2	1 (2)

Mangoes

Dole

Mango, 1/2	1 (2)

Herdez

Sliced mangos, 2 pieces	3

Sunfresh

Mango slices in light syrup, 1/2 cup	2

Tree of Life

Dried mango slices, unsulphured, 1 serving (40 g)	0

Triton International

Mango chunks, 1 cup	1

Tropical Nut & Fruit

Mango slices, 3 slices	3

Melons

Dole

Cantaloupe, 1/4	1 (2)
Honeydew melon, 1 serving (1/10)	1 (2)

Fanci Food

Sweet pickled watermelon rind, 2 Tbsp	1

Oranges

Del Monte

Mandarin oranges in extra light syrup, 1/2 cup	1

Del Monte Fruit Cups

Mandarin oranges in light syrup, 1	1

Dole

Mandarin and crème, 1	2
Mandarin oranges in light syrup, canned, 1/2 cup	1

Dole Fruit Bowls

Mandarin oranges in light syrup, 1 cup	2
Mandarin oranges in light syrup, 1 container	1

Dole Fruit in Gel

Mandarins in orange gel, 1 container	2

Sunfresh

Mandarin oranges in light syrup, 1/2 cup	1
Orange sections in light syrup, 1/2 cup	2

Fruit

	POINTS VALUE	
Sunkist Premium Sweet		
Mandarin oranges, 1/2 cup	0	
Valencia oranges, 1/2 cup	1	
Tree of Life		
Mandarin oranges in light syrup, 2/3 cup	1	
## Papayas		
Brooks		
♦ Caribbean red papaya, 1 cup (cubes)	1	(2)
♦ Caribbean sunrise papaya, 1 cup	1	(2)
Dole		
♦ Papaya, 1/2	1	(2)
Sunfresh		
Papaya chunks in extra light syrup, 1/2 cup	1	
Tree of Life		
Dried papaya spears, unsulphured, 1 serving (100 g)	0	
Triton International		
♦ Papaya chunks, 1 cup	1	(2)
Tropical Nut & Fruit		
Papaya chunks, 1 serving (40 g)	3	
## Peaches & Nectarines		
Cascadian Farm		
♦ Sliced peaches, 1 cup	1	(2)
Del Monte		
♦ Diced peaches - artificially sweetened, 1 can (3 3/4 oz)	0	(2)
Halves, lite peaches in extra light syrup (yellow cling), 1/2 cup	1	
Halves, peaches in heavy syrup (yellow cling), 1/2 cup	2	

	POINTS VALUE	
Halves, peaches in heavy syrup (yellow freestone), 1/2 cup	2	
Peach chunks in extra light syrup, 1/2 cup	1	
Peaches in peach flavored gel, 1 cup	2	
Peaches in raspberry lemonade flavored gel, 1 cup	2	
Peaches in strawberry banana flavored gel - lite, 1 cup	1	
♦ Sliced, fruit natural peaches in pear & peach juices (yellow cling), 1/2 cup	1	(2)
Sliced, peaches in natural raspberry flavored light syrup (yellow cling), 1/2 cup	1	
Sliced, spiced peaches in light syrup (yellow cling), 1/2 cup	1	
Sweet cinnamon chunky-cut peaches in light syrup (yellow cling), 1/2 cup	1	
Whole, spiced peaches in heavy syrup (yellow cling), 1/2 cup	2	
♦ Yellow cling peaches in water, artificially sweetened, 1/2 cup	0	(2)
Del Monte Fruit Cups		
Diced peaches in heavy syrup, 1	1	
♦ Fruit naturals diced peaches in pear and peach juices, 1	1	(2)
Lite diced peaches in extra light syrup, 1	1	
Del Monte Fruit Rageous		
Wild raspberry flavored peaches in light syrup, 1	1	
Del Monte Fruit To-Go		
Peachy peaches in peach-flavored light syrup, 1	1	

	POINTS VALUE	
Del Monte Orchard Select		
Sliced, yellow cling peaches in light syrup, 1/2 cup	2	
Dole		
◆ Fresh frozen sliced peaches with flavor, 3/4 cup	1	(2)
◆ Nectarine, 1	1	(2)
◆ Peach, 1	0	(2)
Sliced peaches in light syrup, 1/2 cup	2	
Dole Fruit Bowls		
Yellow cling diced peaches in light syrup, 1 cup	1	
Yellow cling diced peaches in light syrup, 1 container	1	
Dole Fruit in Gel		
Diced peaches in strawberry gel, 1 container	2	
Sunkist Premium Sweet		
Petite peaches, 1/2 cup	1	

Pears

Del Monte		
Diced pears in light syrup, 1 cup	1	
◆ Halves, fruit naturals pears in pear juice, 1/2 cup	1	(2)
Halves, lite pears in extra light syrup, 1/2 cup	1	
Halves, pear in heavy syrup, 1/2 cup	2	
◆ Pears in water, artificially sweetened, 1/2 cup	1	(2)
Del Monte Fruit Cups		
Diced pears in heavy syrup, 1	1	
Lite diced pears in extra light syrup, 1	1	
Del Monte Orchard Select		
Sliced, bartlett pears in light syrup, 1/2 cup	1	

	POINTS VALUE	
Dole		
◆ Pear, 1	1	(2)
Dole Fruit Bowls		
Diced pears in light syrup, 1 container	1	
Dole Fruit in Gel		
Pears in kiwi-berry gel, 1 container	1	
Tropical Nut & Fruit		
Pears, diced, 1/4 cup	1	

Pineapples

Del Monte		
Chunks, pineapple in heavy syrup, 1/2 cup	2	
Crushed pineapple in heavy syrup, 1/2 cup	2	
◆ Crushed pineapple in its own juice, 1/2 cup	1	(2)
◆ Pineapple chunks - artificially sweetened, 1/2 cup	1	(2)
Pineapple chunks in lightly sweetened pineapple juice, 1/2 cup	1	
◆ Pineapple chunks in pineapple juice, 1/2 cup	1	(2)
◆ Pineapple crushed - artificially sweetened, 1/2 cup	1	(2)
◆ Pineapple sliced - artificially sweetened, 1/2 cup	1	(2)
◆ Pineapple tidbits - artificially sweetened, 1/2 cup	1	(2)
Sliced, pineapple in heavy syrup, 2 slices	2	
◆ Sliced, pineapple in its own juice, 2 slices	1	(2)
Del Monte Fruit Cups		
◆ Pineapple tidbits in pineapple juice, 1	1	(2)

Fruit

	POINTS VALUE

Dole

Fresh frozen pineapple chunks, 3/4 cup	2	(2)
Pineapple, 2 slices	1	(2)
Pineapple chunks in juice, 1/2 cup	1	(2)
Pineapple chunks in syrup, 1/2 cup	2	
Pineapple crushed in juice, canned, 1/2 cup	1	(2)
Pineapple crushed in syrup, canned, 1/2 cup	2	
Pineapple slices in juice, canned, 2 slices	1	(2)
Pineapple slices in syrup, canned, 2 slices	2	
Pineapple tidbits in juice, canned, 1/2 cup	1	(2)
Pineapple tidbits in syrup, canned, 1/2 cup	2	

Dole Fruit Bowls

Pineapple tidbits in pineapple juice, 1 container	1	(2)

Dole Fruit in Gel

Pineapple tidbits in lime gel, 1 container	2	

Dole Snack Jars

Pineapple chunks in light syrup, 1/2 cup	1	

Sunfresh

Pineapple chunks in lightly sweetened pineapple juice, 1/2 cup	1	

Sunkist Premium Sweet

Pineapple, 1/2 cup	1	(2)

Tree of Life

Pineapple rings, unsulphured, 1 Tbsp	4	

Triton International

Pineapple chunks, 1 cup	1	(2)

Tropical Nut & Fruit

Natural pineapple, 1 serving (40 g)	2	
Pineapple wedges sweet, dried, 10 pieces	2	

Plums

Dole

Plum, 2	1	(2)

Sun-Maid

Pitted prunes, 1 oz	1	

Tangerines

Dole

Tangerine, 1 medium	0	(2)

Specialty Fruits

Brooks

Persian limes, 1	0	
Star fruit or carambola, 1/2 cup	0	(2)
Uniq fruit, 1 cup	1	

Dole

Fresh frozen rhubarb chunks, 1 cup	0	(2)
Persimmons, 1 medium	1	(2)

Futuro

Pacaya date palm, 1 oz	0	

Herdez

Whole guavas, 4 pieces	3	

Triton International

Guava chunks, 1 cup	0	(2)

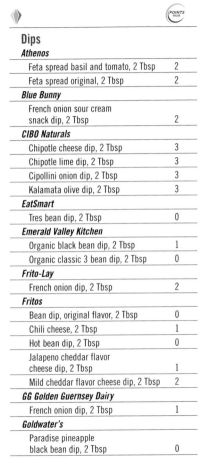

Dips

Athenos

	POINTS VALUE
Feta spread basil and tomato, 2 Tbsp	2
Feta spread original, 2 Tbsp	2

Blue Bunny

French onion sour cream snack dip, 2 Tbsp	2

CIBO Naturals

Chipotle cheese dip, 2 Tbsp	3
Chipotle lime dip, 2 Tbsp	3
Cipollini onion dip, 2 Tbsp	3
Kalamata olive dip, 2 Tbsp	3

EatSmart

Tres bean dip, 2 Tbsp	0

Emerald Valley Kitchen

Organic black bean dip, 2 Tbsp	1
Organic classic 3 bean dip, 2 Tbsp	0

Frito-Lay

French onion dip, 2 Tbsp	2

Fritos

Bean dip, original flavor, 2 Tbsp	0
Chili cheese, 2 Tbsp	1
Hot bean dip, 2 Tbsp	0
Jalapeno cheddar flavor cheese dip, 2 Tbsp	1
Mild cheddar flavor cheese dip, 2 Tbsp	2

GG Golden Guernsey Dairy

French onion dip, 2 Tbsp	1

Goldwater's

Paradise pineapple black bean dip, 2 Tbsp	0

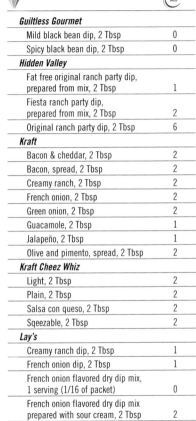

Guiltless Gourmet

	POINTS VALUE
Mild black bean dip, 2 Tbsp	0
Spicy black bean dip, 2 Tbsp	0

Hidden Valley

Fat free original ranch party dip, prepared from mix, 2 Tbsp	1
Fiesta ranch party dip, prepared from mix, 2 Tbsp	2
Original ranch party dip, 2 Tbsp	6

Kraft

Bacon & cheddar, 2 Tbsp	2
Bacon, spread, 2 Tbsp	2
Creamy ranch, 2 Tbsp	2
French onion, 2 Tbsp	2
Green onion, 2 Tbsp	2
Guacamole, 2 Tbsp	1
Jalapeño, 2 Tbsp	1
Olive and pimento, spread, 2 Tbsp	2

Kraft Cheez Whiz

Light, 2 Tbsp	2
Plain, 2 Tbsp	2
Salsa con queso, 2 Tbsp	2
Sqeezable, 2 Tbsp	2

Lay's

Creamy ranch dip, 2 Tbsp	1
French onion dip, 2 Tbsp	1
French onion flavored dry dip mix, 1 serving (1/16 of packet)	0
French onion flavored dry dip mix prepared with sour cream, 2 Tbsp	2

Jams, Spreads, Salsa & Dips

Lay's (cont'd)	POINTS VALUE
Green onion flavored dry dip mix, 1 serving (1/16 of packet)	0
Green onion flavored dry dip mix prepared with sour cream, 2 Tbsp	2
Ranch flavored dry dip mix, 1 serving (1/16 of packet)	0
Ranch flavored dry dip mix prepared with sour cream, 2 Tbsp	2
Litehouse	
Avocado dip, 2 Tbsp	4
Chocolate caramel dip, 2 Tbsp	3
Chocolate dip, 1 serving	1
Chocolate yogurt fruit dip, 2 Tbsp	3
Dilly dip, 2 Tbsp	4
Garden ranch dip, 2 Tbsp	4
Lite ranch veggie dip, 2 Tbsp	2
Low fat caramel dip, 2 Tbsp	2
Onion dip, 2 Tbsp	3
Organic ranch dip, 2 Tbsp	4
Original caramel dip, 2 Tbsp	2
Ranch dip, 2 Tbsp	4
Southwest ranch dip, 2 Tbsp	3
Strawberry yogurt fruit dip, 2 oz	2
Strawberry yogurt fruit dip, 2 Tbsp	1
Toffee caramel, 2 Tbsp	2
Vanilla yogurt fruit dip, 2 oz	3
Vanilla yogurt fruit dip, 2 Tbsp	1
Marzetti	
Blue cheese veggie dip, 2 Tbsp	4
Blue cheese veggie dip, 1 container (3 oz)	12
Caramel apple dip, 1 container (2 oz)	7

	POINTS VALUE
Caramel apple dip, 2 Tbsp	3
Celery and carrot dip, 1 1/2 oz	7
Chocolate fruit dip, 2 Tbsp	2
Cinnamon caramel apple dip, 2 Tbsp	2
Cream cheese fruit dip, 2 Tbsp	2
Cream cheese fruit dip, 1 container (3.75 oz)	5
Cream cheese fruit dip - 100 calorie pack, 1	2
Dill veggie dip, 2 Tbsp	3
Fat free caramel apple dip, 2 oz	2
Fat free dill veggie dip, 2 Tbsp	1
Fat free ranch veggie dip, 2 Tbsp	1
Fat free southwestern veggie dip, 2 Tbsp	1
French onion veggie dip, 2 Tbsp	3
Guacamole dip, 2 Tbsp	4
Horseradish veggie dip, 2 Tbsp	3
Light caramel apple dip, 2 Tbsp	2
Light Creole mustard veggie dip, 2 Tbsp	2
Light dill veggie dip, 2 Tbsp	2
Light French onion veggie dip, 2 Tbsp	2
Light Greek olive veggie dip, 2 Tbsp	2
Light guajillo pepper veggie dip, 2 Tbsp	2
Light ranch veggie dip, 2 Tbsp	2
Light ranch veggie dip - 100 calorie pack, 1	3
Light vanilla yogurt fruit dip, 2 Tbsp	1
Peanut butter caramel apple dip, 2 Tbsp	3

Jams, Spreads, Salsa & Dips

	POINTS VALUE
Ranch veggie dip, 2 Tbsp	3
Ranch veggie dip - singles, 1 container (3 oz)	10
Southwestern ranch veggie dip, 2 Tbsp	3
Spinach veggie dip, 2 Tbsp	4
Strawberry cream cheese dip, 2 Tbsp	2
Morning Glory	
French onion dip, 2 Tbsp	1
Naturally Fresh	
Bleu cheese, 2 Tbsp (individual 4-oz portion cup)	5
Caramel dip, 2 Tbsp	3
Chocolate dip, 2 Tbsp	1
Dijon honey mustard, 2 Tbsp (individual 4-oz portion cup)	4
Honey mustard, 2 Tbsp (individual 4-oz portion cup)	3
Hot sauce, 1 serving (individual 4-oz portion cup)	1
Ranch, 1 Tbsp (individual 4-oz portion cup)	3
Ranch dressing, 2 Tbsp (individual 4-oz portion cup)	3
Strawberry yogurt dip, 2 Tbsp (individual 4-oz portion cup)	1
Sweet and sour sauce, 2 Tbsp (individual 4-oz portion cup)	2
Vanilla yogurt dip, 2 Tbsp (individual 4-oz portion cup)	1
Naturally Fresh Refrigerated	
Ranch dip, 2 Tbsp	4
Ranch vegetable dip, 2 Tbsp	4
Strawberry cream cheese dip, 2 Tbsp	2

	POINTS VALUE
Old El Paso	
Black bean, medium, 2 Tbsp	0
Cheese 'n salsa, low fat, medium, 2 Tbsp	1
Cheese 'n salsa, medium, 2 Tbsp	1
Cheese 'n salsa, mild, 2 Tbsp	1
Ortega	
Guacamole style dip, 2 Tbsp	1
Philadelphia	
Pourovers dip cream cheese spread & salsa, 2 Tbsp	2
Phillips	
Crab & spinach dip, 2 Tbsp	1
Ruffles	
Rich & creamy smoky bacon & cheddar dip, 2 Tbsp	2
Rich & creamy sour cream & chive dip, 2 Tbsp	1
T.G.I. Friday's	
Spinach, cheese & artichoke dip, 2 Tbsp	1
Taco Bell Home Originals	
Black bean con queso - mild, 2 Tbsp	1
Chili con queso, 2 Tbsp	1
Tostitos	
Creamy southwestern ranch dip, 2 Tbsp	1
Creamy spinach dip, 2 Tbsp	1
Monterey Jack queso, 2 Tbsp	1
Spicy queso supreme, 2 Tbsp	1
Zesty bean & cheese dip, 2 Tbsp	1

Jams, Spreads, Salsa & Dips

	POINTS VALUE
Walden Farms	
Bacon dip, 2 Tbsp	0
Bleu cheese dip, 2 Tbsp	0
Caramel dip, 2 Tbsp	0
Chocolate dip, 2 Tbsp	0
French onion dip, 2 Tbsp	0
Marshmallow dip, 2 Tbsp	0
Ranch dip, 2 Tbsp	0

Hummus
Athenos

	POINTS VALUE
Artichoke and garlic, 2 Tbsp	1
Black olive, 2 Tbsp	1
Original, 2 Tbsp	1
Pesto, 2 Tbsp	1
Roasted eggplant, 2 Tbsp	1
Roasted garlic, 2 Tbsp	1
Roasted red pepper, 2 Tbsp	1
Three pepper, 2 Tbsp	1
Emerald Valley Kitchen	
Organic Greek olive hummus, 2 Tbsp	1
Organic hummus, 2 Tbsp	1
Organic red pepper hummus, 2 Tbsp	1
Organic smoked jalapeno & garlic hummus, 2 Tbsp	1
Organic spinach feta hummus, 2 Tbsp	1
Fantastic World Foods	
Original hummus, 2 Tbsp	1
Guiltless Gourmet	
Classic hummus, 2 Tbsp	1
Roasted garlic hummus, 2 Tbsp	1

	POINTS VALUE
Marzetti	
Original hummus, 2 Tbsp	1
Roasted garlic hummus, 2 Tbsp	1
Roasted red pepper hummus, 2 Tbsp	1
Sabra	
Classic hummus, 1 oz	2
Greek olive hummus, 1 oz	2
Hummus roasted red pepper, 1 oz	2
Jalapeno hummus, 1 oz	1
Supremely spicy hummus, 1 oz	2
Sabra To Go	
Classic hummus, 1 serving (1 oz)	2
Swan Gardens	
Organic fresh dill, 1 serving (28 g)	1
Organic green onions & cumin, 1 serving (28 g)	1
Organic hummus, roasted garlic, 2 Tbsp	1
Organic hummus, roasted red peppers, 2 Tbsp	1
Organic hummus, traditional, 2 Tbsp	1
Tribe All Natural Hummus	
Chunky calamata olive, 2 Tbsp	1
Classic, 2 Tbsp	1
Classic organic hummus, 2 Tbsp	1
Cracked chili pepper, 2 Tbsp	1
Dill, 2 Tbsp	1
Eggplant (baba ganoush), 2 Tbsp	1
Forty spices, 2 Tbsp	1
Horseradish, 2 Tbsp	1
Hummus & cracker pack with all natural 40 spices hummus, 1 tray	4

	POINTS VALUE
Hummus & cracker pack with all natural classic hummus, 1 tray	4
Hummus & cracker pack with all natural garlic hummus, 1 tray	4
Hummus & cracker pack with all natural roasted red pepper hummus, 1 tray	3
Jalapeno, 2 Tbsp	1
Lemon, 2 Tbsp	1
Organic hummus with cracked chili pepper, 2 Tbsp	1
Organic hummus with Mediterranean spices, 2 Tbsp	1
Organic hummus with roasted garlic, 2 Tbsp	1
Organic hummus with roasted red peppers, 2 Tbsp	1
Roasted garlic, 2 Tbsp	1
Roasted red peppers, 2 Tbsp	1
Scallion, 2 Tbsp	1
Spicy chipotle, 2 Tbsp	1
Sundried tomato and basil, 2 Tbsp	1
Wholesome Valley Organic	
Classic hummus, 2 Tbsp	1
Garlic hummus, 2 Tbsp	1
Roasted red pepper hummus, 2 Tbsp	1
Spicy chipotle hummus, 2 Tbsp	1

Jam
Cherchies

Cranberry preserve with champagne, 1 Tbsp	1
New England triple berry preserve with merlot, 1 Tbsp	1
Wild Maine blueberry preserve with burgundy, 1 Tbsp	1

	POINTS VALUE
Polaner Sugar Free	
Concord grape jam, 1 Tbsp	0
Smucker's	
Black raspberry (seedless) jam, 1 Tbsp	1
Blackberry jam, 1 Tbsp	1
Blackberry (seedless) jam, 1 Tbsp	1
Boysenberry (seedless) jam, 1 Tbsp	1
Grape jam, 1 Tbsp	1
Red plum jam, 1 Tbsp	1
Red raspberry (seedless) jam, 1 Tbsp	1
Strawberry jam, 1 Tbsp	1
Strawberry (seedless) jam, 1 Tbsp	1
Sugar free blackberry jam, 1 Tbsp	0
Sugar free grape jam, 1 Tbsp	0
Walden Farms	
Strawberry fruit spread, 1 Tbsp	0
Welch's	
Reduced sugar strawberry spread, 1 Tbsp	0

Jelly
Cherchies

Cherry hot pepper jelly, 1 Tbsp	1
Cranberry hot pepper jelly, 1 Tbsp	1
Lem'n hot pepper jelly, 1 Tbsp	1
Roasted garlic hot pepper jelly, 1 Tbsp	1
Muirhead	
Apricot-jalapeno jelly, 1 Tbsp	1
Smucker's	
Apple jelly, 1 Tbsp	1
Black raspberry jelly, 1 Tbsp	1
Blackberry jelly, 1 Tbsp	1

Jams, Spreads, Salsa & Dips

Smucker's (cont'd)	POINTS VALUE
Cherry jelly, 1 Tbsp	1
Cinnamon apple jelly, 1 Tbsp	1
Currant jelly, 1 Tbsp	1
Elderberry jelly, 1 Tbsp	1
Grape jelly, 1 Tbsp	1
Guava jelly, 1 Tbsp	1
Low sugar grape jelly, 1 Tbsp	1
Mint apple jelly, 1 Tbsp	1
Mixed fruit jelly, 1 Tbsp	1
Plum jelly, 1 Tbsp	1
Quince jelly, 1 Tbsp	1
Red raspberry jelly, 1 Tbsp	1
Strawberry jelly, 1 Tbsp	1
Welch's	
Reduced sugar grape jelly, 1 Tbsp	0

Marmalade
Clearbrook Farms
Bitter-sweet orange marmalade, 1 Tbsp	1
Muirhead	
Tomato marmalade, 1 Tbsp	0
Polaner All Fruit	
Orange marmalade, 1 Tbsp	1
Polaner Fancy Fruit	
Orange marmalade, 1 Tbsp	1
Polaner Sugar Free	
Orange marmalade, 1 Tbsp	0
Smucker's	
Low sugar orange marmalade, 1 Tbsp	1
Sugar free orange marmalade, 1 Tbsp	0
Sweet orange marmalade, 1 Tbsp	1

	POINTS VALUE
Smucker's Simply Fruit	
Orange marmalade, 1 Tbsp	1

Peanut Butter
Better'n Peanut Butter
Chocolate peanut spread, 2 Tbsp	2
Low sodium peanut spread, 2 Tbsp	2
Original, 2 Tbsp	2
Fisher	
Creamy peanut butter, 2 Tbsp	5
Crunchy peanut butter, 2 Tbsp	5
Ian's	
PB4Me - creamy, 1 cup (1.5 oz)	6
PB4Me - crunchy, 1 cup (1.5 oz)	6
Joseph's	
Sugar free Valencia creamy peanut butter, 2 Tbsp	5
Sugar free Valencia crunchy peanut butter, 2 Tbsp	5
Laura Scudder's	
Reduced fat peanut butter, 2 Tbsp	5
MaraNatha Natural	
Creamy & roasted peanut butter with salt, 2 Tbsp	5
Creamy & roasted peanut butter, no salt added, 2 Tbsp	5
Crunchy & roasted peanut butter, with salt, 2 Tbsp	5
Crunchy & roasted peanut butter, no salt added, 2 Tbsp	5
No stir creamy & sweet peanut butter, 2 Tbsp	5
No stir crunchy & sweet peanut butter, 2 Tbsp	5

	POINTS VALUE
MaraNatha Organic	
Creamy & roasted peanut butter, no salt added, 2 Tbsp	5
Creamy & roasted peanut butter, with salt, 2 Tbsp	5
Crunchy & roasted peanut butter, no salt added, 2 Tbsp	5
Crunchy & roasted peanut butter, with salt, 2 Tbsp	5
No stir creamy peanut butter, 2 Tbsp	5
No stir crunchy peanut butter, 2 Tbsp	5
Peanut Wonder	
Low fat peanut spread, 2 Tbsp	2
Low fat peanut spread, low sodium, 2 Tbsp	2
Skippy	
Carb options peanut spread, 2 Tbsp	5
Creamy peanut butter, 2 Tbsp	5
Creamy roasted honey nut peanut butter, 2 Tbsp	5
Natural super chunk, 2 Tbsp	5
Reduced fat creamy, 2 Tbsp	4
Reduced fat super chunk, 2 Tbsp	4
Super chunk peanut butter, 2 Tbsp	5
Super chunk roasted honey nut peanut butter, 2 Tbsp	5
Smart Balance	
Omega natural peanut butter and omega-3 from flax oil, chunky, 2 Tbsp	5
Omega natural peanut butter and omega-3 from flax oil, creamy, 2 Tbsp	5

	POINTS VALUE
Smucker's	
Reduced fat natural peanut butter, 2 Tbsp	5
Tree of Life	
Blended organic creamy peanut butter, 2 Tbsp	5
Blended organic crunchy peanut butter, 2 Tbsp	5
Organic creamy peanut butter, 2 Tbsp	5
Organic creamy peanut butter, no salt added, 2 Tbsp	5
Organic crunchy peanut butter, 2 Tbsp	5
Organic crunchy peanut butter, no salt added, 2 Tbsp	5
Tropical Nut & Fruit	
Honey roasted peanut butter, 2 Tbsp	4
Natural peanut butter, 1 Tbsp	5

Preserves
Cherchies

	POINTS VALUE
White tea key lime raspberry preserve, 1 Tbsp	1
White tea pomegranate peach preserve, 1 Tbsp	1
Clearbrook Farms	
California apricot, 1 Tbsp	1
California peach, 1 Tbsp	1
Michigan black cherry, 1 Tbsp	1
Michigan damson plum, 1 Tbsp	1
Michigan red tart cherry, 1 Tbsp	1
Oregon black raspberry, 1 Tbsp	1
Oregon Marion blackberry, 1 Tbsp	1
Oregon red raspberry, 1 Tbsp	1

Jams, Spreads, Salsa & Dips

Clearbrook Farms (cont'd)	POINTS VALUE
Oregon strawberry, 1 Tbsp	1
Seedless Oregon red raspberry, 1 Tbsp	1
Wild Maine blueberry, 1 Tbsp	1
Polaner Fancy Fruit	
Apricot spread, 1 Tbsp	1
Red raspberry preserves, 1 Tbsp	1
Seedless blackberry preserves, 1 Tbsp	1
Strawberry preserves, 1 Tbsp	1
Polaner Sugar Free	
Apricot, 1 Tbsp	0
Blackberry, 1 Tbsp	0
Raspberry, 1 Tbsp	0
Strawberry, 1 Tbsp	0
Smucker's	
Apricot preserves, 1 Tbsp	1
Apricot-pineapple preserves, 1 Tbsp	1
Blueberry preserves, 1 Tbsp	1
Cherry preserves, 1 Tbsp	1
Low sugar apricot preserves, 1 Tbsp	1
Low sugar orange marmalade preserves, 1 Tbsp	1
Low sugar red raspberry preserves, 1 Tbsp	1
Low sugar strawberry preserves, 1 Tbsp	1
Peach preserves, 1 Tbsp	1
Pineapple preserves, 1 Tbsp	1
Plum preserves, 1 Tbsp	1
Red raspberry preserves, 1 Tbsp	1
Strawberry banana preserves, 1 Tbsp	1
Strawberry preserves, 1 Tbsp	1

	POINTS VALUE
Sugar free apricot preserves, 1 Tbsp	0
Sugar free boysenberry preserves, 1 Tbsp	0
Sugar free red raspberry preserves, 1 Tbsp	0
Sugar free strawberry preserves, 1 Tbsp	0

Salsa
Amy's

	POINTS VALUE
Black bean & corn salsa, 2 Tbsp	0
Fire roasted vegetable salsa, 2 Tbsp	0
Medium salsa, 2 Tbsp	0
Mild salsa, 2 Tbsp	0
Spicy chipotle salsa, 2 Tbsp (1 oz)	0
CHI-CHI'S	
All natural medium salsa, 2 Tbsp	0
Fiesta salsa hot, 2 Tbsp	0
Garden salsa, 2 Tbsp	0
Original salsa medium, 2 Tbsp	0
Original salsa mild, 2 Tbsp	0
Salsa con queso, 2 Tbsp	1
Salsa hot, 2 Tbsp	0
Salsa medium, 2 Tbsp	0
Salsa mild, 2 Tbsp	0
EatSmart	
Garden style sweet salsa, 2 Tbsp	0
Salsa con queso, 2 Tbsp	1
EL TORITO	
Fire-roasted tomato salsa - mild, 2 Tbsp	0
Original restaurant salsa - mild, 2 Tbsp	0

	POINTS VALUE
Original restaurant salsa - medium, 2 Tbsp	0
Original restaurant salsa - hot, 2 Tbsp	0

Emerald Valley Kitchen

Organic fiesta salsa, 2 Tbsp	0
Organic green salsa, 2 Tbsp	0
Organic mango, 2 Tbsp	0
Organic salsa - hot, 2 Tbsp	0
Organic salsa - medium, 2 Tbsp	0
Organic salsa - mild, 2 Tbsp	0

Emeril's

Gaaahlic lovers salsa, 2 Tbsp	0
Kicked up chunky salsa, 2 Tbsp	0
Original recipe salsa, 2 Tbsp	0
Southwest style salsa, 2 Tbsp	0

Goldwater's

Cochise corn & black bean salsa, 2 Tbsp	1
Mohave mango salsa, 2 Tbsp	0
Papago peach salsa, 2 Tbsp	0
Paradise pineapple salsa, 2 Tbsp	0
Rio verde tomatillo salsa, 2 Tbsp	0
Ruby raspberry salsa, 2 Tbsp	0
Sedona red hot salsa, 2 Tbsp	0
Sedona red salsa, 2 Tbsp	0

Green Mountain Gringo

Mild salsa, 2 Tbsp	0
Medium salsa, 2 Tbsp	0
Hot salsa, 2 Tbsp	0

Herdez

Salsa casera, 2 Tbsp	0
Salsa casera mild, 2 Tbsp	0
Salsa casera medium, 2 Tbsp	0

	POINTS VALUE
Salsa hot, 2 Tbsp	0
Salsa medium, 2 tsp	0
Salsa ranchera, 2 Tbsp	0
Salsa taquera, 2 Tbsp	0
Salsa verde, 2 Tbsp	0

La Estrellita

Green jalepeno salsa, 2 Tbsp	0
Kid's salsa, extra mild, 2 Tbsp	0
Red hot salsa, 2 Tbsp	0
Red salsa, medium, 2 Tbsp	0
Red salsa, mild, 2 Tbsp	0

Lance

Don Pablo's medium salsa, 2 Tbsp	0
Don Pablo's hot salsa, 2 Tbsp	0

LaTortilla Factory

Fire roasted roma tomato mild salsa, 2 Tbsp	0
Mild salsa, 2 Tbsp	0
Medium salsa, 2 Tbsp	0

Muir Glen Organic

Black bean & corn, 2 Tbsp	0
Garlic cilantro salsa, 2 Tbsp	0
Hot salsa, 2 Tbsp	0
Medium chipotle salsa, 2 Tbsp	0
Medium salsa, 2 Tbsp	0
Mild salsa, 2 Tbsp	0

Naturally Fresh

Salsa, medium, 2 Tbsp	0

Old El Paso

Fiesta taco salsa, 2 Tbsp	0
Fresh Mexican salsa - smooth chipotle, 2 Tbsp	0

Jams, Spreads, Salsa & Dips

Old El Paso (cont'd)

	POINTS VALUE
Fresh Mexican salsa - smooth pineapple chile, 2 Tbsp	0
Garden pepper salsa - mild, 2 Tbsp	0
Garden pepper salsa - medium, 2 Tbsp	0
Green chili salsa, 2 Tbsp	0
Salsa Mexicana - mild, 2 Tbsp	0
Salsa Mexicana - medium, 2 Tbsp	0
Thick 'n chunky salsa - xtra mild, 2 Tbsp	0
Thick 'n chunky salsa - mild, 2 Tbsp	0
Thick 'n chunky salsa - medium, 2 Tbsp	0
Thick 'n chunky salsa - hot, 2 Tbsp	0

Ortega

	POINTS VALUE
Original salsa, mild, 2 Tbsp	0
Restaurant chunky - medium, 2 Tbsp	0
Salsa, garden style mild, 2 Tbsp	0
Salsa, garden style medium, 2 Tbsp	0
Salsa, homestyle mild, 2 Tbsp	0
Salsa, homestyle medium, 2 Tbsp	0
Salsa, Mexican style mild, 2 Tbsp	0
Salsa, roasted garlic medium, 2 Tbsp	0
Salsa, thick & chunky mild, 2 Tbsp	0
Salsa, thick & chunky medium, 2 Tbsp	0
Salsa verde, medium, 2 Tbsp	0
Salsa with green chiles, 2 Tbsp	0

Pace

	POINTS VALUE
Black bean and corn salsa, 2 Tbsp	0
Chipotle chunky salsa, 2 Tbsp	0
Chunky salsa with cilantro, 2 Tbsp	0
Lime & garlic chunky salsa, 2 Tbsp	0

	POINTS VALUE
Mexican four cheese salsa con queso, 2 Tbsp	2
Pico de gallo, 2 Tbsp	0
Roasted red pepper & garlic chunky salsa, 2 Tbsp	0
Salsa con queso, 2 Tbsp	2
Salsa verde, 2 Tbsp	0
Tequila lime salsa, 2 Tbsp	0
Thick & chunky salsa, 2 Tbsp	0
Triple pepper salsa, 2 Tbsp	0

Preciosa

	POINTS VALUE
Salsa picante, 1 Tbsp	0

Sabra

	POINTS VALUE
Mediterranean salsa - mild, 1 oz	1

Taco Bell Home Originals

	POINTS VALUE
Medium salsa con queso, 2 Tbsp	1
Mild salsa con queso, 2 Tbsp	1
Thick 'n chunky mild salsa, 2 Tbsp	0
Thick 'n chunky medium salsa, 2 Tbsp	0

Tostitos

	POINTS VALUE
All natural chunky salsa mild, medium & hot, 2 Tbsp	0
Black bean & corn salsa, 2 Tbsp	0
Pineapple and peach salsa, 2 Tbsp	0
Salsa con queso, 2 Tbsp	1

Zapata

	POINTS VALUE
Fire roasted salsa roja, mild, 2 Tbsp	0
Fire roasted salsa roja, medium, 2 Tbsp	0
Fire roasted salsa roja, hot, 2 Tbsp	0
Fire roasted salsa verde, mild, 2 Tbsp	0
Fire roasted salsa verde, medium, 2 Tbsp	0

Spreads

Polaner All Fruit

Apricot, 1 Tbsp	1
Black cherry, 1 Tbsp	1
Blueberry, 1 Tbsp	1
Boysenberry, 1 Tbsp	1
Grape, 1 Tbsp	1
Peach, 1 Tbsp	1
Pineapple, 1 Tbsp	1
Raspberry, 1 Tbsp	1
Seedless blackberry, 1 Tbsp	1
Seedless raspberry, 1 Tbsp	1
Seedless strawberry, 1 Tbsp	1
Strawberry, 1 Tbsp	1

Smucker's Simply Fruit

Apricot, 1 Tbsp	1
Black cherry, 1 Tbsp	1
Black raspberry (seedless), 1 Tbsp	1
Blackberry (seedless), 2 Tbsp	1
Blueberry, 1 Tbsp	1
Grape, 1 Tbsp	1
Peach, 1 Tbsp	1
Red raspberry, 1 Tbsp	1
Red raspberry (seedless), 1 Tbsp	1
Strawberry, 1 Tbsp	1
Strawberry (seedless), 1 Tbsp	1

Tree of Life

Organic apricot fruit spread, 1 Tbsp	1
Organic blueberry fruit spread, 1 Tbsp	1
Organic cherry fruit spread, 1 Tbsp	1
Organic grape fruit spread, 1 Tbsp	1
Organic peach fruit spread, 1 Tbsp	1
Organic raspberry fruit spread, 1 Tbsp	1
Organic strawberry fruit spread, 1 Tbsp	1

Walden Farms

Apple butter spread, 1 Tbsp	0
Apricot spread, 1 Tbsp	0
Blueberry spread, 1 Tbsp	0
Grape spread, 1 Tbsp	0
Orange spread, 1 Tbsp	0
Raspberry spread, 1 Tbsp	0

Other Spreads & Dips

Apple Time

Apple butter, 1 Tbsp	1

CIBO Naturals

Artichoke & red pepper bruschetta topping, 1 Tbsp	1
Eggplant antipasto bruschetta topping, 2 Tbsp	0
Fig & olive tapenade, 2 Tbsp	3
Kalamata olive Tuscan bean spread, 2 Tbsp	2
Lemon & garlic Tuscan bean spread, 2 Tbsp	1
Olive & garlic tapenade, 2 Tbsp	3
Roasted garlic Tuscan bean spread, 2 Tbsp	1
Roasted red pepper Tuscan bean spread, 2 Tbsp	1

Classico

Basil pesto, 1/4 cup	6
Bruschetta basil & tomato, 1 serving	0
Bruschetta extra garlic, 1 serving	0

Jams, Spreads, Salsa & Dips

	POINTS VALUE
Clearbrook Farms	
Apple butter, 1 Tbsp	1
Cherry butter, 1 Tbsp	1
Peach butter, 1 Tbsp	1
Pear butter, 1 Tbsp	1
Pumpkin butter, 1 Tbsp	1
Red raspberry butter, 1 Tbsp	1
Strawberry butter, 1 Tbsp	1
Triple berry butter, 1 Tbsp	1
Eden Organic	
Apple butter, 1 Tbsp	0
Apple cherry butter, organic, 1 Tbsp	0
Cherry butter (Montmorency tart cherries), 1 Tbsp	1
Kraft	
Sandwich spread, 1 Tbsp	1
Land O Lakes	
Fresh buttery taste spread, soft, 1 Tbsp	2
Fresh buttery taste spread, stick, 1 Tbsp	3
Lucky Leaf	
Apple butter, 1 Tbsp	1
Manischewitz	
Original apple butter spread, 1 Tbsp	0
MaraNatha Natural	
Creamy & raw almond butter, no salt added, 2 Tbsp	4
Creamy & raw sesame tahini, with salt, 2 Tbsp	5
Creamy & roasted almond butter, no salt added, 2 Tbsp	4

	POINTS VALUE
Creamy & roasted cashew butter, no salt added, 2 Tbsp	5
Creamy & roasted cashew macadamia butter, no salt added, 2 Tbsp	5
Creamy & roasted macadamia butter, no salt added, 2 Tbsp	6
Creamy & roasted sesame tahini, 2 Tbsp	5
Crunchy & roasted almond butter, no salt added, 2 Tbsp	4
Honey almond butter, 2 Tbsp	4
Honey peanut spread, 2 Tbsp	4
No stir creamy almond butter, 2 Tbsp	5
No stir crunchy almond butter, 2 Tbsp	5
MaraNatha Organic	
Creamy & raw almond butter, no salt added, 2 Tbsp	4
Creamy & raw sesame tahini, no salt added, 2 Tbsp	5
Creamy & roasted almond butter, no salt added, 2 Tbsp	4
Creamy & roasted sesame tahini, no salt added, 2 Tbsp	5
Crunchy & roasted almond butter, no salt added, 2 Tbsp	4
Marzetti	
Sugar free glaze for strawberries, 3 Tbsp	0
Muirhead	
Banana walnut butter, 1 Tbsp	0
Blueberry butter, 1 Tbsp	1
Cinnamon apple butter, 1 Tbsp	1
Ginger peachy butter, 1 Tbsp	0

	POINTS VALUE
Pear and port butter, 1 Tbsp	0
Pecan pumpkin butter, 1 Tbsp	0
Musselman's	
Apple butter, 1 Tbsp	1
Nasoya	
Dijon vegi-spread, 1 Tbsp	1
Fat-free original vegi-spread, 1 Tbsp	0
Original vegi-spread, 1 Tbsp	1
Oscar Mayer	
Sandwich spread, 2 oz	3
Smucker's	
Cider apple butter, 1 Tbsp	1
Peach butter, 1 Tbsp	1
Spiced apple butter, 1 Tbsp	1
Smucker's Simply Fruit	
Apple butter, 1 Tbsp	1
Soy Wonder	
Creamy, 2 Tbsp	4
Crunchy, 2 Tbsp	4

	POINTS VALUE
Tree of Life	
Natural creamy almond butter, 2 Tbsp	4
Natural creamy cashew butter, 2 Tbsp	5
Natural crunchy almond butter, 2 Tbsp	4
Organic cashew butter creamy, 2 Tbsp	5
Organic creamy almond butter, 2 Tbsp	4
Organic crunchy almond butter, 2 Tbsp	4
Organic or natural raw almond butter creamy, 2 Tbsp	4
Tropical Nut & Fruit	
Cashew butter, 1/4 cup	5
Walden Farms	
Bruschetta, 2 Tbsp	0

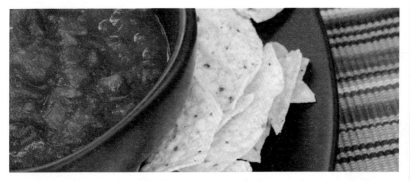

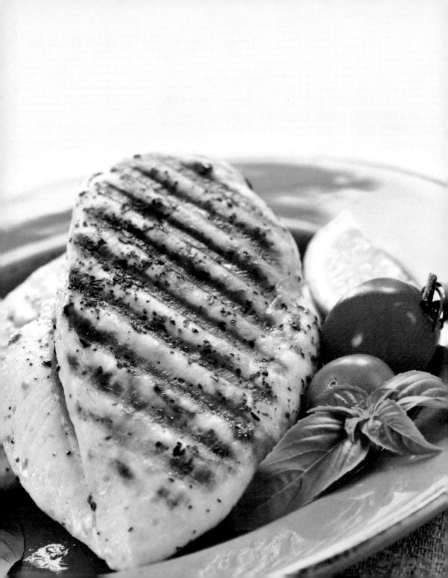

	POINTS VALUE

Bacon

Boar's Head

Canadian style bacon, 2 oz	2	(5)
Imported naturally smoked sliced bacon, 2 slices	2	
Pancetta, 1/2 oz	1	

Farmland

Apple cured sliced cider bacon, 2 slices	2
Butcher's cut extra thick sliced bacon, 1 slice	3
Center cut sliced bacon, 3 slices	2
Fully cooked sliced bacon, 3 1/2 slices	2
Honey maple sliced bacon, 2 slices	2
Sliced bacon, 2 slices	2
Thick sliced bacon, 1 slice	2
Thick sliced hickory smoked stack pack - peppered bacon, 1 slice	2

Hormel

Applewood smoked bacon, 2 slices	3	
Bacon bits, 1 Tbsp	1	
Bacon pieces, 1 Tbsp	1	
Bacon, fully cooked, 2 1/2 slices	2	
Bits, real crumbled bacon, 1 Tbsp	1	
Bits, real crumbled bacon 30% less fat, 1 Tbsp	1	
Canadian style bacon, 2 oz	2	(5)
Country sugar cured bacon, 2 slices	3	
Crumbled bacon 30% less fat, maple, 1 Tbsp	1	
Fully cooked bacon pieces, 1/2 oz	2	
Lower sodium uncured bacon, 2 slices	2	
Maple flavored bacon, 2 slices	2	

	POINTS VALUE

Mesquite sliced bacon, 2 slices	2	
Micro low salt bacon, 2 slices	2	
Microwave bacon, cooked, 2 slices	2	
Original uncured bacon, 2 slices	2	
Real bacon pieces less fat, 1 Tbsp	1	
Real crumbled bacon with picnic bacon 30% less fat, 1 Tbsp	1	

Hormel Black Label

Bacon, cooked, 2 slices	2
Center cut bacon, cooked, 2 slices	2
Low salt bacon, cooked, 2 slices	2

Hormel Old Smokehouse

Bacon, 2 slices	3

Hormel Pillow Pack

Canadian bacon, 22 slices	2	(5)

Hormel Range Brand

Bacon, cooked, 2 slices	3

Jennie-O Turkey Store

Extra lean turkey bacon, 1 serving (15 g)	0
Full flavor turkey bacon, 1 serving (15 g)	1

Jones Dairy Farm

Canadian bacon, 3 slices	1	(5)

Louis Rich

Bacon, turkey, 1 slice	1

Market Day

Fully cooked bacon slices, 3 pieces	2

Oscar Mayer

Bacon bits, real, 1 Tbsp	1
Bacon pieces, real, 1 Tbsp	1
Bacon, center cut, 2 slices	1

Meat & Poultry

Oscar Mayer (cont'd)		POINTS VALUE
Canadian bacon with natural juices, 1 slice	1	(5)
Canadian style bacon made from pork sirloin hips with natural juices, 4 slices	1	(5)
Canadian style bacon made from pork sirloin hips with natural juices, 97% fat free, 1 slice	1	(5)
Hickory country smoked bacon, 2 slices	2	
Natural sliced bacon, 2 slices	2	
Naturally hardwood smoked bacon, 2 slices	2	
Ready to serve bacon, 3 slices	2	
Ready-to-serve thick & hearty bacon, 2 slices	1	
Red Label		
Canadian style bacon, 2 oz	2	(5)
Tyson		
Fully cooked hickory bacon, 2 slices	2	
Hickory bacon, 2 slices	2	

Beef

Boar's Head

	POINTS VALUE
1st cut choice pastrami brisket, 2 oz	2
1st cut cooked choice corned beef brisket, 2 oz	2
All natural cap-off top round oven roasted beef, 2 oz	2
Cajun style seasoned eye round oven roasted beef, 2 oz	2
Choice corned beef brisket - uncooked, 1 serving (2.4 oz)	5
Cooked cap off choice corned beef top round, 2 oz	2
Cooked choice corned beef brisket, 2 oz	3
Deluxe low sodium - all natural cap-off choice top round, 2 oz	2
Italian style seasoned roasted beef with classic braciole seasoning, 2 oz	2
Londonport, top round seasoned roast beef, 2 oz	2
Natural flat cooked corned beef, 2 oz	2
Our deluxe low sodium oven roasted eye round, 2 oz	2
Pepper seasoned eye round - low sodium, 2 oz	2
Seasoned filet of roast beef - cap off top round, 2 oz	2

Fast Classics

	POINTS VALUE
Country fried steaks with gravy, 1 serving (1 steak & 2 Tbsp of gravy)	7
Fully cooked bacon cheeseburgers, 3 oz	5
Fully cooked beef burgers, 3 oz	5

Fast Fixin'

	POINTS VALUE
Ribz for sandwiches, 1 pattie	3
Sirloin beef Philly steak, 1	6

Hormel

	POINTS VALUE
Corned beef, 2 oz	3
Roast beef w/ gravy, 1/2 cup	3
Sliced dried beef, 10 slices	1

Hormel Always Tender

	POINTS VALUE
Beef strip steaks and garlic pepper, 4 oz	5
Beef strips and three pepper blend, 4 oz	5
Peppercorn beef fillet sirloin, 4 oz	3
Tequila lime beef fillet sirloin, 4 oz	3
Teriyaki beef fillet sirloin, 4 oz	3

	POINTS VALUE
Hormel Pillow Pack	
Dried beef, 10 slices	1
Laura's Lean Beef	
96% lean ground round, 4 oz	3
Flank steak, 4 oz	3
Ribeye steak, 4 oz	4
Sirloin steak, 4 oz	3
Market Day	
1/4 pound patties, 1 pattie	7
Bacon wrapped ranch steaks, 1	8
Beef stew meat, 4 oz	6
Filet of sirloin steaks, 1 serving (6 oz)	10
French dip, 2/3 cup	2
Fully cooked pot roast, 3 oz	3
Ground beef, 4 oz (raw)	6
Home style gravy and beef tips, 2/3 cup	3
Marinated sirloin roast (garlic & herb), 4 oz	4
Meatloaf slices, 1 slice	7
Ranch steak, 5 oz (raw)	5
Teriyaki ranch steak, 1 steak	6
Teriyaki steak kabobs, 2 skewers	6
Mary Kitchen	
Corned beef hash, 1 cup	9
Roast beef hash, 1 cup	9
Tyson	
Beef pot roast in gravy, 5 oz	4
Beef steak tips in bourbon sauce, 1 serving (5 oz)	4
Beef tips in gravy, 5 oz	5
Country fried steak, 1 piece	8
Roast beef in brown gravy, 5 oz	3

	POINTS VALUE
Seasoned beef strips (boxed), 3 oz	3
Seasoned steak strip (boxed), 3 oz	3
Steak fingers, 2 pieces	6

Chicken

Alexia	
Chicken nuggets with broccoli, 1 serving (77 g)	5
Chicken nuggets with spinach, 1 serving (77 g)	5
Boar's Head	
Hickory smoked chicken breast, 2 oz	1
Bumble Bee	
Chicken salad with crackers, chicken salad only, 1 can	3
Chicken salad with crackers, crackers only, 6	2
Prime fillet chicken breast lightly seasoned with garlic & herbs, 1 pouch	2
Prime fillet chicken breast with barbeque sauce, 1 pouch	4
Prime fillet chicken breast with southwest seasonings, 1 pouch	2
Bumble Bee Lunch on the Run	
Chicken salad - complete lunch kit, chicken salad only, 1 can	4
Chicken salad - complete lunch kit, crackers only, 6	2
Chicken salad - complete lunch kit, entire kit, 1	10
Chicken salad - complete lunch kit, mixed fruit cup only, 1 serving (4 oz)	1
Chicken salad, complete lunch kit, cookie only, 1	3

Meat & Poultry

	POINTS VALUE
Fast Classics	
Buffalo style chicken breast tenders, 3 oz	5
Buffalo style chicken chunks, 2 pieces	4
Buffalo style chicken wings, 3 oz	4
Chicken breast chunks, 2 pieces	4
Chicken breast tenders, 1 serving (3 oz)	4
Chicken fried chicken breasts, 1 serving (1 breast & 2 Tbsp gravy)	6
Crispy chicken breast strips, 1 serving (3 oz)	4
Flame roasted chicken breasts, 1	4
Honey Bbq chicken wings, 3 oz	5
Tomato basil chicken breasts, 1 piece	3
Fast Fixin'	
Chicken breast nuggets, 6	5
Chicken breast patties, 1 pattie	5
Chicken breast strips, 3	5
Chicken cheese nuggets, 6	6
Dino bites, 4	6
Philly style chicken steaks, 1 piece	3
Popcorn chicken, 14 pieces	6
Fast Fixin' Restaurant Style	
Grilled chicken breast slices, 3 oz	3
Grilled chicken breast strips, 3 oz	3
Italian style chicken breast slices, 3 oz	3
Southwestern style chicken breast slices, 3 oz	3
Foster Farms	
♦ Grilled chicken breast strips, 3 oz	2 (5)
Honey roasted chicken breast strips, 3 oz	3

	POINTS VALUE
Southwestern chicken breast strips, 3 oz	2
Foster Farms Savory Servings	
All natural fire roasted chipotle tenders, 1/2 fillet	3
All natural island teriyaki breast fillets, 1/2 fillet	3
All natural lemon peppercorn turkey tenderloins, 4 oz	2
All natural slow roasted garlic & herb breast fillets, 1/2 fillet	3
All natural true bbq turkey tenderloins, 4 oz	2
All natural zesty lemon herb breast fillets, 1/2 fillet	2
Boneless turkey breast roast, 4 oz	2
Island teriyaki turkey tenderloins, 4 oz	2
Seasoned white/dark boneless turkey roast, 4 oz	4
Hormel	
♦ Chunk breast of chicken, 2 oz	1 (5)
♦ Chunk breast of chicken - no salt, 2 oz	1 (5)
♦ Chunk chicken, 2 oz	1 (5)
Chunk chicken salad lunch kit, 1	5
Ian's	
Buffalo chicken fingers, 3	4
Chicken stix, 1 serving (3 oz)	4
Organic Chicken nuggets, 5	4
Organic Italian chicken tenders, 1 serving (84 g)	5
Wheat free, gluten free chicken nuggets, 5	4
Wheat free/gluten free chicken patties, 1 serving (98 g)	5

	POINTS VALUE
Ian's	
Organic chicken patties, 1	5
Kahiki	
Tempura chicken nuggets, chicken only, 1 serving (85 g)	3
Louis Rich	
Grilled chicken strips, 1 serving (84 g)	2
Honey roasted chicken breast cuts, 2/3 cup	3
Italian style chicken breast strips, 3 oz	2
Oven Roasted chicken breast cuts, 2/3 cup	2
Restaurant style breaded chicken strips, 1 serving (84 g)	4
Southwestern fajita seasoned chicken strips, 1 serving (84 g)	2
Market Day	
Breaded chicken breast patties, 1	5
Broccoli & cheese stuffed chicken, 1 piece	7
Buffalo chicken bites, 3 pieces	4
Chicken bites with Asian sauce, 1 serving (4 bites with 1 1/2 Tbsp sauce)	4
Chicken classics, 1 piece	7
Chicken cordon bleu, 1 piece	8
Chicken fries, 8 pieces	3
Chicken gems, 1 piece	2
Chicken nuggets, 4 pieces	4
Chicken parmesan patties, 1 piece	6
Chicken stir-fry kit, 1 1/3 cups	4
Chicken tenders, 1 piece	4
Chicnsteakes, 1 piece	2
Crispy chicnsteakes, 1 piece	5

	POINTS VALUE	
Diced chicken tenderloin, 3/4 cup	2	
Honey BBQ chicken tenders, 1 piece	4	
Popcorn chicken, 13 pieces	4	
Seasoned chicken breast strips, 1 cup	3	
Southwest chicnsteakes, 1 piece	3	
Spicy buffalo wings, 4 pieces	6	
Teriyaki chicnsteakes, 1 piece	4	
Snow's		
Premium chicken breast, 2 oz	1	(5)
Swanson		
Premium chunk chicken breast in water, 2 oz	1	(5)
Premium chunk mixin' chicken in broth, 2 oz	2	(5)
Premium white & dark chunk chicken in water, 2 oz	1	(5)
T.G.I. Friday's		
Bourbon glazed popcorn chicken, 3 pieces	4	
Buffalo wings, 4 pieces	5	
Honey bbq wings, 3 pieces	5	
Spicy popcorn chicken, 1 serving (86 g)	4	
Tyson		
Boneless skinless breasts, 1 piece	3	(5)
Breaded chicken breast fillets, 1 piece	6	
Breast (all natural), 4 oz	3	(5)
Breast tenderloin (boxed), 1 piece	3	
Buffalo boneless chicken wyngs, 3 pieces	3	
Buffalo strips (bagged), 2 pieces	5	
Buffalo style chicken strips, 2 pieces	5	

Meat & Poultry

Tyson (cont'd)	POINTS VALUE	
Buffalo style hot wings (bone in), 4 pieces	6	
Buffalo style popcorn chicken bites, 5 pieces	4	
Chicken pattie-regular, 1 piece	4	
Chicken pattie-regular, 1 piece	4	
Crispy chicken strips, 2 pieces	5	
Crispy strips (bagged), 2 pieces	5	
Diced chicken breast, 3 oz	2	(5)
Drumsticks (enhanced), 4 oz	4	
Fajita chicken breast strips, 3 oz	3	
Fresh or frozen boneless chicken breast with rib meat, 4 oz	2	(5)
Fresh or frozen chicken tender, 4 oz	2	(5)
Fresh or frozen drumsticks, 4 oz	4	
Fresh or frozen skinless thighs, 4 oz	4	(5)
Fresh or frozen split breast, 4 oz	4	
Fresh or frozen thighs, 4 oz	7	
Fresh or frozen wings, 4 oz	7	
Fresh whole bird, 4 oz	7	
Grilled chicken breast strips, 3 oz	2	
Honey battered breast tenders, 5 pieces	5	
Honey bbq boneless chicken wyngs, 3 pieces	5	
Honey bbq chicken strips, 1 piece	4	
Honey bbq wings (bagged), 4 pieces	6	
Honey bbq wings (bone in), 4 pieces	6	
Hot & spicy chicken wings (bone-in), 3 pieces	6	
Mesquite breast fillets, 1 piece	3	
Nuggets (bagged), 5 pieces	7	

	POINTS VALUE	
Popcorn chicken bites, 6 pieces	6	
Pouch premium chunk chicken breast, 2 oz	2	(5)
Premium chunk chicken breast, 2 oz	1	(5)
Roasted breast halves - skinless, 1 piece	3	(5)
Roasted breast halves-regular, 1 piece	6	
Roasted drumsticks, 2 pieces	5	
Roasted hot and spicy wings, 3 pieces	5	
Roasted thighs, 1 piece	7	
Roasted whole chicken - lemon pepper chicken, 3 oz	3	
Roasted whole chicken-regular, 3 oz	4	
Smokey bbq boneless chicken wyngs, 3 pieces	4	
Southern style breast pattie, 1	6	
Southwestern chicken strip, 3 oz	3	
Tequila lime chicken wings (bone in), 4 pieces	5	
Teriyaki boneless chicken wyngs, 3 pieces	5	
Teriyaki breast fillets, 1 piece	4	
Teriyaki chicken wings (bone-in), 4 pieces	5	
Wings of fire (bone in), 3 pieces	7	

Tyson Any'tizers

	POINTS VALUE	
Barbeque style chicken wings, 3 pieces	5	
Buffalo style boneless chicken wyngs, 3 pieces	4	
Cheddar & bacon chicken bites, 4 pieces	6	
Cheddar & jalapeno chicken bites, 4 pieces	4	

	POINTS VALUE
Homestyle chicken fries, 7 pieces	5
Honey bbq boneless chicken wyngs, 3 pieces	5
Hot 'n spicy chicken wings, 3 pieces	6
Mini chicken bites, 13 pieces	7
Popcorn chicken, 6 pieces	5
Ranch flavored chicken fries, 7 pieces	5

Game Birds

Tyson

Cornish game hen, 4 oz	5

Ground Meat

Aidells

Bacon & cheddar char-broiler, 1 pattie	4
Bacon & cheddar char-broiler, 1 serving (4 oz)	6
Buffalo meatballs, 4	4
Buffalo style meatballs, 4	4
Chipotle meatballs, 4	3
Mushroom char-broiler, 1	5
Spicy bleu cheese char-broiler, 1 pattie	4
Spicy bleu cheese char-broiler, 1 pattie	6
Sun dried tomato & cheese meatballs, 3	4
Sun-dried tomato with Parmesan & Romano cheese meatballs, 3	4
Sweet & sour meatballs, 3	3
Teriyaki meatballs, 4	4
Teriyaki meatballs, 4	4
Vegetable char-broiler, 1	5

Fast Fixin'

Beef meatballs, 3 oz	6
Italian style meatballs, 3 oz	7

	POINTS VALUE
Market Day	
Italian style meatballs, 4 pieces	4
Rosina	
Homestyle meatballs, 3	7
Italian-style meatballs, 3	6
Organic meatballs, 6	4
Swedish meatballs, 6	6
Turkey Italian style meatballs, 1 serving (85 g)	4
Turkey meatballs, 3	4
Tyson	
Italian style chicken meatballs, 6 pieces	4

Jerky

Lance

Beef & cheese, 1 package	4
Beef stick, 1 piece	1
Kippered beefsteak - original, 1 serving (25 g)	1
Kippered beefsteak - peppered, 1 serving (25 g)	1
Kippered beefsteak - teriyaki, 1 serving (25 g)	1
Original beef jerky, 1 piece	1
Peppered beef jerky, 1 piece	1
Spicy beef stick, 1 serving (4 oz)	2
Teriyaki beef jerky, 1 piece	2

Rustlers

Beef jerky, 1 serving (9 g)	1
Spicy stick, 1 package	2

Meat & Poultry

	POINTS VALUE
SnackMasters Natural Gourmet Jerky	
Beef jerky, hot & spicy, 1 oz	2
Beef jerky, original, 1 oz	2
Beef jerky, teriyaki, 1 oz	2
Turkey jerky, hot & spicy, 1 oz	1
Turkey jerky, original, 1 oz	2
Turkey jerky, teriyaki, 1 oz	2
Tasty Eats	
Cajun jerky, 1 oz	2
Ginger jerky, 1 oz	2
Hot n'spicy jerky, 1 oz	2
Jamaican jerky, 1 oz	2
Original jerky, 1 oz	2
Peppered jerky, 1 oz	2
Tandoori jerky, 1 oz	2
Teriyaki jerky, 1 oz	1

Luncheon/Deli Lunches
Armour Healthy Ones

	POINTS VALUE
Browned chicken breast, 1 serving (56 g)	1
Cooked ham, 1 serving (56 g)	1
Deli pre-sliced honey cured ham, 1 serving (57 g)	1
Deli pre-sliced oven roasted chicken breast skinless, 1 serving (57 g)	1
Deli pre-sliced roast beef, 1 serving (57 g)	1
Deli pre-sliced Virginia brand cooked ham, 1 serving (57 g)	1
Deli thin-sliced honey ham, 1 serving (52 g)	1

	POINTS VALUE
Deli thin-sliced honey roasted & smoked turkey breast & white turkey breast, 1 serving	1
Deli thin-sliced mesquite turkey breast & white turkey, 1 serving (52 g)	1
Deli thin-sliced oven roasted turkey, 1 serving (52 g)	1
Deli thin-sliced smoked ham, 1 serving (52 g)	1
Deli thin-sliced smoked turkey breast & white turkey, 1 serving (52 g)	1
Deli thin-sliced variety pack - honey roasted & smoked turkey breast & white, 1 serving (52 g)	1
Deluxe thin-sliced baked cooked ham, 1 serving (56 g)	1
Deluxe thin-sliced honey ham, 1 serving (56 g)	1
Deluxe thin-sliced oven roasted turkey breast & white turkey, 1 serving (56 g)	1
Golden oven roasted turkey breast, 1 serving (56 g)	1
Hardwood smoked ham, 1 serving (56 g)	1
Hearty thick-sliced cooked ham, 1 serving (28 g)	1
Hearty thick-sliced honey ham, 1 serving (28 g)	1
Hearty thick-sliced oven roasted chicken breast, 1 serving (28 g)	1
Hearty thick-sliced oven roasted turkey breast & white turkey, 1 serving (28 g)	1
Honey ham, 1 serving (56 g)	1
Honey maple ham, 1 serving (56 g)	1

	POINTS VALUE
Honey roasted & smoked turkey breast, 1 serving (56 g)	1
Meat franks, 1 (50 g)	1
Medium cooked roast beef, 1 serving (56 g)	1
Medium rare roast beef, 1 serving (56 g)	1
Mesquite smoked chicken breast, 1 serving (56 g)	1
Mesquite smoked honey ham, 1 serving (56 g)	1
Mesquite smoked turkey breast, 1 serving (56 g)	1
Oven roasted turkey breast, 1 serving (57 g)	1
Smoked turkey breast, 1 serving (56 g)	1
Thin sliced baked cooked ham, 1 serving (52 g)	1
Thin sliced oven roasted chicken breast, 1 serving (52 g)	1
Virginia brand ham, 1 serving (56 g)	1

Armour Healthy Ones Sandwich Solutions

Sliced roast beef, 1 serving (57 g)	1
Sliced turkey breast skinless oven roasted, 1 serving (57 g)	1
Sliced turkey breast skinless smoked, 1 serving (57 g)	1
Sliced Virginia ham, 1 serving (57 g)	1

Boar's Head

28% lower sodium bologna, 2 oz	4
Abruzzese hot, 1 oz	3
All American bbq seasoned roasted chicken breast, 2 oz	1

	POINTS VALUE
All natural Italian style seasoned fresh ham, 2 oz	1
All natural salame coated with course black pepper, 1 oz	2
All natural salame coated with herbs, 1 oz	2
Antipasto sopressata & picanti provolone slices, 1 serving	2
Bar b q sauce basted breast of chicken, 2 oz	1
Beef bologna, 2 oz	4
Beef salami, 2 oz	3
Bianco d'oro Italian dry salame, 1 oz	3
Blazing buffalo-style roasted chicken breast, boneless/skinless, 2 oz	1
Bologna (pork & beef), 2 oz	4
Choice pastrami brisket, 2 oz	4
Cooked salami, 2 oz	4
Dutch brand loaf, 2 oz	4
Garlic bologna, 2 oz	4
Genoa salami natural casing, 2 oz	5
Hard salami, 1 oz	3
Head cheese, 2 oz	2
Junior beef salami, 2 oz	3
Lebanon bologna, 2 oz	3
Lite braunschweiger liverwurst, 2 oz	3
Liverwurst paté, 2 oz	4
Maple glazed roasted chicken breast, 2 oz	1
Mortadella (plain), 2 oz	4
Mortadella w/ pistachio nuts, 2 oz	5
Olive loaf, 2 oz	4

Meat & Poultry

Boar's Head (cont'd)	POINTS VALUE
Pastrami navel, 2 oz	5
Pastrami round, 2 oz	2
Porketta, 2 oz	2
Ring bologna, 2 oz	4
Rotisserie seasoned chicken breast, boneless/skinless, 2 oz	1
Salame panino, 1 oz	2
Smoked liverwurst, 2 oz	5
Sopressata calabrese hot, 1 oz	3
Sopressata hot-mini, 1 oz	3
Sopressata pre-cut - mini, 5 slices	3
Sopressata veneta, 1 oz	3
Strassburger brand liverwurst, 2 oz	5
Strassburger liverwurst - natural casing, 2 oz	5
Carl Buddig Deli Cuts	
Brown sugar baked ham, 1 serving (56 g)	2
Honey roasted cured turkey breast & white turkey, 1 serving (56 g)	2
Oven-roasted cured turkey breast & white turkey, 1 serving (56 g)	2
Rotisserie chicken breast, 1 serving (56 g)	2
Smoked ham, 1 serving (56 g)	2
Smoked turkey breast, 2 oz	2
Carl Buddig Original	
Ham with natural juices, 1 package	2
Ham with natural juices, 2 oz	2
Honey ham with natural juices, 1 package	2
Honey ham with natural juices, 2 oz	2

	POINTS VALUE
Honey turkey, 1 package	2
Honey turkey, 2 oz	2
Oven roasted turkey, 2 oz	2
Oven roasted turkey, 1 package	2
Thin sliced beef, 2 oz	2
Thin sliced beef, 1 package	2
Thin sliced chicken, 1 package	2
Thin sliced corned beef, 1 package	2
Thin sliced corned beef, 2 oz	2
Thin sliced pastrami, 1 package	2
Thin sliced pastrami, 2 oz	2
Turkey, 2 oz	2
Turkey, 1 package	2
Casa Italia	
Genoa salami, 1 slice	5
Prosciutto, 1 serving (30 g)	2
Vera mortadella hot, 2 slices	2
Cure 81	
Deviled ham, 4 Tbsp	4
Farmland	
Cooked honey ham, 97% fat free, 1 slice	1
Sliced - oven roasted turkey breast, fat free, 1 oz	1
Sliced cooked - ham - 97% fat free, 1 oz	1
Sliced honey cured turkey breast, 98% fat free, 1 oz	1
Thin shaved cooked ham, 2 oz	1
Thin shaved oven roasted turkey breast, 98% fat free, 2 oz	1

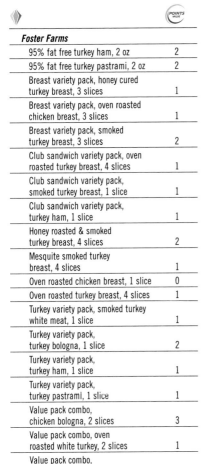

Foster Farms	POINTS VALUE
95% fat free turkey ham, 2 oz	2
95% fat free turkey pastrami, 2 oz	2
Breast variety pack, honey cured turkey breast, 3 slices	1
Breast variety pack, oven roasted chicken breast, 3 slices	1
Breast variety pack, smoked turkey breast, 3 slices	2
Club sandwich variety pack, oven roasted turkey breast, 4 slices	1
Club sandwich variety pack, smoked turkey breast, 1 slice	1
Club sandwich variety pack, turkey ham, 1 slice	1
Honey roasted & smoked turkey breast, 4 slices	2
Mesquite smoked turkey breast, 4 slices	1
Oven roasted chicken breast, 1 slice	0
Oven roasted turkey breast, 4 slices	1
Turkey variety pack, smoked turkey white meat, 1 slice	1
Turkey variety pack, turkey bologna, 1 slice	2
Turkey variety pack, turkey ham, 1 slice	1
Turkey variety pack, turkey pastrami, 1 slice	1
Value pack combo, chicken bologna, 2 slices	3
Value pack combo, oven roasted white turkey, 2 slices	1
Value pack combo, turkey pastrami, 2 slices	1

Hebrew National	POINTS VALUE
Beef bologna, 1 slice	2
Beef salami, 1 slice	2
Lean beef bologna, 4 slices	2
Lean beef salami, 4 slices	2
Hormel	
Black forest ham, 2 oz	1
Black label chopped ham, 2 oz	4
Chicken Vienna sausage, 2 oz	3
Cooked corn beef, 2 oz	1
Cooked ham, 2 oz	1
Cooked pastrami, 2 oz	1
Double smoked ham, 2 oz	1
Homeland hard salami, 1 oz	2
Honey smoked turkey, 2 oz	1
Italian dry salami, 6 slices	3
Oven roasted turkey breast, 2 slices	1
Roasted turkey, 2 oz	1
San Remo genoa salami, 2 oz	6
Seasoned roast beef, 2 oz	1
Sliced honey ham, 2 oz	2
Smoked turkey breast, 2 oz	1
Spiced ham, 2 oz	4
Vienna sausage, 2 oz	4
Vienna sausage hot & spicy, 5 oz	4
Jennie-O Turkey Store	
Lunchmeat hickory smoked, 1 serving (56 g)	1
Lunchmeat honey smoked, 1 serving (56 g)	1

Meat & Poultry

Jennie-O Turkey Store (cont'd)	POINTS VALUE
Lunchmeat pepper grilled, 1 serving (56 g)	1
Lunchmeat sun dried tomato, 1 serving (56 g)	1
Louis Rich	
Chicken, white, oven roasted, 1 slice	1
Naturally smoked turkey breast & white turkey, 98% fat free, 1 slice	1
Oven roasted chicken breast, 3 slices	1
Turkey bologna, 1 slice	1
Turkey breast & white turkey, oven roasted 98% fat free, 1 slice	1
Turkey cotto salami, 1 slice	1
Turkey ham, smoked, chopped, 1 slice	1
Louis Rich Carving Board	
Turkey breast hickory smoked, 3 slices	1
Oscar Mayer	
98% fat free bologna made with turkey, 1 slice	1
All-American variety pak, bologna, 2 slices	4
All-American variety pak, cotto salami, 2 slices	3
All-American variety pak, ham, 2 slices	2
Bologna, beef, 1 slice	2
Bologna, beef, light, 1 slice	2
Bologna, garlic, 1 slice	4
Bologna, light, made with chicken-pork, 1 slice	2
Bologna, made with chicken and pork, 1 slice	2
Braunschweiger, liver sausage, 2 oz	5

	POINTS VALUE
Brown sugar ham, 5 slices	2
Canadian-style bacon, made from pork sirloin hips, 3 slices	1
Chicken breast, 5 slices	1
Chicken breast, oven roasted, 3 slices	2
Chopped honey ham, 1 slice	1
Cooked ham, 2 slices	1
Cooked ham, water added, 96% fat free, 1 slice	1
Cured roast beef, 6 slices	1
Deli shaved beef salami, 4 slices	4
Deli shaved Virginia brand ham, 6 slices	1
Fun pack: beef tacos, 1 package	10
Fun pack: cheesy chip nachos with strawberry-kiwi drink, 1 package	12
Fun pack: nachos with wild cherry drink, 1 package	14
Ham, baked cooked, 3 slices	1
Ham, boiled, 3 slices	1
Ham, chopped, 1 slice	1
Ham, honey, 3 slices	1
Ham, honey & water product, 96% fat free, 3 slices	2
Ham, low sodium, 3 slices	2
Ham, smoked, 3 slices	1
Ham, smoked & water product, 3 slices	1
Hearty thick cut bologna made with chicken & pork, 1 slice	4
Honey ham, water added, thin sliced, 96% fat free, 5 slices	1
Honey smoked turkey, 1 slice	1
Honey smoked turkey breast, 5 slices	1

	POINTS VALUE
Luncheon loaf, spiced, 1 slice	2
Mesquite turkey breast, 5 slices	1
Natural smoked ham, 3 slices	1
Olive loaf, 1 slice	2
Oven roasted turkey breast, 6 slices	1
Oven roasted white turkey & cheese, 1 slice	1
Pickle and pimento loaf, 1 slice	2
Rotisserie style chicken breast, 6 slices	1
Salami cotto, beef, 1 slice	2
Salami cotto, made with chicken, beef and pork, 1 slice	2
Salami genoa, 3 slices	3
Salami, hard, 3 slices	3
Sliced ham & turkey breast, 4 slices	1
Smoked turkey breast, 6 slices	1
Thick cut beef bologna, 1 slice	4
Thick cut meat bologna, 1 slice	4
Thin sliced beef bologna, 3 slices	5
Thin sliced cotto salami, 3 slices	3
Turkey breast, oven roasted, 5 slices	1
Turkey breast, smoked, 5 slices	1
Turkey, white, oven-roasted, 1 slice	1

Oscar Mayer Lunchables

Bologna/American/cookies, no drink, 1 package	9
Deluxe turkey & chicken, 1 package	9
Extra cheesy pizza, no drink, 1 package	6
Extra cheesy pizza/fruit punch, with drink, 1 package	9

	POINTS VALUE
Fun pack: bologna/American cheese, 1 package	10
Fun pack: ham/Swiss, low fat, no drink, 1 package	8
Fun pack: turkey/cheddar, low fat, pudding, 1 package	8
Ham/American cheese/snicker/ fruit punch, 1 package	9
Ham/cheddar, no drink, 1 package	8
Ham/cheddar/cookies, no drink, 1 package	9
Ham/Swiss, no drink, 1 package	8
Pepperoni pizza, no drink, 1 package	7
Pizza cracker stackers, 1 package	10
Turkey/American/cookies, no drink, 1 package	9
Turkey/cheddar, no drink, 1 package	8
White turkey/ham/no drink, 1 package	9

Oscar Mayer Lunchables Fun Pack

Bbq chicken shake up, 1 package	5
Breaded chicken nuggets, 1 package	7
Ham & turkey sub, 1 package	11
Low fat ham and cheddar, 1 package	9
Mini pizzas, 1 package	10
Mini's - cheeseburgers, 1 package	9
Mini's, hot dogs, 1 package	9
Nacho chicken shake up, 1 package	5
Pepperoni & cheese, 1 package	9
Pizza and treatza, 1 package	9
Turkey and American, 1 package	8
Turkey and cheddar, 1 package	8

Meat & Poultry

Oscar Mayer Lunchables Maxed Out

Cheese pizza, 1 package	11
Chicken strips, 1 package	11
Double stacked tacos, 1 package	9
Ham and cheddar, 1 package	15
Nacho, 1 package	13
Pepperoni flavored sausage pizza, 1 package	12
Pizza stix, 1 package	14
Turkey and cheese, 1 package	16

Spam

Classic, 2 oz	5
Classic single, 1 package	7
Garlic, 2 oz	4
Golden honey grail, 2 oz	5
Hot & spicy, 2 oz	5
Less salt, 2 oz	5
Lite, 2 oz	3
Oven roasted turkey, 2 oz	2
Smoked, 2 oz	5
Spread, 4 Tbsp	4
Turkey single, 1 package	3
With bacon, 2 oz	5
With cheese, 2 oz	5

Underwood

Barbeque flavored chicken spread, 1/4 cup	3
Deviled ham spread, 1/4 cup	5
Liverwurst spread, 1/4 cup	3
Roast beef spread, 1/4 cup	3
White meat chicken spread, 1/4 cup	3
White meat turkey spread, 1/4 cup	4

Pork/Ham

Black Label

Canned ham, 3 oz	2

Boar's Head

42% lower sodium branded deluxe ham, 2 oz	1
All natural smoked uncured ham, 2 oz	1
All natural uncured ham, 2 oz	1
Baby maple glazed honey coat ham, 3 oz	2
Black forest brand boneless smoked ham, 2 oz	1
Branded deluxe ham, 2 oz	1
Capocollo, 1 oz	2
Cooked capocollo sweet - natural casing, 2 oz	3
Gourmet pepper ham, 2 oz	1
Honey coat ham, 2 oz	1
Maple glazed honey coat ham, 2 oz	1
Pepper brand ham, 2 oz	2
Pesto parmesan oven roasted ham, 2 oz	2
Prosciutto boneless, skinless/shankless, 1 oz	1
Prosciutto panino, 1 oz	2
Prosciutto piccolo boneless, 1 oz	1
Prosciutto riserva stradolce boneless, 1 oz	1
Ready to eat ham, 3 oz	2
Rosemary & sundried tomato ham, 2 oz	2
Semi-boneless smoked ham, 3 oz	3
Smoked pork shoulder butt roast, 3 oz	4

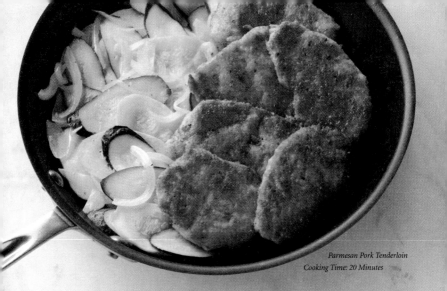

Parmesan Pork Tenderloin
Cooking Time: 20 Minutes

PORK & PARMESAN

Perhaps no food is as sociable as pork. It seems to get along with any seasoning, ingredient or side dish. You'll also find it's agreeable with you – easy to prepare and full of flavor. Ounce for ounce, pork tenderloin is as lean as skinless chicken breast. So visit us online for hundreds of simple, great-tasting recipes. And let your family discover why pork is the big cheese of proteins.

TheOtherWhiteMeat.com/PorkRecipes

Don't be blah.®

©2009 National Pork Board, Des Moines, IA. This message funded by America's Pork Checkoff Program. 2008 National Nutrient Database for Standard Reference, Release 21.

Meat & Poultry

Boar's Head (cont'd)	POINTS
Smoked Virginia ham, 2 oz	1
Spiced ham, 2 oz	3
St. Louis style pork spareribs in gourmet barbecue sauce, 3	11
Sweet slice boneless smoked ham, 3 oz	2
Tavern ham, 2 oz	1
Virginia brand ham, 2 oz	1
Casa Italia	
Grandoro prosciutto cotto, 1 oz	1
Porchetta (oven roasted pork loin), 1 oz	1
Rosemary roasted ham, 1 oz	1
Cure 81	
Half ham, 3 oz	2
Ham with brown sugar, 3 oz	2
Quarter chunk, 3 oz	2
Quarter sliced, 3 oz	2
Curemaster	
Ham, 3 oz	2
Farmland	
Bone-in center cut loins, 4 oz	5
Bone-in commodity trim smoked hams, 3 oz	5
Boneless center cut pork loins, 25% less fat, 4 oz	3
Boneless smoked ham - maple river, 3 oz	3
Boneless smoked ham - pit-style honey cured, 3 oz	3
Boneless smoked ham - special select, 1 slice	1
Boneless smoked ham - tradition, 3 oz	3

	POINTS
Boneless smoked ham & water product, 3 oz	3
Diced ham, 2 oz	2
Extra tender original pork spare ribs - St. Louis style, 4 oz	8
Extra tender pork loin back ribs, 4 oz	8
Extra tender top round fresh boneless ham roast, 4 oz	3
Fresh pork kabob cubes, 4 oz	3
Spiral sliced honey-smoked ham bone-in half, 3 oz	4
Spiral sliced smoked ham - bone-in half, 3 oz	4
Farmland - Special Select	
Boneless smoked ham, 1 slice	1
Farmland Nutrition Wise	
Boneless pork sirloin tip roast, 3 oz	2
Extra tender boneless center-cut pork loins, 4 oz	3
Extra tender pork tenderloin, 4 oz	3
Fresh lean ground pork, 97% fat free, 4 oz	3
Hormel	
Chunk ham, 2 oz	2
Glazed ham with maple & brown sugar, 1 serving	4
Ham & cheese patties, 1	5
Ham patties, 1	5
Jalapeno pigs feet, 2 oz	2
Pickled pigs feet, 2 oz	2
Pickled pork hocks, 2 oz	3
Pickled pork tidbits, 2 oz	3

	POINTS VALUE
Hormel Always Tender	
Adobo pork cubes, 4 oz	3
Apple bourbon pork tenderloin, 4 oz	3
Babyback pork ribs with garlic, 4 oz	6
Babyback ribs, 4 oz	6
Babyback ribs with teriyaki, 4 oz	6
Boneless pork tenderloin, 4 oz	3
Boneless rib ends, 4 oz	4
Center cut boneless pork loin, 4 oz	4
Fajita pork strips, 4 oz	3
Fresh pork roast, 4 oz	4
Garlic pork tenderloin, 4 oz	3
Honey mustard pork loin fillet, 4 oz	3
Loin, 4 oz	5
Mesquite pork tenderloin, 4 oz	3
Mild Thai style, 4 oz	3
Mojo criollo loin filet, 4 oz	3
Onion garlic pork shoulder roast, 4 oz	5
Original pork loin, 4 oz	3
Peppercorn pork tenderloin, 4 oz	3
Picnic, 4 oz	6
Pork - citrus center cut loin fillet, 4 oz	3
Pork - onion garlic roast, 4 oz	5
Pork - original fillet, 4 oz	3
Pork - peppercorn chops, 1	4
Pork - roast flavored roast, 4 oz	4
Pork - sun dried tomato center cut loin fillet, 4 oz	3
Pork - teriyaki chops, 1	4
Pork boneless sirloin roast, 4 oz	3
Pork butts, 4 oz	7

	POINTS VALUE
Pork crown roast, 4 oz	5
Pork medallions applewood smoked bacon, 6 oz	6
Pork medallions double smoked, 6 oz	6
Pork medallions peppered maple bacon, 6 oz	6
Pork shoulder roast, 4 oz	4
Raspberry chipotle tenderloin, 4 oz	3
Sesame ginger pork cubes, 4 oz	4
Spare ribs, 4 oz	8
Teriyaki tenderloin, 4 oz	3
Hormel Pillow Pack	
Diced ham, 2 oz	1
Hormel Spiral Cure 81	
Half ham, 3 oz	3
Jones Dairy Farm	
100 calorie ham sandwich stacks, 6 slices	2
100 calorie ham steak, cherrywood smoked, 1	2
100 calorie ham steaks, 1 steak	2
Market Day	
Baby back ribs, 4 oz	7
BBQ pulled pork, 1/2 cup	6
Bone-in pork chop, 1 chop	4
Boneless pork chops, 1 chop	4
Boneless pork riblets, 7 pieces	10
Deluxe ham steaks, 1	4
Pork tenderloins, 1 serving	3
Rack of pork roast, 1 piece	3
Spiral sliced ham, 3 oz	5
Stuffed pork chop, 1	10

Meat & Poultry

	POINTS VALUE
Tyson	
Bbq seasoned pork mini ribs, 4 pieces	8
Maple & brown sugar glazed ham, 5 oz	4
Pork roast in gravy, 5 oz	3
Teriyaki pork strip, 3 oz	3

Sausage
Aidells

	POINTS VALUE
Andouille dinner, 1 link	4
Andouille mini sausage, 5 links	2
Apricot & ginger breakfast sausage, 2 oz	3
Artichoke & garlic sausage, 1 link	3
Artichoke & garlic sausage, 1 serving (available in club stores)	4
Chicken & apple breakfast sausage, 2 oz	3
Chicken & apple mini sausage, 5 links	3
Chicken & apple sausage, 1 link	4
Chicken & apple sausage, 1 serving (100 g)	5
Chicken apple with Monterey sausage, 1 link	5
Chorizo sausage, 1 link	4
Habanero & green chile sausage, 1 serving (100 g)	4
Habanero & green chile sausage, 1 link	3
Mango sausage, 1 link	4
Maple & bacon breakfast sausage, 2 oz	3
Organic andouille sausage, 1 link	4

	POINTS VALUE
Organic chicken & apple sausage, 1 link	4
Organic spinach & feta, 1 link	3
Organic sun-dried tomato sausage, 1 link	4
Pesto sausage, 1 link	4
Pesto sausage, 1 link	4
Pineapple & bacon sausage, 1 link	6
Portobello mushroom sausage, 1 link	3
Roasted garlic & gruyere cheese sausage, 1 link	5
Roasted red pepper & corn sausage, 1 serving (100 g)	2
Roasted red pepper & corn sausage, 1 link	3
Roasted red pepper sausage, 1 link	2
Spicy mango sausage, 1 link	4
Spicy mango sausage, 1 serving (100 g)	5
Spinach & feta sausage, 1 link	3
Sun-dried tomato with mozzarella cheese sausage, 1 link	3
Sun-dried tomato with mozzarella cheese sausage, 1 serving (100 g)	4
Armour Healthy Ones	
Polska kielbasa, 1 serving (56 g)	2
Smoked sausage, 1 serving (56 g)	2
Boar's Head	
Beef knockwurst, natural casing, 1	8
Cooked bratwurst, natural casing, 1	8
Grande pepperoni, 1 oz	4

	POINTS VALUE
Hot smoked sausage, skinless, 1	7
Italian dry sausage hot, 1 oz	3
Italian dry sausage sweet, 1 oz	3
Kielbasa, 2 oz	3
Pepperoni pre-sliced pouch, 16 slices	4
Pepperoni sandwich style, 1 oz	4
Casa Italia	
Vera mortadella, 1 oz	2
Farmland	
Pork and bacon sausage links, 3	7
Pork sausage links, 2	5
Pork sausage links, 3	6
Pork sausage links, lower sodium, 3	6
Pork sausage patties, 2	6
Pork sausage roll, 2 oz	7
Fluky's	
Fat free skinless wieners, 1 link	1
Hebrew National	
Beef knockwurst, 1 link	7
Hormel	
Chunk pepperoni, 1 oz	4
Mild pepperoni, 15 slices	4
Pepperoni hot & spicy, 15 slices	4
Rosa grande pepperoni, 1 oz	4
Sliced pepperoni, 15 slices	4
Twin pepperoni, 1 oz	4
Hormel Little Sizzlers	
Maple sausage, 3 links	6
Pork sausage hot & spicy, cooked, 3 links	6

	POINTS VALUE
Sausage link, cooked, 3 links	6
Sausage patties, cooked, 2 patties	6
Hormel Pillow Pack	
Giant sliced pepperoni, 5 slices	4
Pepperoni, 14 slices	4
Pepperoni bite size, 1 oz	4
Pepperoni diced, 1 oz	4
Pepperoni hot & spicy, 14 slices	4
Thick slice pepperoni, 8 slices	4
Turkey pepperoni, 17 slices	2
Jennie-O Turkey Store	
Beer brat, 1	6
Bratwurst, 1	4
Breakfast lovers sausage chubs, 1 serving (112 g)	4
Breakfast lovers sausage links, 1 serving (56 g)	4
Breakfast sausage link, mild, 1 serving (56 g)	4
Breakfast sausage pattie, 1 serving (64 g)	4
Cheddar brat, 1	6
Lean Italian sausage link, hot, 1 serving (109 g)	4
Lean Italian sausage link, sweet, 1 serving (109 g)	4
Smoked turkey sausage ring rope, 1 serving (56 g)	2
Sweet Italian dinner sausage, 1 serving (84 g)	4
Turkey kielbasa ring rope, 1 serving (56 g)	2

Meat & Poultry

	POINTS VALUE
Jimmy Dean	
All natural hot sausage, 2 oz (cooked)	6
All natural regular pork sausage, 2 oz (cooked)	5
Fully cooked turkey sausage links, 3	3
Fully cooked turkey sausage patties, 2	3
Jones Dairy Farm	
All natural golden brown sausage and rice links, 3	3
Lance	
Giant hot sausage, 1 serving (1.7 oz)	3
Hot sausage, 1 small piece	2
Hot sausage, 1 large piece	2
Louis Rich	
Turkey polska kielbasa, 2 oz	2
Turkey sausage (original), 2.5 oz	3
Turkey smoked sausage, 2 oz	2
Market Day	
Fully cooked turkey sausage links, 2 pieces	3
Old Smokehouse	
Summer sausage, 2 oz	6
Oscar Mayer	
Pepperoni, 14 slices	4
Pork sausage link, cooked, 2	4
Pork sausage patties, ready to serve, 2	5
Smokies sausage, little, made with pork & turkey, 6	5
Smokies, beef, 1	4

	POINTS VALUE
Summer sausage, 1 slice	2
Summer sausage, beef (thuringer cervelat), 2 slices	4
Rosina	
Sausage meatballs, 6	7

Turkey
Boar's Head

All natural roasted turkey breast, 2 oz	1
All natural smoked turkey breast, 2 oz	1
All natural Tuscan style turkey breast, 2 oz	1
Baby maple glazed honey coat turkey, 2 oz	1
Cracked pepper mill smoked turkey breast, 2 oz	1
Deli dinners ovengold turkey, 3 oz	2
Golden catering style oven roasted skinless turkey breast, 2 oz	1
Hickory smoked black forest turkey breast - 43% lower sodium, 2 oz	1
Maple glazed honey coat cured turkey breast, 2 oz	1
Our premium 47% lower sodium turkey breast - skinless, 2 oz	1
Our premium 50% lower sodium turkey breast - skin on, 2 oz	1
Ovengold roast breast of turkey, 2 oz	1
Ovengold roast breast of turkey - skin-on, 2 oz	1
Salsalito roasted breast of turkey, 2 oz	1

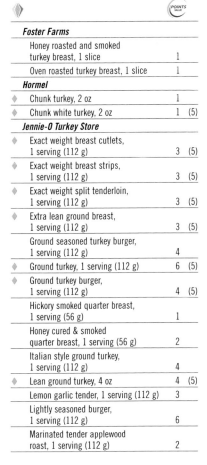

	POINTS VALUE	
Foster Farms		
Honey roasted and smoked turkey breast, 1 slice	1	
Oven roasted turkey breast, 1 slice	1	
Hormel		
Chunk turkey, 2 oz	1	
Chunk white turkey, 2 oz	1	(5)
Jennie-O Turkey Store		
Exact weight breast cutlets, 1 serving (112 g)	3	(5)
Exact weight breast strips, 1 serving (112 g)	3	(5)
Exact weight split tenderloin, 1 serving (112 g)	3	(5)
Extra lean ground breast, 1 serving (112 g)	3	(5)
Ground seasoned turkey burger, 1 serving (112 g)	4	
Ground turkey, 1 serving (112 g)	6	(5)
Ground turkey burger, 1 serving (112 g)	4	(5)
Hickory smoked quarter breast, 1 serving (56 g)	1	
Honey cured & smoked quarter breast, 1 serving (56 g)	2	
Italian style ground turkey, 1 serving (112 g)	4	
Lean ground turkey, 4 oz	4	(5)
Lemon garlic tender, 1 serving (112 g)	3	
Lightly seasoned burger, 1 serving (112 g)	6	
Marinated tender applewood roast, 1 serving (112 g)	2	

	POINTS VALUE	
Marinated tender roast turkey, 1 serving (112 g)	2	
Oven ready bone in breast homestyle, 1 serving (112 g)	3	(5)
Oven ready whole turkey homestyle, 1 serving (112 g)	4	(5)
Oven roasted quarter breast, 1 serving (56 g)	2	(5)
Premium 1/3 pound white turkey, 1 serving (149 g)	6	(5)
Savory seasoned turkey burger, 1 serving (112 g)	4	
Seasoned pepper tender, 1 serving (112 g)	2	
Tequila lime tender, 1 serving (112 g)	2	
Teriyaki tenderloin, 1 serving (112 g)	3	
Turkey breakfast sausage links, 2 (56 g)	4	
Turkey breast tenderloins, 4 oz	2	(5)
Turkey burger, 1 serving (112 g)	4	(5)
Turkey ham, 1 serving (56 g)	2	
Turkey pastrami, 1 serving (56 g)	2	
Jennie-O Turkey Store So Easy		
Cheddar broccoli stuffed turkey breast, 1 serving (168 g)	5	
Slices - homestyle, 1 serving (140 g)	2	
So easy breast roast - homestyle, 1 serving (140 g)	2	
Swiss cheese & ham stuffed turkey breast, 1 serving (168 g)	6	
Traditional herb stuffing stuffed turkey breast, 1 serving (168 g)	6	
White pepper & rice stuffed turkey breast, 1 serving (168 g)	6	

Meat & Poultry

	POINTS VALUE
Louis Rich	
Oven roasted turkey breast, 3 slices	1
Turkey breast & white turkey, oven roasted, 2 slices	1
Turkey patties, white, 1	5
Market Day	
Turkey breast roast, 4 oz	3
Oscar Mayer	
Oven roasted turkey breast, 3 slices	1
Smoked turkey breast, 3 slices	1
Wampler Foods	
Skinless boneless turkey breast roast, 4 oz	3

Other Meats

	POINTS VALUE
Armour Healthy Ones	
Beef franks, 1	1
Ball Park	
Beef fat free franks, 1	1
Beef lite franks, 1	3
Meat fat free franks, 1	1
Meat lite franks, 1	3
Smoke white turkey franks, 1	1
Boar's Head	
All natural salame with white wine, 1 oz	2
Beef frankfurters - skinless, 1	3
Lite beef frankfurters, natural casing, 1	2
Pork & beef frankfurter giants, natural casing, 1	4
Pork & beef frankfurter, skinless, 1	4

	POINTS VALUE
Fluky's	
No fat beef polish, 1 link	2
Foster Farms	
Chicken franks, 1	3
Turkey franks, 1	3
Hebrew National	
97% fat free beef franks, 1	1
Beef franks, 1	4
Jumbo beef franks, 1	7
Quarter pound beef franks, 1	10
Reduced fat beef franks, 1	3
Hormel	
Beef hot dog, 1	5
Cocktail smokies beef, 6	5
Smokies, 1	2
Smokies with cheese, 1	2
Ian's	
Wheat free, gluten free popcorn turkey corn dog, 1	6
Jennie-O Turkey Store	
Turkey wiener, 1	2
Louis Rich	
Bun-length brand turkey franks, 1 link	3
Turkey franks, 1 serving	3
Muirhead	
Green tomato mincemeat, 1 Tbsp	1
Oscar Mayer	
98% fat free wieners made with turkey, 1	1
Cheese hot dogs, made with pork, turkey & chicken, 1	4

	POINTS VALUE
Cheese turkey franks, 1	3
Deli style beef franks, 1	6
Fast franks beef frank with bun, 1	7
Fast franks wiener made with turkey, pork & chicken with bun, 1	7
Fat free wieners made with turkey & beef, 1	1
Franks, beef, 1	4
Franks, beef jumbo, 1	5
Franks, beef, bun-length, 1	5
Franks, beef, light, 1	2
Hot & spicy hot dogs, 1	6
Natural beef franks, 1	4
Premium beef franks, 1	6
Smoked hot dogs, 1	7

	POINTS VALUE
Smokies course ground wieners, 1	4
Turkey frank, 1	3
Wieners, bun-length, made with turkey & pork, 1	5
Wieners, jumbo, made with turkey & pork, 1	5
Wieners, light, made with turkey & pork, 1	2
Wieners, little, made with turkey & pork, 6	5
Wieners, made with turkey & pork, 1	4
Wranglers	
Beef franks, 1	5
Cheese franks, 1	5
Smoked franks, 1	5

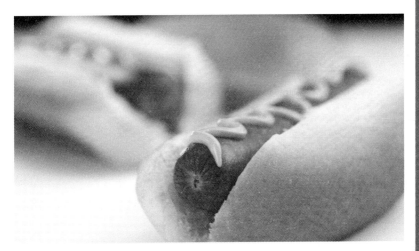

Oils, Dressings & Seasonings

	POINTS VALUE
Cooking Spray	
Gourmé Mist	
Extra virgin olive oil, 1 second spray	0
Organic canola oil, 1 second spray	0
Organic extra virgin olive oil, 1 second spray	0
I Can't Believe It's Not Butter!	
Buttery spray, 1 Tbsp	3
Kernel Season's Gourmet Popcorn Seasoning	
Butter flavored spritzer, 1/3 second spray	0
Manischewitz	
Olive oil cooking spray, 1/3 second spray	0
Olive oil cooking spray, garlic flavored, 1/3 second spray	0
PAM	
Cooking spray, 1/3 second spray	0
Parkay	
Original spray, 1 serving 1 spray	0
Smart Balance	
Buttery burst spray, 1 serving (1 g)	0
Non-stick cooking spray, 1 second spray	0
Spectrum Naturals	
Canola oil with butter flavor, spray, 1/3 second spray	0
Canola oil, baking spray with flour, 1/3 second spray	0
Canola oil, high heat, spray, 1/3 second spray	0

	POINTS VALUE
Grapeseed oil, spray, 1/3 second spray	0
Olive oil, extra virgin, spray, 1/3 second spray	0
Olive oil, organic, extra virgin, spray, 1/3 second spray	0
Sunflower oil, organic, high heat spray, 1/3 second spray	0
Oils	
Bertolli	
Classico olive oil, 1 Tbsp	4
Extra light tasting olive oil, 1 Tbsp	4
Extra virgin olive oil, 1 Tbsp	4
Carapelli	
Extra virgin olive oil, 1 Tbsp	4
Grapeseed oil, 1 Tbsp	4
Light olive oil, 1 Tbsp	4
Mild olive oil, 1 Tbsp	4
Premium extra virgin olive oil, 1 Tbsp	4
Consorzio All Natural	
Basil flavored olive oil, 1 Tbsp	4
Dipping oil, herb flavored olive oil and balsamic vinegar, 1 Tbsp	3
Roasted garlic flavored extra virgin olive oil, 1 Tbsp	4
Roasted pepper flavored olive oil, 1 Tbsp	4
Eden Organic	
Safflower oil, 1 Tbsp	4
Soybean oil, 1 Tbsp	4
Toasted sesame oil - imported, 1 Tbsp	4

	POINTS VALUE
Eden Selected	
Extra virgin olive oil, 1 Tbsp	4
Hot pepper sesame oil, 1 Tbsp	4
Toasted sesame oil, 1 Tbsp	4
Enova	
Cooking & salad oil, 1 Tbsp	4
Faraon	
Olive oil, 1 Tbsp	4
Filippo Berio	
Extra light olive oil, 1 Tbsp	4
Extra virgin olive oil, 1 Tbsp	4
Pure olive oil, 1 Tbsp	4
Hain Pure Foods	
Almond oil, 1 Tbsp	4
Avocado oil, 1 Tbsp	4
Canola oil, 1 Tbsp	4
Extra virgin olive oil, 1 Tbsp	4
Garlic oil, 1 Tbsp	4
Peanut oil, 1 Tbsp	4
Safflower oil, 1 Tbsp	4
Sesame oil, 1 Tbsp	4
Soybean oil, 1 Tbsp	3
Sunflower oil, 1 Tbsp	4
Walnut oil, 1 Tbsp	4
House of Tsang	
Hot chili sesame oil, 1 tsp	1
Mongolian fire oil, 1 tsp	1
Pure sesame oil, 1 tsp	1
Wok oil, 1 Tbsp	4
Kernel Season's Gourmet Popcorn Seasoning	
Popping oil, 1 Tbsp	4

	POINTS VALUE
Lucini	
Delicate lemon extra virgin olive oil, 1 Tbsp	4
Fiery chili extra virgin olive oil, 1 Tbsp	4
Robust garlic extra virgin olive oil, 1 Tbsp	4
Tuscan basil extra virgin olive oil, 1 Tbsp	4
Manischewitz	
Vegetable oil, 1 Tbsp	4
Milpas	
Corn oil, 2 tsp	3
Planters	
Peanut oil, 1 Tbsp	4
PurOliva	
Puroliva, 2 tsp	2
Smart Balance	
Omega oil, 1 Tbsp	4
Spectrum Naturals	
Almond oil, refined, 1 Tbsp	4
Apricot kernel oil, refined, 1 Tbsp	4
Avocado oil, refined, 1 Tbsp	4
Canola oil, high heat, refined, 1 Tbsp	4
Canola oil, organic, refined, 1 Tbsp	4
Canola oil, refined, 1 Tbsp	4
Coconut oil, organic, refined, 1 Tbsp	4
Coconut oil, organic, unrefined, 1 Tbsp	4
Corn oil, unrefined, 1 Tbsp	4
Grapeseed oil, refined, 1 Tbsp	4
Olive oil, extra virgin, unrefined, 1 Tbsp	4
Olive oil, extra virgin, unrefined, Greek, 1 Tbsp	4

Oils, Dressings & Seasonings

Spectrum Naturals (cont'd)	POINTS VALUE
Olive oil, organic, extra virgin, Moroccan, wild harvest, 1 Tbsp	4
Olive oil, organic, extra virgin, unrefined, 1 Tbsp	4
Olive oil, organic, extra virgin, unrefined, California, 1 Tbsp	4
Olive oil, organic, extra virgin, unrefined, Italian, 1 Tbsp	4
Olive oil, organic, extra virgin, unrefined, Mediterranean, 1 Tbsp	4
Olive oil, organic, extra virgin, unrefined, Spanish Arbequina, 1 Tbsp	4
Peanut oil, unrefined, 1 Tbsp	4
Safflower oil, high heat, refined, 1 Tbsp	4
Safflower oil, organic, high heat, refined, 1 Tbsp	4
Sesame oil, organic, unrefined, 1 Tbsp	4
Sesame oil, refined, 1 Tbsp	4
Sesame oil, toasted, organic, unrefined, 1 Tbsp	4
Sesame oil, toasted, unrefined, 1 Tbsp	4
Sesame oil, unrefined, 1 Tbsp	4
Soy oil, organic, refined, 1 Tbsp	4
Sunflower oil, organic, high heat, refined, 1 Tbsp	4
Walnut oil, refined, 1 Tbsp	4
Sunsweet	
Lighter bake butter & oil replacement, 1 Tbsp	1
Tree of Life	
Almond oil, 1 Tbsp	4
Avocado oil, 1 Tbsp	4

	POINTS VALUE
Macadamia nut oil, 1 Tbsp	4
Organic coconut oil, expeller pressed, 1 Tbsp	4
Organic extra virgin olive oil, 1 Tbsp	4
Sesame oil, 1 Tbsp	4
Walnut oil, 1 Tbsp	4

Salad Dressings

A Taste of Thai

Peanut salad dressing mix, 2 Tbsp	1

Annie's Naturals

Artichoke parmesan, 2 Tbsp	4
Balsamic vinaigrette, 2 Tbsp	3
Caesar, 2 Tbsp	3
Cowgirl ranch, 2 Tbsp	3
Goddess, 2 Tbsp	4
Lemon & chive, 2 Tbsp	4
Light Italian, 2 Tbsp	1
Low fat gingerly vinaigrette, 2 Tbsp	1
Low fat honey mustard vinaigrette, 2 Tbsp	1
Low fat raspberry vinaigrette, 2 Tbsp	1
Organic Asian sesame, 2 Tbsp	4
Organic balsamic vinaigrette, 2 Tbsp	3
Organic bbq sweet and spicy, 2 Tbsp	1
Organic buttermilk, 2 Tbsp	2
Organic Caesar, 2 Tbsp	3
Organic cowgirl ranch, 2 Tbsp	3
Organic creamy asiago cheese, 2 Tbsp	2
Organic cucumber yogurt, 2 Tbsp	2
Organic French, 2 Tbsp	3
Organic goddess, 2 Tbsp	4

Oils, Dressings & Seasonings

	POINTS VALUE
Organic green garlic, 2 Tbsp	3
Organic green goddess, 2 Tbsp	4
Organic oil & vinegar, 2 Tbsp	4
Organic papaya poppyseed, 2 Tbsp	4
Organic pomegranate vinaigrette, 2 Tbsp	2
Organic red wine & olive oil, 2 Tbsp	5
Organic roasted garlic vinaigrette, 2 Tbsp	3
Organic sesame ginger with chamomile, 2 Tbsp	3
Organic shiitake and sesame vinaigrette, 2 Tbsp	3
Organic shiitake and sesame vinaigrette, 2 Tbsp	3
Organic thousand island, 2 Tbsp	2
Roasted red pepper, 2 Tbsp	2
Tuscany Italian, 2 Tbsp	2
Woodstock, 2 Tbsp	3
Consorzio	
Balsamic Vinaigrette dressing, 2 Tbsp	2
Mango fat-free dressing & marinade, 1 Tbsp	0
Raspberry & balsamic fat-free dressing, 1 Tbsp	0
Strawberry & balsamic fat-free dressing, 1 Tbsp	0
Earth Island Canada	
Organic creamy ranch dressing, 2 Tbsp	3
Ellen Rose	
Caesar dressing, 2 Tbsp	4
Herb vinaigrette, 2 Tbsp	6

	POINTS VALUE
Lowfat orange ginger dressing, 2 Tbsp	0
Oriental dressing, 2 Tbsp	5
Raspberry vinaigrette, 2 Tbsp	5
Emeril's	
Bacon vinaigrette, 2 Tbsp	3
Bleu cheese, 2 Tbsp	3
Caesar, 2 Tbsp	4
Honey mustard, 2 Tbsp	3
House herb vinaigrette, 2 Tbsp	3
Kicked up French, 2 Tbsp	2
Romano, 2 Tbsp	3
Follow Your Heart	
Creamy garlic dressing, 2 Tbsp	4
Grapeseed oil vegenaise, 1 Tbsp	3
High omega-3 vegenaise, 1 Tbsp	3
Low fat ranch dressing, 2 Tbsp	1
Organic balsamic vinaigrette dressing, 2 Tbsp	1
Organic chipotle-lime ranch dressing, 2 Tbsp	3
Organic chunky bleu cheese dressing, 2 Tbsp	3
Organic creamy Caesar dressing, 2 Tbsp	3
Organic creamy miso ginger dressing, 2 Tbsp	2
Organic creamy ranch dressing, 2 Tbsp	3
Organic Italian vinaigrette dressing, 2 Tbsp	3
Original vegenaise, 1 Tbsp	3
Reduced fat vegenaise with flaxseed & olive oil, 1 Tbsp	1

Oils, Dressings & Seasonings

Follow Your Heart (cont'd)	POINTS VALUE
Sesame dijon dressing, 2 Tbsp	3
Sesame miso dressing, 2 Tbsp	2
Southwestern ranch dressing, 2 Tbsp	2
Thousand island dressing, 2 Tbsp	2
Unforgettables low fat balsamic vinaigrette sauce, 2 Tbsp	1
Unforgettables original balsamic vinaigrette sauce, 2 Tbsp	4
Vegan Caesar dressing, 2 Tbsp	2
Vegan honey mustard dressing, 2 Tbsp	3
Good Seasons	
Asian sesame, prepared, 2 Tbsp	4
Asian sesame mix, 1 serving 1/8 of envelope	0
Asian sesame with ginger, 2 Tbsp	3
Basil vinaigrette, prepared, 2 Tbsp	4
Basil vinaigrette mix, 1/8 envelope	0
Cheese garlic, prepared, 2 Tbsp	4
Cheese garlic dry mix, 1/8 envelope	0
Classic balsamic vinaigrette with extra virgin olive oil, 2 Tbsp	2
Creamy Caesar with aged parmesan, 2 Tbsp	3
Fat free Italian, prepared, 2 Tbsp	0
Fat free Italian dry mix, 1/8 envelope	0
Garlic & herb, prepared, 2 Tbsp	4
Garlic and herb dry mix, 1/8 envelope	0
Gourmet Caesar, prepared, 2 Tbsp	4
Gourmet Caesar dry mix, 1/8 envelope	0
Gourmet parmesan Italian, prepared, 2 Tbsp	4
Gourmet parmesan Italian dry mix, 1/8 envelope	0

	POINTS VALUE
Italian dry mix, 1/8 envelope	0
Italian, prepared, 2 Tbsp	4
Italian vinaigrette with extra virgin olive oil, 2 Tbsp	2
Light Greek vinaigrette with oregano & athenos feta cheese, 2 Tbsp	1
Light honey dijon, 2 Tbsp	1
Light red raspberry vinaigrette with poppyseed, 2 Tbsp	2
Mild Italian dry mix, 1/8 envelope	0
Mild Italian, prepared, 2 Tbsp	4
Roasted garlic, prepared, 2 Tbsp	4
Roasted garlic dry mix, 1/8 envelope	0
Sun dried tomato vinaigrette with roasted red pepper, 2 Tbsp	2
Zesty Italian, prepared, 2 Tbsp	4
Zesty Italian dry mix, 1/8 envelope	0
Heinz	
Creamy Italian, 1 oz	3
Italian, 1 oz	3
Thousand island, 1 oz	4
Henri's	
Fat free French, 2 Tbsp	1
Fat free honey mustard, 2 Tbsp	1
Hidden Valley	
Bacon Ranch, 2 Tbsp	4
Buttermilk recipe original ranch, prepared from mix, 2 Tbsp 1 fl oz	3
Caesar with crushed garlic, 2 Tbsp	3
Coleslaw dressing, 2 Tbsp	4
Fat free ranch, 2 Tbsp	1
Garden vegetable, 2 Tbsp	4

	POINTS VALUE
Light original ranch, 2 Tbsp 1 fl oz	2
Light original ranch with sour cream, 2 Tbsp	2
Milk recipe original ranch, prepared from mix, 2 Tbsp 1 fl oz	3
Original ranch, 2 Tbsp	4

Kraft

	POINTS VALUE
Asian toasted sesame, 2 Tbsp	2
Blue cheese ranch, 2 Tbsp	4
Buttermilk ranch dressing, 2 Tbsp	3
Caesar ranch, 2 Tbsp	3
Caesar with bacon, 2 Tbsp	3
Catalina, 2 Tbsp	3
Cilantro flavored pepper ranch, 2 Tbsp	3
Classic Caesar, 2 Tbsp	3
Coleslaw, 2 Tbsp	3
Coleslaw maker, 2 Tbsp	3
Creamy French, 2 Tbsp	4
Creamy garlic, 2 Tbsp	3
Creamy Italian, 2 Tbsp	3
Cucumber ranch, 2 Tbsp	3
French style fat free salad dressing, 1 serving	1
Garlic ranch, 2 Tbsp	3
House Italian, 2 Tbsp	2
Peppercorn ranch, 2 Tbsp	3
Ranch, 2 Tbsp	3
Ranch with bacon, 2 Tbsp	3
Roasted red pepper Italian with parmesan, 2 Tbsp	1
Roka blue cheese, 2 Tbsp	3
Russian, 2 Tbsp	3
Sour cream & onion ranch, 2 Tbsp	3
Thousand island, 2 Tbsp	2
Thousand island with bacon, 2 Tbsp	3
Three cheese Italian, 2 Tbsp	4
Three cheese ranch, 2 Tbsp	3
Tuna salad maker super easy squeeze, 1 Tbsp	1
Zesty Italian, 2 Tbsp	2

Kraft Carb Well

	POINTS VALUE
Classic Caesar, 2 Tbsp	3
Italian, 2 Tbsp	2
Ranch, 2 Tbsp	3
Roka blue cheese, 2 Tbsp	3

Kraft Free

	POINTS VALUE
Blue cheese flavored, 2 Tbsp	1
Caesar Italian, 2 Tbsp	1
Catalina, 2 Tbsp	1
Classic Caesar, 2 Tbsp	1
Creamy Italian, 2 Tbsp	1
French style, 2 Tbsp	1
Honey dijon, 2 Tbsp	1
Italian, 2 Tbsp	0
Peppercorn ranch, 2 Tbsp	1
Ranch, 2 Tbsp	1
Sour cream & onion ranch, 2 Tbsp	1
Thousand island, 2 Tbsp	1
Zesty Italian, 2 Tbsp	0

Kraft Light Done Right

	POINTS VALUE
Asian toasted sesame, 2 Tbsp	1
Balsamic vinaigrette, 2 Tbsp	1
Catalina, 2 Tbsp	1

Oils, Dressings & Seasonings

Kraft Light Done Right (cont'd)	POINTS VALUE
Classic Caesar, 2 Tbsp	2
Creamy French, 2 Tbsp	2
Cucumber ranch, 2 Tbsp	1
Golden Caesar, 2 Tbsp	2
House Italian, 2 Tbsp	1
Ranch, 2 Tbsp	2
Raspberry vinaigrette, 2 Tbsp	2
Red wine vinaigrette, 2 Tbsp	1
Roka bleu cheese salad dressing, 1 serving	2
Thousand island, 2 Tbsp	1
Three cheese ranch, 2 Tbsp	2
Zesty Italian, 2 Tbsp	1
Kraft Miracle Whip	
Dressing, 1 Tbsp	1
Dressing, hot & spicy, 1 serving	1
Fat free dressing, 1 Tbsp	0
Light dressing, 1 Tbsp	1
Kraft Special Collections	
Caesar Italian with oregano, 2 Tbsp	3
Caesar vinaigrette with parmesan, 2 Tbsp	2
Classic Italian vinaigrette, 2 Tbsp	1
Creamy poppyseed, 2 Tbsp	3
Greek vinaigrette, 2 Tbsp	3
Italian pesto vinaigrette, 2 Tbsp	2
Parmesan Italian with basil, 2 Tbsp	3
Parmesan romano, 2 Tbsp	4
Roasted garlic vinaigrette, 1 serving	1
Sun dried tomato, 2 Tbsp	2
Sweet honey catalina, 2 Tbsp	4
Tangy tomato bacon, 2 Tbsp	3

	POINTS VALUE
Litehouse	
Bacon bleu cheese, 2 Tbsp	4
Balsamic vinaigrette, 2 Tbsp	3
Barbecue ranch, 2 Tbsp	3
Bleu cheese vinaigrette, 2 Tbsp	2
Buttermilk ranch dressing, 2 Tbsp	3
Caesar Caesar, 2 Tbsp	4
Chunky bleu cheese, 2 Tbsp	4
Coleslaw, 2 Tbsp	3
Coleslaw with pineapple, 2 Tbsp	3
Creamy Asian, 2 Tbsp	4
Creamy cilantro, 2 Tbsp	3
Garlic vinaigrette, 2 Tbsp	3
Harvest cranberry vinaigrette, 2 Tbsp	1
Homestyle ranch, 2 Tbsp	3
Honey mustard, 2 Tbsp	4
Huckleberry vinaigrette, 2 Tbsp	1
Jalapeno ranch, 2 Tbsp	3
Lite 1000 island, 2 Tbsp	2
Lite bleu cheese, 2 Tbsp	2
Lite Caesar, 2 Tbsp	2
Lite coleslaw dressing, 2 Tbsp	2
Lite honey dijon vinaigrette, 2 Tbsp	2
Lite ranch, 2 Tbsp	2
Original bleu cheese, 2 Tbsp	4
Original thousand island, 2 Tbsp	4
Pomegranate blueberry vinaigrette, 2 Tbsp	1
Poppyseed, 2 Tbsp	4
Ranch, 2 Tbsp	3
Ranch vinaigrette, 2 Tbsp	3

	POINTS VALUE
Raspberry walnut vinaigrette, 2 Tbsp	3
Red wine olive oil vinaigrette, 2 Tbsp	3
Roquefort, 2 Tbsp	2
Salsa ranch, 2 Tbsp	2
Sesame ginger, 2 Tbsp	1
Soy ginger, 2 Tbsp	3
Spinach salad, 2 Tbsp	1
Sweet French, 2 Tbsp	2
Tangy orange citrus, 2 Tbsp	1
Thai peanut vinaigrette, 2 Tbsp	1
Ultimate premium big bleu, 2 Tbsp	5
Zesty Italian vinaigrette, 2 Tbsp	2
Litehouse Organic	
Balsamic, 2 Tbsp	3
Caesar, 2 Tbsp	3
Ranch, 2 Tbsp	4
Raspberry lime, 2 Tbsp	1
Lucini	
Bold parmesan & garlic, 2 Tbsp	4
Cherry balsamic & rosemary, 2 Tbsp	3
Delicate cucumber & shallot, 2 Tbsp	3
Fig & walnut savory balsamic, 2 Tbsp	3
Roasted hazelnut & extra virgin, 2 Tbsp	3
Tuscan balsamic & extra virgin, 2 Tbsp	3
Maple Grove	
Asiago dressing, 2 Tbsp	1
Blueberry pomegranate vinaigrette, 2 Tbsp	2
Champagne vinaigrette, 2 Tbsp	3
Fat free balsamic vinaigrette, 2 Tbsp	0
Fat free Caesar dressing, 2 Tbsp	0
Fat free cranberry balsamic vinaigrette, 2 Tbsp	0

	POINTS VALUE
Fat free Greek dressing, 2 Tbsp	0
Fat free honey dijon dressing, 2 Tbsp	1
Fat free lime basil vinaigrette, 2 Tbsp	1
Fat free poppyseed dressing, 2 Tbsp	1
Fat free raspberry vinaigrette, 2 Tbsp	1
Fat free vidalia dressing, 2 Tbsp	0
Fat free wasabi dijon dressing, 2 Tbsp	1
Ginger pear vinaigrette, 2 Tbsp	2
Maple fig vinaigrette, 2 Tbsp	1
Organic balsamic vinaigrette dressing, 2 Tbsp	0
Organic dijon vinaigrette dressing, 2 Tbsp	1
Organic Italian herb dressing, 2 Tbsp	1
Organic mandarin sesame dressing, 2 Tbsp	1
Organic raspberry vinaigrette dressing, 2 Tbsp	1
Sesame ginger, 2 Tbsp	1
Strawberry balsamic, 2 Tbsp	1
Sugar free bacon vinaigrette dressing, 2 Tbsp	3
Sugar free balsamic vinaigrette dressing, 2 Tbsp	0
Sugar free dijon dressing, 2 Tbsp	2
Sugar free Italian with balsamic dressing, 2 Tbsp	3
Sugar free ranch, 2 Tbsp	4
Sugar free raspberry vinaigrette, 2 Tbsp	0
Marzetti	
Aged parmesan ranch dressing, 2 Tbsp	4
Asiago peppercorn dressing, 2 Tbsp	4

Oils, Dressings & Seasonings

Marzetti (cont'd)	POINTS VALUE
Balsamic vinaigrette dressing, 2 Tbsp	3
Blue cheese Italian dressing, 2 Tbsp	4
Caesar Dressing, 2 Tbsp	3
California French dressing, 2 Tbsp	4
Country French dressing, 2 Tbsp	4
Cracked peppercorn vinaigrette, 2 Tbsp	4
Creamy Caesar dressing, 2 Tbsp	5
Creamy Italian dressing with peppercorns, 2 Tbsp	4
Fat free honey dijon dressing, 2 Tbsp	1
Fat free Italian, dressing, 2 Tbsp	0
Fat free sweet & sour dressing, 2 Tbsp	1
Honey balsamic dressing, 2 Tbsp	3
Honey dijon dressing, 2 Tbsp	4
House Italian dressing, 2 Tbsp	3
Italian dressing, 2 Tbsp	3
Light balsamic vinaigrette dressing, 2 Tbsp	1
Light slaw dressing, 2 Tbsp	3
Lowfat cole slaw dressing, 2 Tbsp	1
Poppyseed dressing, 2 Tbsp	4
Potato salad dressing, 2 Tbsp	4
Ranch dressing, 2 Tbsp	4
Sesame ginger dressing, 2 Tbsp	3
Slaw dressing, 2 Tbsp	4
Southern recipe slaw dressing, 2 Tbsp	4
Strawberry vinaigrette, 2 Tbsp	3
Sweet and sour dressing, 2 Tbsp	4
Sweet vidalia onion dressing, 2 Tbsp	4
Thousand island dressing, 2 Tbsp	4
Venice Italian dressing, 2 Tbsp	3

Marzetti Refrigerated	POINTS VALUE
Asiago peppercorn dressing, 2 Tbsp	5
Asian ginger dressing, 2 Tbsp	3
Bistro blue cheese dressing, 2 Tbsp	5
Buttermilk ranch dressing, 2 Tbsp	5
Caesar dressing, 2 Tbsp	4
Chunky blue cheese dressing, 2 Tbsp	4
French blue cheese dressing, 2 Tbsp	4
Honey balsamic dressing, 2 Tbsp	3
Honey French dressing, 2 Tbsp	5
Honey mustard dressing, 2 Tbsp	4
Light ancho chipotle ranch dressing, 2 Tbsp	2
Light berry balsamic vinaigrette dressing, 2 Tbsp	1
Light blue cheese dressing, 2 Tbsp	2
Light Caesar dressing, 2 Tbsp	2
Light citrus poppyseed dressing, 2 Tbsp	2
Light honey dijon dressing, 2 Tbsp	2
Light honey French dressing, 2 Tbsp	2
Light ranch dressing, 2 Tbsp	2
Light raspberry cabernet vinaigrette, 2 Tbsp	1
Light slaw dressing, 2 Tbsp	2
Poppyseed dressing, 2 Tbsp	4
Roasted garlic Italian vinaigrette dressing, 2 Tbsp	3
Slaw dressing, 2 Tbsp	4
Spinach salad dressing, 2 Tbsp	2
Strawberry chardonnay vinaigrette, 2 Tbsp	3

Oils, Dressings & Seasonings

	POINTS VALUE
Sweet Italian dressing, 2 Tbsp	4
Thai peanut dressing, 2 Tbsp	4
Thousand island dressing, 2 Tbsp	4
Ultimate blue cheese dressing, 2 Tbsp	5
Ultimate gorgonzola dressing, 2 Tbsp	4
Vinaigrette blue cheese crumbles dressing, 2 Tbsp	3
White balsamic vinaigrette, 2 Tbsp	3

Muirhead

Balsamic vinaigrette, 1 Tbsp	3
Hazel's sweet and sour dressing, 1 Tbsp	1
Herbes de provence vinaigrette, 1 Tbsp	3
Pomegranate vinaigrette, 1 Tbsp	3

Naturally Fresh

Apple cranberry walnut dressing, 2 Tbsp	1
Bacon bleu cheese dressing, 1 Tbsp	5
Bleu cheese vinaigrette, 2 Tbsp	2
Buffalo ranch dressing, 2 Tbsp	3
Caesar dressing, 2 Tbsp	3
Classic bleu cheese dressing, 2 Tbsp	4
Classic Caesar dressing, 2 Tbsp	5
Classic oriental dressing, 2 Tbsp	4
Classic ranch dressing, 2 Tbsp	4
Creamy cilantro dressing, 2 Tbsp	4
Fat-free balsamic vinaigrette, 2 Tbsp	0
Fat-free raspberry vinaigrette, 2 Tbsp	1
Ginger dressing, 2 Tbsp	2
Honey French dressing, 2 Tbsp	3
Honey mustard dressing, 2 Tbsp	4
Jalapeno ranch dressing, 2 Tbsp	3

	POINTS VALUE
Lite bleu cheese dressing, 2 Tbsp	3
Lite peppercorn ranch dressing, 2 Tbsp	2
Lite ranch dressing with msg, 2 Tbsp	2
Mandarin ginger dressing, 2 Tbsp	0
Mixed berry dressing, 2 Tbsp	1
Organic aged balsamic & olive oil vinaigrette, 2 Tbsp	3
Organic Greek feta dressing, 2 Tbsp	3
Organic orange miso dressing, 2 Tbsp	3
Organic peppercorn ranch dressing, 2 Tbsp	3
Organic raspberry vinaigrette, 2 Tbsp	1
Organic sundried tomato and garlic dressing, 2 Tbsp	3
Organic white balsamic vinaigrette, 2 Tbsp	3
Pomango dressing, 2 Tbsp	1
Poppy seed dressing, 2 Tbsp	4
Roasted garlic bleu cheese dressing, 2 Tbsp	5
Slaw dressing, 2 Tbsp	3
Southwestern style ranch dressing, 2 Tbsp	3
Thousand island dressing, 2 Tbsp	4
Wine & cheese dressing, 2 Tbsp	4
Zesty bleu cheese dressing, 2 Tbsp	5

Naturally Fresh Refrigerated

Bleu cheese dressing, all natural, 2 Tbsp	5
Cranberry orange fruit glaze seasonal, 2 Tbsp	1
Cranberry walnut dressing seasonal, 2 Tbsp	3

Oils, Dressings & Seasonings

	POINTS VALUE
Onai's Fresh Miso	
Ginger dressing, 2 Tbsp	1
Original dressing, 2 Tbsp	1
Shiitake sesame dressing, 2 Tbsp	1
Wasabi ginger dressing, 2 Tbsp	1
Regina	
Raspberry balsamic, 1 Tbsp	0
San-J	
Tamari ginger dressing, 2 Tbsp	1
Tamari mustard, 2 Tbsp	1
Tamari peanut, 2 Tbsp	1
Tamari sesame, 2 Tbsp	1
San-J Canada	
Tamari ginger dressing, 2 Tbsp	1
Tamari peanut dressing, 2 Tbsp	1
Tamari sesame dressing, 2 Tbsp	1
Seven Seas	
Creamy Italian, 2 Tbsp	3
Green goddess, 2 Tbsp	4
Red wine vinaigrette, 2 Tbsp	3
Viva Italian, 2 Tbsp	3
Viva robust Italian, 2 Tbsp	3
Seven Seas Free	
Red wine vinaigrette, 2 Tbsp	0
Viva Italian, 2 Tbsp	0
Seven Seas Reduced Fat	
Red wine vinaigrette & oil, 2 Tbsp	1
Viva Italian, 2 Tbsp	1

	POINTS VALUE
Spectrum Naturals	
Omega-3 Asian ginger, organic, 2 Tbsp	4
Omega-3 creamy garlic ranch, organic, 2 Tbsp	3
Omega-3 golden balsamic, organic, 2 Tbsp	3
Omega-3 lemon sesame, organic, 2 Tbsp	4
Omega-3 pomegranate chipotle, organic, 2 Tbsp	4
Omega-3 shiitake sesame, organic, 2 Tbsp	3
Omega-3 vegan Caesar, organic, 2 Tbsp	3
Spin Blend	
Classic, 1 Tbsp	1
Light, 1 Tbsp	1
Walden Farms	
Asian, 2 Tbsp	0
Bacon ranch, 2 Tbsp	0
Balsamic, 2 Tbsp	0
Bleu cheese, 2 Tbsp	0
Caesar, 2 Tbsp	0
Coleslaw mix, 2 Tbsp	0
Creamy bacon, 2 Tbsp	0
French, 2 Tbsp	0
Honey dijon, 2 Tbsp	0
Italian, 2 Tbsp	0
Italian creamy, 2 Tbsp	0
Italian with sun dried tomatoes, 2 Tbsp	0

	POINTS VALUE
Italian zesty, 2 Tbsp	0
Mayo, 1 Tbsp	0
Ranch, 2 Tbsp	0
Ranch, 1 packet	0
Raspberry, 2 Tbsp	0
Russian, 2 Tbsp	0
Sweet onion, 2 Tbsp	0
Thousand island, 2 Tbsp	0
Wish-Bone	
Balsamic basil light, 2 Tbsp	2
Balsamic breeze spritzer, 10 sprays	0
Balsamic Italian vinaigrette, 2 Tbsp	2
Balsamic vinaigrette, 2 Tbsp	1
Berry vinaigrette, 2 Tbsp	1
Blue cheese, 2 Tbsp	4
Cheese Italian, 2 Tbsp	3
Chunky blue cheese, 2 Tbsp	4
Creamy Caesar, 2 Tbsp	5
Creamy Italian, 2 Tbsp	3
Deluxe French, 2 Tbsp	3
Garlic ranch, 2 Tbsp	4
Honey dijon vinaigrette, 2 Tbsp	2
House Italian, 2 Tbsp	3
Italian, 2 Tbsp	2
Italian vinaigrette spritzer, 10 sprays	0
Lemon garlic herb, 2 Tbsp	2
Olive oil vinaigrette, 2 Tbsp	2
Ranch, 2 Tbsp	3
Raspberry hazelnut vinaigrette, 2 Tbsp	2
Raspberry walnut light, 2 Tbsp	2
Red wine mist spritzer, 10 sprays	0
Red wine vinaigrette, 2 Tbsp	2

	POINTS VALUE
Robusto Italian, 2 Tbsp	2
Romano basil vinaigrette, 2 Tbsp	2
Russian, 2 Tbsp	2
Sesame ginger light, 2 Tbsp	2
Skippy natural, 2 Tbsp	5
Spring onion ranch, 2 Tbsp	4
Sweet and spicy French, 2 Tbsp	4
Thousand island, 2 Tbsp	4
Western creamy French, 2 Tbsp	4
Western original, 2 Tbsp	4
Western with bacon, 2 Tbsp	4
Western with blue cheese, 2 Tbsp	4
Wish-Bone Fat Free	
Blue cheese, 2 Tbsp	1
Italian, 2 Tbsp	0
Ranch, 2 Tbsp	0
Red wine vinaigrette, 2 Tbsp	1
Western, 2 Tbsp	1
Wish-Bone Just 2 Good!	
1000 island, 2 Tbsp	1
Blue cheese, 2 Tbsp	1
Country Italian, 2 Tbsp	1
Creamy Caesar, 2 Tbsp	1
Deluxe French, 2 Tbsp	1
Honey dijon, 2 Tbsp	1
Italian, 2 Tbsp	1
Light blue cheese, 2 Tbsp	1
Parmesan/peppercorn ranch, 2 Tbsp	1
Ranch, 2 Tbsp	1
Sweet and spicy French, 2 Tbsp	1
Western, 2 Tbsp	2

Oils, Dressings & Seasonings

	POINTS VALUE
Seasonings	
A1	
Barbecue, 1/4 tsp	0
Classic, 1/4 tsp	0
Garlic & herb, 1/4 tsp	0
Savory pepper, 1/4 tsp	0
A Taste of Thai	
Chicken & rice dinner seasoning, 1/4 packet	1
4C	
Seasoned coating mix for chicken, 1 serving (10 g)	1
Seasoned coating mix for pork, 1 serving (11 g)	1
Ac'cent	
Flavor enhancer, 1/8 tsp	0
Chef Paul Prudhomme's Magic Seasoning Blends	
Blackened redfish magic, 1/4 tsp	0
Blackened steak magic, 1/4 tsp	0
Fajita magic, 1/4 tsp	0
Herbal pizza & pasta magic, 1/4 tsp	0
Hot & sweet pizza & pasta magic, 1/4 tsp	0
Magic barbecue seasoning, 1/4 tsp	0
Magic salt free seasoning, 1/4 tsp	0
Magic seasoning salt, 1/4 tsp	0
Meat magic, 1/4 tsp	0
Pork & veal magic, 1/4 tsp	0
Poultry magic, 1/4 tsp	0
Salmon magic, 1/4 tsp	0

	POINTS VALUE
Seafood magic, 1/4 tsp	0
Vegetable magic, 1/4 tsp	0
Cherchies	
Garlic seasoning, 1/4 tsp	0
Garlic'n herbs seasoning, 1/4 tsp	0
Lem'n dill seasoning, 1 tsp	0
Lem'n dill seasoning, no salt, 1 tsp	0
Lem'n pepper spicy blend, 1 tsp	0
Pepper pizzazz seasoning, 1/4 tsp	0
Salsa seasoning with lime, 1 tsp	0
CHI-CHI'S	
Fajita seasoning mix, 1/4 package	1
Fiesta restaurante seasoning mix, 1 tsp	0
Fiesta taco seasoning mix, 1 serving 1/5 package	0
Durkee	
BBQ buffalo wing, mix, 1 Tbsp	1
Chili seasoning dry mix, 1 Tbsp	0
Meatloaf dry mix, 2 tsp	0
Pot roast dry mix, 2 tsp	0
Sloppy Joe seasoning, 2 tsp	0
Spaghetti dry mix, 1 Tbsp	0
Taco dry mix, 2 tsp	0
Eden	
Dulse flakes - organic, 1 tsp	0
Eden shake furikake - sesame & sea vegetable seasoning, 1/2 tsp	0
Sea salt - French coast, light grey, fine grind, 1/4 tsp	0
Sea salt - Portuguese coast, white, fine grind, 1/4 tsp	0

	POINTS VALUE
Shiso leaf powder pickled beefsteak leaf, 1 tsp	0
Tekka, 1 tsp	0
Eden Organic	
Garlic gomasio sesame salt, 1 tsp	0
Gomasio sesame salt, 1 tsp	0
Kuzu root starch, 1 serving	1
Seaweed gomasio sesame salt, 1 serving	0
Emeril's	
Asian essence, 1/2 tsp	0
Bayou blast!, 1/2 tsp	0
Chicken rub, 1/2 tsp	0
Italian essence, 1/2 tsp	0
Original essence, 1/2 tsp	0
Rib rub, 1/2 tsp	0
Southwest essence, 1/2 tsp	0
Steak rub, 1/2 tsp	0
Fanci Food	
Popcorn salt, finely ground, 1/4 tsp	0
Popcorn seasoning, butter flavor, 1/2 tsp	0
Popcorn seasoning, cheddar flavor, 1/2 tsp	0
Pop'n topper, all natural butter flavor seasoning, 3/4 tsp	0
French's	
Beef stew branded, 2 tsp	0
Beef stew dry mix, 1 Tbsp	0
Buffalo wings, hot, mix, 1 tsp	0
Buffalo wings, mild, mix, 1 1/3 Tbsp	0
Buffalo wings, screaming hot, mix, 1 1/2 Tbsp	0

	POINTS VALUE
Cajun wings, dry mix, 1 Tbsp	0
Chili seasoning dry mix, 1 Tbsp	0
Enchilada seasoning, mix, 2 tsp	0
Meatloaf dry mix, 2 tsp	0
Onion chili-o mix, 1 1/3 Tbsp	0
Pot roast dry mix, 2 tsp	0
Roasting bag, pot roast, mix, 2 tsp	0
Sloppy Joe seasoning, 2 tsp	0
Spaghetti dry mix, 1 Tbsp	0
Taco dry mix, 2 tsp	0
General Mills	
Chex mix seasoning packet, 1/4 tsp	0
Grill Mates	
BBQ seasoning blend, 3/4 tsp	0
Montreal chicken seasoning, 3/4 tsp	0
Montreal steak seasoning, 1/4 tsp	0
Teriyaki dry seasoning mix, 1 tsp	0
Kitchen Bouquet	
Kitchen bouquet, 1 tsp	0
Manischewitz	
Brisket & steak seasoning, 1/4 tsp	0
Fish seasoning, 1/4 tsp	0
Poultry seasoning, 1/4 tsp	0
Marzetti	
Asian sesame salad accents, 1 Tbsp	1
Bac'n almond crunch salad accents, 1 Tbsp	1
Fruit and nut salad accents, 1 Tbsp	1
McCormick	
Celery salt, 1/4 tsp	0
Chili dry seasoning mix, 1 1/3 Tbsp	0
Guacamole dry seasoning mix, 1 tsp	0

Oils, Dressings & Seasonings

McCormick (cont'd)	POINTS VALUE
Lemon & pepper seasoning, 1 1/2 tsp	0
Poultry seasoning, 1/4 tsp	0
Salad supreme seasoning, 2 tsp	0
Season-all, 1/4 tsp	0
Seasoned meat tenderizer, 1/4 tsp	0
Taco dry seasoning mix, 2 tsp	0
Mrs. Dash	
Classic Italiano, 1/4 tsp	0
Extra spicy, 1/4 tsp	0
Garlic & herb, 1/4 tsp	0
Hamburger grilling blend, 1/4 tsp	0
Lemon pepper, 1/4 tsp	0
Onion & herb, 1/4 tsp	0
Original blend, 1/4 tsp	0
Southwest chipotle, 1/4 tsp	0
Table blend, 1/4 tsp	0
Tomato basil garlic, 1/4 tsp	0
Mrs. Dash Grilling Blends	
Mesquite, 1/4 tsp	0
Original chicken blend, 1/4 tsp	0
Original steak blend, 1/4 tsp	0
OLD BAY	
Old bay seasoning, 1/4 tsp	0
Old El Paso	
Burrito seasoning mix, 2 tsp	0
Cheesy taco seasoning mix, 2 tsp	0
Chili seasoning mix, 1 Tbsp	0
Enchilada sauce mix, 2 tsp	0
Fajita seasoning mix, 2 tsp	0
Taco seasoning mix, 2 tsp	0

	POINTS VALUE
Taco seasoning mix, 40% less sodium, 2 tsp	0
Taco seasoning mix, hot and spicy, 2 tsp	0
Taco seasoning mix, mild, 2 tsp	0
Ortega	
Burrito seasoning, 1 1/2 tsp	0
Chipotle seasoning, 1 Tbsp	0
Fajita seasoning, 1 1/2 tsp	0
Hot taco seasoning, 1 Tbsp	0
Oven Fry	
Extra crispy chicken, 1/8 packet	1
Oven Fry Seasoned Coating	
Extra crispy for chicken, 1 serving (15 g)	1
Extra crispy for pork, 1 serving (15 g)	1
Fish fry for fish, 1 serving (11 g)	1
Home style flour for chicken recipe, 1 serving (12 g)	1
Pace	
Taco seasoning mix, 2 tsp	0
Season Brand	
Whole capers, 4 Tbsp	0
Shake 'N Bake	
Barbecue chicken or pork, as packaged, 1 serving 1/8 packet	1
Buffalo wing glazes for chicken, as packaged, 1 serving 1/10 packet	1
Country mild recipe, as packaged, 1 serving 1/8 packet	1
Extra crispy recipe for chicken, as packaged, 1 serving 1/8 packet	1

	POINTS VALUE
Honey mustard chicken or pork, as packaged, 1 serving 1/8 packet	1
Hot & spicy chicken or pork, as packaged, 1 serving 1/8 packet	1
Italian chicken or pork, as packaged, 1 serving 1/8 packet	1
Lemon pepper for chicken or pork, as packaged, 1 serving 1/8 packet	1
Original recipe for chicken, as packaged, 1 serving 1/8 packet	1
Original recipe for fish, as packaged, 1 serving 1/4 packet	2
Original recipe for pork, as packaged, 1 serving 1/8 packet	1
Parmesan crusted for chicken or pork, as packaged, 1 serving 1/8 packet	1
Ranch & herb crusted for chicken or pork, as packaged, 1 serving 1/8 packet	1
Seasoned coating mix garlic & herb, as packaged, 1 serving	1
Tangy honey chicken or pork, as packaged, 1 serving 1/8 packet	1
Spice Islands	
No salt lemon herb seasoning, 1/4 tsp	0
No salt original seasoning, 1/4 tsp	0
No salt spicy pepper seasoning, 1/4 tsp	0
Spice Islands World Flavor	
Calcutta heat seasoning, 1/4 tsp	0
Garam masala seasoning, 1/4 tsp	0
Greek seasoning, 1/4 tsp	0
Herbes de Provence seasoning, 1/4 tsp	0
Jamaican jerk seasoning, 1/4 tsp	0

	POINTS VALUE
Louisiana style Cajun seasoning, 1/4 tsp	0
Mediterranean seasoning, 1/4 tsp	0
Szechuan seasoning, 1/4 tsp	0
Thai seasoning, 1/4 tsp	0
Taco Bell Home Originals	
Fajita seasoning mix, 1 Tbsp	1
Taco seasoning mix, 2 tsp	0
Taco seasoning mix, chipotle flavor, 2 tsp	0
Taco seasoning mix, Santa Fe style flavor, 2 tsp	0
Weber	
Chicago steak, dry mix, 1/4 tsp	0
Gourmet burger, dry mix, 1/4 tsp	0
Kidk'n chicken, dry mix, 1/4 tsp	0
N'Orleans Cajun, dry mix, 1/4 tsp	0
Smokey mesquite, dry mix, 1/4 tsp	0
Sweet & tangy bbq, dry mix, 1/4 tsp	0
Zesty lemon seasoning for seafood & chicken, dry mix, 1/4 tsp	0

Vinegars
Carapelli

	POINTS VALUE
Balsamic vinegar, 1 Tbsp	0
Eden Organic	
Apple cider vinegar, 1 Tbsp	0
Brown rice vinegar, 1 Tbsp	0
Eden Selected	
Red wine vinegar, 1 Tbsp	0
Ume plum vinegar, 1 tsp	0

Oils, Dressings & Seasonings

	POINTS VALUE
Fanci Food	
Malt vinegar, 1 Tbsp	0
Red wine vinegar, 1 Tbsp	0
White wine vinegar, 1 Tbsp	0
White wine vinegar, raspberry, 1 Tbsp	0
White wine vinegar, tarragon, 1 Tbsp	0
Gourmé Mist	
Balsamic vinegar, 1 second spray	0
Balsamic vinegar plus pomegranate, 1 second spray	0
Balsamic vinegar plus raspberry, 1 second spray	0
Barrel aged balsamic vinegar, 1 second spray	0
Heinz	
Apple cider vinegar, 1 Tbsp	0
Balsamic vinegar, 1 Tbsp	0
Distilled white vinegar, 1 Tbsp	0
Gourmet garlic wine vinegar, 1 Tbsp	0
Gourmet malt vinegar, 1 Tbsp	0
Premium tarragon vinegar, 1 Tbsp	0
Red wine vinegar, 1 Tbsp	0
Salad vinegar, 1 Tbsp	0
Lucini	
Dark cherry balsamic, 1 Tbsp	0
Pinot grigio Italian wine vinegar, 1 Tbsp	0
Savory fig balsamic, 1 Tbsp	0
Manischewitz	
Balsamic vinegar, 1 Tbsp	0

	POINTS VALUE
Progresso	
Balsamic vinegar, 1 Tbsp	0
Garlic flavored vinegar, 1 Tbsp	0
Red wine vinegar, 1 Tbsp	0
Regina	
Balsamic vinegar, 1 Tbsp	0
Red wine vinegar, 1 Tbsp	0
Red wine vinegar with garlic, 1 Tbsp	0
White wine vinegar, 1 Tbsp	0
Spectrum Naturals	
Apple cider vinegar, organic filtered, 1 Tbsp	0
Apple cider vinegar, organic unfiltered, 1 Tbsp	0
Balsamic vinegar, 1 Tbsp	0
Balsamic vinegar, organic, 1 Tbsp	0
Brown rice vinegar, organic, 1 Tbsp	0
Brown rice vinegar, organic, seasoned, 1 Tbsp	0
Distilled white vinegar, organic, 1 Tbsp	0
Golden balsamic vinegar, organic, 1 Tbsp	0
Red wine vinegar, organic, 1 Tbsp	0
White wine vinegar, organic, 1 Tbsp	0
Tree of Life	
Apple cider vinegar, 1 Tbsp	0

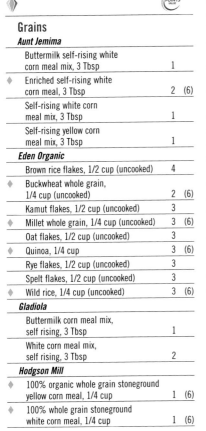

Grains

Aunt Jemima

	POINTS VALUE	
Buttermilk self-rising white corn meal mix, 3 Tbsp	1	
Enriched self-rising white corn meal, 3 Tbsp	2	(6)
Self-rising white corn meal mix, 3 Tbsp	1	
Self-rising yellow corn meal mix, 3 Tbsp	1	

Eden Organic

Brown rice flakes, 1/2 cup (uncooked)	4	
Buckwheat whole grain, 1/4 cup (uncooked)	2	(6)
Kamut flakes, 1/2 cup (uncooked)	3	
Millet whole grain, 1/4 cup (uncooked)	3	(6)
Oat flakes, 1/2 cup (uncooked)	3	
Quinoa, 1/4 cup	3	(6)
Rye flakes, 1/2 cup (uncooked)	3	
Spelt flakes, 1/2 cup (uncooked)	3	
Wild rice, 1/4 cup (uncooked)	3	(6)

Gladiola

Buttermilk corn meal mix, self rising, 3 Tbsp	1	
White corn meal mix, self rising, 3 Tbsp	2	

Hodgson Mill

100% organic whole grain stoneground yellow corn meal, 1/4 cup	1	(6)
100% whole grain stoneground white corn meal, 1/4 cup	1	(6)

	POINTS VALUE	
Wheat bran, unprocessed (millers bran), 1/4 cup	0	
Whole wheat couscous chicken n herb, 1/3 cup (dry)	4	
Whole wheat couscous wild mushroom, 1/3 cup (dry)	4	
Yellow corn meal mix, self-rising, 1/4 cup	1	

Kretschmer

Toasted wheat bran, 1/4 cup	0	

Martha White

Buttermilk corn meal mix, self rising, 3 Tbsp	2	
Plain corn meal, white, 3 Tbsp	2	(6)
Plain corn meal, yellow, 3 Tbsp	2	(6)
White corn meal mix, self rising, 3 Tbsp	2	
Yellow corn meal mix, self rising, 3 Tbsp	2	

Quaker Oats

Enriched white corn meal, 3 Tbsp	2	(6)
Enriched yellow corn meal, 3 Tbsp	1	(6)
Unprocessed bran, 1/3 cup	0	

Seeds of Change

Cuzco whole grain quinoa blend with cilantro, 1/4 cup (1 cup cooked)	3	

Tree of Life

Oat bran, 1/2 cup	2	
Organic oat bran (fine), 1/2 cup	2	
Organic wheat bran, 1/4 cup	5	

Pasta, Rice & Grains

	POINTS VALUE
Noodles	
A Taste of Thai	
Rice noodles, 2 oz	4
Thin rice noodles, 1 serving (2 oz)	4
Vermicelli rice noodles, 1 serving (2 oz)	4
Wild rice noodles, 1 serving (2 oz)	4
Yellow curry noodles quick meal, prepared, 1 cup	7
Manischewitz	
Medium egg noodles, 1 1/4 cups	4
Large egg bows, 1/3 cup	4
Whole grain noodles, 1 1/4 cups	3
Whole grain yolk free extra wide noodles, 1 1/4 cups	3
Wide egg noodles, 1 3/4 cups	4
Thai Kitchen	
Stir-fry rice noodles, 2 oz	3
Thin rice noodles, 1/2 package	8

Pasta
	POINTS VALUE
A Taste of China	
Szechuan noodles, 1 cup (prepared)	5
A Taste of Thai	
Coconut ginger noodles, prepared, 1 cup	6
Fettuccine notta pasta, 1 serving (2 oz)	4
Linguine notta pasta, 1 serving (2 oz)	4
Pad Thai for two, 4 1/2 oz	6
Pad Thai noodles, prepared, 1 cup	5
Peanut noodles, prepared, 1 cup	7
Spaghetti notta pasta, 1 serving (2 oz)	4

	POINTS VALUE
Annie's Homegrown	
Organic curly fettuccine with white cheddar & broccoli sauce, 1/3 cup (about 1 cup prepared)	6
Organic penne pasta with alfredo sauce, 1/3 cup (about 1 cup prepared)	5
Organic rotini pasta with four cheese sauce, 1/3 cup (about 1 cup prepared)	5
Azumaya	
Thin cut noodles, 1 cup	4
Wide-cut noodles, 1 cup	4
Barilla Plus	
Angel hair, 2 oz dry	4
Elbows, 2 oz dry	4
Penne, 2 oz dry	4
Rotini, 2 oz dry	4
Spaghetti, 2 oz dry	4
Thin spaghetti, 2 oz dry	4
Barilla Whole Grain	
Penne, 2 oz dry	3
Rotini, 2 oz dry	3
Spaghetti, 2 oz dry	3
Thin spaghetti, 2 oz dry	3
Dreamfields	
Elbows, 2 oz (dry, 1/2 cup)	3
Lasagna, 2 oz dry	3
Linguine, 2 oz (dry, 1/2-inch circle)	3
Penne rigate, 2 oz (dry, 3/4 cup)	3
Rotini, 2 oz (dry, 2/3 cup)	3
Spaghetti, 2 oz (dry, 1/2-inch circle)	3

Pasta, Rice & Grains

	POINTS VALUE	
Eden		
Japanese brown rice udon, 2 oz	3	
Japanese udon, 2 oz	3	
Lotus root soba, 2 oz	3	
Mugwort soba, 2 oz	3	
Soba, organic, 1/2 cup (1/4 package)	4	
Wild yam soba, 2 oz	3	
Eden Organic		
Artichoke ribbons, 1/2 cup	4	
Flax rice spirals, organic, 60% whole grain, 1 serving	3	
Kamut & buckwheat rigatoni, organic, 100% whole grain, 1/2 cup	3	(6)
Kamut ditalini, 1/2 cup	4	(6)
Kamut elbows, organic 100% whole grain, 1/2 cup	4	(6)
Kamut soba, organic, 1/2 cup	3	(6)
Kamut spaghetti, 1/2 cup	4	(6)
Kamut spirals, 1/2 cup	4	(6)
Kamut udon, 1/2 cup	4	(6)
Kamut vegetable spirals, 1/2 cup	4	(6)
Parsley garlic ribbons, 1/2 cup	4	
Parsley garlic spaghetti, 1/2 cup	3	
Rye spirals, 1/2 cup	3	
Saffron ribbons, 1/2 cup	4	
Small vegetable shells, 1/2 cup	4	
Soba, 1/2 cup	4	
Spaghetti, 100% whole grain, 2 oz	4	(6)
Spelt & buckwheat gemelli, organic, 100% whole grain, 1/2 cup	4	(6)
Spelt ribbons, 1/2 cup	4	(6)

	POINTS VALUE	
Spelt soba, 1/2 cup	4	
Spelt spaghetti, 1/2 cup	4	(6)
Spelt udon, organic, 1/2 cup	4	(6)
Spelt ziti rigati, 1/2 cup	4	(6)
Spinach ribbons, 1/2 cup	3	
Spinach spirals, 1/2 cup	3	
Twisted pair kamute & quinoa, 1/2 cup	4	(6)
Udon, wheat and rice, organic, 1/2 cup	4	
Vegetable alphabets, 1/2 cup	4	
Vegetable alphabets, organic, 60% whole grain, 1/3 cup	4	
Vegetable ribbons, 1/2 cup	4	
Vegetable shells, 1/2 cup	4	
Vegetable spirals, 1/2 cup	4	
Eden Organic Organic		
Whole grain udon, 1/2 cup	4	
Eden Selected		
Bifun (rice) pasta, 2 oz	4	
Harusame (mung bean) pasta, 2 oz	4	
Kuzu pasta, Japanese, 2 oz	4	
Soba - 100% buckwheat, 2 oz	3	(6)
Faraon		
Pasta - alphabet, 1/3 cup	4	
Pasta - elbow, 1/4 cup	5	
Pasta - fettuccini, 1 cup	5	
Pasta - fideo fine cut, 1 cup	5	
Pasta - macaroni, 1 cup	5	
Pasta - ojo perdiz, 1/3 cup	4	
Pasta - pens, 1 cup	5	

Pasta, Rice & Grains

Faraon (cont'd)	POINTS VALUE
Pasta - rings, 1/3 cup	3
Pasta - shells, 1 cup	5
Pasta - small elbow, 1 cup	5
Pasta - small shells, 1/3 cup	5
Pasta - stars, 1/3 cup	3
Pasta - vermicelli, 1/2 cup	4
Pasta - wheel, 1 cup	5
Food for Life	
Ezekiel 4:9, fettuccini, 2 oz	4
Ezekiel 4:9, linguine, 2 oz	4
Ezekiel 4:9, penne, 2 oz	4
Ezekiel 4:9, spaghetti, 2 oz	4
Heartland Naturals	
Penne, 3/4 cup	4
Rotini, 3/4 cup	4
Spaghetti, 2 oz	4
Heartland Perfect Balance	
Elbow macaroni, 1/2 cup	3
Penne, 1/2 cup	3
Rotini, 3/4 cup	3
Spaghetti, 2 oz	3
Thin spaghetti, 2 oz	3
Heartland Plus with ALA Omega-3	
Angel hair, 2 oz	3
Penne, 2/3 cup	3
Rotini, 3/4 cup	3
Spaghetti, 2 oz	3
Heartland Whole Grain	
Penne, 2/3 cup	3
Spaghetti, 2 oz	3

	POINTS VALUE	
Heartland Whole Wheat		
Angel hair, 2 oz	4	
Elbow macaroni, 1/2 cup	4	
Penne, 3/4 cup	4	
Rotini, 3/4 cup	4	
Spaghetti, 2 oz	4	
Hodgson Mill		
Veggie rotini, 2 oz	4	
Whole wheat angel hair pasta, 2 oz	3	(6)
Whole wheat bow tie pasta, 2 oz	3	(6)
Whole wheat egg noodles, 2 oz dry	4	(6)
Whole wheat elbows, 2 oz	3	(6)
Whole wheat fettuccine, 2 oz	3	(6)
Whole wheat lasagna, 2 oz	3	(6)
Whole wheat medium shells, 2 oz	3	(6)
Whole wheat organic angel hair with milled flax seed, 2 oz	3	(6)
Whole wheat organic fettuccine with milled flax seed, 2 oz	4	(6)
Whole wheat organic lasagna with milled flax seed, 2 oz	4	(6)
Whole wheat organic penne with milled flax seed, 2 oz	4	(6)
Whole wheat organic spaghetti with milled flax seed, 2 oz	4	(6)
Whole wheat organic spirals with milled flax seed, 2 oz	4	(6)
Whole wheat penne, 2 oz	3	(6)
Whole wheat spaghetti, 2 oz dry	3	(6)
Whole wheat spinach spaghetti, 2 oz	3	(6)
Whole wheat spirals, 2 oz	3	(6)
Whole wheat thin spaghetti, 2 oz	3	(6)

		POINTS VALUE
◆ Whole wheat veggie bows, 2 oz dry	3	(6)
◆ Whole wheat veggie radiatore, 2 oz	3	(6)
◆ Whole wheat veggie wagon wheels, 2 oz dry	3	(6)
◆ Whole wheat yolkless ribbons, 2 oz	4	(6)

Italian Village
Cavatelli, 1 cup	3

Kraft
Spaghetti with meat sauce, as packaged, 5 1/2 oz	6

Kraft Noodle Classics
Savory chicken, prepared, 1 cup	7

Kraft Spaghetti Classics
Tangy Italian, prepared, 1 cup	4

Manischewitz
Egg noodle flakes, 1/4 cup	4
Egg noodles - fine, medium, extra wide, 2 cups	4
Whole grain noodle style pasta, yolk free extra wide, 1 1/4 cups	3
Yolk free noodles, extra wide, 1 3/4 cups	4
Yolk free noodles, fine, 1 1/2 cups	4
Yolk free noodles, medium, 1 3/4 cups	4
Yolk free noodles, wide, 1 3/4 cups	4

Manischewitz Passover Gold
Egg noodles, fine, 3/4 cup	4
Egg noodles, wide, 3/4 cup	4
Yolk free egg noodles - medium, 3/4 cup	5

Monterey Pasta Company
Organic fettuccine, 1 1/4 cups	5
Organic linguine, 1 1/4 cups	5
Whole wheat linguine with flaxseed, 1 1/4 cups	4

Nasoya
Chinese style noodles, 1 cup	4
Japanese style noodles, 1 cup	4

Near East
Angel hair pasta with spicy tomato, prepared, 1 serving	5
Couscous Moroccan pasta, prepared, 1 1/4 cups	5
Fusilli pasta with parmesan & romano, prepared, 1 serving	6
Gemelli pasta with tomato parmesan, prepared, 1 serving	7
Radiatore pasta basil & herb, prepared, 1 serving	5
Vermicelli pasta with roasted garlic & olive oil, prepared, 1 serving	6

Pasta Roni
Angel hair pasta with herbs, prepared, 1 cup	7
Angel hair pasta with lemon & butter, prepared, 1 cup	8
Angel hair pasta with parmesan cheese, prepared, 1 cup	7
Broccoli au gratin, prepared, 1 cup	6
Broccoli, prepared, 1 cup	7
Chicken & garlic low fat, prepared, 1 cup	7
Chicken, prepared, 1 cup	7

Pasta, Rice & Grains

Pasta Roni (cont'd)	POINTS value
Creamy garlic sauce with corkscrew pasta, prepared, 1 cup	8
Fettuccine alfredo, prepared, 1 cup	11
Fettuccine alfredo, reduced fat, prepared, 1 cup	6
Four cheese sauce with corkscrew pasta, prepared, 1 cup	9
Garlic alfredo, prepared, 1 cup	8
Herb & butter, prepared, 1 cup	8
Homestyle chicken, prepared, 1 cup	5
Linguine with chicken & broccoli, prepared, 1 cup	8
Linguine with creamy chicken parmesan, prepared, 1 cup	9
Mild cheddar, prepared, 1 cup	6
Parmesano, prepared, 1 cup	9
Romanoff, prepared, 1 cup	9
Shells & white cheddar, prepared, 1 cup	7
Stroganoff, prepared, 1 cup	8
Vermicelli with roasted garlic & olive oil, prepared, 1 cup	8
White cheddar & broccoli sauce with rigatoni, prepared, 1 cup	7
Rosetto	
Cheese stuffed shells, 2 pieces	6
Rosina Presents Celentano	
Cavatelli, 1 cup	4
Stuffed shells, 3 (1 tray)	9
Weight Watchers	
Sides - chicken herb whole grain pasta, 1 cup	3
Sides - tomato parmesan whole grain pasta, 1 cup	4

	POINTS value
Rice	
A Taste of India	
Masala rice & lentils, 1 cup (mix)	5
Spiced rice with raisins, 1 cup (prepared)	7
Annie's Homegrown	
Rice pasta & cheddar (gluten free), 3 oz (about 1 cup prepared)	7
Birds Eye Steamfresh	
Long grain white rice, 3/4 cup	3
Long grain white rice with mixed vegetables, 1 cup	3
Rice, chicken flavored, 1 cup cooked	5
Rice, southwestern style, 1 cup cooked	5
Bowl Appetit!	
Cheddar broccoli rice, 1 bowl	6
Herb chicken vegetable rice, 1 bowl	5
Carolina	
Authentic Spanish rice mix, 2 oz (about 1/3 cup rice mix and 1 Tbsp seasoning)	3
Basmati rice, 1/4 cup (uncooked)	3
Broccoli with cheese rice, 1 serving (1/3 cup rice mix and 2 tsp dry seasoning) (2 oz)	4
Brown rice whole grain, uncooked, 1/4 cup	3 (6)
Chicken rice mix, 2 oz (about 1/3 cup rice mix and 1 Tbsp seasoning)	4
Classic pilaf rice mix, 2 oz (about 1/3 cup rice mix and 3/4 tsp seasoning)	4
Jasmine rice, uncooked, 1/4 cup	3

	POINTS VALUE	
Long grain & wild rice mix, 2 oz (about 1/3 cup rice mix and 2 Tbsp seasoning)	4	
Saffron Yellow rice mix, 2 oz (about 1/3 cup rice and 2 tsp seasoning)	4	
Spicy saffron yellow, 2 oz (about 1/4 cup rice mix and 2 Tbsp seasoning)	3	
White rice, uncooked, 1/4 cup	3	
Carolina Gold		
Parboiled rice, uncooked, 1/4 cup	3	
Casbah		
Rice pilaf, 1 serving	3	
Spanish pilaf, 1 serving	3	
Fanci Food		
◆ Wild rice, 1/4 cup (unprepared)	3	(6)
Fantastic World Foods		
Arborio rice, 1/4 cup	3	
Basmati rice, 1/4 cup	3	
Jasmine rice, 1/4 cup	3	
Faraon		
E-Z cook long grain rice, uncooked, 1/4 cup	3	
Long grain rice, uncooked, 1/4 cup	3	
Gourmet House		
◆ All natural brown and wild rice, 1/4 cup (uncooked)	3	(6)
All natural white and wild rice, 1/4 cup (uncooked)	3	
◆ Brown rice, 1/4 cup (uncooked)	3	(6)
◆ Cracked Minnesota cultivated wild rice, 1/4 cup (uncooked)	3	(6)

	POINTS VALUE	
Indian basmati, 1/4 cup (uncooked)	3	
Italian arborio, 1/4 cup (uncooked)	3	
Long grain and wild rice, 1/4 cup (uncooked)	3	
◆ Minnesota cultivated wild rice, 1/4 cup (dry)	3	(6)
◆ Organic brown rice, 1/4 cup (uncooked)	3	(6)
Organic white rice, 1/4 cup (uncooked)	3	
Quick-cooking wild rice, 1/2 cup (uncooked)	3	
Thai jasmine, 1/4 cup (uncooked)	3	
White rice, 1/4 cup (uncooked)	3	
Wild rice garden blend, 1/4 cup (uncooked)	3	
Mahatma		
Authentic Spanish rice mix, 2 oz (about 1/3 cup rice mix and 1 Tbsp seasoning)	3	
Basmati, 1/4 cup (dry)	3	
Broccoli cheese rice mix, 2 1/4 oz (about 1/3 cup rice mix and 1/4 cup seasoning)	5	
◆ Brown rice whole grain, uncooked, 1/4 cup	3	(6)
Chicken rice mix, 2 oz (about 1/3 cup rice mix and 1 Tbsp seasoning)	4	
Classic pilaf rice mix, 2 oz (about 1/3 cup rice mix and 3/4 tsp seasoning)	4	
Jasmine rice, uncooked, 1/4 cup	3	
Long grain & wild rice mix, 2 oz (about 1/3 cup rice mix and 2 Tbsp seasoning)	4	

Pasta, Rice & Grains

Mahatma (cont'd)

<table>
<tr><td></td><td>POINTS VALUE</td></tr>
<tr><td>Spicy yellow rice, 2 oz (about 1/4 cup rice mix and 2 Tbsp seasoning)</td><td>4</td></tr>
<tr><td>Valencia (short grain), 1/4 cup (uncooked)</td><td>3</td></tr>
<tr><td>White rice, uncooked, 1/4 cup</td><td>3</td></tr>
<tr><td>Yellow rice mix, 2 oz (about 1/3 cup rice mix and 2 tsp seasoning)</td><td>4</td></tr>
</table>

Mahatma Gold

Parboiled rice, uncooked, 1/4 cup	3

Manischewitz

Lentil pilaf mix, 1/4 cup	2
Rice pilaf mix, 1/4 cup	3
Spanish pilaf mix, 1/4 cup	3

Market Day

Vegetable fried rice, 1 cup	2
Wild rice blend, 3/4 cup	2

Marrakesh Express

Parmesan cheese, 1 cup	4
Roasted red pepper, 1 cup	4
Sun dried tomato and herb, 1 cup	4
Wild mushroom, 1 cup	4

Minute

Boil-in-bag rice, 1/2 cup dry (1 cup cooked)	3
Brown rice, 1/2 cup dry (2/3 cup cooked)	3 (6)
Enriched pre-cooked boil-in-bag long grain white rice, prepared, 1 cup	4
Instant enriched long grain white rice, prepared, 1 cup	3
Instant enriched premium long grain white rice, prepared, 1 cup	3

Instant whole grain brown rice, prepared, 2/3 cup	3
Premium white rice, 1/2 cup dry (1 cup cooked)	4
White rice, 1/2 cup dry (1 cup cooked)	4

Minute Ready to Serve

Brown & wild rice mix, 1 container (approx. 1 cup)	4
Brown rice, 1 container (approx. 1 cup)	3 (6)
Chicken rice mix, 1 container (approx. 1 cup)	4
White rice, 1 container (approx. 1 cup)	4
Yellow rice mix, 1 container (approx. 1 cup)	4

Near East

Brown rice pilaf mix, prepared, 1 cup	4
Chicken rice pilaf mix, prepared, 1 cup	4
Curry rice pilaf mix, prepared, 1 cup	4
Garlic & herb mix, prepared, 1 cup	4
Lentil pilaf mix, prepared, 1 cup	3
Long grain and wild rice pilaf, prepared, 1 cup	4
Spanish rice pilaf mix, prepared, 1 cup	6
Toasted almond pilaf mix, prepared, 1 cup (2 oz)	4
Wheat pilaf mix, prepared, 1 cup	4

Near East Creative Grains

Chicken & herbs, prepared, 1 cup	5
Creamy parmesan, prepared, 1 cup	6
Roasted garlic, prepared, 1 cup	4
Roasted pecan & garlic, prepared, 1 cup	5

©2009 Riviana Foods Inc.

DAY
TUE WED THU FRI SAT SUN Date

SCHEDULE	ACTION LIST	Ⓐ ✔

Spinning class
Molly to gymnastics / Josh to Karate
Drycleaning
Drop kids off at school
Coffee with Debbie (compliment her haircut)
Car to dealership re: red light won't go away
Client conference call
Training for new phone system

Weekly team-building meeting

Conference call with client
Conference call with field reps
Confirm dinner reservation/call Mom re: babysitting
Shop for anniversary card/new dress?
10-minute power walk
Mandatory workplace safety seminar
Finish 360 evaluations
Presentation to new employees
Crunch numbers for sales meeting
HR meeting re: 401K changes
Interview boss's nephew intern candidate
Finish expense report from sales trip
Retirement party for Ed in Accounting
(stop by to say "hi")
Pick up kids
Mani-pedi
Hair appointment
Take kids to mom's
Anniversary dinner with Jim!

NOTES

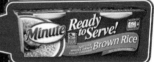

WHEN LUNCH HOUR
IS A LUNCH MINUTE.

Squeezed for time? We can help.™
Minute® Ready to Serve Brown
Rice is delicious, nutritious
and ready in 60 seconds.
It's Minute Rice. Literally.

www.minuterice.com/readytoserve

Pasta, Rice & Grains

Old El Paso

	POINTS VALUE
Cheesy Mexican rice, as packaged, 1/3 package	5
Cheesy Mexican rice, prepared, 1 serving (1/3 package)	6
Spanish rice, as packaged, 1/3 package	5
Spanish rice, prepared, 1 serving (1/3 package)	6

Rice-A-Roni

Beef & mushroom, prepared, 1 cup	6
Beef flavor, 1/3 less salt, prepared, 1 cup	5
Beef flavor, prepared, 1 cup	7
Broccoli au gratin, 1/3 less salt, prepared, 1 cup	7
Broccoli, prepared, 1 cup	6
Chicken & broccoli, prepared, 1 cup	5
Chicken & garlic, prepared, 1 cup	6
Chicken & vegetables, prepared, 1 cup	6
Chicken flavor, 1/3 less salt, prepared, 1 cup	6
Chicken flavor, prepared, 1 cup	7
Chicken teriyaki, prepared, 1 cup	5
Chicken with mushrooms, prepared, 1 cup	8
Chicken, low fat, prepared, 1 cup	4
Fried rice, 1/3 less salt, prepared, 1 cup	5
Fried rice, prepared, 1 cup	7
Garden vegetable rice, prepared, 1 cup	6
Herb & butter, prepared, 1 cup	7
Herb roasted chicken, prepared, 1 cup	6

	POINTS VALUE
Lemon chicken rice, prepared, 1 cup	5
Long grain & wild chicken almonds, prepared, 1 cup	6
Long grain & wild rice original, prepared, 1 cup	5
Long grain & wild rice pilaf, prepared, 1 cup	5
Mexican style, prepared, 1 cup	5
Oriental stir fry, prepared, 1 cup	6
Rice pilaf, prepared, 1 cup	7
Savory chicken vegetable, low fat, prepared, 1 cup	4
Spanish rice, prepared, 1 cup	5
Stroganoff, prepared, 1 cup	8
White cheddar & herbs, prepared, 1 cup	8

Rice-A-Roni Cheesy Pleasers

Country cheddar, prepared, 1 cup	8
Creamy 4 cheese, 1 cup	6
Parmesan chicken rice, prepared, 1 cup	8

Rice-A-Roni Savory Whole Grain

Chicken & herbs rice, prepared, 1 cup	5
Roasted garlic rice, prepared, 1 cup	6
Spanish rice, prepared, 1 cup	5

River

Brown rice, 1/4 cup (uncooked)	3	(6)
Medium grain rice, 1/4 cup (uncooked)	3	

S&W

Natural brown rice, uncooked, 1/4 cup	3	(6)
White rice, uncooked, 1/4 cup	3	

	POINTS VALUE

Seeds of Change

Arroz Hispaniola Caribbean red beans & brown rice, 1 cup	5
Dharamsala aromatic Indian rice blend with mung beans & lentils, 1 cup	4
Persia seven whole grain pilaf, 1/3 cup (1 cup cooked)	4
Rishikesh whole grain brown basmati rice, 1 cup	4
Tapovan white basmati rice, 1 cup	4
Tigris - a mixture of seven whole grains, 1 cup	5
Uyuni quinoa & whole grain brown rice with garlic, 1 cup	5
Velleron French-style herb whole grain blend, 1/3 cup	3

Success

Jasmine rice, 1/4 cup (3/4 cup prepared)	3

Success Rice

◆ Brown rice, 1/2 cup	3	(6)
White rice, 1/2 cup	4	

Sunsun

Enriched long grain rice, uncooked, 1/4 cup	3

Thai Kitchen

Jasmine rice mix, green chili & garlic, prepared, 1 cup cooked	5
Jasmine rice mix, lemongrass & ginger, prepared, 1 cup (prepared)	5
Jasmine rice mix, lemongrass & ginger, prepared, 1 cup (cooked - gluten - free)	5
Jasmine rice mix, roasted garlic & chili, prepared, 1 cup cooked	4

	POINTS VALUE

Jasmine rice mix, spicy Thai chili, prepared, 1 cup cooked	5
Jasmine rice mix, sweet chili & onion, prepared, 1 cup	6
Jasmine rice mix, Thai yellow curry, prepared, 1 cup cooked	5
Jasmine rice select harvest, prepared, 1/2 cup (cooked)	3

Tony Chachere's

Butter and herb rice, 1/3 cup dry mix	3
Chicken rice, 1/3 cup dry mix	3
Creole dirty rice mix, 1/3 cup dry mix	3
Creole gumbo dinner mix, 2 Tbsp dry mix	1
Creole jambalaya dinner mix, 1/4 cup dry mix	3
Creole rice & gravy dinner mix, 1/4 cup dry mix	4
Yellow rice, 1/3 cup dry mix	3

Uncle Ben's

Boil-in-bag enriched long grain rice, 1/3 cup dry (1 cup cooked)	4	
◆ Boil-in-bag whole grain brown rice, 1/4 cup (dry)	3	(6)
◆ Fast & natural brown rice instant whole grain, 1/4 cup dry (1 cup cooked)	3	(6)
Instant rice enriched long grain, 1/2 cup dry (1 cup cooked)	4	
Long grain & wild rice fast cook, butter & herb, 1/2 cup dry (1 cup cooked)	4	
Long grain & wild rice, fast cook recipe, 1/2 cup dry (1 cup cooked)	4	
Long grain & wild rice, original recipe, 1/2 cup dry (1 cup cooked)	4	

Pasta, Rice & Grains

Uncle Ben's (cont'd)	POINTS VALUE
Long grain & wild rice, roasted garlic & olive oil, 1/2 cup dry (1 cup cooked)	3
Long grain & wild rice, vegetable pilaf, 1/2 cup dry (1 cup cooked)	3
Natural whole grain brown rice, 1/4 cup dry (1 cup cooked)	3 (6)
Original converted brand enriched parboiled long grain rice, 1/4 cup dry (1 cup cooked)	3
Whole grain & wild rice, mushroom recipe, 1/2 cup dry (1 cup cooked)	4

Uncle Ben's Country Inn

Broccoli rice au gratin, 1/2 cup dry (1 cup cooked)	4
Chicken, 1/2 cup dry (1 cup cooked)	4
Chicken & broccoli, 1/2 cup dry (1 cup cooked)	4

	POINTS VALUE
Chicken & vegetable, 1/2 cup dry (1 cup cooked)	4
Chicken & wild, 1/2 cup dry (1 cup cooked)	4
Mexican fiesta, 1/2 cup dry (1 cup cooked)	4
Oriental fried rice, 1/2 cup dry (1 cup cooked)	4
Rice pilaf, 1/2 cup dry (1 cup cooked)	4

Water Maid

Medium grain rice, uncooked, 1/4 cup	3

Weight Watchers

Sides - wild mushroom brown & wild rice, 1 cup	3

Zapata

Spanish rice, 2/3 cup	1

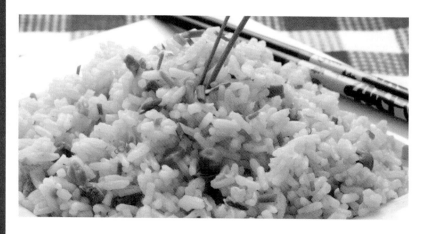

Prepared Foods, Salads & Sides

	POINTS VALUE

Appetizers

Dr. Praeger's

Broccoli bites, 2 pieces	2
Broccoli littles, 2 pieces	1
Pizza bagels, 1	2
Potato bites, 2 pieces	2
Potato littles, 2 pieces	1
Spinach bites, 2 pieces	2
Spinach littles, 2 pieces	1
Sweet potato bites, 2 pieces	2
Sweet potato littles, 2 pieces	1

Jack's Pizza Bursts

Pepperoni, 6 pieces	6
Pepperoni & sausage, 6 pieces	5
Super cheese, 6 pieces	6

Market Day

Li'l bagel dogs, 4	5
Mini chicken cordon bleu bites, 4 pieces	5
Mini cocktail sandwiches, 2 pieces	6
Mozzarella sticks & sauce, 2 pieces (2 oz)	5
Pesto bruschetta, 2 pieces	3
Potato skins, 3 pieces (3.2 oz)	5

Old El Paso Stuffed Nachos

Beef taco flavor, 6	5
Beef, cheese & mild salsa, 6	4
Beef, cheese & hot salsa, 6	4
Chicken, cheese & salsa, 6	5
Nacho cheese, 6	4

Ore-Ida Bagel Bites

Cheese & pepperoni, 4 pieces	4
Cheese, sausage & pepperoni, 4 pieces	4
Nacho cheese, 4 pieces	5
Supreme bagel bites, 4 pieces	4
Ultra five cheese, 4 pieces	5

Ore-Ida Stuffed Bagel Bites

Pepperoni and cheese, 6 pieces	5
Three cheese, 4 pieces	4

Phillips

Crab & shrimp spring rolls, 3 (with 3/4 oz sauce)	6

Poppers

Cheddar cheese stuffed jalapeños, 1 serving (98 g)	7
Cream cheese stuffed jalapeños, 1 serving (77 g)	6
Mozzarella nuggets, 3 pieces	2
Mozzarella sticks, 1 piece	2

T.G.I. Friday's

Broccoli & Cheddar potato skins, 3 pieces	4
Cheddar & bacon potato skins, 2 servings (62 g)	3
Cheddar & bacon potato skins, 3 pieces	5
Four cheese & pepperoni potato skins, 3 pieces	5
Mozzarella sticks with marinara sauce, 1 serving (1 mozzarella stick and 1 Tbsp sauce)	3

Prepared Foods, Salads & Sides

	POINTS VALUE
Thyme & Truffles Hors D'oeuvres	
Cold canape assortment, 1 piece	2
Cranberry pecan spirals, 1 piece	2
Hors d'oeuvres assortment, 1 piece	2
Hors d'oeuvres party assortment, 1 piece	2
Mushroom leek crescent, 1 piece	2
Shrimp puff, 1 piece	2

Egg Entrees
Jimmy Dean

	POINTS VALUE
Ham & cheese omelet, 1	7
Sausage & cheese omelet, 1	7
Three cheese omelet, 1	8
Western style omelet, 1	5

Jimmy Dean Skillets

Bacon, 1/4 package	5
Ham, 1/4 package	3
Sausage, 1/4 package	5

Market Day

Bacon quiche, 1 serving (1/8 quiche)	8
Breakfast casserole, 1/2 cup	4

Ethnic Entrees
Amy's

Asian noodle stir-fry, 1 package	6
Bean & cheese burrito, 1 package	6
Black bean vegetable burrito, 1 package	5
Black bean vegetable enchilada, 1 serving (4.75 oz)	4
Breakfast burrito, 1 package	5
Burrito & rice - non dairy, 1 package	5
Burrito especial, 1 package	5

	POINTS VALUE
Cheese enchilada, 1 serving (4.5 oz)	6
Cheese tamale verde whole meal, 1	8
Indian mattar paneer, 1	6
Indian palak paneer, 1 serving (10 oz)	5
Indian paneer tikka, 1	7
Indian spinach tofu wrap, 1	7
Kids Mexican quesadilla meal, 1	9
Light in sodium Indian mattar paneer, 1	6
Light in sodium Mexican casserole bowl	8
Mexican tamale pie, 1	2
Thai stir-fry, 1	6

Amy's Bowls

Mexican casserole bowl, 1 container	10
Santa Fe enchilada, 1 container	7
Tortilla casserole & black beans bowl, 1	9

Amy's Whole Meals

Black bean enchilada, 1 serving (10 oz)	6
Black bean tamale verde whole meal, 1	7
Cheese enchilada, 1 serving (9 oz)	7

Asian Rhythms

Crab rangoon, 4 pieces	5
Crab rangoon, sweet chili sauce only, 2 Tbsp	1
Crispy dim sum, shrimp money bag, 4 pieces	4
Crispy dim sum, shrimp spring roll, 3 pieces	4

Prepared Foods, Salads & Sides

	POINTS VALUE
Crispy dim sum, shrimp wonton, 4 pieces	4
Crispy dim sum, sweet chili sauce, 2 Tbsp	1
Steamed dim sum, seafood shumai, 4 pieces	2
Steamed dim sum, shrimp hagao, 4 pieces	3
Steamed dim sum, shrimp shumai, 4 pieces	2
Steamed dim sum, vinegar soy sauce, 1 Tbsp	0
Steamed dim sum, vinegar soy sauce, 1 Tbsp	0
Birds Eye Steamfresh	
Meals for two, Asian style chicken vegetable medley with fresh frozen vegetables, 1/2 bag	6
Birds Eye Voila!	
Beef lo mein, 1 cup cooked	4
Chicken fajita, 1 serving (2 1/4 cups frozen, 1 cup cooked)	3
Chicken parmesan, 1 cup cooked	5
Birds Eye Voila! Family Skillets	
Alfredo chicken, 1 cup cooked	6
Cascadian Farm	
◆ Organic Chinese-style stir fry blend, 3/4 cup	0
◆ Organic Thai-style stir fry blend, 3/4 cup	0
Chicken Helper	
Cheesy chicken enchilada, prepared, 1 cup	7

	POINTS VALUE
Ethnic Gourmet Taste of Greece	
Kotopoulo domato ke feta, 1 package	8
Ethnic Gourmet Taste of India	
Bean masala, 1 package	7
Chicken biryani over brown rice, 1 package	8
Chicken korma, 1 package	7
Chicken tandoori with spinach, 1 package	3
Chicken tikka masala, 1 package	4
Eggplant bharta, 1 package	6
Gujarati vegetable curry, 1 package	10
Palak paneer, 1 package	5
Shahi paneer, 1 package	13
Vegetable korma, 1 package	6
Ethnic Gourmet Taste of Malaysia	
Malay chicken curry, 1 package	9
Ethnic Gourmet Taste of Santa Fe	
Chili relleno with mango salsa, 1 package	5
Ethnic Gourmet Taste of Thai	
Chicken pad Thai, 1 package	8
Kaeng kari kai, 1 package	9
Lemongrass & basil chicken, 1 package	8
Pad Thai with shrimp, 1 package	8
Pad Thai with tofu, 1 package	8
Fantastic World Foods	
Falafel, 1/4 cup	2
Fortune of the East	
Sweet and sour chicken, prepared, 1 cup	8

Prepared Foods, Salads & Sides

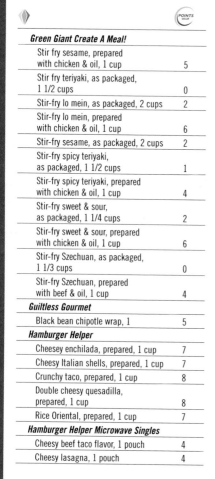

	POINTS VALUE
Green Giant Create A Meal!	
Stir fry sesame, prepared with chicken & oil, 1 cup	5
Stir fry teriyaki, as packaged, 1 1/2 cups	0
Stir-fry lo mein, as packaged, 2 cups	2
Stir-fry lo mein, prepared with chicken & oil, 1 cup	6
Stir-fry sesame, as packaged, 2 cups	2
Stir-fry spicy teriyaki, as packaged, 1 1/2 cups	1
Stir-fry spicy teriyaki, prepared with chicken & oil, 1 cup	4
Stir-fry sweet & sour, as packaged, 1 1/4 cups	2
Stir-fry sweet & sour, prepared with chicken & oil, 1 cup	6
Stir-fry Szechuan, as packaged, 1 1/3 cups	0
Stir-fry Szechuan, prepared with beef & oil, 1 cup	4
Guiltless Gourmet	
Black bean chipotle wrap, 1	5
Hamburger Helper	
Cheesey enchilada, prepared, 1 cup	7
Cheesy Italian shells, prepared, 1 cup	7
Crunchy taco, prepared, 1 cup	8
Double cheesy quesadilla, prepared, 1 cup	8
Rice Oriental, prepared, 1 cup	7
Hamburger Helper Microwave Singles	
Cheesy beef taco flavor, 1 pouch	4
Cheesy lasagna, 1 pouch	4

	POINTS VALUE
Hormel	
Beef tamales, canned, 2	3
Hot-spicy beef tamales, canned, 2	3
Jumbo beef tamales, canned, 2	4
Hormel Individual Canned Servings	
Beef tamales, 1 can	4
Kahiki	
Beef & broccoli, 1 cup	6
Beef & broccoli, 1 package	8
Chicken egg rolls (without sauce), 1	2
Chicken egg rolls, sauce only, 1 packet	0
Chicken fried rice, 1 cup	4
Chicken potstickers (without sauce), 5 pieces	6
Chicken potstickers, sauce only, 1 1/2 Tbsp	1
General Tso's chicken, 1 cup	6
General Tso's chicken, 1 package	8
Pork & shrimp egg rolls, without sauce, 1	2
Pork & shrimp egg rolls, sauce only, 1 packet	0
Sesame orange chicken, 1 cup	6
Sesame orange chicken, 1 package	8
Sweet & sour chicken, 1 cup	6
Sweet & sour chicken, 1 package	8
Vegetable egg rolls, without sauce, 1	1
Vegetable egg rolls, sauce only, 1 packet	0
Kahiki Naturals	
Chicken egg rolls, without sauce, with wheat & flax seed wrapper, 1	1

Prepared Foods, Salads & Sides

	POINTS VALUE
General Tso's chicken, 1 package	6
Mandarin orange chicken, 1 package	7
Szechuan peppercorn beef, 1 package	8
Teriyaki brown rice with mixed vegetables, 1 package	4
Teriyaki mixed vegetables, 1 package	5
Vegetable egg rolls (without sauce), 1	2
Vegetable egg rolls, sauce only, 1 packet	0
Kashi	
Mayan harvest bake, 1	7
Sweet & sour chicken, 1 package	6
Las Palmas	
Taco kit, 1 serving (2 shells, 1/4 package sauce, and 1/4 envelope of seasoning)	3
Manischewitz	
Falafel mix, 2 Tbsp	2
Market Day	
Baked manicotti, 1	6
Carnitas enchiladas, 1 serving (12 oz)	12
Egg rolls with sauce, 3 pieces	7
Vegetable lasagna ratatouille, 1 serving (11.4 oz)	3
Monterey Pasta Company	
Italian sausage borsellini, 1 cup	6
Potato parmesan gnocchi, 1 cup	3
Ravioli made with organic spinach & cheese, 1 cup	5
Ravioli made with organic tomato basil mozzarella ravioli, 1 cup	5
Snow crab ravioli with dill, 1 cup	5
Spinach mushroom tortelloni, 1 cup	5
Tri-color roasted chicken tortelloni, 1 cup	5

	POINTS VALUE
Mrs. T's	
4 cheese pierogies, 3	5
American cheese pierogies, 3	4
Broccoli Cheddar pierogies, 3	4
Cheddar & bacon mini pierogies, 7	3
Jalapeño Cheddar pierogies, 3	3
Potato Cheddar pierogies, 3	3
Potato onion pierogies, 3	3
Sauerkraut pierogies, 3	2
Sour cream & chive pierogies, 3	4
Near East	
Falafel vegetarian patty mix, prepared, 5 patties	3
Old El Paso	
Burrito dinner, prepared, 1	6
Fajita dinner no fuss, prepared, 2	7
Soft taco dinner kit, prepared with chicken breast, 2 taco shells	7
Soft taco dinner kit, prepared with ground beef, 2 taco shells	8
Southwest style taco dinner, prepared with lean ground beef, 2 taco shells	10
Southwest style taco dinner, ranch sauce & seasoning mix, prepared with chicken breast, 2 taco shells	9
Stand 'n stuff taco dinner, prepared tacos with chicken breast, 2 taco shells	7
Stand 'n stuff taco dinner, prepared tacos with lean ground beef, 2 taco shells	8
Taco dinner, prepared tacos with chicken breast, 2 taco shells	5

Prepared Foods, Salads & Sides

Old El Paso (cont'd)	POINTS VALUE
Taco dinner, prepared with ground beef, 2 taco shells	6
Taco dinner, prepared, hard, 2 taco shells	6
Taco dinner, prepared, soft, 2 taco shells	7
Old El Paso Complete Skillet Meal	
Crunchy enchilada style rice & chicken, as packaged, 1 serving (1/5 package)	4
Mexican style cheesy rice & beef, as packaged, 1 serving (1/5 package)	5
Ortega	
Hard & soft taco kit (with taco shells), 1 serving	3
Hard & soft taco kit (with tortillas), 1 serving	5
Seeds of Change	
Spicy Thai peanuts noodles with vegetables and tofu, 1 tray	7
Simply Asia	
Ready in 10 minutes, chili garlic noodles, 1/3 package	6
Ready in 10 minutes, sesame teriyaki noodles, 1/3 package	6
Ready in 10 minutes, soy ginger noodles, 1/3 package	6
Ready in 10 minutes, spicy Kung Pao, 1/3 package	6
Ready in 10 minutes, spicy Szechwan noodles, 1/3 package	6
Ready in 10 minutes, toasted sesame garlic noodles, 1/3 package	7
Ready in 15 minutes, honey teriyaki stir-fry meal, 1/2 cup	5

	POINTS VALUE
Ready in 15 minutes, mandarin orange stir-fry meal, 1/2 cup	4
Ready in 15 minutes, spicy Kung Pao, 1/2 cup	4
Simply Asia Noodle Bowl	
Mandarin orange, 1 bowl	8
Roasted peanut, 1 bowl	11
Sesame teriyaki, 1 bowl	8
Soy ginger, 1 bowl	8
Spicy Kung Pao, 1 bowl	8
Spicy Mongolian, 1 bowl	9
Simply Asia Quick Noodles	
Honey teriyaki, 1 tray	8
Pad Thai, 1 tray	9
Sweet & sour chow mein, 1 tray	8
Szechwan garlic chow mein, 1 tray	9
Simply Asia Take Out	
Honey teriyaki, 1/2 box	5
Pad Thai, 1/2 box	5
Roasted peanut, 1/2 box	7
Spicy Kung Pao, 1/2 box	5
Sweet & sour chow mein, 1/2 box	5
Szechwan garlic chow mein, 1/2 box	6
T.G.I. Friday's	
Chicken quesadilla rolls, 2 pieces	6
Southwestern egg rolls, 1 piece	5
Steak quesadillas, 2 pieces	4
Taco Bell Home Originals	
Cheesy double decker taco dinner, prepared, 1	8
Soft taco dinner, prepared, 2	8

Prepared Foods, Salads & Sides

	POINTS VALUE
Taco dinner, prepared, 2	6
Ultimate nachos, prepared, 1/4 kit	6
Tamarind Tree	
Channa dal masala, 1 package	5
Dal makhani, 1 package	6
Thai Kitchen	
Garlic & roasted pepper rice noodles & sauce, 1/2 package	5
Ginger & sweet chili rice noodles & sauce, 1/2 package	5
Lemongrass & chili stir-fry rice noodles with seasoning, 1/2 package	6
Original pad Thai rice noodles & sauce, 1/2 package	5
Original pad Thai stir-fry rice noodles with sauce, 1/2 package	7
Stir-fry rice noodles with sauce, Thai curry, 1/2 package	6
Tangy sweet & sour rice noodles & sauce, 1/2 package	5
Thai basil & chili rice noodles & sauce, 1/2 package	5
Thai peanut rice noodles & sauce, 1/2 package	6
Thai peanut stir-fry rice noodles with seasoning, 1/2 package	7
Toasted sesame stir-fry rice noodles with seasoning, 1/2 package	7
Thai Kitchen Noodle Cart	
Pad Thai instant rice noodles & sauce, 1 package	5
Roasted garlic instant rice noodles & sauce, 1 package	5

	POINTS VALUE
Thai peanut instant rice noodles & sauce, 1 package	5
Toasted sesame instant rice noodles & sauce, 1 package	5
Thyme & Truffles Hors D'oeuvres	
Mini quesadillas, 1 piece	1
Spanakopita, 1 piece	2
Tyson	
Beef steak fajita kit, 1 serving (1 fajita)	4
Beef steak quesadilla fresh meal kit, 1 serving (1 quesadilla)	6
Chicken enchilada meal kit, 1	5
Chicken fajita meal kit, 1	2
Chicken fried rice meal kit, 2 1/2 cups	9
Chicken quesadillas meal kit, 1	5
Chicken stir fry meal kit, 2 3/4 cups	8
Wanchai Ferry	
Cashew chicken, prepared, 1 cup	7
Kung pao chicken, prepared, 1 cup	7
Sweet & sour chicken, prepared, 1 cup	6
Weight Watchers Smart Ones	
Chicken enchilada Suiza, 1	6
Chicken oriental, 1	4
Spicy Szechuan style vegetables & chicken, 1	4
Weight Watchers Smart Ones Anytime Selections	
Calzone Italiano, 1	6
Chicken and cheese quesadilla, 1	4
Fiesta quesadilla, 1	4

Prepared Foods, Salads & Sides

	POINTS VALUE
Weight Watchers Smart Ones Bistro Selections	
Chicken carbonara, 1	5
Chicken enchiladas Monterey, 1	6
Chicken fettucini, 1	7
Chicken Santa Fe, 1	2
Dragon shrimp lo mein, 1	5
Grilled mandarin chicken, 1	6
Picante chicken and pasta, 1	5
Sweet & sour chicken, 1	3
Thai style chicken & rice noodles, 1	5

Fish & Seafood Entrees
Acme

	POINTS VALUE
Blue Hill Bay baked peppered salmon skin on portion, 2 oz	2
Blue Hill Bay baked salmon skin on portion, 2 oz	2
Blue Hill Bay Pickled herring in wine (all natural), 5 pieces	2
Blue Hill Bay whitefish salad, 4 Tbsp	4
Whitefish salad, 4 Tbsp	4

Annie's Homegrown Organic Skillet Meals

	POINTS VALUE
Creamy tuna spirals, 1 1/2 oz (about 1 cup prepared)	3

Birds Eye Steamfresh

	POINTS VALUE
Meals for two, shrimp alfredo with fresh frozen vegetables, 1/2 bag	9
Meals for two, shrimp pasta primavera with fresh frozen vegetables, 1/2 bag	10

Birds Eye Voila!

	POINTS VALUE
Garlic shrimp, 1 serving (2 cups frozen, 1 cup cooked)	5
Shrimp scampi, 1 serving (1 3/4 cups frozen, 1 cup cooked)	3

Bumble Bee

	POINTS VALUE
Seafood salad with crab and crackers, seafood salad only, 1 can	1
Seafood salad with crab and crackers, crackers only, 6	2
Tuna salad original with crackers, tuna salad only, 1 can	6
Tuna salad original with crackers, crackers only, 6	2

Bumble Bee Easy Peel Sensations

	POINTS VALUE
Lemon & cracked pepper, 1/3 cup	2
Spicy Thai chili, 1/3 cup	4
Sundried tomato & basil, 1/3 cup	2

Chincoteague

	POINTS VALUE
Cape Cod breaded fried clams, 3 oz	6

Dr. Praeger's

	POINTS VALUE
Lightly breaded fish fillets, 1 fillet	2
Lightly breaded fish sticks, 3 sticks	3
Lightly breaded fishies-kids, 3	2
Potato crusted fish fillets, 1	2
Potato crusted fish sticks, 3	3
Potato crusted fishies, 3	2

Gorton's

	POINTS VALUE
Battered dipped fish portions, 1 serving (70 g)	5
Beer batter crispy battered fish fillets, 2 fillets	6
Beer batter tenders, 3 1/2 pieces	7
Crispy battered fish fillets, 2 fillets	6
Crispy battered popcorn fish, 1 serving (about 11 pieces)	7

Prepared Foods, Salads & Sides

	POINTS VALUE
Crunchy golden fish fillets, 2 fillets	6
Crunchy golden fish sticks, 6 sticks	6
Crunchy golden fish sticks breaded minced fish (30 pack), 6	6
Crunchy golden fish sticks breaded minced fish (44 pack), 6	6
Crunchy golden fish sticks breaded minced fish (6 pack), 6	6
Garlic and herb crunchy breaded fish fillets, 2 fillets	6
Grilled tilapia fillets - roasted garlic butter, 1 fillet	2
Lemon herb crunchy breaded fish fillets, 2 fillets	6
Lemon pepper fish fillets, battered, 2 fillets	7
Parmesan crunchy breaded fish fillets, 2 fillets	6
Potato crunch fish fillets, 2 fillets	5
Premium fillets, cod, 1 fillet	6
Ranch crunchy breaded fish fillets, 2 fillets	6
Southern fried country style crunchy breaded fish fillets, 2 fillets	6
Tenders original batter, 3 pieces	5
Tenders, extra crunchy, 3 pieces	5
Tenders, original batter, 3 pieces	5
Gorton's Grilled Salmon	
Classic grilled, 1 fillet	2
Lemon butter, 1 fillet	2
Gorton's Shrimp Bowl	
Alfredo, 1 bowl	5
Fried rice, 1 bowl	7

	POINTS VALUE
Garlic butter, 1 bowl	5
Teriyaki, 1 bowl	6
Ian's	
Baja fish nuggets, 3	4
Fish sticks, 5	4
Wheat free, gluten free fish sticks, 5	4
Wheat free, gluten free lightly battered fish, 1 serving (3.4 oz)	4
Kashi	
Lime cilantro shrimp, 1 package	5
Manischewitz	
Sweet whitefish & pike, 1 piece	1
Market Day	
Fish & chips, 1 serving (2 fillets, 4 oz fries, 2 tbsp tartar sauce)	13
Krispy krunchy cod, 1 piece (3.6 oz)	5
Oven Poppers	
Alaskan pollock qwickies stuffed with wild rice, almonds & cranberries, 1 portion (3 oz)	2
Cod augratin, 1 piece	5
Cod stuffed with broccoli & cheese, 1 piece	3
Crab stuffed flounder, 1 piece	6
Crab stuffed flounder qwickies made with a buttery cracker crumb stuffing, 1 portion (3 oz)	4
Crab stuffed sole, 1 piece	6
Crab stuffed sole qwickies, 1 portion (3 oz)	4
Flounder augratin, 1 piece	5
Flounder stuffed with garlic, shrimp & almonds, 1 piece	6

Prepared Foods, Salads & Sides

Oven Poppers (cont'd) — POINTS VALUE

Salmon qwickies stuffed with spinach & cheese, 1 portion (3 oz)	3
Salmon stuffed with spinach & cheese, 1 piece	7
Sole stuffed with garlic, shrimp & almonds, 1 piece	6
Sole stuffed with lump crabmeat, 1 piece	5
Sole stuffed with shrimp & lobster in newburg sauce, 1 piece	4
Sole stuffed with spinach & cheese, 1/2 container	5
Stuffed tilapia in a ginger teriyaki sauce, 1 piece	6
Stuffed tilapia in a lemon, garlic, butter sauce, 1 piece	6
Tilapia Caribbean, 1 piece (5 oz)	4
Tilapia stuffed with sun dried tomato, shrimp & lobster, 1 piece	4

Phillips

Boardwalk crab cakes, 1	5
Crab & shrimp cake, 1	4
Jalapeno crab slammers, 5 pieces	9
Maryland style crab cakes, 1	3

Tuna Helper

Cheesy pasta, prepared, 1 cup	7
Cheesy pasta, reduced fat recipe, prepared, 1 cup	5
Creamy broccoli, prepared, 1 cup	7
Creamy broccoli, reduced fat recipe, prepared, 1 cup	5
Creamy parmesan, prepared, 1 cup	6

POINTS VALUE

Creamy parmesan, reduced fat recipe, prepared, 1 cup	5
Creamy pasta, prepared, 1 cup	6
Creamy pasta, reduced fat recipe, prepared, 1 cup	5
Creamy roasted garlic, prepared, 1 cup	7
Creamy roasted garlic, reduced fat recipe, prepared, 1 cup	5
Fettuccine alfredo, prepared, 1 cup	7
Fettuccine alfredo, reduced fat recipe, prepared, 1 cup	5
Tetrazzini, prepared, 1 cup	7
Tetrazzini, reduced fat recipe, prepared, 1 cup	5
Tuna melt, prepared, 1 cup	7
Tuna melt, reduced fat recipe, prepared, 1 cup	5

Weight Watchers Fresh Ready Meals

Shrimp fettuccini with vegetables, 1	5

Weight Watchers Smart Ones

Shrimp marinara with linguini, 1	3
Tuna noodle gratin, 1	5

Meat & Poultry Entrees

Annie's Homegrown Organic Skillet Meals

Cheddar chicken, 1 1/2 oz (about 1 cup prepared)	3
Cheeseburger macaroni, 1 serving (1.3 oz, about 1 cup prepared)	3

Betty Crocker Complete Meals

Cheesy beef taco, prepared, 1 cup	5
Chicken & buttermilk biscuit, prepared, 1 serving (1/5 package)	5

	POINTS VALUE
Stroganoff, 1 serving (1/5 package)	4
Stroganoff, prepared, 1 cup	4
Three cheese chicken, 1 serving (1/5 package)	5
Three cheese chicken, prepared, 1 cup	5
Birds Eye Steamfresh	
Meals for two, grilled chicken in roasted garlic sauce with fresh frozen vegetables, 1/2 bag	7
Meals for two, grilled chicken marinara with fresh frozen vegetables, 1/2 bag	7
Meals for two, sweet & spicy chicken with fresh frozen vegetables, 1/2 bag	7
Birds Eye Voila!	
Alfredo chicken, 1 serving (1 1/2 cups frozen, 1 cup cooked)	6
Chicken & shrimp penne with vegetables, 1 serving (1 2/3 cups frozen, 1 cup cooked)	4
Chicken stir-fry, 1 serving (1 3/4 cups frozen, 1 cup cooked)	4
Garden herb chicken, 1 serving (2 cups frozen, 1 cup cooked)	6
Garlic chicken, 1 serving (1 2/3 cups frozen, 1 cup cooked)	5
Pesto chicken primavera, 1 serving (2 cups frozen, 1 cup cooked)	4
Southwestern style chicken, 1 serving (1 2/3 cups frozen, 1 cup cooked)	6
Teriyaki chicken, 1 serving (1 2/3 cups frozen, 1 cup cooked)	4
Three cheese chicken, 1 serving (1 2/3 cups frozen, 1 cup cooked)	4

	POINTS VALUE
Birds Eye Voila! Family Skillets	
Cheesy chicken, 1 serving (1 3/4 cups frozen, 1 cup cooked)	5
Cheesy macaroni & beef, 1 cup cooked	8
Garlic chicken, 1 serving (1 2/3 cups frozen, 1 cup cooked)	5
Birds Eye World Market Blends	
Beef & broccoli stir-fry, 1 serving (2 cups frozen, 1 cup cooked)	3
Boston Market Home Style Meals	
Apple glazed pork with broccoli & rice au gratin, 1 package	7
Beef pot roast, 1 package	10
Chicken pot pie, 1 cup	14
Chicken primavera with penne pasta, 1 package	11
Chicken, broccoli & cheese pot pie, 1 cup	14
Country fried chicken with mashed potatoes & gravy and peas & carrots, 1 package	12
Home style chicken with noodles, 1 package	11
Honey roasted chicken with au gratin potatoes, 1 package	9
Meatloaf with mashed potatoes & gravy, 1 package (340 g)	13
Meatloaf with mashed potatoes & gravy, 1 package (453 g)	16
Roasted pork, 1 package	12
Salisbury steak, 1 package	17
Swedish meatballs, 1 1/2 cups	20

Prepared Foods, Salads & Sides

Boston Market Home Style Meals (cont'd) <small>POINTS VALUE</small>

Turkey breast medallions with mashed potatoes & gravy and green beans & carrots, 1 package	6
Turkey medallions, 1 package	9
Turkey pot pie, 1 cup	14

Chicken Helper

Creamy chicken noodle, prepared, 1 cup	6
Four cheese, prepared, 1 cup	7
Jambalaya, prepared, 1 cup	6

Dinty Moore Hormel

Roast beef & gravy with mashed potatoes, 1 bowl	4

Ethnic Gourmet Taste of Italy

Chicken arrabiata with penne, 1 package	7

Ethnic Gourmet Taste of Santa Fe

Chipotle vegetarian chili lime sauce, 1 package	6
Lime chicken with ancho chile sauce, 1 package	7
Zesty chicken with garlic mashed potatoes, 1 package	7

Fast Classics

Steak fingers, gravy only, 1 serving (1/5 package)	2
Steak fingers, without gravy, 3 pieces	5

Glory

Chicken & dumplings, 1 cup	5
Ham & sausage jambalaya, 1 cup	8
Ham & sausage jambalaya, 1 package	10

	POINTS VALUE
Sausage & rice casserole, 1 cup	7
Turkey & dressing, 1 package	8

Green Giant Complete Skillet Meal

Chicken teriyaki, 1/4 package	4
Creamy chicken parmesan, as packaged, 1/4 package	5
Creamy chicken parmesan, prepared, 1 cup	6
Garlic chicken pasta, as packaged, 1/4 package	4

Hamburger Helper

Bacon cheeseburger, prepared, 1 cup	7
Cheddar cheese melt, prepared, 1 cup	7
Cheeseburger macaroni, prepared, 1 cup	7
Cheesy jambalaya, prepared, 1 cup	7
Cheesy nacho, prepared, 1 cup	8
Cheesy ranch burger, prepared, 1 cup	8
Chili cheese, prepared, 1 cup	7
Italian sausage, prepared, 1 cup	7
Philly cheesesteak, prepared, 1 cup	7
Potatoes stroganoff, prepared, 1 cup	7
Salisbury, prepared, 1 cup	6
Sloppy Joe, prepared, 1 cup	7

Hamburger Helper Microwave Singles

Cheeseburger macaroni, 1 pouch	5
Cheeseburger macaroni flavored, 1 container	4
Megapacks cheeseburger, 1 pouch	7
Stroganoff, 1 pouch	3
Ultimate cheesy burger, 1 container	4

Prepared Foods, Salads & Sides

	POINTS VALUE
Hamburger Helper Wholesome Classics	
Cheeseburger mac, prepared, 1 cup	7
Stroganoff, prepared, 1 cup	7
Hormel	
Beef roast, 5 oz	5
Beef roast family pack, 5 oz	5
Beef tips, 5 oz	4
Beef tips & gravy family pack, 5 oz	4
Chicken breast with gravy, 1	3
Family pack beef tips with gravy, 1 serving	4
Family pack meat loaf with tomato sauce, 5 oz	6
Meat loaf, 5 oz	6
Pork chops with gravy, 5 oz	4
Pork roast, 5 oz	4
Pulled bbq pork, 2 oz	2
Sliced bbq beef brisket, 5 oz	7
Sliced beef steak and gravy, 5 oz	3
Sliced turkey and gravy, 1	3
Southwestern chicken breast strips, 2 oz	1
Southwestern shredded beef, 2 oz	2
Hormel Compleats Microwave Meals	
Beef & beans bbq sauce, 1 bowl	8
Beef pot roast with potatoes & carrots in gravy, 1 bowl	6
Chicken & noodles, 1 bowl	5
Chicken breast & gravy with mashed potatoes, 1 bowl	4
Meat loaf with potatoes & gravy, 1 bowl	6

	POINTS VALUE
Salisbury steak with sliced potatoes & gravy, 1 bowl	6
Turkey & dressing with gravy, 1 bowl	6
Hot Pocket	
Roller stix, egg & sausage with cheese flavor, 1	5
Stuffed sandwich - chicken & Cheddar with broccoli flavor, 1	7
Stuffed sandwich - turkey & ham with cheese flavor, 1	7
Ian's	
Chicken nuggets kid's meal, 8 oz	10
Original chicken pot pie, 1	12
Wheat free, gluten-free chicken fingers kid's meal, 7 oz	7
Jimmy Dean D-Lights	
Turkey sausage breakfast bowl, 1	5
Kashi	
Chicken florentine, 1 package	6
Lemon rosemary chicken, 1 package	7
Lemongrass coconut chicken, 1 package	6
Southwest style chicken, 1 package	4
Market Day	
Beef & broccoli with rice, 1 cup	5
Chicken and dumplings, 1 cup	5
Chicken breast Tuscan, 1 serving	8
Chicken pot pie, 1 cup	13
Individual chicken pot pies, 1 cup	16
Lemon caper chicken, 1 serving	7
Roast turkey with stuffing, 1 serving (12 oz)	6

Prepared Foods, Salads & Sides

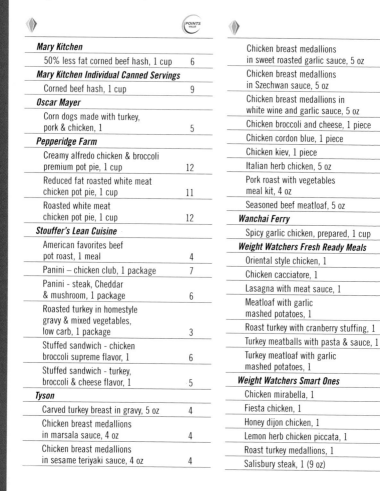

	POINTS VALUE
Mary Kitchen	
50% less fat corned beef hash, 1 cup	6
Mary Kitchen Individual Canned Servings	
Corned beef hash, 1 cup	9
Oscar Mayer	
Corn dogs made with turkey, pork & chicken, 1	5
Pepperidge Farm	
Creamy alfredo chicken & broccoli premium pot pie, 1 cup	12
Reduced fat roasted white meat chicken pot pie, 1 cup	11
Roasted white meat chicken pot pie, 1 cup	12
Stouffer's Lean Cuisine	
American favorites beef pot roast, 1 meal	4
Panini – chicken club, 1 package	7
Panini - steak, Cheddar & mushroom, 1 package	6
Roasted turkey in homestyle gravy & mixed vegetables, low carb, 1 package	3
Stuffed sandwich - chicken broccoli supreme flavor, 1	6
Stuffed sandwich - turkey, broccoli & cheese flavor, 1	5
Tyson	
Carved turkey breast in gravy, 5 oz	4
Chicken breast medallions in marsala sauce, 4 oz	4
Chicken breast medallions in sesame teriyaki sauce, 4 oz	4
Chicken breast medallions in sweet roasted garlic sauce, 5 oz	4
Chicken breast medallions in Szechwan sauce, 5 oz	4
Chicken breast medallions in white wine and garlic sauce, 5 oz	3
Chicken broccoli and cheese, 1 piece	4
Chicken cordon blue, 1 piece	9
Chicken kiev, 1 piece	12
Italian herb chicken, 5 oz	3
Pork roast with vegetables meal kit, 4 oz	8
Seasoned beef meatloaf, 5 oz	8
Wanchai Ferry	
Spicy garlic chicken, prepared, 1 cup	6
Weight Watchers Fresh Ready Meals	
Oriental style chicken, 1	6
Chicken cacciatore, 1	4
Lasagna with meat sauce, 1	6
Meatloaf with garlic mashed potatoes, 1	6
Roast turkey with cranberry stuffing, 1	5
Turkey meatballs with pasta & sauce, 1	6
Turkey meatloaf with garlic mashed potatoes, 1	6
Weight Watchers Smart Ones	
Chicken mirabella, 1	4
Fiesta chicken, 1	5
Honey dijon chicken, 1	4
Lemon herb chicken piccata, 1	4
Roast turkey medallions, 1	4
Salisbury steak, 1 (9 oz)	4

SENSIBLE
yumminess.

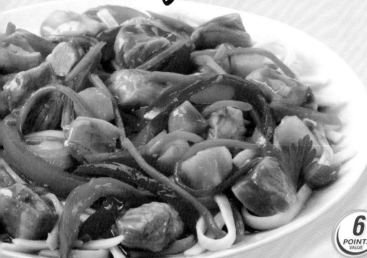

6 POINTS VALUE

Per Serving
**Oriental Style Chicken
With Noodles**

Fresh meals, found in the deli*

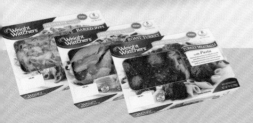

WeightWatchers®
Stop Dieting. Start Living.

Find more information at WeightWatchers.com/freshmeals

WEIGHT WATCHERS on foods and beverages is the registered trademark of WW Foods, LLC and is used under license by Greencore USA. WEIGHT WATCHERS for services and *POINTS®* are the registered trademarks of Weight Watchers International, Inc. and are used under license by Greencore USA.
©2009 Weight Watchers International, Inc. All rights reserved.
*Selection may vary by store. Check your local retailer for availability.

Prepared Foods, Salads & Sides

Weight Watchers Smart Ones (cont'd)	POINTS VALUE
Salisbury steak with macaroni & cheese, 1	6
Santa Fe style rice & beans, 1	6
Swedish meatballs, 1	5
Weight Watchers Smart Ones Artisan Creations	
Grilled flatbread chicken bruschetta, 1 piece	6
Grilled flatbread chicken marinara with mozzarella cheese, 1 piece	6
Grilled flatbread savory steak and ranch, 1 piece	6
Grilled flatbread southwestern style chicken fiesta, 1 piece	6
Weight Watchers Smart Ones Bistro Selections	
Beef pot roast, 1	3
Chicken marsala with broccoli, 1	4
Chicken parmesan, 1	5
Creamy chicken Tuscan with zucchini, 1	4
Creamy parmesan chicken, 1	5
Fire-grilled chicken & vegetables, 1	6
Grilled chicken in garlic herb sauce with zucchini, 1	4
Home-style chicken, 1	5
Meatloaf with mashed potatoes, 1	5
Pepper steak, 1	5
Roast beef with gravy, 1	5
Roast beef with portabello gravy, 1	4
Roasted chicken with sour cream & chive mashed potatoes, 1	4
Salisbury steak and asparagus, 1	4

	POINTS VALUE
Sirloin beef and Asian style vegetables, 1	4
Slow-roasted turkey breast, 1	4
Southwest style adobo chicken, 1	5
Stuffed turkey breast, 1	6
Teriyaki chicken & vegetables, 1	4
Turkey medallions with mushroom gravy and green beans, 1	4
Weight Watchers Smart Ones Fruit Inspirations	
Cranberry turkey medallions, 1	7
Honey mango barbeque chicken, 1	5
Orange sesame chicken, 1	7
Pineapple beef teriyaki, 1	6

Meat Substitutes Entrees
Amy's

	POINTS VALUE
Tofu vegetable lasagna, 1	6
Amy's Whole Meals	
Chili & cornbread, 1	7
Light in sodium veggie loaf, 1	6
Celentano Vegetarian	
Nondairy selects lasagna primavera (organic), 1 tray	5
Linda McCartney	
Butternut squash ravioli, 1 package	9
Fire-grilled vegetarian chicken and vegetables, 1 package	6
Macaroni and cheese, 1 package	9
Spicy peanut pasta with vegetarian chicken, 1 package	8
Mon Cuisine	
Vegan breaded nuggets, IQF, 1 serving (0.8 oz)	1

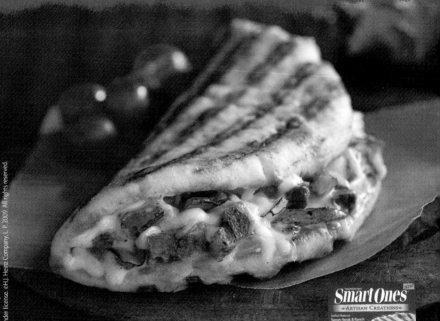

Your microwave has a new setting.

Oven-baked.

When we created new Smart Ones® Artisan Creations Flatbreads, we began with the bread. Which is why it may be the best microwave sandwich ever. And, with a *POINTS* value of just 6, you can relax and enjoy!

SAVE $4.00 at www.eatyourbest.com/food

WEIGHT WATCHERS and ...and beverages is the registered trademark of WW FOODS, LLC and is used under license. WEIGHT WATCHERS for services and POINTS are the UK registered trademarks of WW UK limited. International, Inc. and are used under license. ©H.J. Heinz Company, L.P. 2009. All rights reserved.

Prepared Foods, Salads & Sides

Mon Cuisine (cont'd)	POINTS VALUE
Vegan breaded patties, 2 1/2 oz	2
Vegan meatless Italian shell pasta, 10 oz	4
Vegan Moroccan couscous, 10 oz	5
Vegan pot pie, 9 oz	15
Vegan veal style schnitzel in sauce, 10 oz	6
Vegetarian grilled steak in mushroom gravy, 10 oz	5
Vegetarian salisbury steak in gravy, 10 oz	6
Vegetarian spaghetti & meatballs, 10 oz	7
Vegetarian stuffed cabbage in tomato sauce, 10 oz	4
Tofurky	
Vegetarian feast - roast, stuffing & gravy, 4 oz	4
Vegetarian feast - cranberry-apple potato dumplings only, 2 pieces	3
Vegetarian feast - giblet & mushroom gravy only, 2 Tbsp	1
Vegetarian feast - roast & stuffing only, 4 oz	4
Vegetarian feast - wild rice & mushroom stuffing only, 1/2 cup	2
Vegetarian feast - wishstix only, 1/2 piece	0

Pasta & Vegetable Salads

Annie's Homegrown	
Macaroni & cheese, 1 cup prepared	6
Betty Crocker Suddenly Salad	
Caesar pasta, prepared, 1 cup	6
Chipotle ranch, prepared, 2/3 cup	6

	POINTS VALUE
Classic pasta, prepared, 1 cup	5
Creamy Italian pasta, prepared, 3/4 cup	8
Creamy parmesan pasta, prepared, 1 cup	9
Ranch & bacon pasta, prepared, 3/4 cup	8
DiGiorno	
Basil vinaigrette pasta salad, prepared, 3/4 cup	4
Three cheese Italian for club, as packaged, 1 serving 1/20 box)	5
DiLusso	
Chef salad (small), 1 container	4
Chef salad (large), 1 container	8
Chicken Caesar salad (small), 1 container	4
Chicken Caesar salad (large), 1 container	8
Chicken club salad (small), 1 container	4
Chicken club salad (large), 1 container	8
Chicken fajita salad (large), 1 container	6
Cobb salad (small), 1 container	6
Cobb salad (large), 1 container	11
Greek salad (large), 1 container	6
Ham & broccoli salad (large), 1 container	8
Southwest turkey salad (large), 1 container	6
Dole	
Angel hair cole slaw, 3 oz	0

Prepared Foods, Salads & Sides

	POINTS VALUE
Dole Classic	
♦ Cole slaw, 3 oz	0
♦ Iceberg salad, 3 oz	0
Dole Complete Salads	
Bacon lettuce toss kit - bacon ranch dressing, 1 serving (0.69 fl oz dressing)	2
Fall harvest kit - apple dijon vinaigrette dressing, 1 serving (0.8 fl oz dressing)	2
Family Caesar - Caesar dressing, 1 serving (0.69 fl oz dressing)	3
Garlic Caesar kit - garlic Caesar dressing, 1 serving (0.8 fl oz dressing)	3
Spring garden kit - raspberry vinaigrette dressing, 1 serving (0.7 fl oz dressing)	2
Summer sun kit - tomato herb vinaigrette dressing, 1 serving (0.53 fl oz dressing)	1
Taco toss kit - taco ranch dressing, 1 serving (0.66 fl oz dressing)	2
Winter medley kit - cranberry vinaigrette dressing, 1 serving (0.83 fl oz dressing)	3
Dole Complete Salads with Dressing	
Caesar, 1 serving (3.5 oz)	3
Light Caesar, 1 serving (3.5 oz)	2
Romano, 1 serving (3.5 oz)	2
Sunflower ranch, 1 serving (3.5 oz)	3
Dole Special Blends	
♦ American blend, 3 oz	0
♦ European blend, 3 oz	0
♦ French blend, 3 oz	0
♦ Italian blend, 3 oz	0
♦ Romaine blend, 3 oz	0
Green Giant	
Three bean salad, canned, 1/2 cup	1

	POINTS VALUE
Kashi	
Black bean mango, 1 package	7
Kraft	
Asian sesame, prepared, 1 cup	6
Basil vinaigrette, prepared, 3/4 cup	4
Caesar, prepared, 3/4 cup	9
Classic ranch with bacon, prepared, 3/4 cup	8
Garlic parmesan, prepared, 3/4 cup	9
Harvest ranch peppercorn, prepared, 1 cup	5
Italian, prepared, 3/4 cup	5
Santa Fe style ranch, prepared, 3/4 cup	4
Linsey	
Caesar salad kit, 1 serving (22 g)	3
Italian salad kit, 1 serving (22 g)	3
Light Caesar salad kit, 1 serving (22 g)	2
Linsey ET Tu	
Greek salad kit, 1 serving (1/6 package)	2
Greek salad kit, 1 large serving (100 g)	11
Oriental salad kit, 1 serving (1/6 package)	2
Oriental salad kit, 1 large serving (100 g)	7
Spinach salad kit, 1 serving (1/6 package)	2
Spinach salad kit, 1 large serving (100 g)	11
Vinaigrette salad kit, 1 serving (1/6 package)	3
Vinaigrette salad kit, 1 large serving (100 g)	13

Prepared Foods, Salads & Sides

	POINTS VALUE
Tyson	
Premium chunk chicken salad kit, 1 package	5
Westbrae Natural	
Country style marinated bean salad, 1/2 cup	1
Deli style marinated bean salad, 1/2 cup	1

Pasta Entrees

Amy's

	POINTS VALUE
Cheese lasagna, 1	8
Garden vegetable lasagna, 1	6
Kids baked ziti meal, 1	7
Kids mac n' cheese meal, 1	8
Large size mac & cheese, 1 cup	8
Light in sodium macaroni & cheese, 1	9
Macaroni & cheese, 1	9
Macaroni & soy cheeze, 1	8
Rice mac & cheese, 1 container	9
Vegetable lasagna, 1	6

Amy's Bowls

	POINTS VALUE
Baked ziti bowl, 1	8
Country Cheddar bowl, 1	9
Pesto tortellini bowl, 1	10
Ravioli bowl, 1	8
Stuffed pasta shells bowl, 1	6

Annie's Homegrown

	POINTS VALUE
Arthur mac & cheese, 2 1/2 oz (about 1 cup prepared)	6
Bunny shape pasta & yummy cheese, 2 1/2 oz (about 1 cup prepared)	6

	POINTS VALUE
Deluxe elbow & four cheese, 3.6 oz (about 1 cup prepared)	7
Deluxe rotini & white Cheddar, 3.4 oz (about 1 cup prepared)	6
Deluxe shells & real age Cheddar, 3.6 oz (about 1 cup prepared)	7
Deluxe whole wheat shells & extra cheesy Cheddar, 3 oz (about 1 cup prepared)	5
Micro mac and real age cheese, 1/2 cup packaged (3/4 cup prepared)	5
Micro mac and white Cheddar, 1/2 cup packaged (3/4 cup prepared)	5
Organic alfredo shells & Cheddar, 2 1/2 oz (about 1 cup prepared)	5
Organic peace pasta with parmesan, 2 1/2 oz (about 1 cup prepared)	5
Organic shells & real age Cheddar, 2 1/2 oz (about 1 cup prepared)	5
Organic shells with white Cheddar, 2 1/2 oz (about 1 cup prepared)	5
Organic whole wheat shells & Cheddar, 2 1/2 oz (about 1 cup prepared)	5
Shells & real age Cheddar, 2 1/2 oz (about 1 cup prepared)	6
Shells & white Cheddar, 2 1/2 oz (about 1 cup prepared)	6

Annie's Homegrown Organic Canned Meals

	POINTS VALUE
All stars, 1 cup	3
Arthur loops, 1 cup	3
BernieOs, 1 cup	3
Cheesy ravioli, 1 cup	3
P'sghetti loops with soy meatballs, 1 cup	4

Prepared Foods, Salads & Sides

POINTS VALUE

Annie's Homegrown Organic Skillet Meals

Cheesy lasagna, 1.3 oz (about 1 cup prepared)	2
Stroganoff, 1.3 oz (about 1 cup prepared)	3

Annie's Homegrown Simply Organic Macaroni & Cheese

Macaroni & cheese, 2/3 cup (1 cup prepared)	5
Shells & cheese, 2/3 cup (1 cup prepared)	5

Back To Nature

Back to nature cup, 1 package	4
Crazy bugs macaroni & cheese, as prepared, 1 cup	7
Harvest wheat & Cheddar, as prepared, 1 cup	5
Organic macaroni & cheese, as prepared, 1 cup	7
Organic shells & cheese, as prepared, 1 cup	8
Organic white Cheddar cheese & organic shells, as prepared, 1 cup	7
Original macaroni & cheese, as prepared, 1 cup	7
White Cheddar & spirals, as prepared, 1 cup	7
White Cheddar & whole wheat elbow, as prepared, 1 cup	6

Betty Crocker

Chicken Fettuccine alfredo, prepared, 1 serving (1/5 package)	5

Birds Eye

Pasta & vegetables in a creamy cheese sauce, frozen, 1 cup	3

Birds Eye Voila!

Pasta primavera with chicken, 2 cups frozen (1 cup cooked)	5

Boca

Lasagna - chunky tomato & herb sauce with meatless ground burger, 1 package	5

Boston Market Home Style Meals

Lasagna with meat sauce layered with ricotta & meat sauce, 1 package	11
Macaroni & cheese, 1/2 cup	7

Bowl Appetit!

Cheddar broccoli pasta, 1 bowl	7
Garlic parmesan pasta, 1 bowl	7
Homestyle chicken flavored pasta, 1 bowl	5
Pasta alfredo, 1 bowl	8
Teriyaki rice, 1 bowl	5
Three-cheese rotini, 1 bowl	8

Campbell's

Mini beef ravioli in meat sauce, 1 cup	5
Spaghetti in tomato & cheese sauce, 1 cup	4
Spaghettios, 1 cup	3
Spaghettios a to z's, 1 cup	3
Spaghettios a to z's with meatballs, 1 cup	5
Spaghettios a to z's with sliced franks, 1 cup	5
Spaghettios cars shaped pasta with meatballs, 1 cup	5
Spaghettios dora the explorer shaped pasta, 1 cup	3
Spaghettios in meat sauce, 1 cup	3

Prepared Foods, Salads & Sides

Campbell's (cont'd)	POINTS VALUE
Spaghettios pasta with sliced franks, 1 cup	5
Spaghettios plus calcium, 1 cup	3
Spaghettios raviolio's beef ravioli in meat sauce, 1 cup	5
Spaghettios with meatballs, 1 cup	5
Campbell's Supper Bakes	
Cheesy chicken with pasta, 1 serving (1/7 of box)	3
Creamy stroganoff sauce with pasta, 1 serving (1/6 box)	4
Garlic chicken with pasta, 1 serving (1/7 of box)	4
Herb chicken with rice, 1 serving (1/6 of box)	3
Lemon chicken with herb rice, 1 serving (1/7 of box)	3
Southwestern style chicken with rice, 1 serving (1/6 of box)	3
Traditional roast chicken with stuffing, 1 serving (1/6 box)	3
Carapelli	
Creamy alfredo with penne, 1 cup	4
Four cheese with cavatappi, 1 cup	4
Roasted garlic & fusilli, 1 cup	4
Roasted red pepper radiatore, 1 cup	4
Tomato & basil gemelli, 1 cup	4
Tomato with spiral, 1 cup	4
Celentano	
Manicotti, 1 tray	9
Celentano Light	
Broccoli stuffed shells, 1	6
Cheese ravioli, blanched, 4	4
Manicotti florentine, 1 tray	6

	POINTS VALUE
Celentano Vegetarian	
Organic penne with roasted vegetables, 1 tray	6
Organic spinach & broccoli manicotti with sauce, 1 tray	6
Organic spinach & broccoli stuffed shells, 1 tray	6
Chicken Helper Microwave Singles	
Fettuccine alfredo, 1 pouch	5
Dinty Moore Individual Canned Servings	
Chicken & dumplings, 1 can	4
Dinty Moore Microwave Cups	
Noodles & chicken, 1 cup	4
Ethnic Gourmet Taste of Italy	
Butternut squash ravioli, 1 package (10 oz)	8
Trofie pasta with pesto, 1 package (10 oz)	13
Vegetarian osso bucco with fettucini, 1 package (10 oz)	7
Glory	
Macaroni and cheese, 1 cup	9
Green Giant Complete Skillet Meal	
Cheesy Italian style shells, 1 cup	8
Hamburger Helper	
Beef pasta, prepared, 1 cup	6
Chili macaroni, prepared, 1 cup	6
Double cheeseburger macaroni, prepared, 1 cup	7
Four cheese lasagna, prepared, 1 cup	7
Lasagna, prepared, 1 cup	6
Spaghetti, prepared, 1 cup	6
Three cheese, prepared, 1 cup	7
Tomato basil penne, prepared, 1 cup	7

Prepared Foods, Salads & Sides

	POINTS VALUE
Hodgson Mill	
Whole wheat macaroni & cheese, 2 1/2 oz (about 1/3 box)	4
Hormel Compleats Microwave Bowls	
Chicken & dumplings, 1 bowl	5
Chicken & rice, 1 bowl	6
Spaghetti with meat sauce, 1 bowl	5
Sweet & sour rice, 1 bowl	5
Teriyaki chicken with rice, 1 bowl	5
Hormel Compleats Microwave Meals	
Chicken alfredo chicken with penne pasta in alfredo sauce, 1 bowl	8
Lasagna/meat sauce, 1 bowl	6
Turkey & hearty vegetables, 1 bowl	4
Hormel Individual Canned Servings	
Beans and wieners, 1 can	6
Mac & cheese, 1 cup	6
Hormel Micro Cup Meals	
Lasagna with meat sauce, 1 cup	4
Southwest style rice, 1 cup	3
Spaghetti with meat sauce, 1 cup	4
Teriyaki rice, 1 cup	4
Hormel Pasta Cups	
Cheese tortellini, 1 cup	4
Italian style, 1 cup	5
Lemon pepper, 1 cup	5
Ian's	
Mac & cheese - organic, 1 serving (170 g)	6
Organic pasta kit, 1 serving (6.5 oz)	5
Rotini & mini meatballs, 1 serving (170 g)	5
Wheat free, gluten free mac & meat sauce, 1 bowl	5

	POINTS VALUE
Wheat free, gluten free mac & no cheese, 1 bowl	5
Wheat free, gluten free pasta kit, 1 serving (6.5 oz)	5
Italian Village	
Large round cheese ravioli, 4	4
Mini round cheese ravioli, 13	4
Square cheese ravioli, 9	4
Italian Village Floresta	
Cheese tortellini, 1 cup uncooked	5
Meat tortellini, 1 cup uncooked	6
Square beef ravioli, 6	4
Kashi	
Chicken pasta pomodoro, 1 package	5
Garden vegetable pasta, 1 package	6
Pesto pasta primavera, 1 package	6
Kid's Kitchen	
Beans & wieners, 1 cup	7
Beefy macaroni, 1 cup	3
Cheezy mac & beef, 1 cup	6
Cheezy mac 'n franks, 1 cup	7
Cheezy mac'n cheese, 1 cup	7
Mini beef ravioli, 1 cup	5
Noodle rings & chicken, 1 cup	3
Spaghetti & meatballs, 1 cup	5
Spaghetti rings & franks, 1 cup	6
Kraft	
All shapes, 1 cup	5
Deluxe sharp Cheddar, as packaged, 1 serving (98 g)	7
Easy mac extreme cheese, 1 pouch	5
Easy mac macaroni & cheese, as packaged, 1 serving (61 g)	5

Prepared Foods, Salads & Sides

Kraft (cont'd)	POINTS VALUE
Homestyle macaroni, 3/4 cup	6
Macaroni & cheese spirals, as packaged, 1 serving (70 g)	5
Organic Cheddar cheese & organic elbow pasta dinner, prepared, 1 cup	7
Organic white Cheddar cheese & organic shells dinner, prepared, 1 cup	7
Original, 2 1/2 oz	5
Original, light, prepared, 1 cup	6
Original, prepared using classic recipe, 1 cup	10
Shapes - scooby doo, prepared using classic recipe, 1 cup	9
Spirals, prepared using classic recipe, 1 cup	9
Spirals, prepared using light recipe, 1 cup	6
Supermac original - pasta & sauce, prepared using classic recipe, 1 cup	7
Supermac original - pasta & sauce, prepared using light recipe, 1 cup	4
Three cheese, prepared using classic recipe, 1 cup	9
Three cheese, prepared using light recipe, 1 cup	6
Kraft Bistro Deluxe	
Classic Cheddar, 1 cup	7
Creamy portobello mushroom, 1 cup	7
Sundried tomato parmesan, 1 cup	6
Three cheese italiano, 1 cup	7
Kraft Deluxe	
1/2 the fat made with 2% milk cheese, 3 1/2 oz	6

	POINTS VALUE
Four cheese blend, 1 cup	7
Original, as packaged, 3 1/2 oz	7
Kraft Easy Mac Cups	
Alfredo, 1 package	5
Bacon, 1 package	5
Original, 1 package	5
Triple cheese, 1 package	5
Kraft Premium	
Cheesy alfredo, 1 cup	5
Cheesy alfredo, prepared using classic recipe, 1 cup	8
Cheesy alfredo, prepared using light recipe, 1 cup	6
Mild white Cheddar, prepared using classic recipe, 1 cup	8
Mild white Cheddar, prepared using light recipe, 1 cup	6
Thick 'n creamy, 2 1/2 oz	5
Thick 'n creamy, prepared using classic recipe, 1 cup	8
Thick 'n creamy, prepared using light recipe, 1 cup	6
White Cheddar, mild, 2 1/2 oz	5
Kraft Velveeta	
1/2 the fat, 4 oz	7
Bacon, prepared, 1 cup	8
Original, as packaged, 4 oz	8
Rotini and cheese with broccoli dinner, prepared, 1 cup	9
Market Day	
Cheese lasagna roll-up, 1 serving (3 oz)	3
Cheese ravioli, 7	4

	POINTS VALUE
Chicken fettuccini alfredo, 1 tray (9.5 oz)	9
Florentine lasagna roll-up, 1 serving (3 oz)	2
Mac & cheese singles, 1 pouch	7
Marrakesh Express	
Creamy pearls of pasta, 3 scoops	5
Moroccan pasta, 1 cup	4
Monterey Pasta Company	
Artichoke cheese ravioli with ripe olives, 1 cup	5
Lobster ravioli, 1 cup	5
Rainbow five cheese tortelloni, 1 cup	6
Roasted garlic chicken ravioli, 1 cup	5
Spinach and cheese ravioli, 1 cup	5
Spinach ricotta ravioli, 1 cup	5
Whole wheat chicken and sundried tomato ravioli, 1 cup	4
Whole wheat classic Italian cheese tortellini, 1 cup	5
Whole wheat Spicy chicken pesto ravioli, 1 cup	5
Whole wheat spinach & cheese tortelloni, 1 cup	5
Whole wheat tomato, basil & mozzarella ravioli, 1 cup	5
Whole wheat Tuscan style roasted peppers ravioli, 1 cup	4
Nutritious Living Hi-Lo	
Chicken vegetable parmesan, 1 tray	3
Turkey chili Santa Fe, 1 tray	3

	POINTS VALUE
Old El Paso	
Gordita dinner mix (with ranch sauce), prepared, 1 serving (1 tortilla, 2 Tbsp ranch sauce, 1 tsp seasoning mix)	7
Gordita dinner mix (with red sauce), prepared, 1 serving (1 tortilla, 2 Tbsp red sauce, 1 tsp seasoning mix)	8
Ortega	
Soft taco kit, 2 (2 tortillas, 1 Tbsp sauce, 1/5 envelope seasoning)	5
Taco kit, 2 (2 shells, 1 Tbsp sauce, 1/6 envelope seasoning)	3
Rosetto	
All natural cheese ravioli, 9 pieces	4
All natural whole wheat & cheese ravioli, 9 pieces	4
Beef ravioli, 9 pieces	5
Beef ravioli made with organic durum wheat, 9 pieces	4
Cheese and broccoli ravioli, 4 pieces	5
Cheese manicotti, 2 pieces	6
Cheese ravioli, 9 pieces	5
Cheese tortellini, 1 cup	5
Chicken and herb ravioli, 9 pieces	4
Gourmet butternut squash ravioli, 9 pieces	4
Gourmet pesto ravioli with walnuts, 9 pieces	6
Italian style ravioli with sausage, 9 pieces	5
Small round cheese ravioli, 13 pieces	5
Large round cheese ravioli, 5 pieces	4

Prepared Foods, Salads & Sides

	POINTS VALUE
Rosina	
Non dairy vegetarian selects penne with roasted vegetables (made with organic ingredients), 1 tray	6
Non dairy vegetarian selects spinach & broccoli manicotti (organic), 1 tray	6
Non dairy vegetarian selects spinach & broccoli stuffed shells (organic), 1 tray	6
Rosina Presents Celentano	
Beef ravioli, 3	4
Cheese tortellini, 1 cup	5
Four cheese baked ziti, 8 oz	7
Lasagne with sauce, 1/2 tray	6
Manicotti, 1 tray	9
Manicotti with sauce, 1 (10 oz)	9
Manicotti without sauce, 1/2 tray	8
Mini cheese ravioli, 12	4
Round cheese ravioli, 4	5
Stuffed shells with sauce, 1 tray	9
Stuffed shells without sauce, 4	7
Rosina Presents Celentano Light	
Light broccoli stuffed shells with sauce, 1 tray	6
Light cheese ravioli, 4	4
Light lasagna, 1 tray	7
Light manicotti florentine with sauce, 1 tray	6
Light stuffed shells with sauce, 1 tray	7
Manicotti, 1 tray	6
Seeds of Change	
Fettuccine alfredo di roma made with soy protein & broccoli, 1 tray	6
Hanalei vegetarian chicken teriyaki, 1 tray	5
Lasagna calabrese, 1 tray	5

	POINTS VALUE
Spinach lasagna di parma, 1 tray	7
Venetian penne marinara, 1 tray	6
Stouffer's Lean Cuisine	
Ravioli Cheese, 1 package	5
Spaghetti with Meat Sauce, 1 package	5
Swanson	
Chicken a la king, 1 can	7
Chicken and dumplings, 1 cup	5
T.G.I. Friday's	
Four cheese toasted ravioli (toasted ravioli with sauce), 1 serving	5
Weight Watchers Fresh Ready Meals	
Baked ziti, 1	6
Fettuccini primavera, 1	4
Three cheese macaroni, 1	4
Vegetable lasagna, 1	5
Weight Watchers Smart Ones	
Angel hair marinara, 1	4
Creamy rigatoni with broccoli & chicken, 1	6
Fettuccini alfredo, 1	4
Lasagna bolognese, 1	5
Lasagna florentine, 1	6
Macaroni & cheese, 1	5
Pasta primavera, 1	5
Ravioli florentine, 1	5
Spaghetti bolognese, 1	6
Three cheese macaroni, 1	6
Three cheese ziti marinara, 1	6
Traditional lasagna with meat sauce, 1	6
Weight Watchers Smart Ones Bistro Selections	
Penne pollo, 1	6

Guess who's layer after layer of delicious?

International, Inc. and are used under license. ©H.J. Heinz Company L.P. 2009. All rights reserved.

Weight Watchers® Smart Ones® Lasagna Florentine layers fresh pasta with creamy ricotta, zucchini, spinach, and garden-style marinara — all topped with real mozzarella and parmesan. And with a *POINTS*® value of only 6, it's delizioso and smart!

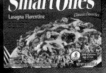

SAVE $4.00 at www.eatyourbest.com/food

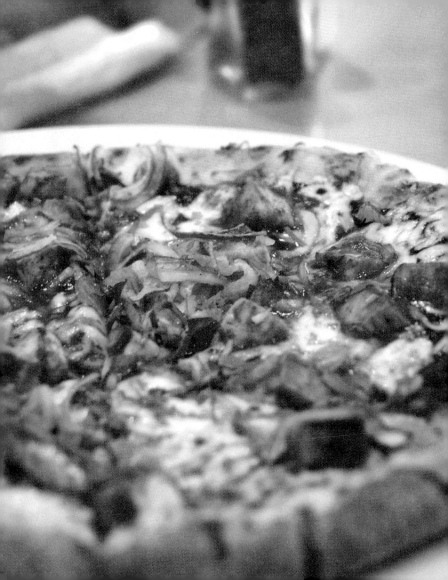

Prepared Foods, Salads & Sides

Pizza

A.C. LaRocco

Item	POINTS
Cheese & garlic thin crust vegetarian pizza, 1/3 pizza	5
Garden vegetarian pizza, 1/3 pizza	5
Greek sesame vegetarian pizza, 1/3 pizza	5
Quattro formaggio thin crust vegetarian pizza, 1/3 pizza	4
Spinach & artichoke thin crust vegetarian pizza, 1/3 pizza	4
Tomato & feta vegetarian pizza, 1/3 pizza	5
Ultra thin bruschetta style pizza, 1/2 pizza	3
Ultra thin garlic chicken parmesan, 1/2 pizza	4

Amy's

Item	POINTS
3 cheese pizza with cornmeal crust, 1 serving (4.83 oz)	9
Cheese & pesto pizza with whole wheat crust, 1 serving (4.66 oz)	8
Cheese pizza, 1 serving (4.33 oz)	7
Cheese pizza snacks, 1 serving (5-6 pieces)	4
Margherita pizza, 1/3 pizza	6
Mediterranean pizza with cornmeal crust, 1 serving (5.83 oz)	8
Mushroom and olive pizza, 1 serving (4.33 oz)	5
Pesto pizza, 1 serving (4.5 oz)	7
Rice crust cheese pizza, 1 serving (4 oz)	7
Rice crust spinach pizza, 1/3 pizza	8
Roasted vegetable pizza, 1 serving (4 oz)	6
Single serve cheese pizza, 1	9
Single serve light in sodium spinach pizza, 1	10
Single serve margherita pizza, 1	8
Single serve mushroom & olive pizza, 1	10
Single serve non-dairy rice crust cheeze pizza, 1	11
Single serve pesto pizza, 1	10
Single serve roasted vegetable pizza, 1	9
Single serve spinach pizza, 1	10
Soy cheeze pizza, 1 serving (4.33 oz)	6
Spinach pizza, 1 serving (4.66 oz)	7
Spinach pizza snack, 1 serving (5-6 pieces)	4
Veggie combo pizza, 1 serving (5.33 oz)	7

Boboli

Item	POINTS
100% whole wheat pizza crust, 12", 1 serving (1/6 crust)	2
8" mini 100% whole wheat twin pizza crusts, 1/2	3
8" mini original twin pizza crusts, 1/2 crust	4
Original pizza crust, 12", 1 serving (1/6 crust)	4
Thin pizza crust, 12", 1 serving (1/6 crust)	3

Bravissimo

Item	POINTS
7" cheese pizza, 1/2	6
7" spinach pizza, 1/2	6

425

Prepared Foods, Salads & Sides

Bravissimo (cont'd)	POINTS VALUE
7" vegetable pizza, 1/2	5
9" cheese pizza, 1/3	6
9" pepperoni pizza, 1/3	6
9" roasted vegetable pizza, 1/3	4
9" spinach mushroom pizza, 1/3	6
California Pizza Kitchen	
Barbecue chicken, 1/3 pizza	6
Cajun recipe, 1/3	6
Five cheese and tomato, 1/3 pizza	7
Garlic chicken, 1/3 pizza	6
Hawaiian recipe, 1/3	6
Jamaican jerk chicken recipe pizza, 1/3 pizza	6
Sausage, pepperoni and mushroom, 1/3 pizza	6
Thai chicken, 1/3 pizza	6
California Pizza Kitchen Thin Crust	
BBQ recipe chicken, 1/3	6
Cajun recipe, 1/3	6
Garlic chicken, 1/3	6
Margherita, 1/3	6
Sicilian recipe, 1/3	7
Sweet and spicy Italian, 1/3	6
White, 1/3	6
Celeste For One	
Cheese, 1	8
Vegetable, 1	8
DiGiorno Garlic Bread	
Four cheese, 1 serving (1/6 pizza)	8
Pepperoni, 1 serving (1/6 pizza)	8
Supreme, 1 serving (1/8 pizza)	7

	POINTS VALUE
DiGiorno Harvest Wheat	
Four cheese, 1 serving (1/6 pizza)	5
Pepperoni, 1 serving (1/6 pizza)	6
DiGiorno Harvest Wheat Thin Crust	
Pepperoni, 1 serving (1/5 pizza)	5
Supreme, 1 serving (1/5 pizza)	5
DiGiorno Microwave Rising Crust	
Just cheese, 1 serving (1/2 pizza)	7
Pepperoni, 1 serving (1/2 pizza)	8
Supreme, 1 serving (1/2 pizza)	8
Three meat, 1 serving (1/2 pizza)	9
DiGiorno Microwave Thin Crust	
Four cheese (dual serve), 1/2 small	7
Four cheese (dual serve), 1	13
Grilled chicken & vegetable (dual serve), 1/2 small	6
Grilled chicken & vegetable (dual serve), 1	12
Pepperoni (dual serve), 1/2 small	7
Pepperoni (dual serve), 1	14
Supreme, 1/2	7
DiGiorno Rising Crust	
Four cheese, 1 serving (1/6 pizza)	7
Four cheese, 8", 1/3 pizza	6
Italian sausage, 1 serving (1/6 pizza)	8
Meatball marinara, 1 serving (1/6 pizza)	7
Pepperoni, 1 serving (1/6 pizza)	7
Pepperoni (2 or 3 pack), 1 serving (1/6 pizza)	8
Pepperoni, 8", 1/3 pizza	6

	POINTS
Sausage and pepperoni, 1 serving (1/6 pizza)	8
Spicy chicken supreme, 1 serving (1/6 pizza)	7
Spinach, mushroom, & garlic, 1 serving (1/6 pizza)	6
Supreme, 1 serving (1/6 pizza)	8
Supreme, 8", 1/3 pizza	7
Three meat, 1 serving (1/6 pizza)	8
Three meat, 8", 1/3 pizza	7
DiGiorno Rising Crust Half & Half	
Cheese and pepperoni (cheese half), 1 serving (1/6 pizza)	7
Pepperoni/supreme (pepperoni half), 1 serving (1/6 pizza)	9
DiGiorno Rising Crust Microwave	
Cheese, 1	15
Pepperoni, 1	17
Supreme, 1	17
Three meat, 1	18
DiGiorno Stuffed Crust	
Four cheese, 1 serving (1/5 pizza)	8
Pepperoni, 1 serving (1/5 pizza)	8
Supreme, 1 serving (1/8 pizza)	8
Three meat, 1 serving (1/6 pizza)	8
DiGiorno Thin Crust	
Cheese, made with organic flour and cheese, 1 serving (1/4 of pizza)	7
Four cheese, 1 serving (1/5 of pizza)	7
Four meat, 1 serving (1/5 pizza)	7
Grilled chicken tomato & spinach, 1 serving (1/5 pizza)	6
Mushroom, pepperoni and bacon, 1 serving (1/5 pizza)	7

	POINTS
Pepperoni, 1 serving (1/5 pizza)	7
Spinach & garlic, made with organic flour, tomatoes and spinach, 1 serving (1/4 of pizza)	7
Spinach, mushroom, & garlic, 1 serving (1/5 pizza)	5
Supreme, 1 serving (1/5 pizza)	7
DiGiorno Ultimate	
Four cheese, 1 serving (1/5 pizza)	7
Four meat, 1 serving (1/5 pizza)	9
Pepperoni, 1 serving (1/5 pizza)	8
Supreme, 1 serving (1/5 pizza)	8
Healthy Choice	
Italian style pepperoni pizza, 1 (6 oz)	7
Ian's	
Organic pizza kit, 1 serving (4.5 oz)	5
Organic Whole grain French bread pizza, 1 serving (4 oz)	5
Wheat free, gluten free pizza kit, 1 serving (7.25 oz)	1
Wheat free, gluten free soy cheesy French bread pizza, 1 slice (4 oz)	4
Jack's Naturally Rising Crust	
Cheese, 1 serving (1/5 pizza)	7
Combination, 1 serving (1/6 pizza)	7
Pepperoni, 1 serving (1/6 pizza)	7
Sausage, 1 serving (1/6 pizza)	7
The works, 1 serving (1/6 pizza)	7
Three meat, 1 serving (1/6 pizza)	7
Jack's Naturally Rising Pizza	
Bacon cheeseburger, 1 serving (1/6 pizza)	7

Prepared Foods, Salads & Sides

	POINTS value
Jack's Original	
Bacon cheeseburger, 1/4 pizza	6
Canadian style bacon, 1/3 pizza	7
Cheese, 1/3 pizza	7
Hamburger, 1/4 pizza	6
Mexican, 1/4 pizza	6
Pepperoni, 1/3 pizza	9
Pepperoni, 1/2 pizza	8
Pepperoni & mushroom, 1/4 pizza	7
Pepperoni & sausage, 9", 1/2 pizza	8
Sausage, 1/4 pizza	6
Sausage & mushroom, 1/4 pizza	6
Sausage & pepperoni, 1/4 pizza	7
Spicy Italian sausage, 1/3 pizza	8
Supreme, 1/4 pizza	7
Jack's Original Half & Half	
Pepperoni/cheese (cheese half), 1/3 pizza	7
Pepperoni/cheese (pepperoni half), 1/3 pizza	10
Sausage/pepperoni (pepperoni half), 1/4 pizza	7
Sausage/pepperoni (sausage half), 1/4 pizza	6
Jack's Supercheese	
Cheese, 1/4	7
Jeno's Crisp 'N Tasty	
Canadian style bacon, 1 serving	9
Cheese, 1 serving	10
Combination, 1 serving	11
Hamburger, 1 serving	11
Pepperoni, 1 serving	12
Sausage, 1 serving	11

	POINTS value
Supreme, 1 serving	11
Three meat, 1 serving	11
Kashi	
Five cheese & tomato pizza, 1/3 pizza	6
Mediterranean pizza, 1/3 pizza	6
Mexicali black bean thin crust pizza, 1/3 pizza	4
Mushroom trio & spinach pizza, 1/3 pizza	5
Roasted garlic chicken pizza, 1/3 pizza	6
Roasted vegetable pizza, 1/3 pizza	5
Tomato garlic cheese pizza, 1/3 pizza	5
Vegan Italian pizza, 1/3 pizza	4
Kid's Kitchen	
Pizza wedges pepperoni, 1 cup	6
Linda McCartney	
Cheese pizza, 1/2	6
Mushroom and spinach pizza, 1/2	6
Market Day	
Cheese pizza, 1/4	6
Cheese pizza eat-zzas, 1	8
Chicken club grilling pizzas, 1/2	12
Chicken pico de gallo pizzas, 1/2	9
Mediterranean pizzas, 1/2	9
Pepperoni pizza eat-zzas, 1	10
Taco pizza, 1/4	7
Martha White	
Pizza crust mix, deep pan, prepared, 1 serving (1/5 package)	3
Pizza crust mix, prepared, 1 serving (1/4 package)	3

	POINTS VALUE
Palermo's Primo Thin Crust Pizza	
6 cheese, 1/3 pizza	7
BBQ recipe chicken, 1/3 pizza	7
Cheddar & tomato, 1/3 pizza	7
Greek, 1/3 pizza	7
Grilled chicken caesar, 1/3 pizza	7
Ham & pineapple, 1/4 pizza	5
Margherita, 1/3 pizza	6
Sausage, 1/4 pizza	8
Special edition pepperoni, 1/3 pizza	9
Supreme, 1/3 pizza	8
Palermo's Primo Thin Pizza	
Primavera alfredo, 1/4 pizza	7
Vegetables & goat cheese, 1/3 pizza	6
Paraclete	
5" pizza shells, 1	1
7" pizza shells, 1	1
Pillsbury	
Classic pizza crust, refrigerated, 1 serving (1/5 loaf)	3
Stouffer's Lean Cuisine	
4 cheese pizza, 1	7
Brick oven style bbq chicken pizza, 1	7
Pepporoni pizza, 1	7
Roasted vegetable pizza, 1	6
Tombstone	
Brickoven style pepperoni, 1 serving (1/4 pizza)	7
Brickoven style sausage & pepperoni, 1 serving (1/4 pizza)	8
Brickoven style supreme, 1 serving (1/4 pizza)	7

	POINTS VALUE
Tombstone Brick Oven Style	
Cheese, 1/3	8
Classic sausage, 1/4	6
Deluxe, 1/4	6
Tombstone Garlic Bread	
Cheese, 1 serving (1/6 pizza)	8
Pepperoni, 1 serving (1/6 pizza)	8
Supreme, 1 serving (1/6 pizza)	8
Tombstone Light	
Vegetable pizza, 1 serving (1/5 pizza)	4
Tombstone Mini Deep Dish	
Cheese, 1 pizza	9
Pepperoni, 1 pizza	10
Supreme, 1 pizza	10
Tombstone Original	
Canadian style bacon, 1/4 pizza	7
Cheese, 1/4 pizza	7
Cheese, 9", 1/2 pizza	8
Deluxe, 1/5 pizza	6
Deluxe, 9", 1/3 pizza	6
Four meat, 1/5 pizza	7
Hamburger, 1/5 pizza	7
Pepperoni, 1/4 pizza	9
Pepperoni & sausage, 1/4 pizza	8
Pepperoni & sausage, 9", 1/3 pizza	6
Pepperoni, 9", 1/3 pizza	6
Sausage, 1/5 pizza	6
Sausage & mushroom, 1/5 pizza	6
Sausage, 9", 1/3 pizza	6
Supreme, 1/5 pizza	7

Prepared Foods, Salads & Sides

	POINTS VALUE
Tombstone Original Half and Half	
Cheese/pepperoni (cheese half), 1/4 pizza	7
Cheese/pepperoni, 12" (pepperoni half), 1/4 pizza	9
Pepperoni/sausage (pepperoni half), 1/4 pizza	8
Pepperoni/sausage, sausage half, 1/4 pizza	8
Supreme/pepperoni (pepperoni half), 1/5 pizza	7
Supreme/pepperoni (supreme half), 1/5 pizza	7
Tombstone Pizza Bursts	
Pepperoni & sausage, 6 pieces	5
Tombstone Stuffed Crust Pizza	
Pepperoni, 1 serving (1/6 pizza)	7
Three meat, 1 serving (1/6 pizza)	7
Tombstone Thin Crust	
Cheese, 1/4	7
Sausage, 1/4	7
Totino's Mexican Style Rolls	
Cheesy taco, 6	5
Totino's Party Pizza	
Canadian style bacon, 1/2	7
Cheese, 1/2	7
Classic pepperoni, 1/2	9
Combination (sausage), 1/2	9
Hamburger, 1/2	9
Mexican style taco beef, 1/2	9
Mini meatball, 1/2	8
Pepperoni, 1/2	9

	POINTS VALUE
Pepperoni trio, 1/2	9
Sausage, 1/2	9
Supreme (sausage & pepperoni), 1/2	9
Three cheese, 1/2	8
Three meat, 1/2	8
Totino's Pizza Rolls	
Cheese, 6 rolls	4
Combination (sausage & pepperoni), 6 rolls	5
Pepperoni, 6 rolls	5
Pepperoni trio pizza rolls, 6	5
Sausage, 6 rolls	5
Supreme, 6 rolls	5
Three meat, 6 rolls	5
Totino's Reduced Fat Pizza Rolls	
Pepperoni, 6	4
Totino's Ultimate Pizza Rolls	
Cheese, 3	4
Combination (sausage & reduced fat pepperoni), 3	4
Pepperoni & reduced fat pepperoni, 3	5
Weight Watchers Smart Ones	
Fajita chicken pizza, 1	7
Weight Watchers Smart Ones Anytime Selections	
Cheese pizza minis, 1 tray	5
Pepperoni pizza minis, 1 tray	5
Vegetable pizza minis, 1 tray	5
Weight Watchers Smart Ones Bistro Selections	
Four cheese pizza, 1	7
Pepperoni pizza, 1	8

Delicious pizza: Now in mini size

WEIGHT WATCHERS on foods and beverages is the registered trademark of WW Foods, LLC and is used under license. WEIGHT WATCHERS for services and *POINTS* are the registered trademarks of Weight Watchers International, Inc. and are used under license. ©H.J. Heinz Company, L.P. 2009. All rights reserved.

Smart Ones® Pizza Minis start with zesty tomato sauce, then add real pepperoni and melty mozzarella. With a *POINTS®* value of only 5, they offer big pizza flavor in a fun snack size.

SAVE $4.00 at www.eatyourbest.com/food

Prepared Foods, Salads & Sides

Potato, Rice & Grain Sides

A Taste of China

Sweet and sour rice, 1 cup (prepared)	5

A Taste of Thai

Coconut ginger rice, prepared, 3/4 cup (dry)	4
Garlic basil coconut rice, prepared, 3/4 cup (5.2 oz)	4
Jasmine rice, uncooked, 1/4 cup	3
Yellow curry rice, prepared, 3/4 cup (5.4 oz)	4

Alexia

Country reds mashed potato & parmesan, 1 serving (140 g)	3
Crinkles with sea salt, 1 serving (85 g)	2
Julienne with sea salt, 1 serving (85 g)	3
Organic Yukon gold julienne fries, 1 serving (85 g)	3
Oven crinkles with onion & garlic, 1 serving (85 g)	2
Oven crinkles with salt & pepper, 1 serving (85 g)	2
Oven fries - olive oil & sea salt, 1 serving (85 g)	2
Oven fries - rosemary & garlic, 1 serving (85 g)	2
Oven fries with rosemary and garlic, 1 serving (85 g)	2
Oven reds - sun-dried tomatoes & pesto, 1 serving (85 g)	2
Oven reds with parmesan and roasted garlic, 1 serving (85 g)	2
Potato - parmesan & roasted garlic, 1 serving (85 g)	2
Sweet potato fries, 1 serving (85 g)	3
Yukon gold creamy mashed potatoes, 1 serving (140 g)	3

Amy's

Brown rice & vegetables bowl, 1	5
Light in sodium brown rice & vegetable bowl, 1	5
Light in sodium shepherd's pie, 1	3

Amy's Bowls

Brown rice & vegetables bowl, 1 serving	5

Betty Crocker

Russet harvest creamy butter mashed potatoes, prepared, 2/3 cup	3

Betty Crocker Deluxe Potatoes

Cheesy Cheddar au gratin, prepared, 1/2 cup	4
Cheesy Cheddar au gratin, reduced-fat recipe, prepared, 1/2 cup	3
Creamy scalloped, prepared, 2/3 cup	3
Loaded au gratin, prepared, 1/2 cup	3
Mashed potato bake three cheese, prepared, 2/3 cup	4

Betty Crocker Mashed Potatoes

Butter & herb mix, 2/3 cup	4
Four cheese mix, prepared, 1/2 cup	4
Four cheese mix, reduced-fat recipe, prepared, 1/2 cup	3

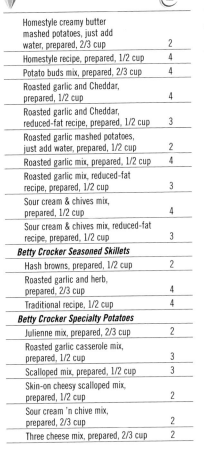

	POINTS VALUE
Homestyle creamy butter mashed potatoes, just add water, prepared, 2/3 cup	2
Homestyle recipe, prepared, 1/2 cup	4
Potato buds mix, prepared, 2/3 cup	4
Roasted garlic and Cheddar, prepared, 1/2 cup	4
Roasted garlic and Cheddar, reduced-fat recipe, prepared, 1/2 cup	3
Roasted garlic mashed potatoes, just add water, prepared, 1/2 cup	2
Roasted garlic mix, prepared, 1/2 cup	4
Roasted garlic mix, reduced-fat recipe, prepared, 1/2 cup	3
Sour cream & chives mix, prepared, 1/2 cup	4
Sour cream & chives mix, reduced-fat recipe, prepared, 1/2 cup	3
Betty Crocker Seasoned Skillets	
Hash browns, prepared, 1/2 cup	2
Roasted garlic and herb, prepared, 2/3 cup	4
Traditional recipe, 1/2 cup	4
Betty Crocker Specialty Potatoes	
Julienne mix, prepared, 2/3 cup	2
Roasted garlic casserole mix, prepared, 1/2 cup	3
Scalloped mix, prepared, 1/2 cup	3
Skin-on cheesy scalloped mix, prepared, 1/2 cup	2
Sour cream 'n chive mix, prepared, 2/3 cup	2
Three cheese mix, prepared, 2/3 cup	2

	POINTS VALUE
Birds Eye	
Rice pilaf in herbed butter sauce, frozen, 1 cup	4
Boston Market Home Style Meals	
Glazed rotisserie white meat chicken with mashed potatoes & gravy and green beans & carrots, 1 package (283 g)	3
Glazed rotisserie white meat chicken with mashed potatoes & gravy and green beans & carrots, 1 package (453 g)	5
Carolina	
Black beans & rice mix, 2 oz (about 1/3 cup rice mix and 1 Tbsp seasoning)	3
Red beans & rice mix, 2 oz (about 1/3 cup rice mix and 1 Tbsp seasoning)	3
Casbah	
Couscous pilaf, 1 serving (45 g)	3
Toasted couscous - original, 1 serving (45 g)	3
Toasted couscous - Thai Cuban, 1 serving (45 g)	3
Cascadian Farm	
Crinkle cut French fries, 18 pieces	2
Shoe string fries, 30 pieces	2
Straight cut French fries, 18 pieces	3
Wedge cut oven fries, 8 pieces	2
Dinty Moore Microwave Cups	
Rice with chicken, 1 cup	4
Scalloped potatoes. ham, 1 cup	5

Prepared Foods, Salads & Sides

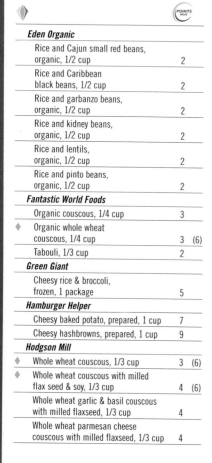

	POINTS VALUE
Eden Organic	
Rice and Cajun small red beans, organic, 1/2 cup	2
Rice and Caribbean black beans, 1/2 cup	2
Rice and garbanzo beans, organic, 1/2 cup	2
Rice and kidney beans, organic, 1/2 cup	2
Rice and lentils, organic, 1/2 cup	2
Rice and pinto beans, organic, 1/2 cup	2
Fantastic World Foods	
Organic couscous, 1/4 cup	3
◆ Organic whole wheat couscous, 1/4 cup	3 (6)
Tabouli, 1/3 cup	2
Green Giant	
Cheesy rice & broccoli, frozen, 1 package	5
Hamburger Helper	
Cheesy baked potato, prepared, 1 cup	7
Cheesy hashbrowns, prepared, 1 cup	9
Hodgson Mill	
◆ Whole wheat couscous, 1/3 cup	3 (6)
◆ Whole wheat couscous with milled flax seed & soy, 1/3 cup	4 (6)
Whole wheat garlic & basil couscous with milled flaxseed, 1/3 cup	4
Whole wheat parmesan cheese couscous with milled flaxseed, 1/3 cup	4

	POINTS VALUE
Hungry Jack	
Au gratin, mix, 1/2 cup	2
Au gratin, prepared, 1 serving (1/8 package)	2
Cheddar & bacon, mix, 1 serving	2
Cheddar & bacon, prepared, 1/2 cup (1/8 package)	3
Mashed potato flakes, prepared, 1/2 cup	3
Ian's	
Alphatots - alphabet shaped fun fries, 3 1/2 oz	4
Kashi	
Pilaf, 7 whole grain, 1/2 cup (cooked)	3
Pilaf, fiery fiesta, 1 cup	4
Pilaf, Moroccan curry, 1 cup	4
Pilaf, original, 1 cup	4
Ranchero beans and pilaf, 1	7
Mahatma	
Black beans & rice mix, 2 oz (about 1/3 cup rice mix and 1 Tbsp seasoning)	3
Red beans & rice mix, 2 oz (about 1/3 cup rice mix and 1 Tbsp seasoning)	3
Market Day	
Quick 'n' crispy fries, 42 (3 oz)	4
Marrakesh Express	
Chicken with vegetables, 1 cup	3
Curry, 1 cup	3
Mango salsa, 1 cup	4
Plain, 1 cup	4
Sun dried tomato, 1 cup	3

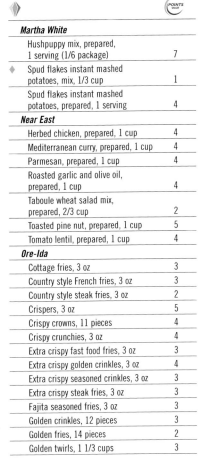

	POINTS VALUE
Martha White	
Hushpuppy mix, prepared, 1 serving (1/6 package)	7
Spud flakes instant mashed potatoes, mix, 1/3 cup	1
Spud flakes instant mashed potatoes, prepared, 1 serving	4
Near East	
Herbed chicken, prepared, 1 cup	4
Mediterranean curry, prepared, 1 cup	4
Parmesan, prepared, 1 cup	4
Roasted garlic and olive oil, prepared, 1 cup	4
Taboule wheat salad mix, prepared, 2/3 cup	2
Toasted pine nut, prepared, 1 cup	5
Tomato lentil, prepared, 1 cup	4
Ore-Ida	
Cottage fries, 3 oz	3
Country style French fries, 3 oz	3
Country style steak fries, 3 oz	2
Crispers, 3 oz	5
Crispy crowns, 11 pieces	4
Crispy crunchies, 3 oz	4
Extra crispy fast food fries, 3 oz	3
Extra crispy golden crinkles, 3 oz	4
Extra crispy seasoned crinkles, 3 oz	3
Extra crispy steak fries, 3 oz	3
Fajita seasoned fries, 3 oz	3
Golden crinkles, 12 pieces	3
Golden fries, 14 pieces	2
Golden twirls, 1 1/3 cups	3

	POINTS VALUE
Oven chips, 3 oz	3
Pixie crinkles, 3 oz	3
Shoestrings, 32 pieces	3
Steak fries, 7 pieces	2
Texas crispers, 3 oz	3
Waffle fries, 3 oz	3
Zesties, 3 oz	3
Zesty twirls, 1 1/4 cups	3
Rice-A-Roni	
Red beans & rice, prepared, 1 cup	6
Seeds of Change	
Siena Tuscan style whole grain rice & beans, 1/4 cup (1 cup cooked)	3
Turkish seven grain pilaf, 1 tray	5
Stouffer's Lean Cuisine	
Santa fe-style rice and beans, 1 (10.375 oz)	6
Tony Chachere's	
Creole red beans and rice dinner mix, 1/4 cup (dry mix)	2
Uncle Ben's Ready Rice Pouch	
Butter & garlic flavored rice, 1 cup cooked	4
Cajun style with red beans & bell peppers, 1 cup cooked	4
Chicken flavored whole grain brown, 1 cup cooked	4
Creamy four cheese flavored with vermicelli, 1 cup cooked	4
Garden vegetable with peas, carrots & corn, 1 cup cooked	4

Prepared Foods, Salads & Sides

Uncle Ben's Ready Rice Pouch (cont'd)	POINTS VALUE
Long grain & wild with 23 herbs & seasonings, 1 cup cooked	4
Original enriched long grain white rice, 1 cup cooked	4
Original long grain enriched (family size package), 1 cup cooked	5
Rice pilaf with orzo pasta, 1 cup cooked	4
Roasted chicken flavored (family size package), 1 cup cooked	5
Roasted chicken flavored with carrots & herbs, 1 cup cooked	4
Spanish style with tomatoes & peppers, 1 cup cooked	4
Teriyaki style with peas & carrots, 1 cup cooked	4
Whole grain brown rice, 1 cup cooked	5

Uncle Ben's Ready Whole Grain Medley Pouch

Brown & wild brown rice, wild rice & red rice perfectly seasoned with herbs & spices, 1 cup cooked	4
Santa Fe brown rice, red & white wheat, black beans, corn, peppers, cilantro & seasonings, 1 cup cooked	4
Vegetable harvest, 1 cup cooked	4

Weight Watchers Smart Ones

Broccoli & Cheddar roasted potatoes, 1	5

Sandwiches
Alexia

	POINTS VALUE
Tuscan style panini - 4 cheese, 1	8
Tuscan style panini - grilled chicken pesto, 1	9
Tuscan style panini - grilled steak, 1	8
Tuscan style panini - smoked chicken, 1	9

Amy's

Broccoli & cheese in a pocket sandwich, 1	7
Cheese pizza in a pocket sandwich, 1	6
Indian samosa wrap, 1 serving (5 oz)	5
Roasted vegetables in a pocket sandwich, 1	4
Soy cheeze pizza in a pocket sandwich, 1	6
Spinach feta in a pocket sandwich, 1	5
Tofu rancheros breakfast, 1 container (9 oz)	8
Tofu scramble breakfast, 1 container (9 oz)	7
Tofu scramble in a pocket sandwich, 1	4
Vegetable pie in a pocket sandwich, 1	6

Fast Fixin'

On the go bbq rib sandwiches, 1	6
On the go cheeseburgers, 1	5
On the go chipotle chicken sandwiches, 1	7

Prepared Foods, Salads & Sides

	POINTS VALUE
Guiltless Gourmet	
California veggie wrap, 1	5
Four bean chili wrap, 1	6
Mediterranean spinach wrap, 1	5
Hot Pocket	
Lean pocket stuffed sandwich, chicken, broccoli and cheese flavor, 1	5
Lean pocket stuffed sandwich, turkey, broccoli and cheese flavor, 1	5
Ian's	
Mini cheeseburgers, 1	5
Mini chicken patty sandwiches, 1	4
Jimmy Dean D-Lights	
Canadian bacon muffin sandwich, 1	5
Turkey sausage muffin sandwich, 1	5
Turkey sausage reduced fat croissant sandwich, 1	6
Kangaroo	
Cheese omelet pita, 1	4
Santa Fe omelet pita, 1	4
Kashi	
Chicken rustico 7 whole grains & sesame pocket bread, 1	6
Turkey fiesta 7 whole grains & sesame pocket bread, 1	5
Veggie medley 7 whole grains & sesame pocket bread, 1	5
Lightlife Smart Tortilla Wrap	
Breakfast scramble with smart bacon, 1	6

	POINTS VALUE
Market Day	
Breakfast bundles, 1 piece	4
Breakfast pizzas, 1	11
Breakfast quesadilla, 1 serving (106 g)	7
Chop house cheeseburger, 1	10
Honey wheat pretzel turkey sandwich, 1	6
PB&J squarewiches, 1	6
Philly cheese steak kit, 1	15
Oscar Mayer	
Honey ham and Swiss melt, 1 package	9
Monterey turkey melt, 1 package	10
Oven baked ham and Cheddar melt, 1 package	9
Smoked turkey breast/bacon/mayonnaise, 1 package	5
Steakhouse Cheddar melt, 1 package	10
Turkey Cheddar dijon melt, 1 package	9
Oscar Mayer Deli Creations	
Smoked ham water added/natural mild Cheddar cheese/mayonnaise, 1 package	6
Smoked ham water added/natural Swiss cheese/dijon mustard, 1 package	4
Smoked turkey breast/natural mild Cheddar cheese/mayonnaise, 1 package	6

Prepared Foods, Salads & Sides

	POINTS VALUE
Pillsbury Frozen Sunrise Skillet Meal	
Sunrise skillet (potatoes, peppers, onions, sausage, biscuits), as packaged, 1 serving (1/8 package)	9
Sunrise skillet (potatoes, peppers, onions, sausage, biscuits), prepared with fat-free egg product including biscuit, 1 1/3 cups	11
Weight Watchers Smart Ones Morning Express	
Breakfast quesadilla, 1	4
Canadian style bacon English muffin sandwich, 1	4
English muffin sandwich, 1	4
Stuffed breakfast sandwich, 1	5

Vegetable Entrees
Amy's

Black bean vegetable enchilada - light in sodium, 1	3
Broccoli pot pie, 1	10
Country vegetable pie, 1	8
Indian mattar tofu, 1	5
Indian vegetable korma, 1	6
Non-dairy vegetable pot pie, 1	7
Shepherd's pie, 1	3
Vegetable lasagna - light in sodium, 1	6
Vegetable pot pie, 1	9

Amy's Bowls

Brown rice, black-eyed peas & veggies bowl, 1 container	6
Teriyaki, 1 container	5

	POINTS VALUE
Amy's Whole Meals	
Country dinner, 1	8
Veggie loaf, 1	6
Celentano Vegetarian	
Eggplant parmigiana, 1 tray	11

Vegetable Sides
Alexia

Onion rings, 1 serving (85 g)	5

Amy's

Spinach feta in a pocket sandwich, 1 container	5
Vegetable pie in a pocket sandwich, 1 container	6

Amy's Whole Meals

Southern meal with cornbread and beans, 1	7

Boar's Head

◆ Sauerkraut, 2 Tbsp	0

Celentano Vegetarian

Eggplant rollettes, 1 tray	9

Del Monte

◆ Sauerkraut, 2 Tbsp	0

Dr. Praeger's

Broccoli pancakes, 1	1
Potato pancakes, 1	2
Spinach pancakes, 1	2
Sweet potato pancakes, 1	2

Eden Organic

◆ Sauerkraut, 1/2 cup	0

Garden Lite

Broccoli souffle, 1 container (7 oz)	2

Guess who's making oatmeal jealous?

WEIGHT WATCHERS and POINTS are the registered trademarks of Weight Watchers International, Inc. and are used under license. © H.J. Heinz Company, L.P. 2009. All rights reserved.

Our Breakfast Quesadilla has fluffy eggs, turkey bacon and three delicious cheeses, wrapped in a toasty flour tortilla. With a **POINTS**® value of 4, it's a tasty alternative to your regular breakfast.

SAVE $4.00 at www.eatyourbest.com/food

Prepared Foods, Salads & Sides

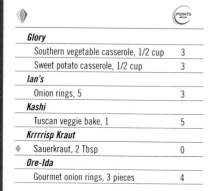

	POINTS VALUE
Glory	
Southern vegetable casserole, 1/2 cup	3
Sweet potato casserole, 1/2 cup	3
Ian's	
Onion rings, 5	3
Kashi	
Tuscan veggie bake, 1	5
Krrrrisp Kraut	
♦ Sauerkraut, 2 Tbsp	0
Ore-Ida	
Gourmet onion rings, 3 pieces	4

	POINTS VALUE
Peas of Mind	
Black bean polenta puffet, 1	3
Carrot risotto puffet, 1	3
Eat your greens puffet, 1	3
Mamma's pasta puffet, 1	1
Nanna's banana puffet, 1	2
The Dalai lentil puffet, 1	1
Rosina Presents Celentano	
Eggplant parmigiana, 1 tray	9
Silver Floss	
♦ Sauerkraut, 2 Tbsp	0

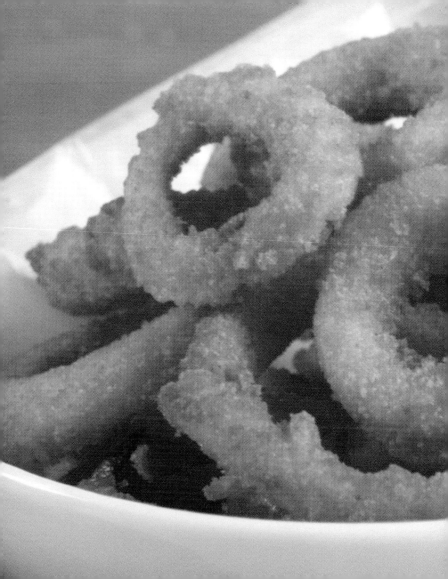

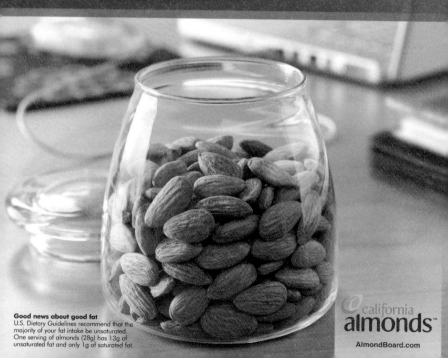

How to take the sneaking out of snacking.

Step 1: Get a bowl.

Step 2: Fill with whole, roasted California Almonds.

Step 3: Place out in the open at home, at work or anywhere that allows you to grab some anytime of day.

Step 4: Smile knowing that studies show you're getting lots of nutritious, heart-healthy benefits in a tasty, delicious snack.

Step 5: Repeat daily.

Remember: A handful of almonds a day in place of foods higher in saturated fat can help you maintain a healthy cholesterol level.

Good news about good fat
U.S. Dietary Guidelines recommend that the majority of your fat intake be unsaturated. One serving of almonds (28g) has 13g of unsaturated fat and only 1g of saturated fat.

california
almonds
AlmondBoard.com

POINTS VALUE

Cheese Snacks

Baked! Cheetos

Crunchy cheese flavored snacks, 34 pieces	3
Flamin' hot cheese flavored snacks, 1 package	3

Baked! Cheetos Crunchy

Cheese flavored snacks (100 calorie mini bites), 1 package	2

Cheetos

Asteroids crunchy cheese flavored snacks (100 calorie mini bites), 1 package	2
Asteroids flamin' hot cheese flavored snacks convenient cups, 1 cup	4
Bacon Cheddar on cheese flavored crackers, 1 package	4
Cheddar bbq flavored crunchy snacks, 19 pieces	4
Cheddar jalapeno cheese flavored snacks, 21 pieces	4
Cheesy enchilada flavored snacks, 20 pieces	4
Chili limon flavored snacks, 21 pieces	4
Cracker trax, cheesy Cheddar flavored baked snack crackers, 25 pieces	3
Cracker trax, spicy Cheddar flavored baked snack crackers, 25 pieces	3
Crunchy, 21 pieces	4
Double cheese flavored cheese flavored snacks, 19 pieces	4
Fantastix, chili cheese flavored baked corn & potato snack, 1 serving (28 g)	3
Flamin' hot, 21 pieces	4

POINTS VALUE

Flamin' hot jumbo puffs cheese flavored snacks, 13 pieces	4
Flamin' hot limon cheese flavored snacks, 28 pieces	4
Jumbo puffs cheese flavored snacks, 13 pieces	4
Natural white Cheddar puffs cheese flavored snacks, 32 pieces	4
Puffs, 29 pieces	4
Twisted cheese flavored snacks, 7 pieces	3
White Cheddar flavored crunchy snacks, 20 pieces	4
Xxtra flamin' hot cheese flavored snacks, 21 pieces	4

Garden of Eatin'

Cheddar puffs, 32 pieces	4
Crunchitos, 35	3

Little Bear

Crunchitos, 1 cup	3
Lite Cheddar puffs, 2 cups	3
Original Cheddar puffs, 2 cups	3

Market Day

Italian four cheese dipper, 1 slice	6

Michael Season's

Hot chili pepper curls, 1 cup	3
White Cheddar pops, 2 1/2 cups	3

Snyder's of Hanover

Cheese twist, 1 serving (1 oz)	3
Multigrain aged Cheddar puffs, 1 1/2 cups	3
Multigrain white Cheddar puffs, 25	3

Weight Watchers

Cheddar twists, 1 pouch	2

Snacks

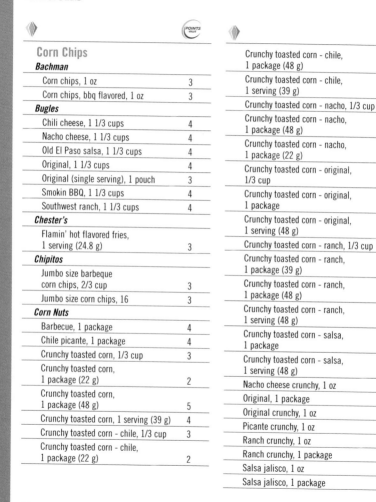

POINTS VALUE

Corn Chips

Bachman

Corn chips, 1 oz	3
Corn chips, bbq flavored, 1 oz	3

Bugles

Chili cheese, 1 1/3 cups	4
Nacho cheese, 1 1/3 cups	4
Old El Paso salsa, 1 1/3 cups	4
Original, 1 1/3 cups	4
Original (single serving), 1 pouch	3
Smokin BBQ, 1 1/3 cups	4
Southwest ranch, 1 1/3 cups	4

Chester's

Flamin' hot flavored fries, 1 serving (24.8 g)	3

Chipitos

Jumbo size barbeque corn chips, 2/3 cup	3
Jumbo size corn chips, 16	3

Corn Nuts

Barbecue, 1 package	4
Chile picante, 1 package	4
Crunchy toasted corn, 1/3 cup	3
Crunchy toasted corn, 1 package (22 g)	2
Crunchy toasted corn, 1 package (48 g)	5
Crunchy toasted corn, 1 serving (39 g)	4
Crunchy toasted corn - chile, 1/3 cup	3
Crunchy toasted corn - chile, 1 package (22 g)	2

Crunchy toasted corn - chile, 1 package (48 g)	5
Crunchy toasted corn - chile, 1 serving (39 g)	4
Crunchy toasted corn - nacho, 1/3 cup	3
Crunchy toasted corn - nacho, 1 package (48 g)	4
Crunchy toasted corn - nacho, 1 package (22 g)	2
Crunchy toasted corn - original, 1/3 cup	3
Crunchy toasted corn - original, 1 package	4
Crunchy toasted corn - original, 1 serving (48 g)	5
Crunchy toasted corn - ranch, 1/3 cup	3
Crunchy toasted corn - ranch, 1 package (39 g)	4
Crunchy toasted corn - ranch, 1 package (48 g)	5
Crunchy toasted corn - ranch, 1 serving (48 g)	2
Crunchy toasted corn - salsa, 1 package	2
Crunchy toasted corn - salsa, 1 serving (48 g)	5
Nacho cheese crunchy, 1 oz	3
Original, 1 package	4
Original crunchy, 1 oz	2
Picante crunchy, 1 oz	3
Ranch crunchy, 1 oz	3
Ranch crunchy, 1 package	4
Salsa jalisco, 1 oz	2
Salsa jalisco, 1 package	4

POINTS VALUE

Fritos

Bar-b-que, 29 pieces	4
Chili cheese, 31 pieces	4
Corn chips, 32 pieces	4
Flamin' hot flavor corn chips, 28 pieces	4
Flavor twists Cheddar ranch flavored corn snacks, 23 pieces	4
Flavor twists honey bbq flavored, 23 pieces	4
Lime & salt flavored corn chips, 33 pieces	4
Pinch of salt low sodium corn chips, 34 pieces	4
Scoops!, 10 pieces	4
Spicy jalapeno naturally & artificially flavored corn chips, 28 pieces	4

Garden of Eatin'

Blue corn chips, 42 chips	4

Good Health Polenta Chips

Barbecue chips, 1 serving (5 oz)	3
Guacamole chips, 1 serving (5 oz)	3
Mediterranean lime, 1 serving (5 oz)	3
Sea salt chips, 1 serving (5 oz)	3

Lance

BBQ corn chips (blastin), 35	5
Hot fries, 1 oz	4

Sun Chips

Cinnamon flavor multigrain snacks, 15	3
French onion multigrain, 15	3
Garden salsa flavor multigrain snacks, 15	3
Harvest Cheddar 100 calorie mini bites multigrain snacks, 1 package	2
Harvest Cheddar multigrain, 15	3
Original multigrain, 16	3

Crackers

Annie's Homegrown

Cheddar bunnies, 50 pieces	3
Cheddar bunnies, 1 packet	3
Chocolate bunny grahams, 24 pieces	3
Chocolate chip bunny grahams, 24 pieces	3
Cinnamon bunny grahams, 24 pieces	3
Honey bunny grahams, 24 pieces	3
Organic bunny classics buttery rich, 10 pieces	2
Organic bunny classics Cheddar, 9 pieces	2
Organic bunny classics saltine, 13 pieces	2
Sour cream & onion Cheddar bunnies, 55 pieces	3
White Cheddar blonde bunnies, 55 pieces	3
Whole wheat Cheddar bunnies, 50 pieces	3

Austin

Cheese crackers with Cheddar cheese (sandwich), 1 package	4
Cheese crackers with Cheddar cheese reduced fat (sandwich), 1 package	4

Snacks

 Austin (cont'd) POINTS VALUE

Cheese crackers with Cheddar Jack (sandwich), 1 package	5
Cheese crackers with megastuffed peanut butter (sandwich), 1 package	5
Cheese crackers with peanut butter (sandwich), 1 package	4
Cheese crackers with peanut butter reduced fat (sandwich), 1 package	4
Chocolatey peanut butter, 1 package	4
Dolphins & friends, 60	3
Grilled cheese flavored crackers (sandwich), 1 package	4
Toast and pb&J sandwich crackers, 1 package	4
Toasty crackers with peanut butter (sandwich), 1 package	4
Toasty crackers with peanut butter reduced fat (sandwich), 1 package	4
Wafer on Cheddar cheese, 1 package	4
Wheat crackers with Cheddar cheese (sandwich), 1 package	4
Wheat crackers with Cheddar cheese reduced fat (sandwich), 1 package	4
Bachman	
Baked jax, 23	3
Back to Nature	
Classic rounds - flaky, buttery baked crackers, 5	2
Crispy wheats baked snack crackers, 1 pouch	3
Crispy wheats baked snack crackers, 17	3
Harvest whole wheats crackers, 6	2

  POINTS VALUE

Barbara's Bakery	
Barbara's wheatines, original, 1 large square	1
Cheese puffs, bakes - original, 1 1/2 cups	4
Cheese puffs, jalapeno, 3/4 cup	4
Cheese puffs, original, 3/4 cup	4
Cheese puffs, white Cheddar, 1 1/2 cups	4
Original rite lite rounds, 5	1
Barnum's Animals	
Animal crackers, 1 serving	2
Be Happy & Healthy	
Reggae rice crackers, 1/2 cup	2
Berkshire Bakehouse	
Cinnamon snack toast, 1 slice	1
Harvest wheat snack toast, 1 slice	1
Wild blueberry snack toast, 1 slice	1
Carr's	
Rosemary crackers, 7 pieces	3
Cheetos	
Cheddar cheese on golden toast crackers, 1 package	5
Chippers	
Ranch baked snack crackers, 12	3
Crown Pilot	
Crackers, 1	2
Devonsheer	
Classic melba rounds, 5 pieces	1
Classic melba toast, 3 pieces	1
Garlic melba rounds, 5 pieces	1
Garlic melba toast, 3 pieces	1

	POINTS VALUE
Onion melba rounds, 3 pieces	1
Rye melba toast, 3 pieces	1
Sesame melba rounds, 5 pieces	1
Sesame melba toast, 3 pieces	1
Unsalted classic melba toast, 3 pieces	1
Unsalted wheat melba toast, 3 pieces	1
Wheat melba toast, 3 pieces	1
Doritos	
Jalapeño cheese! on golden toast flavored crackers, 1 package	5
Nacho cheesier! on golden toast flavored crackers, 1 package	5
EatSmart	
Cheddairs, 1 oz	3
Eden	
Brown rice crackers, 1 serving	2
Nori maki rice crackers, 15	2
Finn Crisp	
Caraway, 1 serving (13 g)	0
Coriander, 1 serving (13 g)	0
Crispbread - fiber, 1 slice	0
Crispbread - multigrain, 1 slice	0
Crispbread - traditional, 1 slice	0
Multigrain, 1 serving	0
Multigrain round crispbread, 1 serving (13 g)	0
Original, 1 serving (13 g)	0
Rounds - multigrain, 1 slice	0
Rounds - sesame, 1 slice	1
Sesame round crispbread, 1 serving (13 g)	1
Thin crisps - caraway, 2 slices	0

	POINTS VALUE
Thin crisps - multigrain, 2 slices	0
Thin crisps - original, 2 slices	0
Thin crisps - roast onion, 2 slices	0
Flat Earth	
Ranch carrot & green bean medley crunchy, 33 pieces	3
Frito-Lay	
Cream cheese & chive on toast flavored crackers, 1 package	5
Peanut butter on cheese crackers, 1 package	4
Peanut butter on toast crackers, 1 package	4
GeniSoy Smart Hearts	
Garlic parmesan, 3/4 cup	2
Lightly salted, 3/4 cup	2
White Cheddar, 3/4 cup	2
Good Health Guppies	
Cheddar crackers, 42	2
Health Valley	
Amaranth graham crackers, 6	2
Organic bruschetta vegetable crackers, 4	2
Organic cracked pepper crackers, 4	2
Organic garden herb crackers, 4	2
Organic sesame crackers, 4	1
Organic stoned wheat, 4	1
Organic whole wheat crackers, 4	1
Original rice bran graham crackers, 6	2
Ian's	
Organic Cheddar crackers, 1 pouch	2
Organic wheat crackers, 1 pouch	2

Snacks

Jacobsen's

Blueberry, 1 slice	1
Cinnamon, 1 slice	1
Cinnamon-raisin, 1 slice	1
Honey maple, 1 slice	1
Original, 1 slice	1
Raspberry, 1 slice	1

JJ Flats

7 grain flatbread, 6 pieces	2
Everything flatbread, 6 pieces	2
Roasted garlic flatbread, 6 pieces	2
Sesame flatbread, 6 pieces	3

KA-ME

Rice crunch cracker, black sesame & soy sauce, 1 serving (28 g)	2
Rice crunch cracker, seaweed, 1 serving (28 g)	2
Rice crunch crackers, cheese, 1 serving (28 g)	2
Rice crunch crackers, plain, 1 serving (28 g)	2
Rice crunch crackers, sesame, 1 serving (28 g)	2
Rice crunch crackers, wasabi, 1 serving (28 g)	2

Kashi TLC

Asiago cheese crackers, 15	3
Country Cheddar, 18	3
Entertain party cracker stoneground 7-grain, 4	2
Entertainer party crackers bruschetta, 4	2
Entertainer party crackers roasted garlic & thyme, 4	2
Fire roasted vegetable, 15	2
Honey sesame, 15	2
Natural ranch, 15	2
Original 7-grain, 15	2

Keebler

Animal crackers dora the explorer, 9	3
Animal crackers hot wheels, 9	3
Cheese & peanut butter sandwich crackers, 1 package	4
Cheese on club sandwich crackers, 1 package	4
Cheese on wheat sandwich crackers, 1 package	5
Club cracker sticks butter herb, 12	3
Club cracker sticks honey wheat, 12	3
Club cracker sticks original, 12	3
Club crackers multigrain, 4	1
Club crackers, buttery garlic, 4	1
Club crackers, multigrain puffed, 24	3
Club crackers, original, 4	1
Club crackers, puffed original, 24	3
Club, reduced fat, 5	1
Graham, cinnamon crisp, 8	3
Graham, cinnamon crisp, low fat, 8	2
Graham, honey, 8	3
Graham, original, 8	3
Sandwich crackers - toast & peanut butter, 1 package	4
Special k Italian tomato & herb crackers, 24	2
Special k multigrain crackers, 24	2

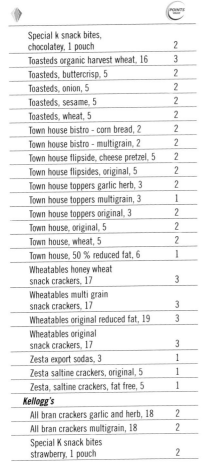

	POINTS VALUE
Special k snack bites, chocolatey, 1 pouch	2
Toasteds organic harvest wheat, 16	3
Toasteds, buttercrisp, 5	2
Toasteds, onion, 5	2
Toasteds, sesame, 5	2
Toasteds, wheat, 5	2
Town house bistro - corn bread, 2	2
Town house bistro - multigrain, 2	2
Town house flipside, cheese pretzel, 5	2
Town house flipsides, original, 5	2
Town house toppers garlic herb, 3	2
Town house toppers multigrain, 3	1
Town house toppers original, 3	2
Town house, original, 5	2
Town house, wheat, 5	2
Town house, 50 % reduced fat, 6	1
Wheatables honey wheat snack crackers, 17	3
Wheatables multi grain snack crackers, 17	3
Wheatables original reduced fat, 19	3
Wheatables original snack crackers, 17	3
Zesta export sodas, 3	1
Zesta saltine crackers, original, 5	1
Zesta, saltine crackers, fat free, 5	1
Kellogg's	
All bran crackers garlic and herb, 18	2
All bran crackers multigrain, 18	2
Special K snack bites strawberry, 1 pouch	2

	POINTS VALUE
Kraft Cheese Nips	
Baked snack crackers - Cheddar, 1 package (35 g)	4
Baked snack crackers - Cheddar, 1 serving (47 g)	5
Baked snack crackers - spongebob squarepants, 25	3
Big crackers, 1 serving (31 g)	3
Cheddar, 29	3
Four cheese, 1 serving (30 g)	3
Mini, 1 package	2
Peanut butter crackers, 1 package	4
Real cheese crackers, 1 package	5
Reduced fat Cheddar, 31	3
Kraft Handi-Snacks	
Cheez'n breadsticks, 1	3
Cheez'n crackers, 1	2
Cheez'n pretzels, 1	2
Teddy graham bearwiches n' crème, 1	4
Lance	
Captain's wafers, 2 packages	2
Cheddar charged cheese ball, 27 pieces	4
Cheddar charged cheese puffs, 9 pieces	4
Cheese-on-wheat, 6	5
Cream cheese & chives on capt. Wafer, 6	5
Crushed saltines, 1 oz	3
Gold-n-chees, 1 package	4
Graham crackers, 3	2
Nekot smores, 6	6

Snacks

Lance (cont'd)	POINTS VALUE
Nip chee, 6	5
Oblong melba toast, 4 slices	1
Oyster crackers, 1 package	1
Peanut butter wheat, 6	5
Peanut butter with honey on captain's. wafers, 6	5
Reduced fat toastchee, 6	4
Saltines, 2 packages	1
Sesame twins, 2 packages	1
Smoked Swiss cheese on wheat, 6	5
Smokehouse Cheddar on captain's. wafers, 6	4
Snack mix, gold-n-cheese, 1 package	5
Toastchee, 6	5
Toasty, 6	5
Triple cheese twisters cheese twists, 30 pieces	5
Wheat twins, 2 packages	1
Lay's	
Original baked cracker crisps, 38 pieces	3
Rosemary & garlic flavored baked cracker crisps, 38 pieces	3
Smooth Cheddar flavored baked cracker crisps, 38 pieces	3
Zesty herb & parmesan flavored baked cracker crisps, 38 pieces	3
Little Debbie	
Cheddar on cheese crackers, 1 serving (26 g)	3
Peanut butter cheese crackers, 4	3
Peanut butter toasty crackers, 4	3

	POINTS VALUE
Manischewitz	
Concord grape matzo, 1	2
Egg & onion matzo, 1	2
Egg matzo, 1	2
Everything matzo, 1	2
Matzos, unsalted, 1	2
Saltine matzo, 1	2
Savory garlic matzo, 1	2
Thin matzo, unsalted, 1	2
Thin matzo, salted, 1	2
Thin tea matzo, 1	2
Wheat matzo, 1	2
Yolk free egg matzo, 1	2
Market Day	
Cheddar cheese guppies, 1 pouch	2
Colby Jack cheese sticks, 1 stick	3
Giant cinnamon goldfish grahams, 1 pouch	3
Michael Season's	
Baked cheese curls - Cheddar, 1 cup	3
Baked cheese puffs - Cheddar, 2 cups	3
Mi-Del	
Honey grahams, 4	2
Nabisco	
Chicken in a biskit, 1 serving (31 g)	4
Grahams, 8 (2 full cracker sheets)	3
Sociables baked savory crackers, 1 serving (14 g)	2
Vegetable thins baked snack crackers, 1 serving (31 g)	4
Whole grain chips - apple, 16	2
Whole grain chips - banana, 16	2
Whole grain chips - tomato basil, 16	2

Snacks

	POINTS VALUE
Nabisco 100 Calorie Packs	
Cheese nips thin crisps, 1 pouch	2
Honey maid cinnamon roll thin crisps, 1 pouch	2
Ritz toasted chips minis sour cream & onion, 1 pouch	2
Wheat thins toasted chips minis, 1 pouch	1
Nabisco Cheese Nips	
Crackers with real cheese, 1 pouch	3
Nabisco Honey Maid	
Chocolate grahams, 8	3
Chocolate sticks, 1 serving (31 g)	3
Cinnamon grahams, 8	3
Cinnamon grahams, lowfat, 8 (2 full cracker sheets)	2
Cinnamon sticks, 1 package (49 g)	4
Cinnamon sticks, 14	3
Cinnamon sticks packs 2 go, 1 packet	2
Graham sticks - honey, 14	3
Honey grahams, 8	3
Honey grahams, lowfat, 8 (2 full cracker sheets)	2
Nabisco Kid Sense Fun Packs	
Teddy grahams cubs cinnamon, 1 serving (22 g)	2
Nabisco Premium	
Gold crackers, 1 serving (15 g)	2
Low sodium saltine, 5	1
Original saltine, 5	1
Original saltine, 1 large packet (4-crackers)	1
Original saltine, 3 packets (2 crackers)	1
Soup & oyster crackers, 1 serving (15 g)	1
Unsalted tops saltine, 5	1
Unsalted tops saltine, 2 packages (12 g)	1
Nabisco Ritz	
Baseball crackers, 1 serving (16 g)	2
Cheddar oven-toasted chips, 1 package (21 g)	2
Cheddar oven-toasted chips, 1 serving (28 g)	3
Cracker sandwiches with real cheese, 1 package (38 g)	5
Crackers, 1 serving (16 g)	2
Football shape crackers, 1 serving (16 g)	2
Garlic butter crackers, 1 serving (16 g)	2
Holiday crackers, 5 (16 g)	2
Low sodium crackers, 1 serving (16 g)	2
Mini original bite size, 1 serving (30 g)	4
Original chips, 1 serving (28 g)	3
Reduced fat crackers, 1 serving (15 g)	2
Toasted chips - sour cream & onion, 1 small package (21 g)	2
Toasted chips - sour cream & onion, 1 package (49 g)	5
Toasted chips - sour cream & onion, 14 (28 g)	3
Whole grain chips - vegetable medley, 5 (16 g)	2
Whole wheat crackers, 1 serving (15 g)	1

Snacks

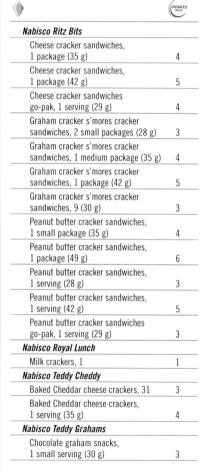

POINTS VALUE

Nabisco Ritz Bits

Cheese cracker sandwiches, 1 package (35 g)	4
Cheese cracker sandwiches, 1 package (42 g)	5
Cheese cracker sandwiches go-pak, 1 serving (29 g)	4
Graham cracker s'mores cracker sandwiches, 2 small packages (28 g)	3
Graham cracker s'mores cracker sandwiches, 1 medium package (35 g)	4
Graham cracker s'mores cracker sandwiches, 1 package (42 g)	5
Graham cracker s'mores cracker sandwiches, 9 (30 g)	3
Peanut butter cracker sandwiches, 1 small package (35 g)	4
Peanut butter cracker sandwiches, 1 package (49 g)	6
Peanut butter cracker sandwiches, 1 serving (28 g)	3
Peanut butter cracker sandwiches, 1 serving (42 g)	5
Peanut butter cracker sandwiches go-pak, 1 serving (29 g)	3

Nabisco Royal Lunch

Milk crackers, 1	1

Nabisco Teddy Cheddy

Baked Cheddar cheese crackers, 31	3
Baked Cheddar cheese crackers, 1 serving (35 g)	4

Nabisco Teddy Grahams

Chocolate graham snacks, 1 small serving (30 g)	3
Chocolate graham snacks, 1 serving (35 g)	3
Chocolatey chip graham snacks, 1 serving (30 g)	3
Cinnamon graham snacks, 1 small serving (30 g)	3
Cinnamon graham snacks, 1 serving (35 g)	3
Dora the explorer graham snacks, 1 serving (31 g)	3
Graham snacks - chocolate, 1 package (35 g)	3
Graham snacks - chocolate, 24 pieces (30 g)	3
Graham snacks - cinnamon, 1 package (21 g)	2
Graham snacks - honey, 2 packages (28 g)	3
Honey graham snacks, 1 small serving (30 g)	3
Honey graham snacks, 1 serving (35 g)	3
Honey graham snacks go-pak, 1 serving (30 g)	3
Honey graham snacks mini snak saks, 1 serving (30 g)	3
Mini chocolatey chips graham snacks snak saks, 1 serving (30 g)	3

Nabisco Triscuit

Baked whole wheat crackers - low sodium, 6 crackers	2
Baked whole wheat crackers - original, 1 package (55 g)	5
Baked whole wheat crackers - original, 6	2

	POINTS VALUE
Cheddar, 1 serving (28 g)	2
Deli-style rye, 1 serving (28 g)	2
Garden herb, 1 serving (28 g)	2
Reduced fat baked whole wheat crackers, 7	2
Roasted garlic, 1 serving (28 g)	2
Thin crisps, 1 serving (30 g)	2
Nabisco Uneeda	
Biscuit, 2	1
Nabisco Wheat Thins	
Baked snack crackers - big, 1 package (44 g)	4
Baked snack crackers - big, 1 serving (31 g)	3
Baked snack crackers - tomato and basil, 15	3
Baked snack crackers 100% whole grain, 16	3
Harvest crisps five grain baked snack crackers, 13	3
Honey, 1 serving (31 g)	3
Low sodium, 1 serving (31 g)	3
Multi-grain, 1 serving (30 g)	3
Original flavor baked snack crackers, 1 serving (35 g)	4
Original flavor baked snack crackers, 16	3
Original flavor baked snack crackers, 1 package (50 g)	5
Original packs 2 go, 1 packet	4
Ranch, 1 serving (29 g)	3
Reduced fat baked snack crackers, 16	3

	POINTS VALUE
Natural Nectar Cracklebred	
Multigrain crackers, 3	1
Original crackers (gluten free), 3	1
Sundried tomato & oregano crackers (gluten free), 3	1
New Morning	
Mini-bites, chocolate graham snacks, 1 packet	2
Mini-bites, honey graham snacks, 1 packet	2
Old London	
Classic melba toast, 3 pieces	1
Roasted garlic melba snacks, 5 pieces	1
Rye melba toast, 3 pieces	1
Salt free whole grain melba toast, 3 pieces	1
Sesame melba snacks, 5 pieces	1
Sesame melba toast, 3 pieces	1
Wheat melba toast, 3 pieces	1
Whole grain melba snacks, 5 pieces	1
Whole grain melba toast, 3 pieces	1
Old London	
American classic toast, 1 serving	1
Cheddar melba snacks, 4 pieces	1
Italia toast, 1 serving	1
Mediterranean toast, 1 serving	1
Sea salt melba snacks, 4 pieces	1
Sourdough melba toast, 3 pieces	1
Spicy 3 pepper melba snacks, 4 pieces	1
Peek Freans	
Signature ovals - sesame, 5	1

Snacks

	POINTS VALUE
Pepperidge Farm	
Baked naturals artisan Cheddar snack sticks, 11	3
Baked naturals savory Cheddar pretzel thins, 11	3
Baked naturals simply pretzel pretzel thins, 11	2
Baked naturals toasted sesame snack sticks, 12	3
Baked naturals toasted wheat wheat crisps, 17	3
Baked naturals zesty tomato herb wheat crisps, 16	3
Classic water distinctive crackers, 4	1
Distinctive butter flavored thins, 4	2
Distinctive harvest wheat crackers, 3	2
Entertaining quartet distinctive crackers, 4	1
Golden butter distinctive crackers, 4	2
Harvest wheat distinctive crackers, 3	2
Pumpernickel snack sticks, 15	2
Sesame snack sticks, 12	3
Three cheese snack sticks, 11	3
Xtra Cheddar flavor blasted goldfish, 51	3
Pepperidge Farm Goldfish	
100 calorie pack Cheddar goldfish, 1 packet	2
100 calorie pack chocolate graham goldfish, 1 packet	2
100 calorie pack cinnamon graham goldfish, 1 packet	2

	POINTS VALUE
100 calorie pack pretzel goldfish, 1 packet	2
100 calorie pack xtra Cheddar flavor blasted goldfish, 1 packet	2
Baby Cheddar goldfish, 89 pieces	3
Blazin' buffalo wing flavor blasted goldfish, 51 pieces	3
Cheddar goldfish, 55 pieces	3
Cheddar goldfish made with whole grains, 55 pieces	3
Cheddar goldfish multi-pack, 1 packet	3
Cheddar goldfish with calcium, 55 pieces	3
Cinnamon goldfish graham snacks, 1 packet	5
Goldfish colors, 55 pieces	3
Jalapeno queso flavor blasted goldfish, 51 pieces	3
Nothin' but nacho flavor blasted goldfish, 51 pieces	3
Original goldfish, 55 pieces	3
Parmesan goldfish, 60 pieces	3
Pizza goldfish, 55 pieces	3
Pretzel goldfish, 43 pieces	3
Reduced sodium Cheddar goldfish, 60 pieces	3
Starfish goldfish, 53 pieces	3
Xplosive pizza flavor blasted goldfish, 51 pieces	3
Xtra Cheddar flavor blasted goldfish multipack, 1 packet	3
Red Oval Farms	
Sesame and onion crackers, 2	1

	POINTS VALUE
Red Oval Farms Stoned Wheat Thins	
Crackers (oval shape) - seeds & grains, 4	2
Ry-Krisp	
California onion dill, 2 whole crackers	1
Light, 2 whole crackers	1
Multi-grain (fat free), 2 whole crackers	0
Natural, 2 whole crackers	0
New York deli rye, 2 whole crackers	1
Seasoned, 2 whole crackers	1
Sesame, 2 whole crackers	1
Sabritones	
Lime & chili flavored wheat snacks, 23	4
Sesmark	
Ancient grains - garlic hummus, 1 serving (30 g)	2
Ancient grains - parmesan herb, 1 serving (30 g)	3
Ancient grains - sea salt, 1 serving (30 g)	3
Multigrain chips - buttery caramel, 1 serving (30 g)	2
Multigrain chips - cinnamon sugar, 1 serving (30 g)	2
Multigrain chips - hickory Cheddar, 1 serving (30 g)	2
Multigrain chips - original, 1 serving (30 g)	2
Multigrain chips - roasted garlic & herbs, 1 serving (30 g)	2
Rice minis - lightly salted, 1 serving (30 g)	3
Rice minis - sesame/garlic, 1 serving (30 g)	3

	POINTS VALUE
Rice thins - brown rice, 1 serving (30 g)	2
Rice thins - Cheddar, 1 serving (30 g)	3
Rice thins - sesame, 1 serving (30 g)	3
Rice thins - teriyaki, 1 serving (30 g)	3
Savory thins - black sesame & garlic, 1 serving (30 g)	3
Savory thins - cracked wheat and sesame, 1 serving (30 g)	2
Savory thins - original, 1 serving (30 g)	3
Savory thins - teriyaki, 1 serving (30 g)	3
Savory thins - three cheese & tomato, 1 serving (30 g)	3
Savory thins - toasted onion & garlic, 1 serving (30 g)	2
Sesame thins - Cheddar, 1 serving (30 g)	2
Sesame thins - garlic, 1 serving (30 g)	3
Sesame thins - original, 1 serving (30 g)	3
Sunshine	
Krispy saltines with whole wheat, 5	1
Krispy, soup & oyster, 16	1
Krispy, unsalted tops, 5	1
Zesta saltines with whole wheat, 5	1
Sunshine Cheez-It	
Big, 13	3
Cheddar Jack, 25	3
Cheez-its, 27	3
Duoz sharp Cheddar parmesan, 25	3
Duoz zesty queso Cheddar blanco, 25	3
Gripz, 1 pouch	3
Gripz nacho micro, 1 pouch	3
Hot & spicy, 25	3

Snacks

Sunshine Cheez-It (cont'd)	POINTS VALUE
Parmesan garlic, 25	3
Pasteurized cheese snack aerosol - Cheddar, 2 Tbsp	2
Pasteurized cheese snack aerosol - white Cheddar, 2 Tbsp	2
Pepper Jack, 25	3
Reduced fat, 1 pouch	3
Reduced fat, 29	3
Reduced fat white Cheddar, 25	3
Right bites extra cheesy party mix, 1 pouch	2
Right bites reduced fat 100 calorie, 1 pouch	2
Rotational, 26	3
Sponge Bob, 1 pouch	4
Sponge Bob, 30	3
Stix Cheddar, 35	3
Stix white Cheddar, 35	3
Twisterz Cheddar and cool ranch, 17	3
Twisterz Cheddar and more Cheddar, 17	3
White Cheddar, 25	3
Tree of Life	
Organic classic golden crackers, 6	2
Organic cracked pepper crackers, 10	2
Organic garden vegetable crackers, 10	2
Organic herb & garlic crackers, 10	2
Organic sesame & flax seed crackers, 10	3
Organic toasted onion crackers, 10	2
Organic water cracker cracked pepper, 4	1

	POINTS VALUE
Organic water cracker original, 4	1
Organic water cracker sesame, 4	2
Sesame sticks, salted, 1/3 cup	4
Weight Watchers	
Multigrain crisps - original, 1 pouch	2
World of Grains	
Garden vegetable crackers, 1 package (30 g)	2
Garlic herb crackers, 1 package (30 g)	2
Multigrain crackers, 1 package (30 g)	2
Rosemary crackers, 1 package (30 g)	2
Tomato basil crackers, 1 package (30 g)	2

Dried Fruit
Sun-Rype

	POINTS VALUE
100% fruit strip, cherry, 1 (0.5 oz)	1
100% fruit strip, strawberry, 1 (0.5 oz)	1
100% fruit strip, wildberry, 1 (0.5 oz)	1
Sun-Rype FruitSource	
Blueberry pomegranate, 1 (1.3 oz)	2
Mini bites, mixed berry, 1/4 cup (6 oz)	2
Plus veggie mini bites, tropical, 1/4 cup (6 oz)	2
Plus veggie raspberry, 1 (1.3 oz)	2
Strawberry, 1 (1.3 oz)	2
Sun-Rype Squiggles	
100% fruit twist, raspberry citrus, 1 (0.63 oz)	1
100% fruit twist, strawberry, 1 (0.63 oz)	1

Tropical Nut & Fruit

	POINTS VALUE
Blueberries, natural, 1 serving (40 g)	2
Cantaloupe, 1 serving (40 g)	3
Cherries & berries, 1 serving (40 g)	2
Chilean flame raisins, 1/4 cup	2
Date coconut roll, 1 serving (40 g)	2
Date pieces with oat flour, 2 Tbsp	2
Deglet noor pitted dates, 1 serving (5-8)	2
Dehydrated apple rings, 1/3 cup	2
Diced peaches, 1/4 cup	1
Dried blueberries, 1/4 cup	2
Dried cantaloupe, 3 1/2 pieces	3
Dried cherries, 1/3 cup	2
Dried cranberries, 1/3 cup	2
Dried raspberries, 1/3 cup	2
Dried razz cherries, 1/3 cup	3
Dried strawberry, 1/2 cup	2
Medjool dates, 1 serving (2-5)	2
Papaya spears, 1 serving (40 g)	3
Papaya spears, unsulfured, 2 slices	3
Peaches, sulfured, 1/4 cup	1
Pears, sulfured, 1/4 cup	1
Pineapple rings, 1 serving (40 g)	2

Fruit Snacks

Be Happy & Healthy

Blueberry soft twisters, 4	2
Green apple soft twisters, 4	2
Strawberry soft twisters, 4	2
Watermelon soft twisters, 4	2

Flat Earth

	POINTS VALUE
Crispy apple crunchy fruit snacks, 22 pieces	3
Luscious pineapple flavored crunchy fruit snacks, 35 pieces	3

Kellogg's

Fruit flavored snacks optimized gelatin (all inclusive), 1 pouch	2

Welch's Fruit Snacks

Berries n cherries, 1 pouch	2
Concord grape, 1 pouch	2
Fruit punch, 1 pouch	2
Mixed fruit, 1 pouch	2
Strawberry, 1 pouch	2

Welch's Reduced Sugar Fruit Snacks

Mixed fruit, 1 bag	1

Nuts

Almond Accents

Butter toffee, 1 serving (7 g)	1
Garlic Caesar, 1 serving (7 g)	1
Honey roasted, 1 serving (7 g)	1
Italian parm, 1 serving (7 g)	1
Original oven roast, 1 serving (7 g)	1
Ranch, 1 serving (7 g)	1

Be Happy & Healthy

All about almonds, 23 pieces	4
Calypso cashews, 1/4 cup	4
Got nuts?, 1/4 cup	4
Power pistachios, 1/2 cup	6

Snacks

	POINTS VALUE
Blue Diamond	
Oven roasted cinnamon brown sugar almonds, 24 nuts	4
Oven roasted no salt almonds, 24 nuts	4
Oven roasted sea salt almonds, 24 nuts	4
Oven roasted vanilla bean almonds, 24 nuts	4
Whole almonds, 1 bag (18 g)	2
Brookside	
Milk chocolate almonds, 9 pieces	5
Chocolate Bowl	
Milk chocolate cashews, 12 pieces	5
DrSoy	
Barbecue, 1 oz	3
Original, 1 oz	3
Ranch, 1 oz	3
Eden	
Tamari almonds, dry roasted, 3 Tbsp	3
Estee	
Candy coated peanuts, 1/4 cup	4
Everybody's Nuts	
European roast pistachios, 1/2 cup (without shells)	4
Roasted no salt pistachios, 1/2 cup (without shells)	4
Salt & pepper pistachios, 1/2 cup (without shells)	4
South of the border pistachios, 1/2 cup (without shells)	4
Fisher	
Almonds, hickory smoked flavor, 1/4 cup	4
Almonds, roasted & salted, 1/4 cup	4
Butter toffee peanuts, 1 oz	3

	POINTS VALUE
Cashews, halves & pieces, 1 oz	4
Chopped walnuts, 1 oz	5
Deluxe mixed nuts, no peanuts, 1 oz	4
Fancy pecans, roasted & salted, 1 oz	5
Honey roasted peanuts, 1/4 cup	4
Honey roasted peanuts, dry roasted, 1 oz	4
Lightly salted mixed nuts, less than 50% peanuts, 1 oz	4
Macadamias, halves & pieces, 1 oz	5
Mixed nuts, less than 50% peanuts, 1 oz	4
Nature's nut mix, 1 oz	4
Party peanuts, 1/4 cup	4
Peanuts, dry roasted, 1/4 cup	4
Peanuts, salted in-shell, dry roasted, 1 oz (shelled peanuts)	4
Peanuts, unsalted in-shell, 1 oz (shelled peanuts)	4
Pistachios, natural, 1 package (1 bag shelled nuts)	3
Premium whole cashews, 1 oz	4
Raw peanuts, 1 oz	4
Spanish peanuts, redskin, 1 oz	4
Whole natural almonds, 1 oz	4
Fisher Chef's Naturals	
Blanched sliced almonds, 1 oz	4
Chopped hazelnuts, 1 oz	4
Chopped macadamias, 1 oz	5
Chopped pecans, 1 oz	5
Pecan halves, 1 oz	5
Pine nuts, 1 oz	5
Slivered almonds, 1 oz	4

MORE
THAN A SNACK.®

Eating almonds as part of your healthy lifestyle provides you with a satisfying snack that may help with weight management.

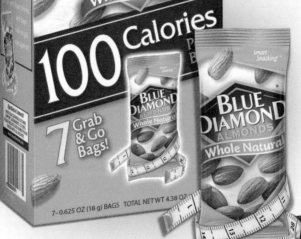

NEW!

Smart Snacking!™

BLUE DIAMOND ALMONDS
Whole Natural

100 Calories

7 Grab & Go Bags!

7–0.625 OZ (18 g) BAGS TOTAL NET WT 4.38 OZ

100 CALORIES PER PACK

BLUE DIAMOND ALMONDS

A handful of almonds a day is a healthy snacking choice.

©2009 Blue Diamond Growers. All rights reserved.

Snacks

POINTS VALUE

Fisher Golden Roast

Lightly salted peanuts, dry roasted, 1 oz	4
Peanuts, dry roasted, 1 oz	4
Unsalted peanuts, dry roasted, 1 oz	4

Frito-Lay

Deluxe mixed nuts, 1/4 cup	4
Dry roasted peanuts, 1 serving (49.6 g)	7
Honey roasted cashews, 1 serving (42.5 g)	7
Honey roasted peanuts, 1 serving (30 g)	4
Hot peanuts, 1 serving (49.6 g)	7
Jumbo salted peanuts, 3 Tbsp	4
Praline pecans, 1 serving (56.7 g)	8
Salted almonds, 1 serving (42.5 g)	7
Salted cashews, 3 Tbsp	6
Salted in-shell peanuts, 1 serving (28 g)	4
Salted in-shell pistachio nuts, 1 serving (25 g)	3
Salted peanuts, 1 package (49.6 g)	7
Smoked almonds, 1 serving (46.6 g)	7

GeniSoy

BBQ, 1/4 cup	2
Chocolate soy nuts, 1/4 cup	5
Deep sea salted, 1/4 cup	2
Unsalted, 1/4 cup	2

Lance

Cashews, 1 package	5
Honey toasted peanuts, 1 package	5

POINTS VALUE

Hot & spicy peanuts, 1 package	7
Roasted peanuts (unsalted), 3/4 cup	4
Salted in shell roasted peanuts, 2/3 cup	4
Salted peanuts, 1 package	4

Nut Harvest

Natural honey roasted peanuts, 2 Tbsp	4
Natural lightly roasted almonds, 2 Tbsp	5
Natural sea salted peanuts, 3 Tbsp	5
Natural sea salted whole cashews, 3 Tbsp	5

Planters

Almonds, 1 oz	4
Black walnuts, 1 bag (56 g)	9
Cashew halves & pieces lightly salted, 1 oz	4
Cashew halves with pieces, 1 oz	4
Cashew sesame mix with peanuts, 1 oz	4
Cocktail peanuts, 1 oz	4
Deluxe mixed nuts, 1 package (63 g)	10
Deluxe mixed nuts, 1 oz	4
Deluxe mixed nuts, lightly salted, 20 pieces	4
Dry roasted almonds, 23 pieces	4
Dry roasted cashews, 19 pieces	4
Dry roasted mixed nuts, 1 oz	4
Dry roasted peanuts, 1 package (28 g)	4
Dry roasted peanuts, 1 oz	4
Dry roasted peanuts lightly salted, 1 oz	4
Dry roasted peanuts lightly salted, 1 package (56 g)	8

	POINTS VALUE
Dry roasted peanuts unsalted, 1 oz	4
Dry roasted pistachios (uncolored), 1/2 cup	4
Dry roasted pistachios (uncolored), 1 small package (30 g)	4
Dry roasted pistachios (uncolored), 1 large package (32 g)	5
Fancy cashews, 1 oz	4
Hazelnuts, chopped, 1 serving (56 g)	9
Honey roasted cashews, 1 oz	4
Honey roasted cashews, 1 small package (42 g)	6
Honey roasted cashews, 1 large package (56 g)	8
Honey roasted mixed nuts (oil roasted), 1 oz	4
Honey roasted peanuts, dry roasted, 1 oz	4
Honey roasted peanuts, dry roasted, 1 package (28 g)	4
Honey roasted peanuts, dry roasted, 1 package (49 g)	6
Honey roasted peanuts, dry roasted, 1 package (56 g)	7
Honey roasted peanuts, dry roasted, 1 package (70 g)	10
Lightly salted cocktail peanuts, 1 oz	4
Lightly salted mixed nuts, 1 oz	4
Lovers mix - cashew, 17 pieces	5
Lovers mix - macadamia, 22 pieces	5
Lovers mix - pecans, 24 pieces	5
Lovers mix - pistachio, 35 pieces	4
Macadamia nuts, 3 Tbsp	5

	POINTS VALUE
Macadamias, chopped, 1 bag (56 g)	11
Mix cashews with almonds and macadamias, 1 oz	5
Mix cashews with almonds and pecans, 1 oz	4
Old fashioned peanuts (grandstand), 30 pieces	4
Pecan chips, 1 bag (56 g)	10
Pecan halves, 1 oz	5
Pecan pieces, 1 oz	5
Pecan pieces, 1 package (56 g)	11
Pine nuts, 1 bag (56 g)	9
Raw Spanish peanuts, 1 oz	3
Regular mixed nuts, 30 pieces	4
Salted peanuts, 35 pieces	4
Salted peanuts, 1 package (28 g)	4
Salted peanuts, 1 package (49 g)	7
Salted peanuts, 1 package (56 g)	8
Seasonuts bbq peanuts, 1 serving (70 g)	10
Seasonuts bbq peanuts, 1 package (49 g)	7
Seasonuts honey mustard peanuts, 43 pieces	4
Seasonuts honey mustard peanuts, 1 package (70 g)	10
Select mix lightly salted cashews with almonds and pecans, 21 pieces	4
Select mix lightly salted cashews with almonds and pecans, 1 package (63 g)	10
Sliced almonds, 1 serving (33 g)	4
Slivered almonds, 1/3 cup	5

Snacks

Planters (cont'd)

	POINTS VALUE
Slivered almonds, 1 bag (56 g)	8
Slivered almonds, 1 serving (34 g)	5
Smoked almonds, 1 package (42 g)	6
Spicy nuts & Cajun, 1 package (56 g)	7
Sweet 'n crunchy peanuts, 1 oz	3
Tavern nuts - coated redskin peanuts, 36 pieces	4
Unsalted cocktail peanuts, 1 oz	4
Unsalted mixed nuts, 1 oz	4
Walnut halves, 1 serving (30 g)	5
Walnut pieces, 1 serving (29 g)	5
Whole cashews, 1 oz	4
Whole lightly salted cashews, 1 oz	4

Planters NUTrition

Energy mix, 1/4 cup	4
Lightly salted almonds, 1 serving (28 g)	4
Lightly salted smoked almonds, 1 serving (25 g)	4
Mixed nuts, lightly salted, 1 oz	4
Mixed nuts, roasted, lightly salted, 1 package (42 g)	6
South beach diet mix, 21 pieces	4

Planters Sweet Roasts

Cinnamon (almonds, peanuts & pecans), 1 oz	4
Honey roasted (peanuts & cashews), 1 oz	4
Vanilla (almonds, cashews & peanuts), 1 oz	4

Sabra

Pine nuts, 1 oz	2

(Planters)

	POINTS VALUE

Sabritas

Picante peanuts, 1 package	7
Salt & lime peanuts, 1 package	7

Sunkist

Roasted & salted pistachios, 1/2 cup (with shells)	4

Sunkist Almond Accents

Butter toffee, 1 Tbsp	1
Garlic Caesar, 1 Tbsp	1
Honey roasted, 1 Tbsp	1
Italian parmesan, 1 Tbsp	1
Original oven roast, 1 Tbsp	1
Ranch style, 1 Tbsp	1
Roasted no salt, 1 Tbsp	1

Tree of Life

Almonds, whole raw, 1/4 cup	4
Carob almonds, 1 serving (40 g)	6
Carob peanuts, 1 serving (40 g)	6
Cashew pieces, raw, 1/4 cup	4
Cashews, roasted and salted, 1/4 cup	5
Cashews, roasted no salt, 1/4 cup	5
Just nuts trail mix, 1 serving (30 g)	5
Macadamia nuts, raw, 1/4 cup	6
Organic Brazils, 1/4 cup	6
Organic cashews, large raw, 1/4 cup	4
Organic raw almonds, 1/4 cup	5
Pecan halves, 1 serving (26.4 g)	5
Pistachios, roasted and salted, 1/4 cup	4
Pistachios, roasted, no salt, 1/4 cup	5
Raw hazel nuts (filberts), 1/4 cup	5

	POINTS VALUE
Soy nuts, roasted and salted, 1 serving (38 g)	3
Soy nuts, roasted, no salt, 1 serving (30 g)	3
Walnut halves and pieces, 1/4 cup	5
Whole cashews, raw, 1/4 cup	4
Yogurt almonds, 1 serving (40 g)	5
Yogurt peanuts, 1 serving (40 g)	5

Tropical Nut & Fruit

	POINTS VALUE
Ale nuts, 23 pieces	3
Almonds, whole, natural roasted, no salt, 1/4 cup	4
Almonds, whole, natural roasted, salted, 1/4 cup	4
Black sesame seeds, 3/4 cup	12
Black walnuts, 1 oz	5
Blanched hazelnuts, 1/4 cup	5
Blanched peanuts, raw, 1/4 cup	3
Blanched peanuts, roasted, no salt, 1/4 cup	4
Blanched peanuts, roasted, salted, 1/4 cup	4
Blanched sliced almonds, 1/4 cup	4
Blanched slivered almonds, 1 oz	4
Bourbon praline pecans, 2 Tbsp	3
Brazil nuts, roasted, salted, 1 oz	5
Brazils, 6 pieces	6
Buffalo nuts, 1/4 cup	3
Butter toffee almonds, 14 pieces	3
Butter toffee peanuts, 18 pieces	3
Cajun peanuts, 3 Tbsp	4
Cashew butts, roasted and salted, 1 oz	5

	POINTS VALUE
Cashew butts, roasted, no salt, 1 oz	5
Cashew pieces, raw, 1/4 cup	4
Cashew pieces, roasted, salted, 1 oz	5
Cashew splits, roasted and salted, 1 oz	5
Cashew splits, roasted, no salt, 2 Tbsp	5
Cashews, roasted, salted, 1/4 cup	5
Cashews, whole, raw, 1/4 cup	4
Cashews, whole, roasted, no salt, 2 Tbsp	5
Cashews, whole, roasted, salted, 2 Tbsp	5
Chili lemon pistachios, 1/4 cup	4
Cinnamon pecans, 2 Tbsp	3
Cinnamon spiced pecans, 10 pieces	3
Deluxe mixed nuts, roasted and salted, 1 oz	5
Deluxe mixed nuts, roasted, no salt, 1/3 cup	5
Dry roasted almonds, 1/4 cup	4
Five star deluxe nut, 1/4 cup	5
Garlic onion pistachios, 1/4 cup	4
Granulated peanuts, 1 oz	4
Habanaro pistachios, 1/4 cup	4
Hammons black walnut, 1 serving (30 g)	3
Hickory pistachios, 1/4 cup	4
Hickory smoked 5 star mix, 1/4 cup	5
Hickory smoked almonds, 1 oz	4
Honey pecans, 2 Tbsp	3
Honey roast almonds, 24 pieces	4
Honey roasted cashews, 2 Tbsp	4

Snacks

Tropical Nut & Fruit (cont'd) POINTS VALUE

Honey roasted peanuts, 1 oz	4
Honey roasted pecan pieces, 1 oz	5
Imperial macadamia, 2 Tbsp	5
In-shell peanuts, roasted, salted, 1 oz	4
Kettle peanuts, jalapeno, 1 oz	4
Kettle peanuts, roasted, salted, 1 oz	4
Kettle peanuts, salt & pepper, 1 oz	4
Macadamia nuts, raw, 1 oz	5
Mixed nuts with peanuts, roasted and salted, 1/4 cup	4
Mixed nuts with peanuts, roasted, no salt, 1/4 cup	4
Nacho peanuts, 3 Tbsp	4
Natural hazelnuts, 1/4 cup	5
Natural pistachios, 1/4 cup (edible part)	4
Natural pistachios, 1/4 cup	4
Natural sesame seeds, 1/4 cup	5
Natural sliced almonds, 1 oz	4
NY Deli blend, 4 Tbsp	3
Peach pecans, 1 oz	3
Peanut butter stock, 1 oz	4
Pecan crusting deluxe, 1 serving (15 g)	2
Pecan halves, raw, 1 oz	5
Pecan halves, roasted & salted, 1 oz	6
Pecan pieces, raw, 1 oz	5
Pine nuts (pignolias), 1/4 cup	4
Pistachios, roasted, salted, 1/2 cup	4
Pistachios, shelled, roasted, salted, 3 Tbsp	4
Praline pecans, 2 Tbsp	3

	POINTS VALUE
Praline pecans, 1/4 cup	4
Raw cashew butts, 1/4 cup	4
Raw cashew splits, 1/4 cup	4
Raw Spanish peanuts, 1/4 cup	4
Red pistachios, 1/4 cup	4
Redskin peanuts, raw, 1 oz	4
Redskin peanuts, roasted and salted, 1 oz	5
Redskin peanuts, roasted, no salt, 2 Tbsp	5
Roasted, no salt pecan halves, 1 oz	6
Salted peanuts, 2/3 cup	4
Select mixed nuts, 1 serving	5
Sesame tahini, 2 Tbsp	5
Shelled raw pistachios, 3 Tbsp	4
Shelled roasted, no salt pistachios, 1 oz	4
Spanish peanuts, roasted, no salt, 3 Tbsp	5
Spanish peanuts, roasted, salted, 1 oz	5
Sunflower seeds, in shell, roasted, salted, 3/4 cup	4
Sunflower seeds, roasted, no salt, 3 Tbsp	5
Sweet & nutty, 2 Tbsp	5
Tamari almonds, 28 pieces	4
Tamari seasoned cashews, 1/4 cup	4
Walnut combination - halves & pieces, 1/4 cup	5
Walnut combination medium pieces, 1/4 cup	5
Walnut light halves/pieces, 1/4 cup	5
Walnut pieces, 1/4 cup	5

	POINTS VALUE
Wasabi soy sauce cashews, 1/3 cup	4
Whole raw almonds, 1/4 cup	4
True North	
Almond clusters, 7	4
Almond crisps, 15	3
Almonds pistachios walnuts & pecans, 3 Tbsp	4
Honey wheat peanut crunches, 1/4 cup	3
Peanut clusters, 6	4
Peanut crisps, 15	3
Peanut, almond & pecan clusters, 8	4
Pistachio crisps, 12	3
Sesame peanut crunches, 1/4 cup	3
Wonderful	
Roasted & salted pistachios, 1/2 cup (with shells)	4

Other Chips

	POINTS VALUE
Bachman	
Treat party mix, 1/2 cup	3
Baken-ets	
Fried pork skins, 9 pieces	2
Hot n' spicy fried pork skins, 9 pieces	2
Salt & vinegar fried pork skins, 9 pieces	2
Funyuns	
Flamin' hot onion flavored snacks, 13 pieces	3
Good Health Humbles	
Olive oil lemon feta baked hummus chips, 1 serving (5 oz)	3
Roasted red pepper baked hummus chips, 1 serving (5 oz)	3

	POINTS VALUE
Sesame garlic baked hummus chips, 1 serving (5 oz)	3
Old London	
Garlic bagel snacks, 5 pieces	1
Original bagel snacks, 5 pieces	1
Poppy seed bagel snacks, 5 pieces	1
Stacy's	
Everything bagel chips, 12	3
Soy thin crisps simply cheese flavored baked, 18	3
Soy thin crisps sticky bun flavored baked soy crisps, 18	2
Soy thin crisps sweet bbq flavored baked soy crisps, 18	2
Toasted garlic flavored bagel chips, 9	3
Whole wheat bagel chips, 11	3
Terra	
Parsnips chips, 12	3
Stripes & blues gourmet bbq, 14	3
Stripes & blues sea salt, 14	3
Sweets and beets chips, 12	4

Pita Chips

	POINTS VALUE
Athenos	
Pita chips, garlic & herb, 11	3
Pita chips, original, 11	3
Pita chips, whole wheat, 11	2
Garden of Eatin'	
Pita chips, Asian spice, 9 pieces	2
Pita chips, brown sugar & cinnamon, 8 pieces	2
Pita chips, Greek isle, 9 pieces	2
Pita chips, sea salt, 9 pieces	2

Snacks

Kangaroo

Cinnamon sugar pita chips, 10 (1 oz)	3
Garlic herb pita chips, 10 (1 oz)	2
Sea salt pita chips, 10 (1 oz)	2
Whole grain French onion pita chips, 10 (1 oz)	2

Kettle Brand

Baked pita chips, salt & pepper, made with organic flour, 1 oz	2
Baked pita chips, salt kissed, made with organic flour, 1 oz	2

Snyder's of Hanover

Multigrain baked pita chips parmesan garlic & herb, 1 serving (1 oz)	3
Multigrain baked pita chips sea salt, 1 serving (1 oz)	3
Multigrain baked pita chips sundried tomato & herb, 1 serving (1 oz)	3

Stacy's

Cinnamon sugar pita chips, 7 pieces	3
Hot & spicy flavored pita chips, 9 pieces	3
Multigrain seasoned with sea salt pita chips, 9	3
Parmesan garlic & herb pita chips, 9 pieces	3
Simply naked pita chips, 10 pieces	3
Tuscan herb flavored pita chips, 7 pieces	3

Popcorn

Bachman

Asiago peppercorn flavored popcorn, 2 cups	3
Buffalo wing & bleu cheese flavored popcorn, 2 cups	3
Cheese popcorn, 3 cups	3
Garlic & herb flavored popcorn, 2 cups	3
Lite popcorn, 5 cups	2
Regular popcorn, 2/3 cup	3
Super premium white Cheddar popcorn, 2 1/2 cups	3
White Cheddar popcorn, 2 1/2 cups	3

Bearitos

50% less fat popcorn, 3 1/2 cups	3
Buttery popcorn, 2 1/2 cups	4
♦ Microwave popcorn no oil added, 5 cups	2
♦ Microwave popcorn no salt/no oil, 5 cups	2
♦ No salt/no oil popcorn, 5 cups	2
White Cheddar popcorn, 2 1/3 cups	4

Boston's

Homestyle popcorn, 3 1/2 cups	3
Lite popcorn, 1 package (30 g)	2

Chester's

Butter flavored puffcorn snacks, 3 cups	4
Cheese flavored popcorn snacks, 3 cups	3
Cheese flavored puffcorn snacks, 3 cups	4

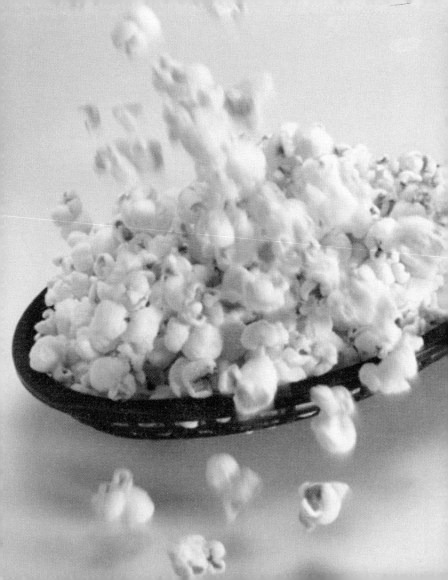

Snacks

Chester's (cont'd)

Flamin' hot flavored popcorn, 1 package (24.5 g)	3

Cracker Jack

Caramel-coated popcorn and peanuts snack, 1/2 cup	2

Eden Organic

◆ Popcorn, yellow, unpopped, 2 Tbsp	1

Garden of Eatin'

Microwave popcorn butter flavor, 2 cups	3
Microwave popcorn no oil added, 2 1/2 cups	2

Good Health

Half naked popcorn, 1 serving (4 oz)	2
Organic popcorn, 1 serving (3.5 oz)	3

JOLLY TIME

Butter 3 pack, 5 cups	1
Caramel apple 3 pack, 5 cups	1
Kettle corn 100 cal mini bag, 1 bag	1
Kettle corn 3 pack, 4 cups	1

JOLLY TIME American's Best

◆ 94% fat free butter flavor microwave pop corn, popped, 5 cups	1

JOLLY TIME Big Cheez

Ultimate Cheddar microwave pop corn, popped, 3 1/2 cups	3

JOLLY TIME Blast O Butter

Light ultimate theatre style microwave pop corn, popped, 4 cups	2
Ultimate theatre style microwave pop corn, popped, 3 1/2 cups	3
Ultimate theatre style, mini bags, popped, 3 1/2 cups	3

JOLLY TIME Butter-Licious

Light original butter microwave pop corn, popped, 5 cups	2
Original butter microwave pop corn, popped, 4 cups	3

JOLLY TIME Crispy 'N White

Light natural flavor crispy 'n white microwave pop corn, popped, 5 cups	2
Natural flavor crispy 'n white microwave pop corn, popped, 4 cups	3

JOLLY TIME Healthy Pop

◆ 100 calorie healthy pop butter 94% fat free, popped, 5 cups	1
100 calorie healthy pop kettle corn, 94% fat free, 4 cups	1
◆ 100 calorie healthy pop low sodium, butter, 94% fat free, popped, 5 cups	1
94% fat free, butter flavor microwave pop corn, popped, 5 cups	1
94% fat free, caramel apple flavor microwave pop corn, popped, 5 cups	1
94% fat free, kettle corn microwave pop corn, popped, 4 cups	1

JOLLY TIME Kettle Mania

Kettle corn microwave pop corn, popped, 3 cups	3

JOLLY TIME White & Buttery

Buttery, white microwave pop corn, popped, 4 cups	3

Kernel Season's Gourmet Popcorn

◆ Raw popcorn, 2 Tbsp (5 cups air popped)	2

Healthy Pop... the ONLY Microwave Pop Corn Endorsed By Weight Watchers.

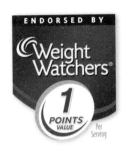

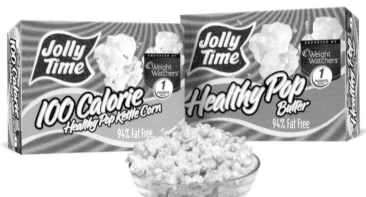

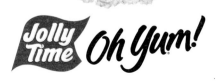

GHT WATCHERS for services and *POINTS*® are the registered trademarks of Weight Watchers International, Inc. and are used with permission.

jollytime.com ©APCC2009

Snacks

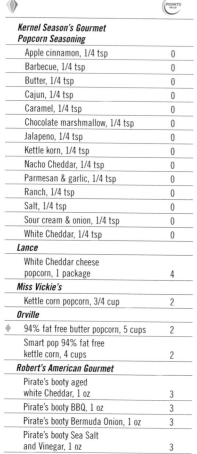

Kernel Season's Gourmet Popcorn Seasoning

	POINTS VALUE
Apple cinnamon, 1/4 tsp	0
Barbecue, 1/4 tsp	0
Butter, 1/4 tsp	0
Cajun, 1/4 tsp	0
Caramel, 1/4 tsp	0
Chocolate marshmallow, 1/4 tsp	0
Jalapeno, 1/4 tsp	0
Kettle korn, 1/4 tsp	0
Nacho Cheddar, 1/4 tsp	0
Parmesan & garlic, 1/4 tsp	0
Ranch, 1/4 tsp	0
Salt, 1/4 tsp	0
Sour cream & onion, 1/4 tsp	0
White Cheddar, 1/4 tsp	0

Lance

White Cheddar cheese popcorn, 1 package	4

Miss Vickie's

Kettle corn popcorn, 3/4 cup	2

Orville

94% fat free butter popcorn, 5 cups	2
Smart pop 94% fat free kettle corn, 4 cups	2

Robert's American Gourmet

Pirate's booty aged white Cheddar, 1 oz	3
Pirate's booty BBQ, 1 oz	3
Pirate's booty Bermuda Onion, 1 oz	3
Pirate's booty Sea Salt and Vinegar, 1 oz	3

Smart Balance

	POINTS VALUE
Light butter, popped, 4 cups	2
Light popcorn (minibag), 1	3
Low fat, low sodium, 5 cups	2
Movie style, 3 1/2 cups	4

Smartfood

Reduced fat white Cheddar cheese flavored popcorn, 1 package (28 g)	3
White Cheddar cheese flavored popcorn, 1 3/4 cups	4

Snyder's of Hanover

Butter flavored popcorn, 1 serving (0.63 oz)	2

Tree of Life

Organic butter flavored popcorn, popped, 4 cups	3
Organic lightly salted popcorn, popped, 4 cups	1

Potato Chips

Baked! Lay's

Cheddar & sour cream flavored potato crisps, 14 pieces	2

EatSmart

Potato chips, french onion, 1 serving (1 oz)	3
Potato chips, lightly salted, 1 serving (1 oz)	3
Potato chips, sweet barbeque, 1 serving (1 oz)	3

El Isleno

Plantains chips, 32 pieces	3

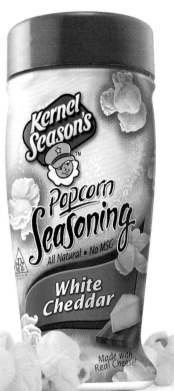

Topping with taste that won't go to your waist.
0 Fat · 2 Calories Per Serving* · All Natural · No MSG

Kernel Season's

Popcorn **Seasoning**

All Natural · No MSG

White Cheddar

Made with Real Cheese!

Fourteen delicious flavors including Butter, Nacho Cheddar, Kettle Corn, Parmesan & Garlic and more. Find Kernel Season's in your grocer's popcorn aisle.

To order online or find a store location near you, visit www.NoMoreNakedPopcorn.com or call 1-866-328-7672.

*per 1/4 teaspoon of White Cheddar

Snacks

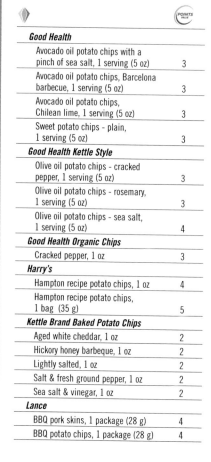

Good Health

	POINTS VALUE
Avocado oil potato chips with a pinch of sea salt, 1 serving (5 oz)	3
Avocado oil potato chips, Barcelona barbecue, 1 serving (5 oz)	3
Avocado oil potato chips, Chilean lime, 1 serving (5 oz)	3
Sweet potato chips - plain, 1 serving (5 oz)	3

Good Health Kettle Style

Olive oil potato chips - cracked pepper, 1 serving (5 oz)	3
Olive oil potato chips - rosemary, 1 serving (5 oz)	3
Olive oil potato chips - sea salt, 1 serving (5 oz)	4

Good Health Organic Chips

Cracked pepper, 1 oz	3

Harry's

Hampton recipe potato chips, 1 oz	4
Hampton recipe potato chips, 1 bag (35 g)	5

Kettle Brand Baked Potato Chips

Aged white cheddar, 1 oz	2
Hickory honey barbeque, 1 oz	2
Lightly salted, 1 oz	2
Salt & fresh ground pepper, 1 oz	2
Sea salt & vinegar, 1 oz	2

Lance

BBQ pork skins, 1 package (28 g)	4
BBQ potato chips, 1 package (28 g)	4

	POINTS VALUE
Boomin bbq potato chips, 22 chips	3
Buffalo wing & blue cheese potato chips, 22 chips	3
Chargin Cheddar sour cream potato chips, 22 chips	4
Hot & spicy pork skins, 19 pieces	4
Hot and spicy potato chips, 1 oz	3
Plain pork skins, 1 package (28 g)	4
Plain potato chips, 1 package (28 g)	4
Salt & vinegar (stormy), 1 serving (28 g)	3
Wild sour cream and onion potato chips, 22 chips	4

Lay's

Baked! barbecue flavor crisps, 14	2
Baked! potato crisps, 15	2
Baked! sour cream & onion flavored potato crisps, 14	2
Barbecue flavor potato chips, 15	4
California cool dill flavored potato chips, 15	4
Cheddar & sour cream artificially flavored potato chips, 15	4
Chili limon potato chips, 15	4
Classic potato chips, 15	4
Crab spice flavored potato chips, 15	4
Deli style original potato chips, 17	4
Dill pickle flavored potato chips, 17	4
Flamin' hot flavor potato chips, 17	4
Hot'n spicy barbecue flavored potato chips, 15	4

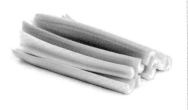
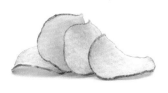

Tastes natural.   Tastes great...naturally.

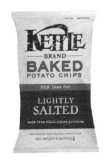

All natural never tasted so good.

How can a baked potato chip taste so good? It's simple: start with a real potato, slice it thick and leave the skin on it. The result is an all-natural chip with a hefty crunch and the great taste of real potatoes.

Kettle Brand® Baked Potato Chips.
Just 120 calories, 3 grams of fat and 2 grams of fiber per serving.

kettlefoods.com   great taste...naturally™

Snacks

Lay's (cont'd)

	POINTS value
Jalapeno Cheddar flavored potato chips, 15	4
Kettle cooked creamy queso & salsa flavored potato chips, 16	3
Kettle cooked jalapeño potato chips, 15	3
Kettle cooked Maui onion potato chips, 15	3
Kettle cooked mesquite bbq potato chips, 18	3
Kettle cooked original potato chips, 16	3
Kettle cooked reduced fat original flavored potato chips, 18	3
Kettle cooked sea salt & malt vinegar potato chips, 18	3
Kettle cooked sweet chili & sour cream flavored potato chips, 15	3
Lightly salted potato chips, 20	4
Limon tangy lime potato chips, 17	4
Loaded potato skins flavored potato chips, 15	4
Natural kettle cooked sea salt and vinegar potato chips, 16	4
Natural kettle cooked sea salted potato chips, 16	4
Pinch of salt low sodium potato chips, 15	4
Salt & vinegar potato chips, 17	4
Sour cream & onion potato chips, 17	4

	POINTS value
Southwestern jalapeno & Cheddar flavored potato chips, 15	4
Sweet & spicy teriyaki flavored potato chips, 15	4
Lay's Light	
Original potato chips, 20	1
Lay's Natural	
Country BBQ thick cut potato chips, 14	4
Sea salted thick cut potato chips, 17	4
Lay's Stax	
Cheddar flavored potato crisps, 12	4
Hot'n spicy barbecue flavored potato crisps, 12 pieces	4
Italian tomato basil flavor potato crisps, 12 pieces	4
Mesquite barbecue flavored potato crisps, 12 pieces	4
Original flavor potato crisps, 13	4
Ranch flavored potato crisps, 12 pieces	4
Salt & vinegar flavored potato crisps, 12 pieces	4
Spicy buffalo wings flavored potato crisps, 12 pieces	4
Sweet Thai chili flavor potato crisps, 12 pieces	4

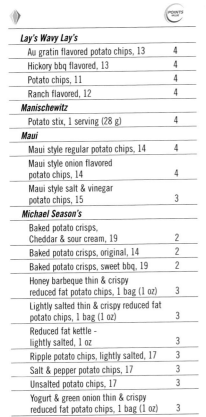

Lay's Wavy Lay's

Au gratin flavored potato chips, 13	4
Hickory bbq flavored, 13	4
Potato chips, 11	4
Ranch flavored, 12	4

Manischewitz

Potato stix, 1 serving (28 g)	4

Maui

Maui style regular potato chips, 14	4
Maui style onion flavored potato chips, 14	4
Maui style salt & vinegar potato chips, 15	3

Michael Season's

Baked potato crisps, Cheddar & sour cream, 19	2
Baked potato crisps, original, 14	2
Baked potato crisps, sweet bbq, 19	2
Honey barbeque thin & crispy reduced fat potato chips, 1 bag (1 oz)	3
Lightly salted thin & crispy reduced fat potato chips, 1 bag (1 oz)	3
Reduced fat kettle - lightly salted, 1 oz	3
Ripple potato chips, lightly salted, 17	3
Salt & pepper potato chips, 17	3
Unsalted potato chips, 17	3
Yogurt & green onion thin & crispy reduced fat potato chips, 1 bag (1 oz)	3

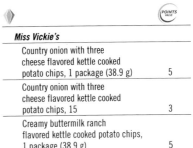

Miss Vickie's

Country onion with three cheese flavored kettle cooked potato chips, 1 package (38.9 g)	5
Country onion with three cheese flavored kettle cooked potato chips, 15	3
Creamy buttermilk ranch flavored kettle cooked potato chips, 1 package (38.9 g)	5
Creamy buttermilk ranch flavored kettle cooked potato chips, 15	3
Hand-picked jalapeno flavored kettle cooked potato chips, 15	3
Hand-picked jalapeno flavored kettle cooked potato chips, 1 package (38.9 g)	5
Sea salt & vinegar flavored potato chips, 1 package (38.9 g)	4
Simply salted nine grain chips, 15	3
Simply sea salt kettle cooked potato chips, 22	3
Simply sea salt kettle cooked potato chips, 1 package (38.9 g)	5
Smokehouse bbq flavored potato chips, 1 package (38.9 g)	5

Munchos

Potato crisps, 16	4
Shrimp flavored potato crisps, 17	3

Snacks

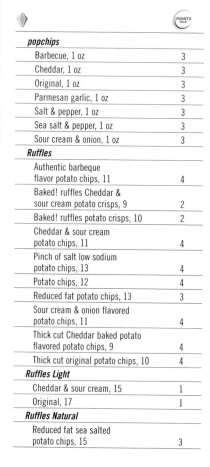

POINTS VALUE

popchips

Barbecue, 1 oz	3
Cheddar, 1 oz	3
Original, 1 oz	3
Parmesan garlic, 1 oz	3
Salt & pepper, 1 oz	3
Sea salt & pepper, 1 oz	3
Sour cream & onion, 1 oz	3

Ruffles

Authentic barbeque flavor potato chips, 11	4
Baked! ruffles Cheddar & sour cream potato crisps, 9	2
Baked! ruffles potato crisps, 10	2
Cheddar & sour cream potato chips, 11	4
Pinch of salt low sodium potato chips, 13	4
Potato chips, 12	4
Reduced fat potato chips, 13	3
Sour cream & onion flavored potato chips, 11	4
Thick cut Cheddar baked potato flavored potato chips, 9	4
Thick cut original potato chips, 10	4

Ruffles Light

Cheddar & sour cream, 15	1
Original, 17	1

Ruffles Natural

Reduced fat sea salted potato chips, 15	3

POINTS VALUE

Snyder's of Hanover

100 calorie pack multigrain French onion sunflower chips, 1 serving (0.74 oz)	2
100 calorie pack multigrain southwest Cheddar sunflower chips, 1 serving (0.74 oz)	2
Hot buffalo wing potato chips, 1 oz	3
Jalapeño potato chips, 1 oz	3
Kosher dill potato chips, 1 oz	3
Malt vinegar & sea salt café fries, 1 serving (1 oz)	3
Original potato chips, 1 oz	3
Ripple potato chips, 1 oz	3
Salt & vinegar potato chips, 1 oz	3
Smokey barbeque potato chips, 1 serving (1.5 oz)	4
Sour cream & onion potato chips, 1 oz	3
Tangy tomato & spices café fries, 1 serving (1 oz)	3

Terra

Blue potato chips, 15	3
Crinkles blues jalapeno chili potato chips, 14	3
Crinkles candied sweet potato chips, 17	4
Crinkles red bliss potato chips bloody Mary, 12	3
Crinkles yukon golds garlic mashed potato chips, 17	3

love. without the handles.

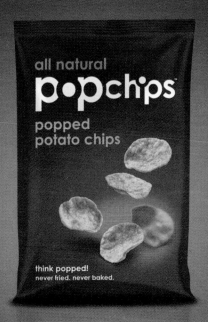

never fried (unhealthy). never baked (undelicious). we take a little heat, add some pressure, and pop! it's a chip so delicious and crispy you won't notice it's (we hesitate to say) healthier. and with a craving-crushing 20 chips per serving, 120 calories and 4 grams of fat, who wouldn't want to pop one in their mouth?

©2009 popchips.com

Snacks

Terra (cont'd)	POINTS VALUE
Potpourri potato chips, 13	3
Red bliss olive oil & fine herbs potato chips, 12	3
Red bliss olive oil & roasted garlic parmesan potato chips, 12	3
Red bliss olive oil and sun-dried tomatoes potato chips, 12	3
Red bliss olive oil potato chips, 12	3
Spiced sweet potato chips, 17	4
Spiced taro chips, 10	3
Sweet potato chips, 1 small bag (34 g)	4
Sweet potato chips, 1 bag (42 g)	4
Sweet potato chips, 17	3
Unsalted potato chips au naturel, 18	3
Unsalted potato chips hickory bbq, 16	4
Unsalted potato chips lemon pepper, 16	4
Yukon gold onion & garlic potato chips, 9	3
Yukon gold original potato chips, 9	3
Yukon gold salt & pepper potato chips, 9	3
Yukon gold salt & vinegar potato chips, 9	3

Terra Kettles

Chesapeake Bay & beer potato chips, 15	3
General Tso potato chips, 15	3
Pesto & smoked mozzarella potato chips, 15	3
Potato chips, Arrabiata, 15	3
Sea salt & pepper potato chips, 15	4

	POINTS VALUE
Sea salt & vinegar potato chips, 15	4
Sea salt with russets & blues potato chips, 15	4
Sea salt with russets and sweet potato chips, 15	4

Pretzels
Bachman

Butter tray stix, 1 oz	2
Butter twist pretzel, 5	2
Kidzels, 19	2
Low sodium petite pretzels, 17	2
Mini pretzels, 17	2
Nutzel, 1/2 cup	2
Original twist pretzel, 5	2
Pita pretzel squares, 11	2
Pretzel stix, 1 oz	2
Puzzle pretzels, 15	2
Rolled rods, 2	2
Sourdough bites, 10	2
Specials, 5	2
Thin 'n rights pretzels, 12	2
Wheat & honey pretzelsnack, 9	2

Combos

Cheddar cheese cracker, 1 oz	3
Cheddar cheese cracker, 1 bag (48.9 g)	6
Cheddar cheese pretzel, 1 oz	3
Cheddar cheese pretzel, 1 bag (51 g)	5
Nacho cheese pretzel, 1 bag (51 g)	5
Nacho cheese pretzel, 1 oz	3
Pepperoni pizza, 1 oz	3
Pepperoni pizza, 1 bag (48.2 g)	6

	POINTS VALUE
Pizzeria pretzel, 1 bag (51 g)	5
Pizzeria pretzel, 1 oz	3
Hanover	
Soft pretzels, 1	3
Harry's	
Everything sourdough, 1	2
Sourdough pretzels, 1	2
Unsalted sourdough pretzels, 1	2
Wheat honey pretzels, 1	2
Whole wheat honey, 1	2
Ian's	
Organic grilled cheese stuffed pretzel, 1	3
Organic nacho cheese stuffed pretzel, 1	3
Organic original whole grain pretzel, 1	3
Kettle Brand	
Honey dijon, made with organic flour, 1 oz	2
Kidzels	
Kidzels, 19	2
Market Day	
Traditional pretzels with salt packets, 1	3
Nabisco 100 Calorie Packs	
Mr. salty milk chocolate covered pretzels, 1 pouch	2
Otis Spunkmeyer	
Pretzel (with salt), 1	6
Rold Gold	
Baked cinnamon flavored braided, 8	2
Baked garlic flavored braided twists, 8	2

	POINTS VALUE
Cheddar cheese flavor tiny twists, 20	2
Classic sticks, 48	2
Classic style rods, 3	2
Classic thins, 9	2
Classic tiny twists, 17	2
Fat free tiny twists, 18	2
Hard sourdough, 1	2
Heartzels, 1 package (28 g)	2
Honey mustard, 20	2
Honey wheat braided twists pretzels, 8	2
Rold Gold Pretzel Waves	
Cheddar blend flavored pretzel snacks, 9 pieces	3
Dark chocolate drizzle pretzel snacks, 7 pieces	3
Parmesan garlic flavored pretzel snacks, 9 pieces	2
Vanilla yogurt drizzle pretzel snacks, 6 pieces	3
Sabra	
Pretzel crisps, 4	1
Snyder's of Hanover	
100 calorie pack mini pretzels, 1 package (0.9 oz)	2
100 calorie pack snaps pretzels, 1 package (0.9 oz)	2
100 calorie pack sticks pretzels, 1 package (0.9 oz)	2
Butter sesame pretzel crackers, 1 oz	2
Butter sesame sticks, 1 oz	2
Butter snaps, 1 oz	2
Buttermilk ranch pieces, 1 oz	3

Snacks

	POINTS VALUE
Cheddar cheese pieces, 1 oz	3
Cheddar cheese pretzel sandwich lunch pack, 1 oz	3
Cheddar cheese sandwiches, 1 oz	3
Dipping sticks, 1 oz	2
Garlic bread nibblers, 1 oz	3
Garlic bread pieces, 1 oz	3
Hard sourdough pretzel, 1 oz	2
Homestyle pretzels, 1 oz	2
Honey bbq pretzel pieces, 1 oz	3
Honey mustard & onion nibblers, 13	3
Honey mustard & onion pretzel pieces, 1 oz	3
Honey wheat sticks, 1 oz	2
Hot buffalo wing pieces, 1/3 cup	3
Jalapeno Cheddar sandwiches, 1 oz	3
Jalapeño pretzel pieces, 1 oz	3
Milk chocolate pretzel dips, 1 oz	3
Mini pretzels, 1 oz	2
Multigrain lightly salted pretzel sticks, 7	2
Olde tyme pretzels, 1 oz	2
Olde tyme sticks, 1 oz	2
Organic honey wheat sticks, 1 oz	3
Organic oat bran sticks, 1 oz	2
Organic pumpernickel and onion sticks, 1 oz	2
Original pretzel crackers, 1 oz	2
Peanut butter pretzel sandwich lunch pack, 1 oz	3
Peanut butter sandwiches, 1 oz	3

	POINTS VALUE
Pumpernickel & onion pretzel crackers, 1 oz	2
Pumpernickel and onion sticks, 1 oz	2
Rods, 1 oz	2
Snaps, 1 oz	2
Sourdough fat free nibblers, 1 oz	2
Special dark pretzel dips, 1 oz	3
Special edition fudge covered peanut butter sandwiches, 1 oz	4
Steakhouse onion pretzel pieces, 1/3 cup	3
Thins, 1 oz	2
Unsalted mini pretzels, 1 oz	2
White chocolate pretzel dips, 1 oz	3
Superpretzel	
Soft pretzel bites with 1/7 salt pak, 5	3
Soft pretzel bites without added salt, 5	3
Soft pretzel with 1/6 salt pak, 1	3
Soft pretzels without added salt, 1	3
Superpretzel Pretzelfils	
Mozzarella, 2 sticks	3
Pepperjack, 2 sticks	3
Pizza, 2 sticks	2
Superpretzel Softstix	
Cheese filled soft pretzel sticks, Cheddar, 2	3
Tree of Life	
Peanut butter pretzel nuggets, 8	5
Yogurt mini pretzels, 1 serving (40 g)	5
Weight Watchers	
Pizza pretzel thins, 1 pouch	2

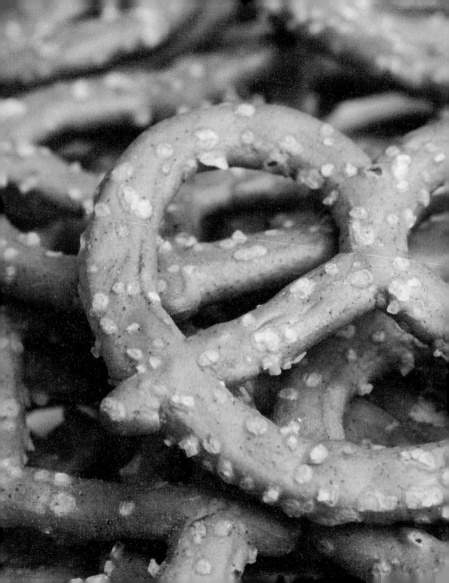

Snacks

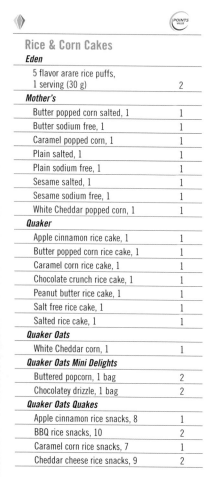

Rice & Corn Cakes
Eden

5 flavor arare rice puffs, 1 serving (30 g)	2

Mother's

Butter popped corn salted, 1	1
Butter sodium free, 1	1
Caramel popped corn, 1	1
Plain salted, 1	1
Plain sodium free, 1	1
Sesame salted, 1	1
Sesame sodium free, 1	1
White Cheddar popped corn, 1	1

Quaker

Apple cinnamon rice cake, 1	1
Butter popped corn rice cake, 1	1
Caramel corn rice cake, 1	1
Chocolate crunch rice cake, 1	1
Peanut butter rice cake, 1	1
Salt free rice cake, 1	1
Salted rice cake, 1	1

Quaker Oats

White Cheddar corn, 1	1

Quaker Oats Mini Delights

Buttered popcorn, 1 bag	2
Chocolatey drizzle, 1 bag	2

Quaker Oats Quakes

Apple cinnamon rice snacks, 8	1
BBQ rice snacks, 10	2
Caramel corn rice snacks, 7	1
Cheddar cheese rice snacks, 9	2
Chocolate crunch rice snacks, 7	1
Creamy ranch rice snacks, 10	2
Nacho rice snacks, 7	2
Sour cream & onion rice snacks, 10	2

Tree of Life

Oriental rice snacks, 1 serving (30 g)	2

Seeds, Snack & Trail Mixes
Be Happy & Healthy

Buzzworthy banana, 1/3 cup	3
Chocolate twisted bliss, 7	4
Cool beans, 1 serving (63 g)	7
Debbie loves fruit, 1/4 cup	2
Energy mix, 1 serving (30 g)	2
Hit the road Jack, 3 Tbsp	3
Honey, I ate the peanuts, 35	4
Hot 'n sweet nuts, 1/4 cup	3
Nacho chips - they're mine, 33	2
Raisin' health, 1 serving (30 g)	3
Rockin raisins, 22	4
Rocky mountain munch, 1/4 cup	2
Soy glad you're healthy, 1/4 cup	3
Swinging sesame stix, 1/3 cup	4
Tropical mix, 1 serving (30 g)	3
Whassup wasabi, 1/3 cup	3
Yogurt twisted bliss, 7	4
You've got trail!, 3 Tbsp	3
Zydeco Cajun mix, 1/3 cup	4

Boston's

Snack mix, 1/2 cup	2

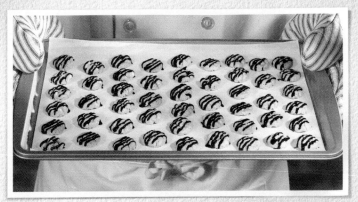

RICE CAKES GET
AN EXTREME BAKE-OVER.

Quaker rice snacks have changed for the better. They're now
made with the goodness of wheat, brown rice and corn,
which we bake to crispy, crunchy perfection. Then we top
them off with incredible flavors, like chocolatey
drizzle. In all, there are 25 sweet and
savory flavors to enjoy. Yes, rice snacks have
changed. And the result is extremely delicious.

Good stuff made delicious

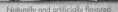
Naturally and artificially flavored.

Snacks

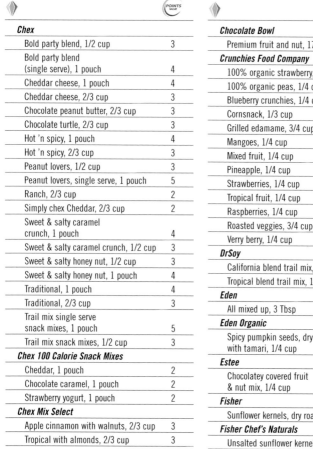

	POINTS VALUE
Chex	
Bold party blend, 1/2 cup	3
Bold party blend (single serve), 1 pouch	4
Cheddar cheese, 1 pouch	4
Cheddar cheese, 2/3 cup	3
Chocolate peanut butter, 2/3 cup	3
Chocolate turtle, 2/3 cup	3
Hot 'n spicy, 1 pouch	4
Hot 'n spicy, 2/3 cup	3
Peanut lovers, 1/2 cup	3
Peanut lovers, single serve, 1 pouch	5
Ranch, 2/3 cup	2
Simply chex Cheddar, 2/3 cup	2
Sweet & salty caramel crunch, 1 pouch	4
Sweet & salty caramel crunch, 1/2 cup	3
Sweet & salty honey nut, 1/2 cup	3
Sweet & salty honey nut, 1 pouch	4
Traditional, 1 pouch	4
Traditional, 2/3 cup	3
Trail mix single serve snack mixes, 1 pouch	5
Trail mix snack mixes, 1/2 cup	3
Chex 100 Calorie Snack Mixes	
Cheddar, 1 pouch	2
Chocolate caramel, 1 pouch	2
Strawberry yogurt, 1 pouch	2
Chex Mix Select	
Apple cinnamon with walnuts, 2/3 cup	3
Tropical with almonds, 2/3 cup	3

	POINTS VALUE
Chocolate Bowl	
Premium fruit and nut, 17 pieces	4
Crunchies Food Company	
100% organic strawberry, 1/3 cup	0
100% organic peas, 1/4 cup	0
Blueberry crunchies, 1/4 cup	0
Cornsnack, 1/3 cup	2
Grilled edamame, 3/4 cup	2
Mangoes, 1/4 cup	0
Mixed fruit, 1/4 cup	0
Pineapple, 1/4 cup	0
Strawberries, 1/4 cup	0
Tropical fruit, 1/4 cup	0
Raspberries, 1/4 cup	0
Roasted veggies, 3/4 cup	2
Verry berry, 1/4 cup	0
DrSoy	
California blend trail mix, 1 oz	2
Tropical blend trail mix, 1 oz	2
Eden	
All mixed up, 3 Tbsp	3
Eden Organic	
Spicy pumpkin seeds, dry roasted with tamari, 1/4 cup	5
Estee	
Chocolatey covered fruit & nut mix, 1/4 cup	5
Fisher	
Sunflower kernels, dry roasted, 1 oz	4
Fisher Chef's Naturals	
Unsalted sunflower kernels, 1 oz	4

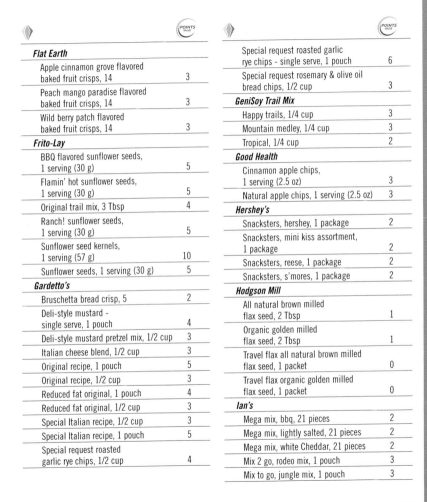

Flat Earth

Apple cinnamon grove flavored baked fruit crisps, 14	3
Peach mango paradise flavored baked fruit crisps, 14	3
Wild berry patch flavored baked fruit crisps, 14	3

Frito-Lay

BBQ flavored sunflower seeds, 1 serving (30 g)	5
Flamin' hot sunflower seeds, 1 serving (30 g)	5
Original trail mix, 3 Tbsp	4
Ranch! sunflower seeds, 1 serving (30 g)	5
Sunflower seed kernels, 1 serving (57 g)	10
Sunflower seeds, 1 serving (30 g)	5

Gardetto's

Bruschetta bread crisp, 5	2
Deli-style mustard - single serve, 1 pouch	4
Deli-style mustard pretzel mix, 1/2 cup	3
Italian cheese blend, 1/2 cup	3
Original recipe, 1 pouch	5
Original recipe, 1/2 cup	3
Reduced fat original, 1 pouch	4
Reduced fat original, 1/2 cup	3
Special Italian recipe, 1/2 cup	3
Special Italian recipe, 1 pouch	5
Special request roasted garlic rye chips, 1/2 cup	4
Special request roasted garlic rye chips - single serve, 1 pouch	6
Special request rosemary & olive oil bread chips, 1/2 cup	3

GeniSoy Trail Mix

Happy trails, 1/4 cup	3
Mountain medley, 1/4 cup	3
Tropical, 1/4 cup	2

Good Health

Cinnamon apple chips, 1 serving (2.5 oz)	3
Natural apple chips, 1 serving (2.5 oz)	3

Hershey's

Snacksters, hershey, 1 package	2
Snacksters, mini kiss assortment, 1 package	2
Snacksters, reese, 1 package	2
Snacksters, s'mores, 1 package	2

Hodgson Mill

All natural brown milled flax seed, 2 Tbsp	1
Organic golden milled flax seed, 2 Tbsp	1
Travel flax all natural brown milled flax seed, 1 packet	0
Travel flax organic golden milled flax seed, 1 packet	0

Ian's

Mega mix, bbq, 21 pieces	2
Mega mix, lightly salted, 21 pieces	2
Mega mix, white Cheddar, 21 pieces	2
Mix 2 go, rodeo mix, 1 pouch	3
Mix to go, jungle mix, 1 pouch	3

Snacks

	POINTS value
Kids Chex	
Cheddar snack mixes, 2/3 cup	3
Lance	
Sunflower seed kernels, 1 package (32 g)	5
Sunflower seeds, in shell, 1 small package (43 g)	3
Sunflower seeds, in shell, 1 package (53 g)	4
Market Day	
Munch packs, 1 pouch	5
Munchies	
Cheese fix snack mix, 3/4 cup	3
Flamin' hot snack mix, 3/4 cup	3
Totally ranch snack mix, 3/4 cup	3
Nabisco 100 Calorie Packs	
Ritz snack mix, 1 pouch (0.78 oz)	2
Nature's Path	
Snack mix - bbq, 1 serving (30 g)	3
Snack mix - original, 1 serving (30 g)	3
Nut Harvest	
Natural nut & fruit mix, 2 Tbsp	4
Pepperidge Farm	
Pumpernickel snack sticks, 15	2
Sesame snack sticks, 12	3
Wheat snack sticks, 9	3
Philadelphia Snack Bites	
Turtle snack bites, 1	3
Planters	
Berry, nut and chocolate, 3 Tbsp	3
Dry roasted sunflower kernels, 1/4 cup	4
Honey nut medley, 4 Tbsp	4

	POINTS value
Mixed nuts and raisins, 3 Tbsp	4
Mixed nuts and raisins, 1 package (48 g)	6
Nut and chocolate mix, 3 Tbsp	4
Nut and chocolate mix, 1 package (56 g)	6
Oil roasted sunflower kernels, 1/4 cup	4
Oil roasted sunflower kernels, 1 small package (49 g)	7
Oil roasted sunflower kernels, 1 medium package (56 g)	8
Oil roasted sunflower kernels, 1 large package (70 g)	10
Pumpkin seeds, 1 package (61 g)	5
Sesame nut mix, 1 oz	4
Spicy party mix with peanuts, 1/3 cup	4
Sunflower seeds, 3/4 cup	4
Sunflower seeds, 1 small package (25 g)	4
Sunflower seeds, 1 medium package (28 g)	4
Sunflower seeds, 1 large package (43 g)	7
Trail mix golden nut crunch, 3 Tbsp	4
Trail mix sweet & nutty, 3 Tbsp	3
Planters Trail Mix	
Fruit & nut mix, 3 Tbsp	3
Nut & chocolate mix, 1 small package (28 g)	3
Nut & chocolate mix, 1 medium package (35 g)	4
Nut & chocolate mix, 1 large package (48 g)	6

	POINTS VALUE
Nuts, seeds & raisins, 3 Tbsp	4
Spicy nuts & Cajun sticks, 1 serving (29 g)	4
Quaker	
Baked Cheddar snack mix, 3/4 cup	3
Kids snack mix, 1 cup	3
Traditional snack mix, 1/2 cup	3
Quaker Oats Whole Grain Granola Bites	
Chocolate, 1 bag	2
Cinnamon, 1 bag	2
Peanut butter, 1 bag	2
Ruth's Foods	
Chia goodness, apple almond cinnamon, 2 Tbsp	2
Chia goodness, cranberry ginger, 2 Tbsp	2
Chia goodness, original, 2 Tbsp	3
Chia raw goodness, 1 heaping Tbsp	1
Snyder's of Hanover	
Multigrain French onion sunflower chips, 16	3
Multigrain lightly salted sunflower chips, 16	3
Multigrain southwestern Cheddar sunflower chips, 16	3
Sunshine Cheez-It	
Party mix, 1/2 cup	3
Tree of Life	
Everyday trail mix, 1 serving (30 g)	3
Flax seed, 3 Tbsp	3
Nutty deluxe, trail mix, 1/4 cup	3
Organic golden flax seed, 3 Tbsp	3

	POINTS VALUE
Organic trail mix, 1/4 cup	3
Pumpkin seeds, roasted and salted, 1/4 cup	7
Sunflower seed kernels, raw, 1/4 cup	5
Tropical Nut & Fruit	
Ah soy!, 1 oz	3
Ball park, 1 oz	3
Banana split, 1 oz	3
Bartender's blend, 1 serving (30 g)	3
Bazaar mix, 1/3 cup	2
Berry good, 1 oz	3
Berry natural, 1 serving (30 g)	2
Berry-ific (organic), 1/3 cup (1 oz)	3
Blueberry thrill, 1 oz	3
Cajun harvest, 1 oz	4
California mix, 1/3 cup	3
California mix, 1 oz	3
California natural mix, 1 oz	2
Capitol crunch, 4 Tbsp	4
Capitol crunch II, 3 Tbsp	4
Champion's choice, 1 oz	4
Checkmate, 1 oz	3
Cinnamon splash, 3 Tbsp	2
Cinnamon splendor, 1 serving (30 g)	2
Continental blend, 3 Tbsp	4
Convention mix, 1/3 cup	4
Country club, 1 oz	5
Diet delight, 1/4 cup	3
Distant lands, 3 Tbsp	4
Fall sweet tooth, 1/4 cup	3
Festival mix, 1 oz	3

Snacks

Tropical Nut & Fruit (cont'd)	
Firecracker hot & spicy, 1/2 cup	4
French quarter, 1 oz	4
Fruit bowl, 1 serving (40 g)	2
Fruit flashers harvest, 3 pieces	1
Fruitful bounty, 2 Tbsp	3
Gold nugget crunch, 3 Tbsp	3
Hawaiian mix, 1 oz	2
Hi-energy mix, 1 oz	2
Indian summer mix, 1 serving (23 g)	2
Indian summer mix, 1 serving (30 g)	3
Just nutty (organic), 1/3 cup	5
Kona coffee crunch, 1/3 cup	3
Mexicali fire, 1 oz	4
Mulligan mix, 4 Tbsp	3
Native south, 1 serving (30 g)	3
Neptune's choice, 1 oz	3
Nutty tyme, 1 oz	4
Oriental delight, 1 oz	3
Oriental delight natural, 1 oz	4
Pasta prima, 1 oz	4
Pastel sunburst, 1/3 cup	4
PB&J mix, 1/4 cup	3
Pistachio berry blend, 1 oz	3
Poppin' nut crunch, 3 Tbsp	4
Red, white, and blue sunburst, 1/3 cup	4
Rise 'n shine, 1/3 cup	3
Salty dog, 1 oz	4
Santa's snack, 1 oz	4
Sesame nut mix, 1 oz	4
Sesame seeds, hulled, 1/4 cup	6

	POINTS VALUE
Sienna cream crunch, 1 serving (30 g)	3
South of the border, 1 oz	4
Student mix, 1 oz	4
Sunburst mix, 1 oz	4
Sunflower seeds, raw, 1 oz	3
Sunflower seeds, roasted and salted, 1 oz	5
Sweet & salty, 1 oz	4
Sweet caroline, 1 oz	4
Sweet heat, 3 Tbsp	4
Sweet tooth, 1 oz	3
Tahitian gold, 1/4 cup	3
The big cheese, 1 oz	4
Trail mix, 1 oz	3
Tropical's treasure, 1 oz	1
Wild about wasabi, 1/3 cup	4
Yogurt ambrosia, 1/4 cup	2
World of Grains	
Cranberry almond clusters, 1 package (20 g)	1
Oatmeal raisin clusters, 1 package (20 g)	1
Vanilla nut clusters, 1 package (20 g)	1

Tortilla Chips

Bachman

Multigrain tortilla chips, 14	3
White restaurant style tortilla chips, 11	3

Bearitos

Blue tortilla chips, 15	3
Blue tortilla chips, unsalted, 15	3
White tortilla chips, 15	3

	POINTS VALUE
White tortilla chips, unsalted, 15	3
Yellow tortilla chips, 15	3
Yellow tortilla chips, unsalted, 15	3
Chipitos	
Black bean & salsa tortilla chips, 8	3
Nacho tortilla chips, 12	3
Nacho tortilla chips, 12	3
Sweet chile lime tortilla chips, 12	3
Thai barbecue tortilla chips, 12	3
Doritos	
Blazin' buffalo & ranch flavored tortilla chips, 12	3
Collisions, zesty taco flavored tortilla chips, 11	3
Collisons, hot wings flavored tortilla chips, 11	3
Cool ranch tortilla chips, 12 pieces	3
Fiery habanero flavored tortilla chips, 11	3
Nacho cheese 100 calorie mini bites flavored tortilla chips, 1 pouch	2
Nacho cheese tortilla chips, 11	3
Quest for the flavor tortilla chips, 12	3
Reduced fat cool ranch flavored tortilla chips, 1 pouch	3
Reduced fat nacho cheese flavored tortilla chips, 1 pouch	3
Salsa verde tortilla chips, 12	3
Smokin' Cheddar bbq flavored tortilla chips, 12	3
Spicy nacho tortilla chips, 12	3
Spicy sweet chili flavored tortilla chips, 11	3

	POINTS VALUE
Taco tortilla chips, 12	3
Toasted corn tortilla chips, 13	3
Doritos Baked!	
Baked nacho cheese, 15 pieces	2
Food Should Taste Good	
Buffalo chips, 12 chips	3
Chocolate chips, 10 chips	3
Cinnamon chips, 12 chips	2
Jalapeno chips, 10 chips	3
Lime chips, 12 chips	3
Multigrain chips, 10 chips	3
Olive chips, 10 chips	3
Potato chive chips, 12 chips	3
Sweet potato chips, 12 chips	3
The works, 10 chips	3
Yellow corn chips, 12 chips	3
Garden of Eatin'	
Baked blue tortilla chips, 19	2
Baked yellow tortilla chips, 19	2
Blue chips unsalted, 15	3
Little soy blues, 13	3
Mini white rounds, 18	3
Mini white strips, 18	3
Multigrain tortilla chips, everything, 16	3
Multigrain tortilla chips, sea salt, 16	3
Red hot blues, 15 chips	3
Red tortilla chips, 15	3
Salsa reds tortilla chips, 15 chips	3
Sesame blues, 9 chips	3
Sunny blues chips, 9 chips	3

Snacks

Garden of Eatin' (cont'd)

	POINTS VALUE
Three pepper blue tortilla chips, 13	3
White tortilla chips, chili & lime, 10	3
White tortilla chips, guacamole, 10	3
White tortilla chips, key lime jalapeno, 15	3
White tortilla chips, pico de gallo, 7	3
White tortilla chips, salted, 15	3
White tortilla chips, tamari, 9	3
Yellow corn chips, 42	4
Yellow tortilla chips, black bean, 13	3
Yellow tortilla chips, black bean chili, 13	3
Yellow tortilla chips, foccacia, 15	3
Yellow tortilla chips, Maui style, 15	3
Yellow tortilla chips, nacho cheese, 9	3
Yellow tortilla chips, salted, 13	3

GeniSoy

	POINTS VALUE
Lightly salted, 1 serving (28 g)	2
Nacho, 1 serving (28 g)	2

Guiltless Gourmet Baked, Not Fried

	POINTS VALUE
Blue corn tortilla chips, 18	2
Chili lime tortilla chips, 18	2
Chili verde corn tortilla chips, 18	2
Chipotle, 18	2
Mucho nacho tortilla chips, 18	2
Spicy black bean tortilla chips, 18	2
Unsalted yellow corn tortilla chips, 18	2
Yellow corn tortilla chips, 18	2

Lance

	POINTS VALUE
Don Pablos bite size round white tortilla chips, 1 oz	3
Don Pablo's restaurant style white tortilla chips, 1 oz	3

LaTortilla Factory

	POINTS VALUE
Bolsa grande tortillas, 2	2
King size yellow corn tortillas, 2	2
Restaurant style yellow corn chips, 12	3
Safflower white corn, 1 serving (1 oz)	3
Super size white corn tortillas, 2	2
Traditional yellow corn, 1 serving (1 oz)	3

Little Bear

	POINTS VALUE
Yellow corn chips, 42	4
Yellow tortilla chips, 15	3

Mexi-Snax

	POINTS VALUE
Multigrain blue chips, 1 oz	3
Multigrain white chips, 1 oz	3
Stoneground nacho tortilla chips, 15	3
Stoneground pico de gallo tortilla chips, 15	3
Stoneground salsa picante tortilla chips, 15	3
Stoneground salted original tortilla chips, 15	3
Stoneground sesame tortilla chips, 15	3
Stoneground tamari tortilla chips, 15	3

Santitas

	POINTS VALUE
100% white corn, 9	3
Tortilla chips, 9	3
Tortilla strips, 11	3

Snyder's of Hanover

	POINTS VALUE
Lightly salted tortillas, 1 oz	2
Restaurant style tortillas, 1 oz	2

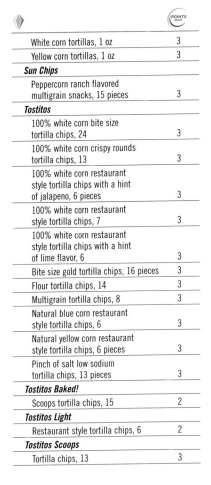

	POINTS VALUE
White corn tortillas, 1 oz	3
Yellow corn tortillas, 1 oz	3
Sun Chips	
Peppercorn ranch flavored multigrain snacks, 15 pieces	3
Tostitos	
100% white corn bite size tortilla chips, 24	3
100% white corn crispy rounds tortilla chips, 13	3
100% white corn restaurant style tortilla chips with a hint of jalapeno, 6 pieces	3
100% white corn restaurant style tortilla chips, 7	3
100% white corn restaurant style tortilla chips with a hint of lime flavor, 6	3
Bite size gold tortilla chips, 16 pieces	3
Flour tortilla chips, 14	3
Multigrain tortilla chips, 8	3
Natural blue corn restaurant style tortilla chips, 6	3
Natural yellow corn restaurant style tortilla chips, 6 pieces	3
Pinch of salt low sodium tortilla chips, 13 pieces	3
Tostitos Baked!	
Scoops tortilla chips, 15	2
Tostitos Light	
Restaurant style tortilla chips, 6	2
Tostitos Scoops	
Tortilla chips, 13	3

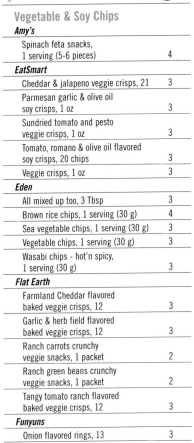

	POINTS VALUE
Vegetable & Soy Chips	
Amy's	
Spinach feta snacks, 1 serving (5-6 pieces)	4
EatSmart	
Cheddar & jalapeno veggie crisps, 21	3
Parmesan garlic & olive oil soy crisps, 1 oz	3
Sundried tomato and pesto veggie crisps, 1 oz	3
Tomato, romano & olive oil flavored soy crisps, 20 chips	3
Veggie crisps, 1 oz	3
Eden	
All mixed up too, 3 Tbsp	3
Brown rice chips, 1 serving (30 g)	4
Sea vegetable chips, 1 serving (30 g)	3
Vegetable chips, 1 serving (30 g)	3
Wasabi chips - hot'n spicy, 1 serving (30 g)	3
Flat Earth	
Farmland Cheddar flavored baked veggie crisps, 12	3
Garlic & herb field flavored baked veggie crisps, 12	3
Ranch carrots crunchy veggie snacks, 1 packet	2
Ranch green beans crunchy veggie snacks, 1 packet	2
Tangy tomato ranch flavored baked veggie crisps, 12	3
Funyuns	
Onion flavored rings, 13	3

Snacks

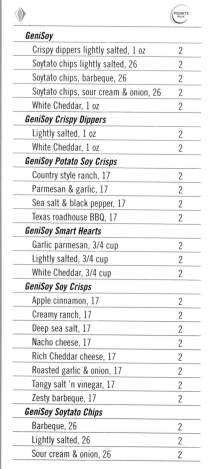

	POINTS VALUE
GeniSoy	
Crispy dippers lightly salted, 1 oz	2
Soytato chips lightly salted, 26	2
Soytato chips, barbeque, 26	2
Soytato chips, sour cream & onion, 26	2
White Cheddar, 1 oz	2
GeniSoy Crispy Dippers	
Lightly salted, 1 oz	2
White Cheddar, 1 oz	2
GeniSoy Potato Soy Crisps	
Country style ranch, 17	2
Parmesan & garlic, 17	2
Sea salt & black pepper, 17	2
Texas roadhouse BBQ, 17	2
GeniSoy Smart Hearts	
Garlic parmesan, 3/4 cup	2
Lightly salted, 3/4 cup	2
White Cheddar, 3/4 cup	2
GeniSoy Soy Crisps	
Apple cinnamon, 17	2
Creamy ranch, 17	2
Deep sea salt, 17	2
Nacho cheese, 17	2
Rich Cheddar cheese, 17	2
Roasted garlic & onion, 17	2
Tangy salt 'n vinegar, 17	2
Zesty barbeque, 17	2
GeniSoy Soytato Chips	
Barbeque, 26	2
Lightly salted, 26	2
Sour cream & onion, 26	2

	POINTS VALUE
Good Health	
Veggie chips, 1 serving (7.5 oz)	3
Good Health Veggie Stix	
Veggie stix, 1 serving (7 oz)	3
Morningstar Farms	
Veggie bites broccoli Cheddar, 3 pieces	4
Veggie bites spinach artichoke, 3 pieces	4
Quaker Oats Soy Crisps	
BBQ, 26	3
White Cheddar, 26	4
Robert's American Gourmet	
Veggie Booty, 1 oz	3
Terra	
Mediterranean exotic vegetable chips, 14	3
Original exotic vegetable chips, 14	3
Stix, original, 1 oz	3
Taro chips, 10	3
Zesty tomato exotic vegetable. chips, 14	3
Tree of Life	
Malt sweetened carob chips, 50	2
Peas, wasabi, 1/4 cup	2

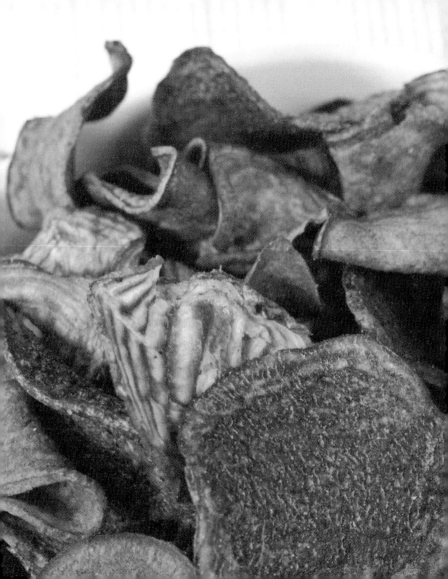

Soups, Stews & Chilis

	POINTS VALUE
Chili	
Amy's	
Black bean chili, 1 cup	3
Light in sodium medium chili, 1 cup	5
Light in sodium spicy chili, 1 cup	5
Medium chili, 1 cup	5
Medium chili with vegetables, 1 cup	4
Southwestern black bean chili, 1 cup	4
Spicy chili, 1 cup	5
Austex American Originals	
Chili, no beans, 1 cup	7
Chili, with beans, 1 cup	6
Boca	
Chili, 1 package	2
Bush's	
Chili magic - Texas, mix, 1/2 cup	2
Chili magic - traditional recipe, mix, 1/2 cup	1
Homestyle chili, chunky with beans, 1 cup	5
Homestyle chili, hot with beans, 1 cup	5
Homestyle chili, no beans, 1 cup	5
Homestyle chili, original with beans, 1 cup	5
Campbell's Chunky	
Firehouse hot & spicy beef & bean chili, 1 cup	4
Hold the beans chili, 1 cup	5
Roadhouse beef & bean chili, 1 cup	4
Sizzlin' steak - grilled steak chili with beans, 1 cup	3

	POINTS VALUE
Campbell's Chunky Microwavable Bowls	
Firehouse hot & spicy beef & bean chili, 1 cup	4
Roadhouse beef & bean chili, 1 cup	4
Castleberry's American Originals	
Chili, no beans, 1 serving (1 oz)	3
Chili, no beans, 1 cup	7
Chili, with beans, 1 cup	6
Cattle Drive Gold	
Chicken chili with beans, 1 cup	6
Chili with beans, 1 cup	6
Cherchies	
9 spice red bean chili mix, 1 serving (56 g)	3
White bean chili mix, 1 serving (1.77 oz)	3
Fantastic World Foods	
♦ Vegetarian chili, 1/2 cup	3
Goldwater's	
Senator's chili mix, 1 serving (0.25 oz)	0
Hormel	
Chili no beans less salt, canned, 1 cup	5
Chili no beans, canned, 1 cup	5
Chili with beans less salt, canned, 1 cup	5
Chili with beans, canned, 1 cup	5
Chunky chili no beans, canned, 1 cup	4
Chunky chili with beans, canned, 1 cup	5
Homestyle chili with beans, canned, 1 cup	8

	POINTS VALUE
Hot & spicy chili, no beans, canned, 1 cup	5
Hot & spicy chili, with beans, canned, 1 cup	5
Hot chili no beans, canned, 1 cup	5
Hot chili with beans, canned, 1 cup	5
Turkey chili no beans, canned, 1 cup	3
Turkey chili with beans, canned, 1 cup	4
◆ Vegetarian chili, canned, 1 cup	3
Hormel Individual Canned Servings	
Chili with beans, 1 can	4
Hot chili with beans, 1 can	4
Hormel Micro Cup Meals	
Chili no beans, 1 cup	4
Chili with beans, 1 cup	4
Hot chili with beans, 1 cup	4
Nalley	
Hot chili con carne with beans, 1 cup	5
Original chili con carne with beans, 1 cup	5
Original vegetarian 99% fat free vegetarian chili with beans, 1 cup	4
Really hearty chili con carne with beans, 1 cup	7
Thick chili con carne with beans, 1 cup	5
Turkey chili con carne with beans, 1 cup	4
Old El Paso	
Black bean with chipotle, 1 cup	2
Stagg	
Chunkero chili with beans, 1 cup	7
Classic chili, 1 cup	7

	POINTS VALUE
Country brand chili, with beans, 1 cup	7
Dynamite hot chili, with beans, 1 cup	7
Fiesta grille chili with beans, 1 cup	5
Laredo chili with beans, 1 cup	7
Quickdraw chili with beans, 1 bowl	5
Ranch house chicken chili, with beans, 1 cup	5
Santa Fe chicken chili with beans, 1 cup	4
Silverado beef 97% fat free chili, 1 cup	4
Silverado beef chili, with beans, 1 cup	5
Steak house chili, no beans, 1 cup	8
Turkey ranchero chili, with beans, 1 cup	4
◆ Vegetable garden 4-bean chili, 1 cup	3
White chicken chili with beans, 1 cup	5
Wyler's Mrs. Grass	
◆ Homestyle three bean chili mix, 1/4 carton	2

Beef Soups
Campbell's

	POINTS VALUE
◆ Beef consommé, 1/2 cup	0
Beef noodle soup, 1/2 cup	1
◆ Beef with vegetables and barley soup, 1/2 cup	1
Beefy mushroom soup, 1/2 cup	1
◆ Vegetable beef, 1/2 cup	1
Campbell's Chunky	
Baked potato with steak & cheese, 1 cup	4
Beef burgundy soup, 1 cup	3

Soups, Stews & Chilis

◆ Campbell's Chunky (cont'd)

	POINTS VALUE
Beef rib roast with potatoes & herbs, 1 cup	2
Beef stew soup, 1 cup	3
◆ Beef with country vegetables, 1 cup	2
Beef with white and wild rice, 1 cup	3
◆ Grilled sirloin steak with hearty vegetables, 1 cup	2
◆ Hearty beef barley, 1 cup	3
◆ Old fashioned vegetable beef, 1 cup	2
◆ Pepper steak, 1 cup	2
Rigatoni & meatballs soup, 1 cup	4
Salisbury steak with mushrooms & onions, 1 cup	3
◆ Savory pot roast, 1 cup	2
Sirloin burger with country vegetable, 1 cup	3
◆ Slow roasted beef with mushrooms, 1 cup	2
Steak 'n potato, 1 cup	2
Stroganoff-style beef soup, 1 cup	5

Campbell's Chunky Healthy Request
◆ Old fashioned vegetable beef, 1 cup	2

Campbell's Chunky Microwavable Bowls
◆ Beef with country vegetables, 1 cup	2
◆ Old fashioned vegetable beef, 1 cup	2
Sirloin burger with country vegetables, 1 cup	3

Campbell's Healthy Request
Beef barley soup, 1 cup	2
◆ Vegetable beef, 1/2 cup	1

Campbell's Microwavable Bowls
Vegetable beef soup, 1 cup	1

◆ Campbell's Select

	POINTS VALUE
◆ Beef with roasted barley, 1 cup	2
◆ Slow roasted beef and vegetables, 1 cup	2
Zesty Azteca meatball & rice soup, 1 cup	2

Campbell's Soup at Hand
◆ Vegetable beef, 1 container	1

Cherchies
Hearty beef & pasta soup mix, 1 serving	1

Hormel Micro Cup Soups
◆ Beef vegetable, 1 cup	2

Muir Glen Organic Soup Chef Inspirations
◆ Beef & vegetable soup, 1 cup	2

Progresso
◆ Beef & baked potato, 1 cup	2
◆ Beef & vegetable, 1 cup	2
◆ Beef barley, 1 cup	3
◆ Beef barley 99% fat free, 1 cup	2
Chickarina with meatballs, 1 cup	2

Progresso Light Soups
Beef pot roast soup, 1 cup	1
Italian style meatball soup, 1 cup	1

Progresso Microwavable Soups
◆ Beef & vegetable, 1 cup	2

Progresso Reduced Sodium Soups
Beef & vegetable soup, 1 cup	2
Italian-style wedding soup with meatballs, 1 cup	2

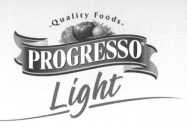

Try Our Two Newest Flavors!
Chicken & Dumpling
Italian Style Meatball

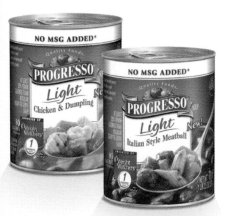

- 1 *POINTS*® value and 80 calories per serving
- No MSG added†
- No artificial flavors
- Low fat
- Endorsed by Weight Watchers®

Progresso Light is the *only* nationally branded soup endorsed by Weight Watchers!

*Except that which occurs naturally in yeast extract and hydrolyzed vegetable proteins.

At least 33% fewer calories than regular ready-to-serve soup.
©2009 General Mills A18556
Weight Watchers for services and *POINTS*® are the registered trademarks of Weight Watchers International, Inc. and are used with permission.

Soups, Stews & Chilis

POINTS VALUE

Progresso Rich & Hearty Soups

	POINTS VALUE
Beef pot roast with country vegetables, 1 cup	2
Savory beef barley vegetable, 1 cup	2
Sirloin steak & vegetables, 1 cup	2
Steak & homestyle noodles, 1 cup	2
Steak & roasted russet potatoes, 1 cup	3
Steak & sauteed mushrooms, 1 cup	2
Vegetable beef slow cooked, 1 cup	2

Wyler's Mrs. Grass

Homestyle beef vegetable mix, 1/4 carton	1

Wyler's Soup Starter Homestyle Soup Mix

Beef vegetable, prepared with water, 1 cup (1/7 package)	1
Hearty beef stew, prepared with water, 1 cup (1/8 package)	1

Bouillon, Broth & Stocks
A Taste of Thai

Coconut ginger soup base, 1 tsp	0

Campbell's

Beef broth, 1/2 cup	0
Chicken broth, 1/2 cup	0
Scotch broth, 1/2 cup	1

Campbell's Low Sodium Soup

Chicken broth, 1 can	1

Glory Seasoned

Cooking base - beef, 1 tsp	0
Cooking base - chicken, 1 tsp	0
Cooking base - vegetable, 1 tsp	0

Health Valley

Fat-free beef flavored broth, 8 oz	0
Fat-free beef flavored broth no salt, 8 oz	0
Fat-free chicken broth, 8 oz	1
Fat-free vegetable broth, 8 oz	0
Low fat chicken broth, 8 oz	1
Low fat chicken broth no salt, 8 oz	1

Herb-Ox

Beef bouillon cubes, 1	0
Beef instant bouillon powder, 1 tsp	0
Beef instant broth & seasoning, 1 packet	0
Beef instant broth & seasoning low sodium packet, 1	0
Chicken bouillon cubes, 1	0
Chicken instant bouillon powder, 1 tsp	0
Chicken instant broth & seasoning, 1 packet	0
Chicken instant broth & seasoning low sodium packet, 1	0
Garlic chicken bouillon cubes, 1	0
Vegetable bouillon cubes, 1	0

Home Again

Beef base, 1 tsp	0
Chicken base, 1 tsp	0
Chicken base, no msg, 1 tsp	0
Chicken flavor stock, 1 tsp	0
Ham base, 3/4 tsp	0

Preciosa

Bacon bouillon, 1 tablet	0
Chicken bouillon, 1 tsp	0
Chicken/onion bouillon, 1 tsp	0

Progresso

Beef broth flavored, 1 cup	0
Chicken broth, 1 cup	0
Reduced sodium chicken broth, 1 cup	0

	POINTS VALUE
Swanson	
50% less sodium beef broth, 1 cup	0
Beef broth, 1 cup	0
Certified organic beef broth, 1 cup	0
Certified organic chicken broth, 1 cup	0
Certified organic vegetable broth, 1 cup	0
Chicken broth, 1 cup	0
Natural goodness chicken broth, 1 cup	1
Seasoned beef broth with onion, 1 cup	0
Seasoned chicken broth with roasted garlic, 1 cup	0
Vegetable broth, 1 cup	1
Wyler's	
Reduced sodium beef, 1 cube	0
Reduced sodium chicken, 1 cube	0
Sodium free beef, 1 tsp	0
Sodium free chicken, 1 tsp	0
Zesty garlic beef, 1 cube	0
Zesty garlic chicken, 1 cube	0

Chicken Soups

4C

Noodle soup with real chicken broth, 1 serving	1

Campbell's

25% less sodium chicken noodle, 1/2 cup	1
Chicken alphabet, 1/2 cup	1
Chicken and dumplings, 1/2 cup	1
Chicken and stars, 1/2 cup	1
Chicken gumbo, 1/2 cup	1

	POINTS VALUE
Chicken mushroom barley soup, 1/2 cup	1
Chicken noodle, 1/2 cup	1
Chicken noodle o's, 1/2 cup	2
Chicken noodle soup with white chicken meat, dry soup mix, prepared, 1/2 cup	2
Chicken vegetable, 1/2 cup	1
Chicken with rice, 1/2 cup	1
Chicken with white and wild rice, 1/2 cup	1
Chicken won ton, 1/2 cup	1
Cream of chicken - 98% fat free, 1/2 cup	1
Cream of chicken and mushroom, 1/2 cup	1
Cream of chicken condensed soup, 1/2 cup	3
Cream of chicken with herbs, 1/2 cup	1
Creamy chicken noodle, 1/2 cup	2
Dora the explorer, kid shapes, 1/2 cup	1
Double noodle in chicken broth, 1/2 cup	2
Double noodle in chicken broth, dry soup mix, 1/2 cup	3
Goldfish pasta with chicken in chicken broth, 1/2 cup	1
Goldfish pasta with meatball in chicken broth, 1/2 cup	1
Homestyle chicken noodle, 1/2 cup	1
Mega noodle in chicken broth, 1/2 cup	2
Noodle soup with real chicken broth, dry soup mix, 1 serving	2

Soups, Stews & Chilis

Campbell's (cont'd)	POINTS VALUE
Select harvest light savory chicken with vegetables, 1 cup	1
Shrek shaped pasta with chicken in chicken broth, 1/2 cup	1
Southwestern style chicken vegetable, 1/2 cup	1
Campbell's Chunky	
Chicken and dumplings, 1 cup	3
Chicken broccoli cheese & potato, 1 cup	5
Chicken corn chowder, 1 cup	4
Chicken mushroom chowder, 1 cup	5
Classic chicken noodle, 1 cup	2
Fajita chicken with rice & beans soup, 1 cup	2
Grilled chicken & sausage gumbo, 1 cup	2
Grilled chicken with vegetables & pasta, 1 cup	2
Hearty chicken with vegetables, 1 cup	2
Savory chicken with white & wild rice, 1 cup	2
Campbell's Chunky Healthy Request	
Chicken noodle soup, 1 cup	2
Classic chicken noodle soup, 1 cup	2
Grilled chicken & sausage gumbo, 1 cup	2
Grilled chicken & sausage gumbo, 1 cup	2
Campbell's Chunky Microwavable Bowls	
Chicken & dumplings, 1 cup	4
Chicken noodle, 1 cup	2
Grilled chicken & sausage gumbo, 1 cup	2

	POINTS VALUE
Campbell's Healthy Request	
Chicken noodle, 1/2 cup	1
Chicken rice, 1/2 cup	1
Cream of chicken, 1/2 cup	2
Homestyle chicken noodle, 1/2 cup	1
Campbell's Low Sodium Soup	
Chicken with noodles, 1 can	3
Campbell's Microwavable Bowls	
Chicken noodle soup, 1 cup	1
Campbell's Select	
Chicken vegetable medley, 1 cup	2
Chicken with egg noodles, 1 cup	2
Creamy chicken alfredo, 1 cup	4
Herbed chicken with roasted vegetables, 1 cup	2
Mexican style chicken tortilla, 1 cup	2
Roasted chicken with rotini & penne pasta, 1 cup	2
Savory chicken and long-grain rice, 1 cup	2
Campbell's Select Healthy Request	
Chicken with egg noodles, 1 cup	2
Mexican style chicken tortilla, 1 cup	2
Mexican style chicken tortilla, 1 cup	2
Savory chicken and long grain rice, 1 cup	2
Campbell's Select Microwavable Bowls	
Chicken with egg noodles, 1 cup	2
Mexican style chicken tortilla soup, 1 cup	2
Savory chicken and long grain rice, 1 cup	2

	POINTS VALUE
Campbell's Soup at Hand	
25% less sodium chicken with mini noodles, 1 container	1
Chicken & stars, 1 container	1
Chicken with mini noodles, 1 container	1
Creamy chicken, 1 container	3
Cherchies	
Chicken pot pie soup mix, 1/4 cup	2
Fantastic World Foods	
New England vegetarian chicken simmer soup, 1 oz (dry mix)	2
Vegetarian chicken noodle, 1/4 cup (dry mix)	2
Health Valley	
Chicken flavored noodles with vegetables soup cup, 1 serving (.99 oz)	2
Chicken noodle, 8 oz	2
Chicken rice, 8 oz	2
Organic cream of chicken, 8 oz	3
Hormel Micro Cup Soups	
Chicken & rice, 1 cup	2
Chicken noodle, 1 cup	2
Imagine Foods	
Creamy chicken, 1 cup	1
Manischewitz	
Original chicken noodle soup, 1 cup	1
Zesty chicken noodle soup, 1 cup	2
Market Day	
Chicken & dumpling soup, 1/2 cup	3
Chicken tortilla soup, 1 cup	5
Chicken with wild rice soup, 1 cup	2

	POINTS VALUE
Progresso	
Chicken & sausage gumbo soup, 1 cup	3
Chicken & wild rice, 1 cup	2
Chicken barley, 1 cup	2
Chicken herb dumpling, 1 cup	2
Chicken noodle, 1 cup	2
Chicken noodle, 99% fat free, 1 cup	2
Chicken rice with vegetables, 1 cup	2
Hearty chicken & rotini, 1 cup	2
Homestyle chicken with vegetables & pasta, 1 cup	2
Minestrone with chicken, 1 cup	2
Roasted chicken rotini, 1 cup	2
Southwestern style chicken chowder, 1 cup	2
Traditional roasted garlic chicken, 1 cup	2
Progresso 100% Natural Soups	
Chicken noodle, 1 cup	2
Hearty chicken & rotini, 1 cup	2
Progresso Carb Monitor Soups	
Chicken cheese enchilada flavor, 1 cup	4
Progresso Light Soups	
Chicken & dumpling, 1 cup	1
Chicken noodle, 1 cup	1
Chicken vegetable rotini, 1 cup	1
Roasted chicken & vegetable, 1 cup	1
Santa Fe style chicken, 1 cup	1
Progresso Microwavable Soups	
Chicken noodle, 1 cup	2
Chicken wild rice, 1 cup	2

Soups, Stews & Chilis

	POINTS VALUE
Progresso Reduced Sodium Soups	
Chicken & wild rice soup, 1 cup	2
Chicken gumbo, 1 cup	2
Chicken noodle, 1 cup	2
Progresso Rich & Hearty Soups	
Chicken & homestyle noodles, 1 cup	2
Chicken corn chowder, 1 cup	4
Chicken pot pie style, 1 cup	3
Creamy chicken wild rice, 1 cup	3
Progresso Vegetable Classic	
Hearty penne in chicken broth, 1 cup	1
Wyler's Mrs. Grass	
Chicken with white and wild rice mix, 1/4 carton	1
Homestyle chicken noodle mix, 1/4 carton	1
◆ Homestyle chicken vegetable mix, 1/4 carton	1
Wyler's Soup Starter Homestyle Soup Mix	
Chicken noodle, prepared with water, 1 cup	1
Chicken with white & wild rice, prepared with water, 1 cup	3

Other Meat Soups
Campbell's

	POINTS VALUE
Bean with bacon soup, 1/2 cup	3
Split pea with ham and bacon, 1/2 cup	3
Campbell's Chunky	
Hearty bean 'n ham, 1 cup	3
Old fashioned potato ham chowder, 1 cup	4
◆ Split pea 'n' ham, 1 cup	3

	POINTS VALUE
Campbell's Select	
Italian sausage with pasta & pepperoni, 1 cup	3
Mediterranean meatball with bowtie pasta, 1 cup	2
◆ Savory white bean with roasted ham, 1 cup	3
◆ Split pea with roasted ham, 1 cup	2
Campbell's Select Microwavable Bowls	
Italian sausage pasta & pepperoni, 1 cup	3
Cherchies	
Cajun sausage soup mix, 1/3 cup	2
Hormel Micro Cup Soups	
Bean & ham soup, 1 cup	3
Progresso	
◆ Split pea with ham, 1 cup	2

Seafood Soups
Campbell's

	POINTS VALUE
Cream of shrimp, 1/2 cup	2
◆ Manhattan clam chowder, 1/2 cup	1
New England clam chowder, 1/2 cup	2
Select harvest light Maryland-style crab, 1 cup	1
Campbell's Chunky	
◆ Manhattan clam chowder, 1 cup	2
New England clam chowder, 1 cup	4
Campbell's Chunky Microwavable Bowls	
New England clam chowder, 1 cup	3
Campbell's Healthy Request	
New England clam chowder, 1 cup	2

	POINTS VALUE
Campbell's Select	
98% fat free New England clam chowder, 1 cup	2
New England clam chowder, 1 cup	3
Campbell's Select Microwavable Bowls	
98% fat free New England clam chowder, 1 cup	2
Campbell's Soup at Hand	
New England clam chowder, 1 container	3
Cape Cod	
99% Fat Free New England style clam chowder (condensed), 1/2 cup	1
Chincoteague	
Chesapeake Bay crab & Cheddar soup (condensed), 1/2 cup	2
Chesapeake bay cream of crab soup, 1 cup	5
Clam bisque (condensed), 1/2 cup	2
Lobster and Cheddar bisque (condensed), 1/2 cup	3
Lobster bisque (condensed), 1/2 cup	2
◆ Manhattan clam chowder (condensed), 1/2 cup	2
New England clam chowder (condensed), 1/2 cup	2
She crab soup (condensed), 1/2 cup	2
Shrimp bisque (condensed), 1/2 cup	2
◆ Vegetable red crab soup, 1 cup	2
Health Valley	
◆ Seafood Manhattan clam chowder, 8 oz	2
Seafood New England clam chowder, 8 oz	3

	POINTS VALUE
Hormel Micro Cup Soups	
New England clam chowder, 1 cup	3
Market Day	
Supreme lobster bisque, 1 cup (8 fl oz)	8
Phillips	
Crab & corn chowder, 1 cup	5
Crab & shrimp chowder, 1 cup	4
Cream of crab soup, 1 cup	9
Lobster bisque, 1 cup	8
Maryland style crab soup, 1 cup	2
New England clam chowder, 1 cup	4
Shrimp bisque, 1 cup	7
Progresso	
◆ Manhattan clam chowder, 1 cup	2
New England clam chowder, 1 cup	4
New England clam chowder 99% fat free, 1 cup	2
Progresso Rich & Hearty Soups	
New England clam chowder, 1 cup	4
Snow's	
Authentic New England clam chowder, 1 cup	2
New England clam chowder, 1/2 cup	2
New England corn chowder, 1/2 cup	2
Snow's 98% Fat Free	
Authentic New England clam chowder, 1 cup	2

Stews

	POINTS VALUE
Austex American Originals	
Beef stew, classic, 1 cup	6
Campbell's	
Oyster stew, 1/2 cup	2

Soups, Stews & Chilis

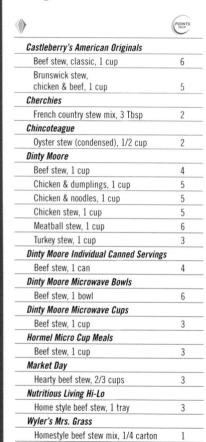

	POINTS VALUE
Castleberry's American Originals	
Beef stew, classic, 1 cup	6
Brunswick stew, chicken & beef, 1 cup	5
Cherchies	
French country stew mix, 3 Tbsp	2
Chincoteague	
Oyster stew (condensed), 1/2 cup	2
Dinty Moore	
Beef stew, 1 cup	4
Chicken & dumplings, 1 cup	5
Chicken & noodles, 1 cup	5
Chicken stew, 1 cup	5
Meatball stew, 1 cup	6
Turkey stew, 1 cup	3
Dinty Moore Individual Canned Servings	
Beef stew, 1 can	4
Dinty Moore Microwave Bowls	
Beef stew, 1 bowl	6
Dinty Moore Microwave Cups	
Beef stew, 1 cup	3
Hormel Micro Cup Meals	
Beef stew, 1 cup	3
Market Day	
Hearty beef stew, 2/3 cups	3
Nutritious Living Hi-Lo	
Home style beef stew, 1 tray	3
Wyler's Mrs. Grass	
Homestyle beef stew mix, 1/4 carton	1

	POINTS VALUE
## Turkey Soups	
Campbell's Chunky	
Turkey pot pie soup, 1 cup	4
Progresso	
Turkey noodle, 1 cup	2
## Vegetable & Other Soups	
4C	
Recipe mix, onion, 1 serving (7 g)	0
Amy's	
Alphabet soup, 1 cup	1
Butternut squash - light in sodium, 1 cup	2
Chunky tomato bisque, 1 cup	2
Chunky tomato bisque - light in sodium, 1 cup	2
Chunky vegetable soup, 1 cup	1
Corn chowder, 1 cup	4
Cream of mushroom soup, 3/4 cups	3
Cream of tomato soup, 1 cup	2
Cream of tomato - light in sodium, 1 cup	2
Curried lentil soup, 1 cup	5
Fire roasted southwestern vegetable soup, 1 cup	2
Lentil soup, 1 cup	3
Lentil vegetable - light in sodium, 1 cup	3
Minestrone, 1 cup	1
Minestrone soup, 1 cup	1
No chicken noodle soup, 1 cup	2
Organic minestrone - light in sodium, 1 cup	1

Soups, Stews & Chilis

	POINTS VALUE
◆ Organic vegetable barley soup, 1 cup	1
Pasta & 3 bean, 1 cup	2
Potato leek soup, 1 cup	4
◆ Split pea soup, 1 cup	1
◆ Split pea soup – light in sodium, 1 cup	1
Summer corn & vegetable soup, 1 cup	3
Thai coconut soup (tom kha phak), 1/2 can	5
Bush's	
Lentil soup, 1/2 cup	2
Campbell's	
25% less sodium cream of mushroom soup, 1/2 cup	2
◆ 25% less sodium tomato soup, 1/2 cup	2
Broccoli cheese, 1/2 cup	2
Broccoli cheese - 98% fat free, 1/2 cup	1
Cars fun shapes, 1/2 cup	1
Cheddar cheese, 1/2 cup	2
Cream of asparagus, 1/2 cup	2
Cream of broccoli, 1/2 cup	2
Cream of broccoli - 98% fat free, 1/2 cup	1
Cream of celery, 1/2 cup	2
Cream of celery - 98% fat free, 1/2 cup	1
Cream of mushroom, 1/2 cup	2
Cream of mushroom - 98% fat free, 1/2 cup	1
Cream of mushroom with roasted garlic, 1/2 cup	1

	POINTS VALUE
Cream of onion, 1/2 cup	2
Cream of potato, 1/2 cup	2
Curly noodle, 1/2 cup	2
Fiesta nacho cheese, 1/2 cup	3
◆ French onion, 1/2 cup	1
Golden mushroom, 1/2 cup	2
◆ Green pea, 1/2 cup	3
Italian-style wedding soup, 1/2 cup	1
Minestrone, 1/2 cup	1
Old fashioned tomato rice, 1/2 cup	2
Old fashioned vegetable, 1/2 cup	1
◆ Onion soup mix, 1 Tbsp	0
Pepper pot, 1/2 cup	2
Select harvest light Italian-style vegetable, 1 cup	1
◆ Select harvest light southwest-style vegetable, 1 cup	1
Southwest-style pepper Jack, 1/2 cup	2
◆ Tomato, 1/2 cup	2
Tomato bisque, 1/2 cup	3
Vegetable, 1/2 cup	1
Vegetarian vegetable, 1/2 cup	1
Campbell's Chunky	
Baked potato with Cheddar & bacon bits, 1 cup	3
Hearty vegetable with pasta, 1 cup	2
◆ Savory vegetable, 1 cup	1
Campbell's Chunky Healthy Request	
Vegetable, 1 cup	2
Campbell's Healthy Request	
Cream of celery, 1/2 cup	1
Cream of mushroom, 1/2 cup	1

Soups, Stews & Chilis

 Campbell's Healthy Request (cont'd)   POINTS VALUE

Minestrone, 1/2 cup	1
◆ Tomato, 1/2 cup	2
Vegetable, 1/2 cup	1

Campbell's Microwavable Bowls

Creamy tomato soup, 1 cup	3
◆ Tomato soup, 1 cup	2
◆ Vegetable soup, 1 cup	2

Campbell's Select

Creamy potato with roasted garlic, 1 cup	4
Creamy tomato parmesan soup, 1 cup	4
Harvest tomato with basil soup, 1 cup	1
Italian style wedding, 1 cup	2
Minestrone, 1 cup	1
Potato broccoli cheese, 1 cup	2
Tomato garden, 1 cup	2
◆ Vegetable medley, 1 cup	1

Campbell's Select Gold Label Soup

Blended red pepper black bean soup, 1 cup	2
Creamy portobello mushroom soup, 1 cup	2
Golden butternut squash soup, 1 cup	1
◆ Italian tomato with basil & garlic soup, 1 cup	1
Southwestern corn, 1 cup	4

Campbell's Select Healthy Request

Italian-style wedding, 1 cup	2

Campbell's Select Microwavable Bowls

Italian-style wedding soup, 1 cup	2
Minestrone, 1 cup	1

POINTS VALUE

Campbell's Soup at Hand

25% less sodium classic tomato, 1 container	2
◆ Blended vegetable medley, 1 container	1
◆ Classic tomato, 1 container	2
Cream of broccoli, 1 container	3
Creamy tomato, 1 container	3
Italian-style wedding, 1 container	2
Velvety potato, 1 container	3

Cherchies

Barley & red lentil soup mix, 1 serving (2 oz)	3
Black & navy bean soup mix, 1 serving (2 oz)	3
Corn chowder, 1/3 cup dry mix	2
Cuban black beans soup mix, 1 serving (62 g)	3
French potato soup, 1 serving (1/7 package)	1
Gumbo mix with filé seasoning, 1 serving (1/9 package)	2
Italian wedding soup mix, 1/4 cup	1
Mexican tortilla soup, 1 serving (23 g)	1
Minestrone soup mix, 1/4 cup	2
Mixed bean soup mix, 1 serving (2 oz)	3
Mushroom chowder, 1/2 cup dry mix	1
Pasta e fagioli soup mix, 1 serving (2 oz)	3
Spicy Southwest bean soup mix, 1 serving (2 oz)	3
Split pea & lentil soup mix, 1 serving (2 oz)	3
Vegetable chowder, 1 oz dry mix	2

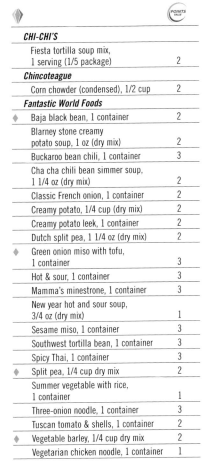

	POINTS VALUE
CHI-CHI'S	
Fiesta tortilla soup mix, 1 serving (1/5 package)	2
Chincoteague	
Corn chowder (condensed), 1/2 cup	2
Fantastic World Foods	
Baja black bean, 1 container	2
Blarney stone creamy potato soup, 1 oz (dry mix)	2
Buckaroo bean chili, 1 container	3
Cha cha chili bean simmer soup, 1 1/4 oz (dry mix)	2
Classic French onion, 1 container	2
Creamy potato, 1/4 cup (dry mix)	2
Creamy potato leek, 1 container	2
Dutch split pea, 1 1/4 oz (dry mix)	2
Green onion miso with tofu, 1 container	3
Hot & sour, 1 container	3
Mamma's minestrone, 1 container	3
New year hot and sour soup, 3/4 oz (dry mix)	1
Sesame miso, 1 container	3
Southwest tortilla bean, 1 container	3
Spicy Thai, 1 container	3
Split pea, 1/4 cup dry mix	2
Summer vegetable with rice, 1 container	1
Three-onion noodle, 1 container	3
Tuscan tomato & shells, 1 container	2
Vegetable barley, 1/4 cup dry mix	2
Vegetarian chicken noodle, 1 container	1

	POINTS VALUE
Health Valley	
Black bean microwaveable bowl soup, 8 oz	2
Cream potato with broccoli soup cup, 1 serving (0.83 oz)	1
Fat-free 5 bean vegetable soup, 8 oz	2
Fat-free 14 garden vegetable soup, 8 oz	1
Fat-free black bean & vegetable soup, 8 oz	2
Fat-free corn & vegetable soup, 8 oz	1
Fat-free lentil & carrots soup, 8 oz	1
Fat-free minestrone, 8 oz	1
Fat-free pasta Italiano soup cup, 1 serving (1.34 oz)	2
Fat-free pasta parmesan soup cup, 1 serving (.97 oz)	2
Fat-free split pea & carrots soup, 8 oz	1
Fat-free tomato vegetable soup, 8 oz	1
Fat-free vegetable barley soup, 8 oz	1
Lentil microwaveable bowl soup, 8 oz	2
Lentil with couscous soup cup, 1 serving (1.33 oz)	2
Minestrone microwaveable bowl soup, 8 oz	1
Organic black bean soup, 8 oz	2
Organic black bean soup no salt, 8 oz	2
Organic cream of celery soup, 8 oz	2
Organic cream of mushroom soup, 8 oz	2
Organic lentil soup, 8 oz	1
Organic lentil soup no salt, 8 oz	1
Organic minestrone soup, 8 oz	1
Organic minestrone soup no salt, 8 oz	1

Soups, Stews & Chilis

Health Valley (cont'd)	POINTS VALUE
Organic mushroom barley soup, 8 oz	1
Organic mushroom barley soup no salt, 8 oz	1
Organic potato & leek soup, 8 oz	1
Organic potato & leek soup no salt, 8 oz	1
Organic split pea soup, 8 oz	1
Organic split pea soup no salt, 8 oz	1
Organic tomato soup, 8 oz	1
Organic tomato soup no salt, 8 oz	1
Organic vegetable soup, 8 oz	1
Organic vegetable soup no salt, 8 oz	1
Spicy black bean with couscous soup cup, 1 serving (1.33 oz)	2
Split pea microwaveable bowl soup, 8 oz	2
Tomato bisque microwaveable bowl soup, 8 oz	2
Vegetable soup, 1 cup	0
Vegetable microwaveable bowl soup, 8 oz	2
Zesty black bean with rice soup cup, 1 serving (1.03 oz)	1
Imagine Foods	
Acorn squash & mango soup, 1 cup	1
Corn chipotle bisque, 1 cup	2
Creamy broccoli, 1 cup	1
Creamy butternut squash, 1 cup	2
Creamy potato leek, 1 cup	2
Creamy sweet corn, 1 cup	2
Creamy tomato, 1 cup	1
Creamy tomato basil, 1 cup	2
Cuban black bean bisque, 1 cup	3

	POINTS VALUE
Fire roasted tomato bisque, 1 cup	2
Sweet pea soup, 1 cup	1
Sweet potato, 1 cup	2
Lucini	
Roman tomato cream soup, 1 cup	3
Rustic Italian minestrone soup, 1 cup	3
Tuscan tomato & basil soup, 1 cup	1
Umbrian lentil soup, 1 cup	3
Manischewitz	
Borscht with shredded beets, 1 cup	1
Clear borscht, 1 cup	1
Matzo ball soup mix, 1 Tbsp (1 cup prepared)	1
Reduced sodium borscht, 1 cup	2
Schav, 1 cup	0
Manischewitz Homestyle Soup Mix	
Mediterranean black bean, 1 serving (1/6 package)	3
Market Day	
Broccoli & cheese soup singles, 1 pouch	5
Italian wedding soup, 1/2 cup	3
Loaded baked potato soup, 1/2 cup	4
Minestrone soup, 1 cup	2
Muir Glen Organic Soup	
Creamy tomato soup, 1 cup	4
Garden vegetable, 1 cup	1
Hearty tomato, 1 cup	2
Lentil, 1 cup	2
Minestrone, 1 cup	2
Southwest black bean soup, 1 cup	2
Split pea, 1 cup	3

	POINTS VALUE
Progresso	
Italian style wedding soup, 1 cup	2
Lentil, 99% fat free, 1 cup	2
Minestrone, 99% fat free, 1 cup	1
Potato broccoli & cheese chowder, 1 cup	4
Progresso Light Microwave Bowls	
Homestyle vegetable & rice soup, 1 cup	0
Italian-style vegetable soup, 1 cup	0
Vegetable & noodle soup, 1 cup	0
Progresso Light Soups	
Homestyle vegetable & rice soup, 1 cup	0
Italian-style vegetable soup, 1 cup	0
Reduced sodium vegetable soup, 1 cup	0
Savory vegetable barley soup, 1 cup	0
Southwestern-style vegetable soup, 1 cup	0
Vegetable & noodle soup, 1 cup	0
Progresso Microwavable Soups	
Italian-style wedding, 1 cup	3
Lentil, 1 cup	2
Minestrone, 1 cup	1
Vegetable, 1 cup	1
Progresso Reduced Sodium Soups	
Garden vegetable, 1 cup	1
Minestrone soup, 1 cup	2
Progresso Vegetable Classic	
Creamy mushroom, 1 cup	3
French onion, 1 cup	1
Garden vegetable, 1 cup	1

	POINTS VALUE
Green split pea, 1 cup	3
Hearty black bean, 1 cup	2
Hearty tomato, 1 cup	2
Lentil, 1 cup	2
Macaroni & bean, 1 cup	3
Minestrone, 1 cup	1
Tomato basil, 1 cup	3
Tomato rotini, 1 cup	2
Vegetable, 1 cup	1
Vegetable Italiano, 1 cup	2
Vegetarian vegetable with barley, 1 cup	1
San-J	
Vegan wakame soup envelope, 1 package	1
White miso soup envelope, 1 package	1
Simply Asia Rice Noodle Soup Bowl	
Garlic sesame, 1	5
Sesame chicken flavor, 1	5
Shiitake mushroom, 1	5
Spring vegetable, 1	5
Simply Asia Soup Bowl	
Miso soup, 1	4
Sesame chicken soup, 1	8
Spring vegetable soup, 1	3
Szechwan hot & sour soup, 1	5
Thai Kitchen	
Instant rice noodle soup, Bangkok curry, 1 package	3
Instant rice noodle soup, garlic & vegetable, 1 package	3

Soups, Stews & Chilis

Thai Kitchen (cont'd)	POINTS VALUE
Instant rice noodle soup, lemongrass & chili, 1 package	3
Instant rice noodle soup, spring onion, 1 package	4
Instant rice noodle soup, Thai ginger, 1 package	3
Rice noodle soup bowl, hot & sour, 1	5
Rice noodle soup bowl, lemongrass & chili, 1	5
Rice noodle soup bowl, mushroom, 1	5
Rice noodle soup bowl, roasted garlic, 1	5
Rice noodle soup bowl, spring onion, 1	5
Rice noodle soup bowl, Thai ginger, 1	5

	POINTS VALUE
Uncle Ben's Hearty Soup	
Broccoli cheese & rice, 1/4 cup (cooked)	2
Wyler's Mrs. Grass	
Cheddar broccoli mix, 1/4 carton	2
Potato, garlic and chives mix, 1/4 carton	2
Wyler's Soup Starter Homestyle Soup Mix	
Cheddar broccoli, prepared with water, 1 cup	2
♦ Hearty chicken vegetable, prepared with water, 1 cup	1
♦ Hearty three bean chili, prepared with water, 1 cup	2
Potato, garlic & chives, prepared with water, 1 cup	2

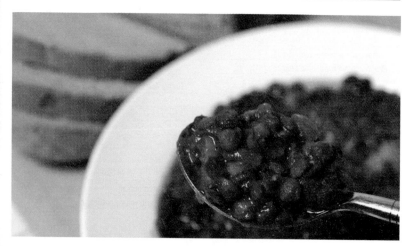

	POINTS VALUE

Meat Substitutes

Amy's

◆ All American veggie burger, 1	2	(5)
Bistro veggie burger, 1 serving (2.5 oz)	2	
Breakfast patties, 1 serving (1.33 oz)	2	
◆ California veggie burger, 1	2	(5)
Cheddar veggie burger, 1	3	
◆ Quarter pound veggie burger, 1	4	(5)
◆ Texas veggie burger, 1	2	(5)

Betty Crocker

Bac Os chips or bits, 1 1/2 Tbsp	1	

Boca

◆ All American flame grilled burger, 1	1	(5)
◆ All-American classic burger (made with organic soy), 1	2	(5)
Bratwurst sausage, meatless, 1	3	
Breakfast links, 2	1	
Breakfast links (made with organic soy), 2	2	
Breakfast patties, 1	1	
Cheeseburger, 1	2	
Cheeseburger (made with organic soy), 1	2	
Chick'n hot & spicy buffalo wings, 1 serving (87 g)	3	
◆ Garden burger, 1	2	(5)
◆ Grilled vegetable burger, 1	1	(5)
◆ Ground burger, 1/2 cup	1	(5)
Italian sausage, meatless, 1	3	
Original chik'n nuggets, 4	4	
Original chik'n patties, 1	3	
Original chik'n patties, 1	3	

	POINTS VALUE

◆ Original ground burger, 1/2 cup	1	(5)
◆ Original vegan burger, 1	1	(5)
◆ Original vegan burger (15-lb box), 1	2	(5)
◆ Original vegan burger (3 1/2-lb box), 1	1	(5)
◆ Roasted garlic burger, 1	1	(5)
◆ Roasted garlic burger (naturally flavored, made with organic soy), 1	2	(5)
◆ Roasted onion burger, 1	1	(5)
◆ Roasted onion burger (naturally flavored, made with organic soy), 1	2	(5)
Smoked sausage, meatless, 1	3	
Spicy chik'n patties, 1	3	
◆ Vegan burger, 1	1	(5)

Dr. Praeger's

◆ Bombay veggie burgers, 1 burger	2	(5)
◆ California veggie burgers, 1 burger	2	(5)
California veggieballs, 2 pieces	1	
◆ Gluten free California veggie burgers, 1	2	(5)

Fantastic World Foods

◆ Nature's burger, 1/4 cup	3	(5)
Sloppy Joe mix, 1/4 cup	1	
Taco filling, 1/4 cup	1	
◆ Tofu burger, 3 Tbsp	2	(5)

Garden Burger

BBQ riblets, 1 serving (1 riblet with sauce)	4	
Breaded chik'n veggie patties, 1	3	
Breakfast sausage veggie pattie, 1	1	
◆ California burger, 1	2	(5)
Chik'n grill veggie patties, 1	1	

Soy & Meat Substitutes

Garden Burger (cont'd)	POINTS VALUE	
Eating right homestyle burger, 1	1	(5)
Eating right veggie pattie, 1	2	(5)
Flame griller burger, 1	1	(5)
Garden tenders, 5	2	
Garden vegan, 1	1	(5)
Gourmet baja steak, 1	2	(5)
Gourmet fire dragon steak, 1	3	(5)
Gourmet hula steak, 1	5	(5)
Gourmet Tuscany steak, 1	4	(5)
Hamburger style classic, 1	1	(5)
Herb crusted cutlet, 1	3	
Homestyle classic veggie burger, 1	2	(5)
Malibu burger, 1	3	
Mama mia meatless meatballs, 6	3	
Original, 1	1	(5)
Savory portabella veggie burger, 1	1	(5)
Sun-dried tomato basil burger, 1	2	(5)
Veggie medley burger, 1	1	(5)
Lightlife		
Gimme lean, ground sausage style, 2 oz	1	
Light burgers, 1/3 cup	1	(5)
Mushroom burgers, 5 oz	3	(5)
Smart dogs, 1 link	1	
Smart pretzel dog, 1	7	
Tofu pups, 1	1	
Veggie burger, 5 oz	2	(5)
Veggie dogs, 1 link	2	
Lightlife Smart Bacon		
Smart bacon, 2 strips	1	

	POINTS VALUE	
Lightlife Smart BBQ		
Smart bbq, 1/4 cup	1	
Lightlife Smart Breakfast		
Breakfast patties, 1 pattie	1	
Lightlife Smart Chili		
Smart chili, 1 cup	4	
Lightlife Smart Cutlets		
Chick'n fillet style veggie protein cutlets, 1	3	
Lightlife Smart Deli		
Bologna, 4 slices	1	
Ham, 4 slices	1	
Pepperoni, 13 slices	1	
Turkey, 4 slices	1	
Lightlife Smart Dogs		
Jumbos, 1	1	
Lightlife Smart Ground		
Original, 1/3 cup	1	(5)
Taco & burrito, 1/3 cup	1	(5)
Lightlife Smart Links		
Breakfast, 2 links	1	
Lightlife Smart Menu		
Garlic teriyaki chick'n, 1 package	5	
Meatless meatballs, 6	3	
Orange sesame chick'n, 1 package	5	
Veggie Bolognese, 1 package	4	
Lightlife Smart Patties		
Burger style, 1 burger	3	(5)
Chick'n style, 1 pattie	3	
Mushroom burgers veggie protein patties, 1	3	(5)

	POINTS VALUE
Lightlife Smart Sausages	
Chorizo veggie protein sausages, 1 link	3
Italian style veggie protein sausages, 1 link	3
Lightlife Smart Strips	
Chick 'n strips, 3 oz	1
Steak strips, 3 oz	1
Lightlife Smart Stuffer	
Chick'n broccoli melt, 1	4
Chick'n cordon melt, 1	4
Turk'y with cranberry stuffing, 1	4
Lightlife Smart Tenders	
Lemon pepper chick'n veggie protein tenders, 3	3
Savory chick'n veggie protein tenders, 3	3
Lightlife Smart TexMex	
Smart Texmex, 1/4 cup	1
Lightlife Smart Tortilla Wrap	
Chick'n ranchero, 1	6
Mexican beef style, 1	7
Mon Cuisine	
Vegan beef steak in cherry sauce, 1 serving (4 oz)	2
Vegan bologna chub style, 1 serving (4 oz)	3
Vegan breaded & spicy strips, 1 serving (1.76 oz)	2
Vegan breaded chicken style cutlet, 1 serving (10 oz)	6
Vegan breaded cutlet, 1 serving (3.2 oz)	3

	POINTS VALUE	
Vegan breaded drumstick, 1 serving (2.5 oz)	2	
Vegan breaded nuggets with sesame, 1 serving (0.8 oz)	1	
◆ Vegan burger, 1 serving (2.5 oz)	2	(5)
Vegan chicken chub style, 1 serving (4 oz)	3	
Vegan chicken nuggets, 1 serving (9 oz)	1	
Vegan chicken patties, 1 serving (10 oz)	2	
Vegan cutlet, 1 serving (2.2 oz)	1	
Vegan cutlet in curry sauce, 1 serving (4 oz)	2	
Vegan diced stir fry, 1 serving (3.5 oz)	3	
Vegan falafel balls, 1 serving (1 oz)	1	
◆ Vegan garden vegetable patty, 1 serving (2.5 oz)	2	(5)
Vegan giant chicken style patty, 1 serving (4 oz)	3	
Vegan ginger egg roll, 1 serving (5 oz)	3	
Vegan Hawaiian nuggets with pineapple in sauce, 1 serving (4 oz)	2	
Vegan kebab (Middle Eastern style), 1 serving (1.5 oz)	1	
Vegan kebab (Romanian style), 1 serving (1.5 oz)	1	
Vegan Moroccan style chicken with cous cous, 1 serving (4 oz)	2	
Vegan ravioli, 1 serving (0.5 oz)	0	
Vegan ravioli in tomato sauce, 1 serving (4 oz)	2	
Vegan salami style chub, 1 serving (4 oz)	3	

Soy & Meat Substitutes

Mon Cuisine (cont'd)

	POINTS VALUE	
Vegan stuffed cabbage in tomato sauce, 1 serving (8 oz)	4	
Vegan stuffed Kiev, 1 serving (4.5 oz)	3	
Vegan stuffed shell pasta, 1 serving (1.5 oz)	2	
Vegan stuffed shell pasta in tomato sauce, 1 serving (8 oz)	4	
Vegetarian breakfast links, 1 serving (1.21 oz)	1	
Vegetarian burger, 1 serving (3.2 oz)	3	(5)
Vegetarian cocktail franks, 1 serving (0.32 oz)	0	
Vegetarian cocktail franks, 1 serving (0.32 oz)	0	
Vegetarian crumbles, 1 serving (2.5 oz)	1	(5)
Vegetarian grill burger, 1 serving (3 oz)	2	(5)
Vegetarian grilled steak, 1 serving (3.2 oz)	3	
Vegetarian grilled steak in mushroom sauce, 1 serving (8 oz)	4	
Vegetarian Hawaiian nuggets with pineapple in sauce, 1 serving (4 oz)	2	
Vegetarian meatball, 1 serving (1 oz)	0	
Vegetarian meatballs in tangy sauce, 1 serving (1 oz)	1	
Vegetarian okra patties, 1 serving (2.8 oz)	1	(5)
Vegetarian pepperoni chubs, 1 serving (1 oz)	1	
Vegetarian pepperoni sliced, 1 serving (1 oz)	1	
Vegetarian salisbury steak, 1 serving (4 oz)	4	
Vegetarian salisbury steak in brown sauce, 1 serving (8 oz)	5	

	POINTS VALUE	
Vegetarian stuffed cabbage in tomato sauce, 1 serving (8 oz)	4	
Vegetarian stuffed pepper in marinara sauce, 1 serving (8 oz)	4	
Vegetarian veal style cutlet in marinara sauce, 1 serving (9.6 oz)	6	
Vegetarian vegetable patties, 1 serving (3.5 oz)	3	(5)

Morningstar Farms

	POINTS VALUE	
America's original veggie dog, frozen, 1	1	
Asian veggie patties, 1	2	(5)
Breakfast pattie with organic soy, 1	2	
Chik patties, frozen, 1	3	
Chik'n nuggets, frozen, 4	4	
Country scramble breakfast bites, 3 pieces	4	
Garden veggie patties, frozen, 1	2	(5)
Ginger teriyaki veggie cakes, 1	2	
Grillers burger style recipe crumbles, frozen, 2/3 cup	1	(5)
Grillers original, frozen, 1	3	(5)
Grillers prime, frozen, 1 pattie	4	(5)
Grillers vegan, 1	1	(5)
Italian herb chik pattie, 1	3	
Italian herb chik'n pattie, 1	3	
Meal starters chik'n, 12 strips	3	
Meal starters steak strips, 12	3	
Meatfree buffalo wings, frozen, 5	4	
Meatfree corn dog, frozen, 1	3	
Meatfree mini corn dogs, frozen, 4	4	
Mushroom lover's burger, 1	3	(5)
Original chik'n tenders, 2	4	

Soy & Meat Substitutes

	POINTS VALUE
Roasted herb chik'n, with organic soy, frozen, 1 pattie	2
Sausage style recipe crumbles, frozen, 2/3 cup	2
Southwest veggie cakes, 1	2
◆ Spicy black bean burger, frozen, 1	2 (5)
◆ Tomato basil pizza burger, frozen, 1 pattie	2 (5)
◆ Vegan burger, with organic soy, frozen, 1 pattie	1 (5)
Veggie breakfast bacon strips, frozen, 2	1
Veggie breakfast sausage links, frozen, 2	1
Veggie breakfast sausage patties, 1 pattie	2
Veggie corn dog made with natural ingredients, 1	4
Veggie Italian style sausage, 1 link	3
◆ Veggie medley burger with organic soy, 1	2 (5)
Veggie sausage patties maple flavored, 1	2

Quorn

	POINTS VALUE
Chick'n nuggets, 1 serving (65 g)	4
Chick'n tenders, 1 cup	1
Chik'n patties, 1	3
Cranberry & goat cheese chik'n cutlet, 1	6
Garlic & herb chick'n cutlets, 1	4
◆ Grounds, 2/3 cup	1 (5)
Gruyere chick'n cutlets, 1	6
Meatless meatballs, 4	2

	POINTS VALUE
Naked chick'n cutlets, 1	1
Southwestern chik'n wing, 1 serving (3-4 pieces)	4
Turk'y roast, 1 serving (1/5 roast)	1

SuperBurgers

	POINTS VALUE
◆ Original, 1 pattie	2 (5)

Tofurky

	POINTS VALUE
"Philly-style" steak deli slices, 5 slices	2
Beer brats, 3 1/2 oz	6
Breakfast links, 1	2
Chipotle franks, 1	1
Cranberry & stuffing deli slices, 5 slices	2
Foot long veggie dog, 3 1/2 oz	3
Franks, 1	1
Hickory smoked deli slices, 5 slices	2
Italian deli deli slices, 5 slices	2
Italian sausage, 3 1/2 oz	6
Kielbasa, 3 1/2 oz	5
Oven roasted deli slices, 5 slices	2
Peppered deli slices, 5 slices	2
Vegetarian roast, 4 oz	4

Veggie Patch

	POINTS VALUE
Apple spice meatless sausage, 1 link	3
Artichokes & sundried tomato meatless sausage, 1 link	2
◆ California veggie burgers, 1	1 (5)
Chick'n cutlets, 1	3
Chick'n nuggets, 4 nuggets	4
Garlic portabella burgers, 1	2

Soy & Meat Substitutes

Veggie Patch (cont'd)	POINTS VALUE	
Garlic portabella burgers (club store size), 1	3	(5)
Jalapeno & cheddar meatless sausage, 1 link	2	
Meatless buffalo wings, 4 wings	4	
Meatless garlic portabella meatballs, 4	3	
Meatless meatballs, 4	2	
Spinach nuggets, 4 nuggets	3	
Veggie dog, 1	2	
Worthington		
Chic-ketts, 2 slices (3/8" slices)	2	
Chili, 1 cup	6	
Choplets, 2 slices	1	
Diced chik, 1/4 cup (drained)	1	
Dinner roast, 1 slice (3/4" slice)	4	
FriChik original, 2 pieces	3	
FriPats, 1 pattie	3	
Leanies, 1 link	2	
Low fat frichik, 2 pieces	2	
Low fat veja-links, 1 link	1	
Meatless chicken style roll, 1 slice (3/8" slice)	2	
Meatless chicken style slices, 3 slices	2	
Meatless corned beef (roll), 1 slice (3/8" slice)	3	
Multigrain cutlets, 2 slices	1	
Prime stakes, 1 piece	3	
Prosage links, 2	1	
Prosage roll, 1 slice (5/8" slice)	3	
Saucettes, 1 link	2	
Smoke turkey (roll), 1 slice (3/8" slice)	3	

	POINTS VALUE	
Stakelets, 1 piece	3	
Stripples, 2 strips	1	
Super links, 1	3	
Vegetable skallops, 1/2 cup	1	
Vegetable steaks, 2 slices	1	
Vegetarian burger, 1/4 cup	1	(5)
Veja-links, 1 link	1	
Wham (roll), 1 slice (3/8" slice)	3	

Soy
Azumaya

Extra firm tofu, 1 serving (79 g)	2	(5)
Firm tofu, 1 serving (79 g)	1	(5)
Lite extra firm tofu, 1 serving (79 g)	1	(5)
Lite silken tofu, 1 serving (91 g)	1	(5)
Oriental spice tofu, 3 oz	2	
Silken tofu, 1 serving (1/5 block)	1	(5)
Super firm cubed tofu, 1 serving (2.8 oz)	2	(5)
Zesty garlic tofu, 3 oz	2	

Eden

Dried tofu, 1 serving	1	

House Foods

Organic tofu - extra firm, 3 oz	2	(5)
Organic tofu - firm, 3 oz	1	(5)
Organic tofu - medium firm (regular), 3 oz	1	(5)
Organic tofu - soft (silken), 3 oz	1	(5)
Premium tofu, extra firm, 3 oz	2	(5)
Premium tofu, extra soft, 3 oz	1	(5)
Premium tofu, firm, 3 oz	2	(5)
Premium tofu, medium firm, 3 oz	1	(5)

Soy & Meat Substitutes

	POINTS VALUE
Premium tofu, soft (silken), 3 oz	1 (5)
Tofu cutlet (Atsu-age), 2 1/2 oz	2
Tofu shirataki - fettuccine shape, 4 oz	0
Tofu shirataki - spaghetti shape, 4 oz	0
Tofu shirataki angel hair shaped noodle substitute, 1 serving (4 oz)	0
Tofu steak - garlic & pepper, 1/4 package	2
Tofu steak (Cajun), 1 serving (3 oz)	2
Tofu steak (grilled), 1 serving (3 oz)	2

Lightlife
	POINTS VALUE
Flax tempeh, 4 oz	4
Garden veggie tempeh, 4 oz	5
Smoky tempeh strips, 3 slices	1
Soy tempeh, 4 oz	4
Three grain tempeh, 4 oz	5
Wild rice tempeh, 4 oz	4

Nasoya
	POINTS VALUE
Chinese spice tofu, 1 serving (1/4 package)	2
Cubed super firm tofu, 1 serving (2.8 oz)	2 (5)
Extra firm tofu, 1 serving (1/5 package)	2 (5)
Firm tofu, 1 serving (1/5 package)	1 (5)
Garlic onion tofu, 1 serving (1/4 package)	2
Lite firm tofu, 1 serving (1/5 package)	0 (5)
Lite silken tofu, 1 serving (1/5 package)	1 (5)
Silken tofu, 1 serving (1/5 package)	1 (5)
Soft tofu, 1 serving (1/5 package)	1 (5)

Silk
	POINTS VALUE
Cultured soy - peach, 1 container	3
Cultured soy - raspberry, 1 container	3
Cultured soy - strawberry, 1 container	3

Toby's Tofu Paté
	POINTS VALUE
Jalapeno, 2 Tbsp	2
Lite, 2 Tbsp	1
Lite jalapeño, 2 Tbsp	1
Original, 2 Tbsp	2

Tofurky
	POINTS VALUE
Jurky - original, 4 pieces	2
Jurky - peppered, 4 pieces	2
Organic five grain tempeh, 3 oz	3
Organic soy tempeh, 3 oz	3
Spicy veggie tempeh, 3 oz	3

Tree of Life
	POINTS VALUE
Firm style tofu, 1 serving (1/5 package)	2 (5)
Organic tofu, 1 serving (1/5 package)	2 (5)
Reduced fat tofu, 1 serving (1/5 package)	2 (5)
Smoked tofu, hot & spicy, 1 serving	3
Smoked tofu, original, 1 serving	3
Water pack tofu, 1 serving (1/5 package)	2 (5)

Vegetables

Artichokes

Birds Eye
Artichoke hearts, 12 pieces	0

Dole
Artichoke, 1 medium	0

Fanci Food
Artichoke bottoms, 3 pieces	0
Artichoke hearts quartered & marinated, 1 oz	0
Artichoke hearts, quarters, 3 pieces	0
Extra small artichoke hearts, 3 pieces	0
Hot artichoke hearts quartered & marinated, 1 oz	0
Marinated artichoke salad, 1 oz	0
Small artichoke hearts, 3 pieces	0

Progresso
Artichoke hearts (in brine), 1 serving (130 g)	0
Artichoke hearts (marinated), 1 serving with liquid (32 g)	1

Asparagus

Birds Eye
Asparagus spears, 7	0
Asparagus stir fry, frozen, 2 cups (1 cup cooked)	1

Cascadian Farm
Asparagus cuts, 2/3 cup	0

Del Monte
Green asparagus hand selected, 1/2 cup	0

Dole
Asparagus, 5 spears	0

Fanci Food
White asparagus spears, peeled, 1/2 cup	0

Green Giant
Cut spears asparagus, 50% less sodium, canned, 1/2 cup	0
Cut spears asparagus, canned, 1/2 cup	0
Extra long asparagus spears, canned, 5 spears	0

Green Giant Simply Steam
Asparagus cuts, 2/3 cup	0

Hanover
Asparagus cuts and tips, 3/4 cup	0

Hanover The Gold Line
Petite asparagus spears, 14 spears	0

Kounty Kist
Cut spears asparagus, 1/2 cup	0
Long green asparagus spears, 5	0
Long green xl asparagus spears, 3	0

LeSueur
Extra large asparagus spears, canned, 3 spears	0

Market Day
Asparagus spears, 19 pieces	0

Triton International
Gourmet asparagus spears, 5 spears	0
Gourmet asparagus tips and cuts, 1/2 cup	0

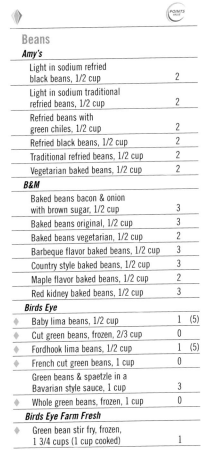

Beans

Amy's

	POINTS VALUE
Light in sodium refried black beans, 1/2 cup	2
Light in sodium traditional refried beans, 1/2 cup	2
Refried beans with green chiles, 1/2 cup	2
Refried black beans, 1/2 cup	2
Traditional refried beans, 1/2 cup	2
Vegetarian baked beans, 1/2 cup	2

B&M

Baked beans bacon & onion with brown sugar, 1/2 cup	3
Baked beans original, 1/2 cup	3
Baked beans vegetarian, 1/2 cup	2
Barbeque flavor baked beans, 1/2 cup	3
Country style baked beans, 1/2 cup	3
Maple flavor baked beans, 1/2 cup	2
Red kidney baked beans, 1/2 cup	3

Birds Eye

Baby lima beans, 1/2 cup	1 (5)
Cut green beans, frozen, 2/3 cup	0
Fordhook lima beans, 1/2 cup	1 (5)
French cut green beans, 1 cup	0
Green beans & spaetzle in a Bavarian style sauce, 1 cup	3
Whole green beans, frozen, 1 cup	0

Birds Eye Farm Fresh

Green bean stir fry, frozen, 1 3/4 cups (1 cup cooked)	1

Birds Eye Steamfresh

	POINTS VALUE
Cut green beans, 2/3 cup	0
Whole premium selects green beans, 1 cup	0

Bush's

Baby butter beans, 1/2 cup	1
Black beans, 1/2 cup	1 (5)
Bold & spicy baked beans, 1/2 cup	1
Boston recipe baked beans, 1/2 cup	2
Cannellini beans, 1/2 cup	1 (5)
Chili beans - hot (pinto), 1/2 cup	1
Chili beans - hot (red beans), 1/2 cup	1
Chili beans - medium (pinto), 1/2 cup	1
Chili beans - medium (red beans), 1/2 cup	1
Chili beans - mild (pinto bean), 1/2 cup	1
Chili beans - mild (red beans), 1/2 cup	1
Country style baked beans, 1/2 cup	2
Dark red kidney beans, 1/2 cup	1 (5)
Garbanzo beans, 1/2 cup	1 (5)
Great northern beans, 1/2 cup	1 (5)
Grillin' beans bourbon and brown sugar, 1/2 cup	3
Grillin' beans smokehouse tradition, 1/2 cup	3
Grillin' beans southern pit barbecue, 1/2 cup	3
Grillin' beans steakhouse recipe, 1/2 cup	3
Homestyle baked beans, 1/2 cup	2

Vegetables

Bush's (cont'd)

POINTS VALUE

Honey baked beans, 1/2 cup	2
Large butter beans, 1/2 cup	1
Light red kidney beans, 1/2 cup	1 (5)
Maple cured bacon baked beans, 1/2 cup	2
Mixed beans (pinto & great northern), 1/2 cup	1 (5)
Navy beans, 1/2 cup	1 (5)
Onion baked beans, 1/2 cup	2
Original baked beans, 1/2 cup	2
Pinto beans, 1/2 cup	1 (5)
Pinto beans with bacon, 1/2 cup	1
Red beans, 1/2 cup	1 (5)
Refried beans - fat free, 1/2 cup	2
Refried beans - traditional, 1/2 cup	2
Seasoned recipe black beans, 1/2 cup	1
Seasoned recipe dark red kidney beans, 1/2 cup	1
Seasoned recipe pinto beans, 1/2 cup	1
Speckled butter beans, 1/2 cup	1
Vegetarian baked beans, 1/2 cup	2

Campbell's

Baked beans, brown sugar & bacon flavored, 1/2 cup	3
Pork and beans, 1/2 cup	2

Cascadian Farm

Green beans (cut), 3/4 cup	0
Green beans (petite whole), 1 cup	0
Green beans with toasted almonds (French-cut), 2/3 cup	1

Del Monte

POINTS VALUE

Cut, Italian green beans, 1/2 cup	0
Cut, no salt added green beans, 1/2 cup	0
Dilled green beans, 1/2 cup	1
French style green beans, 1/2 cup	0
French style, no salt added green beans, 1/2 cup	0
Green & wax beans, 1/2 cup	0
Lima beans, 1/2 cup	1 (5)
Organic cut green beans, 1/2 cup	0
Seasoned green beans, 1/2 cup	0
Whole green beans, 1/2 cup	0

Eden Organic

Aduki beans, 1/2 cup	1
Baked beans (navy) with sorghum, 1/2 cup	2
Black beans, 1/2 cup	1 (5)
Black eyed peas, 1/2 cup	1 (5)
Black soybeans, 1/2 cup	2 (5)
Butter beans, 1/2 cup	1
Cannellini (white kidney) beans, 1/2 cup	1 (5)
Chili beans (dark red kidney), 1/2 cup	2
Garbanzo beans (chick peas), 1/2 cup	2 (5)
Great northern beans, 1/2 cup	1 (5)
Navy beans, 1/2 cup	1 (5)
Pinto beans, 1/2 cup	1 (5)
Refried black beans, 1/2 cup	2
Refried blacksoy & black beans, 1/2 cup	1

	POINTS VALUE	
Refried kidney beans, 1/2 cup	1	
Refried pinto beans, 1/2 cup	1	
◆ Small red beans, 1/2 cup	1	(5)
◆ Spicy pinto beans, 1/2 cup	2	
Spicy refried black beans, 1/2 cup	2	
Spicy refried pinto beans, 1/2 cup	1	
Fantastic World Foods		
◆ Instant black beans, 1/4 cup	2	
Instant refried beans, 1/4 cup	2	
Faraon		
◆ Black beans, canned, 1/2 cup	1	(5)
◆ Black beans, uncooked, 1/2 cup	1	(5)
◆ Garbanzo beans, canned, 1/4 cup	2	(5)
◆ Garbanzo beans, uncooked, 1/2 cup	1	(5)
◆ Great northern beans, uncooked, 1/4 cup	1	(5)
◆ Lima beans, uncooked, 1/4 cup	1	(5)
◆ Mayocoba beans, uncooked, 1/4 cup	0	
◆ Mexican haba beans, uncooked, 1/4 cup	3	
◆ Pink beans, uncooked, 1/4 cup	1	(5)
◆ Pinto beans, canned, 1/2 cup	1	(5)
◆ Pinto beans, uncooked, 1/4 cup	0	(5)
◆ Red kidney beans, uncooked, 1/4 cup	1	(5)
Refried pinto beans, 1/2 cup	2	
◆ Small red beans, uncooked, 1/4 cup	0	(5)
Glory		
Black beans with rice, 1/2 cup	2	
Butter beans, 1/2 cup	1	
Crock pot beans, 1/2 cup	2	
Lima beans, 1/2 cup	1	
Northern beans, 1/2 cup	1	
Pinto beans, 1/2 cup	1	
Red beans with rice, 1/2 cup	1	
String beans with potatoes, 1/2 cup	0	
Glory Seasoned		
New Orleans red beans, 1/2 cup	1	
Pole beans, 1/2 cup	0	
String beans, 1/2 cup	0	
Glory Sensibly Seasoned		
Black beans, 1/2 cup	1	
Pinto beans, 1/2 cup	1	
Red beans, 1/2 cup	1	
String beans, 1/2 cup	0	
Goya		
◆ Black beans, 1/2 cup	1	(5)
◆ Cannellini, 1/2 cup	1	(5)
◆ Chick peas, 1/2 cup	1	(5)
◆ Dark kidney beans, 1/2 cup	1	(5)
◆ Great Northern beans, 1/2 cup	1	(5)
◆ Lentils, 1/2 cup	1	(5)
◆ Pink beans, 1/2 cup	1	(5)
◆ Pinto beans, 1/2 cup	1	(5)
◆ Red kidney beans, 1/2 cup	1	(5)
◆ Small white beans, 1/2 cup	1	(5)
Green Giant		
◆ Black beans (frijoles negro), canned, 1/2 cup	1	(5)
◆ Butter beans, canned, 1/2 cup	1	
◆ Cut green beans, 50% less sodium, canned, 1/2 cup	0	
◆ Cut green beans, canned, 1/2 cup	0	

Vegetables

◇ *Green Giant (cont'd)* — POINTS VALUE

Cut green beans, frozen, 3/4 cup	0
French style green beans, canned, 1/2 cup	0
Garbanzo beans (chick peas), canned, 1/2 cup	1 (5)
Great northern beans, canned, 1/2 cup	1 (5)
Green bean casserole, 2/3 cup	3
Kidney (dark) red beans, canned, 1/2 cup	1 (5)
Kidney (light) red beans, canned, 1/2 cup	1 (5)
Kitchen sliced green beans 1/2-inch diagonal cut, 1/2 cup	0
Kitchen sliced green beans, canned, 1/2 cup	0
Pinto beans, canned, 1/2 cup	1 (5)
Red beans, canned, 1/2 cup	1 (5)
Select whole green beans, frozen, 1 cup	0
Spicy chili beans, canned, 1/2 cup	1

Green Giant Butter Sauce Vegetables

Baby lima beans, frozen, 2/3 cup	2 (5)

Green Giant Simply Steam

Baby lima beans, 1/2 cup	1 (5)
Green beans & almonds, 2/3 cup	1

Hanover

Canned black beans in brine, 1/2 cup	1 (5)
Canned cut and whole green beans, 1/2 cup	0
Cut golden beans, 3/4 cup	0
Cut green beans, 3/4 cup	0
Cut Italian green beans, 3/4 cup	0

Fordhook lima beans, 1/2 cup	1 (5)
French style green beans, 1 cup	0
Garbanzo beans in brine (chick peas), 1/2 cup	1 (5)
Great Northern beans "9" brine, 1/2 cup	1 (5)
Light & dark red kidney beans "9" brine, 1/2 cup	1 (5)
Pinto beans in "9" sauce, 1/2 cup	1
Whole green beans, 1 cup	0

Hanover The Gold Line

Baby lima beans, 1/2 cup	1 (5)
Petite green beans, 3/4 cup	0

Heinz

Vegetarian beans, 1 cup	4
Vegetarian beans, no meat, 1/2 cup	2

Joan of Arc

Black beans, 1/2 cup	1 (5)
Butter beans, 1/2 cup	1
Dark red kidney beans, 1/2 cup	1 (5)
Garbanzo beans, 1/2 cup	2 (5)
Great northern beans, 1/2 cup	1 (5)
Light red kidney beans, 1/2 cup	1 (5)
Pinto beans, 1/2 cup	1 (5)
Red beans, 1/2 cup	1 (5)
Spicy chili beans, 1/2 cup	2

Las Palmas

Refried beans, 1/2 cup	2

Market Day

Gourmet green beans, 1 cup	0

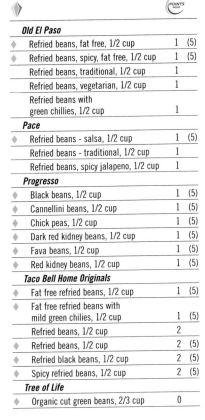

Old El Paso

	POINTS
Refried beans, fat free, 1/2 cup	1 (5)
Refried beans, spicy, fat free, 1/2 cup	1 (5)
Refried beans, traditional, 1/2 cup	1
Refried beans, vegetarian, 1/2 cup	1
Refried beans with green chillies, 1/2 cup	1

Pace

Refried beans - salsa, 1/2 cup	1 (5)
Refried beans - traditional, 1/2 cup	1
Refried beans, spicy jalapeno, 1/2 cup	1

Progresso

Black beans, 1/2 cup	1 (5)
Cannellini beans, 1/2 cup	1 (5)
Chick peas, 1/2 cup	1 (5)
Dark red kidney beans, 1/2 cup	1 (5)
Fava beans, 1/2 cup	1 (5)
Red kidney beans, 1/2 cup	1 (5)

Taco Bell Home Originals

Fat free refried beans, 1/2 cup	1 (5)
Fat free refried beans with mild green chilies, 1/2 cup	1 (5)
Refried beans, 1/2 cup	2
Refried beans, 1/2 cup	2 (5)
Refried black beans, 1/2 cup	2 (5)
Spicy refried beans, 1/2 cup	2 (5)

Tree of Life

Organic cut green beans, 2/3 cup	0

Zapata

	POINTS
Black beans, 1/2 cup	1 (5)
Garbanzo beans, 2/3 cup	2 (5)
Refried beans, 1/2 cup	2 (5)
Refried black beans, 1/2 cup	2 (5)
Spicy refried beans, 1/2 cup	2 (5)

Broccoli & Cauliflower

Birds Eye

Baby broccoli florets, 1 cup	0
Baby broccoli spears, frozen, 4 spears	0
Broccoli & cauliflower mixture, 1 serving (90 g)	0
Broccoli & cheese sauce, frozen, 1/2 cup	2
Broccoli cuts, tender, 1 serving (87 g)	0
Broccoli florets, 1 cup	0
Broccoli spears, 1 serving (89 g)	0
Broccoli stir fry, frozen, 1 cup	0
Cauliflower florets, frozen, 4 pieces	0
Chopped broccoli, frozen, 3/4 cup	0

Birds Eye Farm Fresh

Broccoli florets & cauliflower, 1 cup	0

Birds Eye Steamfresh

Broccoli cuts, 1 cup	0
Broccoli florets, 1 cup	0
Garlic cauliflower, specially seasoned, 1 cup	1

Cascadian Farm

Broccoli & cheese sauce, 2/3 cup	1
Broccoli cuts, 2/3 cup	0
Broccoli florets, 1 1/3 cups	0

Vegetables

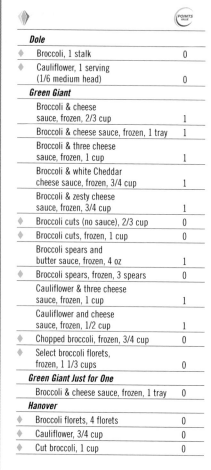

Dole

Broccoli, 1 stalk	0
Cauliflower, 1 serving (1/6 medium head)	0

Green Giant

Broccoli & cheese sauce, frozen, 2/3 cup	1
Broccoli & cheese sauce, frozen, 1 tray	1
Broccoli & three cheese sauce, frozen, 1 cup	1
Broccoli & white Cheddar cheese sauce, frozen, 3/4 cup	1
Broccoli & zesty cheese sauce, frozen, 3/4 cup	1
Broccoli cuts (no sauce), 2/3 cup	0
Broccoli cuts, frozen, 1 cup	0
Broccoli spears and butter sauce, frozen, 4 oz	1
Broccoli spears, frozen, 3 spears	0
Cauliflower & three cheese sauce, frozen, 1 cup	1
Cauliflower and cheese sauce, frozen, 1/2 cup	1
Chopped broccoli, frozen, 3/4 cup	0
Select broccoli florets, frozen, 1 1/3 cups	0

Green Giant Just for One

Broccoli & cheese sauce, frozen, 1 tray	0

Hanover

Broccoli florets, 4 florets	0
Cauliflower, 3/4 cup	0
Cut broccoli, 1 cup	0

Hanover The Gold Line

Broccoli mini florets (petit), 1 cup	0

Market Day

Broccoli florets, 1/2 cup	0

Tree of Life

Organic broccoli cuts, 1 cup	0

Veggie Patch

Broccoli bites with real Cheddar cheese, 3	3

Brussels Sprouts

Birds Eye Steamfresh

Baby brussels sprouts, 10	0
Brussels sprouts, 1 serving (83 g)	0

Dole

Brussels sprouts, 4	0

Green Giant

Baby brussels sprouts & butter sauce, 1 cup	1

Green Giant Butter Sauce Vegetables

Baby brussels sprouts, frozen, 1/2 cup	1

Hanover The Gold Line

Brussels sprouts, 1/2 cup	0

Cabbage

Dole

Shredded red cabbage, 3 oz	0

Glory

Country cabbage, 1/2 cup	0

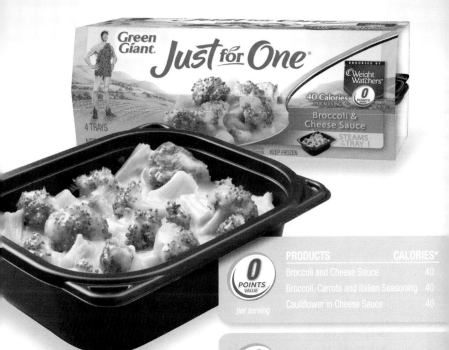

Green Giant.

Endorsed By

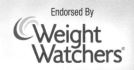

Weight Watchers

Great taste you can count on!
with only **0** or **1 POINTS** value per tray

	PRODUCTS	CALORIES*
0 POINTS VALUE *per serving*	Broccoli and Cheese Sauce	40
	Broccoli, Carrots and Italian Seasoning	40
	Cauliflower in Cheese Sauce	40

	PRODUCTS	CALORIES*
1 POINTS VALUE *per serving*	Corn and Butter Sauce	80
	Peas & Corn in a Basil Butter Sauce	80

*per serving

Weight Watchers for services and *POINTS®* are the registered trademarks of Weight Watchers International, Inc. and are used with permission.
©2009 General Mills
A#18495

Vegetables

Carrots

Del Monte

Carrots, 1/2 cup	0	
Carrots, organic, 1/2 cup	0	

Dole

Carrots, 1	0	
Peeled mini carrots, 3 oz	0	
Shredded carrots, 3 oz	0	

Glory

Glazed carrots, 1/2 cup	1	

Green Giant

Honey glazed carrots, frozen, 1 cup	1	

Hanover

Frozen sliced carrots, 1/2 cup	0	

Hanover The Gold Line

Baby whole carrots, 2/3 cup	0	

LeSueur

Tender baby whole carrots, canned, 1/2 cup	0	

Celery

Dole

Celery, 2 stalks	0	

Corn

Birds Eye

Baby gold & white corn, 2/3 cup	2	(6)
Baby white corn kernels, 2/3 cup	1	(6)
Corn on the cob, sweet mini, 1 serving (85 g)	2	(6)
Super sweet kernel corn, 2/3 cup	1	(6)
Sweet corn & bacon in a creamy cheese sauce, 1/2 cup	3	
Sweet corn & butter sauce, 1/2 cup	2	
Sweet corn on the cob, frozen, 1 ear	3	(6)
Sweet kernel corn, frozen, 2/3 cup	2	(6)

Birds Eye Steamfresh

Gold & white corn, 2/3 cup	1	(6)
Super sweet corn, 2/3 cup	1	(6)
Super sweet corn, single serve, 1 serving (92 g)	1	(6)
Sweet mini corn on the cob, 1 ear	2	(6)

Cascadian Farm

Super sweet corn, 3/4 cup	1	(6)

Del Monte

Cream style corn - supersweet, no salt added, 1/2 cup	1	
Fiesta corn, whole kernel supersweet, 1/2 cup	1	(6)
Gold & white, whole kernel supersweet, 1/2 cup	1	(6)
Golden, cream style, 1/2 cup	1	
Golden, cream style supersweet, 1/2 cup	1	
Golden, cream style, no salt added, 1/2 cup	1	
Golden, whole kernel, 1/2 cup	1	(6)
Golden, whole kernel supersweet/vac pack, 1/2 cup	1	(6)
Golden, whole kernel supersweet/vac pack, no sugar added, 1/2 cup	1	(6)
Organic whole kernel golden corn, 1/2 cup	1	(6)
Organic whole kernel golden corn super sweet, 1/2 cup	1	(6)
Santa Fe corn, 1/2 cup	1	(6)

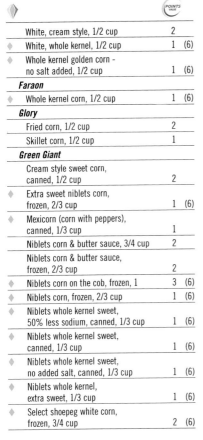

	POINTS VALUE	
White, cream style, 1/2 cup	2	
White, whole kernel, 1/2 cup	1	(6)
Whole kernel golden corn - no salt added, 1/2 cup	1	(6)
Faraon		
Whole kernel corn, 1/2 cup	1	(6)
Glory		
Fried corn, 1/2 cup	2	
Skillet corn, 1/2 cup	1	
Green Giant		
Cream style sweet corn, canned, 1/2 cup	2	
Extra sweet niblets corn, frozen, 2/3 cup	1	(6)
Mexicorn (corn with peppers), canned, 1/3 cup	1	
Niblets corn & butter sauce, 3/4 cup	2	
Niblets corn & butter sauce, frozen, 2/3 cup	2	
Niblets corn on the cob, frozen, 1	3	(6)
Niblets corn, frozen, 2/3 cup	1	(6)
Niblets whole kernel sweet, 50% less sodium, canned, 1/3 cup	1	(6)
Niblets whole kernel sweet, canned, 1/3 cup	1	(6)
Niblets whole kernel sweet, no added salt, canned, 1/3 cup	1	(6)
Niblets whole kernel, extra sweet, 1/3 cup	1	(6)
Select shoepeg white corn, frozen, 3/4 cup	2	(6)

	POINTS VALUE	
Shoepeg white corn and butter sauce, frozen, 3/4 cup	2	(6)
Supersweet yellow & white whole kernel, canned, 1/3 cup	1	(6)
White shoepeg corn, canned, 1/3 cup	1	(6)
Whole kernel sweet corn, 50% less sodium, canned, 1/2 cup	1	(6)
Whole kernel sweet corn, canned, 1/2 cup	1	(6)
Green Giant Just for One		
Niblets corn & butter sauce, frozen, 1 tray	1	
Green Giant Simply Steam		
Niblets corn, 2/3 cup	1	(6)
Shoepeg white corn, 1/2 cup	1	(6)
Hanover		
Sweet corn, 2/3 cup	1	(6)
Hanover The Gold Line		
Shoepeg corn, 3/4 cup	0	(6)
White sweet corn, 2/3 cup	1	(6)
Kounty Kist		
Whole kernel golden sweet corn, 1/3 cup	1	(6)
Whole kernel sweet corn, 1/2 cup	1	(6)
Market Day		
Supersweet corn, 1/2 cup	1	(6)
Tree of Life		
Organic sweet corn, 2/3 cup	2	(6)
Veggie Patch		
Sweet corn bites with real mozzarella cheese, 3	3	

Vegetables

Lentils

Eden Organic

Lentils (green) with onion & bay leaf, 1/2 cup	1

Faraon

Lentils, uncooked, 1/4 cup	2 (5)

Lettuce/Leafy Greens

Dole

Classic & romaine blend, 3 oz	0
Iceberg lettuce, 3 oz	0
Lettuce (iceburg), 1 serving (1/6 medium head)	0
Lettuce (leaf), 1 1/2 cups shredded	0
Lettuce (romaine), 6 leaf/leaves	0

Glory

Collard greens, 1/2 cup	0
Cut collard greens, 1/2 cup	1
Mixed greens, 1/2 cup	0
Mustard greens, 1/2 cup	1
Turnip greens, 1/2 cup	0
Turnips with roots, 1/2 cup	0

Glory Seasoned

Kale, 1/2 cup	1

Glory Sensibly Seasoned

Collard greens, 1/2 cup	0
Mixed greens, 1/2 cup	0
Turnip greens, 1/2 cup	0

Mushrooms

Eden

Maitake mushrooms, dried sliced, 10 pieces	0
Shiitake mushrooms, dried sliced, 6 slices	0
Shiitake mushrooms, whole dried, 3	0

Fanci Food

Pickled cocktail mushrooms, 1 serving (1 oz)	0

Green Giant

Pieces & stems, canned, 1/2 cup	0
Sliced mushrooms broiled in butter, canned, 1/2 cup	0
Sliced mushrooms with garlic, canned, 1/2 cup	0
Sliced mushrooms, canned, 1/2 cup	0
Whole mushrooms, canned, 1/2 cup	0

Herdez

Champinones, 2 Tbsp	0

Poppers

Breaded mushrooms, 6 pieces	4

Veggie Patch

Portabello bites with real mozzarella cheese, 3	3

Onions

Birds Eye

Pearl onions in real cream sauce, frozen, 1/2 cup	1
White pearl onions, frozen, 2/3 cup	0

Boar's Head

Sweet vidalia onions in sauce, 1 Tbsp	0

	POINTS VALUE
Dole	
Green onions, 1/4 cup chopped	0
McCormick	
Minced onions, 1/4 tsp	0
Ore-Ida	
Diced IQF onions 3/8", 3/4 cup	0
Onion ringers, 5 pieces	4
Vidalia o's, 4 pieces	4
Season Brand	
Cocktail onions, 2 Tbsp	0
Vidalia	
Vidalia onions, 1 cup	0
Vidalia onions, 1 medium	1

Other Vegetables

	POINTS VALUE
B&G	
Giardiniera, 2 pieces	0
Birds Eye	
Asian vegetables in sesame ginger sauce, 1 cup	1
Baby corn & vegetable blend, 2/3 cup	0
Baby corn, bean & pea mix, 3/4 cup	1
Baby mixed beans and carrots, 1 cup	0
Baby pea & vegetable blend, 3/4 cup	0
Baby sweet peas & pearl onions, 2/3 cup	1
California blend & Cheddar cheese sauce, frozen, 1/2 cup	2
Classic mixed vegetables, frozen, 2/3 cup	1
Green beans & lightly toasted almonds, 3/4 cup	1

	POINTS VALUE
Pepper stir fry, frozen, 1 cup	0
Roasted potatoes & broccoli in savory real cheese sauce, frozen, 2/3 cup	2
Rotelle & vegetables in herbed garlic sauce, 1 cup	2
Stir-fry, teriyaki, 1 serving (211 g)	3
Stir-fry, Thai, 1 serving (126 g)	0
Sugar snap stir fry, frozen, 1 cup	0
Szechuan vegetables in a sesame sauce, frozen, 1 cup	1
Tender peas & pearl onions in lightly seasoned sauce, frozen, 2/3 cup	1
Tuscan vegetables in herbed tomato sauce, 1 cup	1
Vegetables & shells in garlic butter sauce, frozen, 1 package	6
Zucchini & squash mixture, 3/4 cup	0
Birds Eye Farm Fresh	
Broccoli florets & peppers & onions & mushrooms, 1 cup	0
Broccoli florets, carrots & water chestnuts, 1 cup	0
Broccoli florets, cauliflower, carrots, frozen, 1 cup	0
Broccoli florets, corn, & peppers, frozen, 3/4 cup	1
Brussels sprouts, cauliflower & carrots, 3/4 cup	0
Cauliflower, carrots, snow pea pods, 1 cup	0
Italian blend, 3/4 cup	0

Vegetables

	POINTS VALUE
Birds Eye Steam & Serve	
Asian vegetables with roasted cashews, 1 cup	2
Beans with a twist, 1 cup	2
Italian herb harvest vegetables, 1 1/4 cups	2
Lemon pepper vegetables, 1 cup	2
Spring vegetables in citrus sauce, 1 serving	1
Birds Eye Steamfresh	
Asian medley, specially seasoned, 1 cup	1
Asparagus, gold & white corn, baby carrots, 2/3 cup	1
Baby broccoli blend, 1 serving (96 g)	1
Baby potato & vegetable blend, 1 serving (74 g)	1
Broccoli & cauliflower, 1 cup	0
Broccoli, carrots, sugar snap peas & water chestnuts, 3/4 cup	0
Broccoli, cauliflower & carrots, 3/4 cup	0
Garlic baby peas & mushrooms, specially seasoned, 3/4 cup	1
Mixed vegetables, 2/3 cup	1
Bush's	
Golden hominy, 1/2 cup	1
White hominy, 1/2 cup	1
Cascadian Farm	
Organic purely steam broccoli & carrots lightly seasoned, 1 1/2 cups	1
Premium gardener's blend, 3/4 cup	1

	POINTS VALUE
Premium mixed vegetables: carrots, corn, peas, 2/3 cup	1
Premium peas & carrots, 2/3 cup	0
Chiquita	
Avocado, California, 1 serving (1/5 medium)	1
Crunchies Food Company	
Edamame, 3/4 cup	2
Salted edamame, 1/4 cup	2
Del Monte	
Mixed vegetables with corn, 1/2 cup	0
Mixed vegetables with corn, no sugar added, 1/2 cup	0
Peas and carrots, 1/2 cup	1
Eden	
Agar agar flakes, 1 Tbsp	0
Arame, 1/2 cup	0
Hiziki, 1/2 cup	0
Kombu, 1 serving (1/2 of 7" piece)	0
Mekabu, 1 tsp	0
Pickled ginger - sliced, with shiso leaves, 1 Tbsp	0
Spicy nori strips, 1 packet (5 sheets)	0
Toasted nori krinkles, 1/2 cup	0
Wakame, 1/2 cup	0
Wakame flakes - instant, for miso soup, 1 tsp	0
Eden Selected	
Agar agar bars, 1 bar	0
Lotus root, dried, sliced, 1 serving (10 g)	0

	POINTS VALUE
Fanci Food	
◆ Hearts of palm, 2 sticks	0
Hearts of palm, marinated, 1/2 cup	0
Faraon	
◆ Frozen yuca, 1/2 cup	4
◆ Mixed vegetables, 1/2 cup	1
◆ Tender cactus, 1/2 cup	0
◆ White hominy, 1/2 cup	1
Glory Sensibly Seasoned	
Tomatoes and okra, 1/2 cup	0
Tomatoes/okra/corn, 1/2 cup	0
Green Giant	
Alfredo vegetables, frozen, 1 cup	1
Baby vegetable medley, seasoned, frozen, 3/4 cup frozen (1/2 cup prepared)	0
Broccoli & carrots with garlic & herbs, frozen, 1 1/4 cups	0
Broccoli, carrots, cauliflower & cheese sauce, frozen, 1 cup	1
Broccoli, cauliflower & carrots and cheese sauce, frozen, 2/3 cup	1
◆ Garden medley vegetables, canned, 1/2 cup	1
Garden vegetable medley: peas, potatoes, peppers & herbs, frozen, 1 cup	1
Italian-style vegetables, seasoned, frozen, 1 cup (frozen, 1/2 cup prepared)	1
◆ Mixed vegetables, frozen, 2/3 cup	1

	POINTS VALUE
Parmesan asiago sauce: select peas, cauliflower, pepper, frozen, 1/2 cup	1
Pasta, broccoli, carrots, sugar snap peas & garlic sauce, 1 cup	4
Roasted garlic & herb sauce: select broccoli & cauliflower, frozen, 1 1/4 cups	1
Roasted potatoes with broccoli & cheese sauce, frozen, 1 cup (frozen, 1.2 cup prepared)	2
Super sweet corn, peas & herb butter sauce, frozen, 3/4 cup	1
◆ Sweet peas with tiny pearl onions, canned, 1/2 cup	1
Tuscan herb sauce: select cauliflower, broccoli, beans, carrots, low-fat sauce, frozen, 1 1/4 cups	1
Green Giant Just for One	
Broccoli, carrots & Italian seasoning, frozen, 1 tray	0
Cauliflower & cheese sauce, frozen, 1 tray	0
Peas & corn in a basil butter sauce, frozen, 1 tray	1
Green Giant Simply Steam	
Broccoli & carrots (lightly seasoned with garlic & herbs), 3/4 cup	1
◆ Garden medley, 1/2 cup	1
◆ Sweet peas & pearl onions, 1/2 cup	1
Hanover	
◆ 5-way mixed vegetables, 2/3 cup	1
◆ Crinkle cut yellow & zucchini squash blend, 2/3 cup	0

Vegetables

	POINTS VALUE
Garden medley, 3/4 cup	0
Green & red peppers & onion strips, 2/3 cup	0
Latino blend, 1/2 cup	1
Oriental blend, 3/4 cup	0
Soup vegetables, 2/3 cup	1
Succotash, 2/3 cup	1

Hanover The Gold Line

Petite green beans, petite golden beans, baby whole carrot blend, 3/4 cup	0
Shoepeg corn & petite peas, 1/2 cup	1
White corn, asparagus, red peppers, 3/4 cup	1
White sweet corn, petite broccoli florets, red peppers, 3/4 cup	1

LeSueur

Early peas with mushrooms & pearl onions, canned, 1/2 cup	1

Market Day

Gemelli pasta & vegetable blend, 1 cup	1
Prince Edward vegetable medley, 1 cup	0
Stir fry blend, 1 cup	1

Milpas

Nixtamal hominy, 1 cup	2

Port Arthur

Water chestnuts, sliced and peeled, 1/2 cup	1
Water chestnuts, whole, peeled, 1/2 cup	1

Sardo

Pickled mild mixed vegetables, 1 oz	0

Season Brand

	POINTS VALUE
Sliced bamboo shoots, 1/2 cup	0
Sliced water chestnuts, 1/2 cup	1
Whole water chestnuts, 1/2 cup	1

Sunfresh

Whole hearts of palm, 1 serving (2-3 sticks plus liquid)	0

Tree of Life

Organic California blend, 3/4 cup	0
Organic garden blend, 2/3 cup	1
Organic mixed vegetables, 1/2 cup	1
Organic mixed vegetables, 1/2 cup	1

Peas

Birds Eye

Baby sweet peas, 1 serving (87 g)	1	(6)
Garden peas, frozen, 2/3 cup	1	(6)
Sweet garden peas, 2/3 cup	1	(6)

Birds Eye Steamfresh

Premium sugar snap peas, 2/3 cup	0	(6)
Sweet peas, 2/3 cup	1	(6)
Sweet peas, single serve, 1 serving (92 g)	1	(6)

Bush's

Blackeye peas, 1/2 cup	1	(5)
Blackeye peas with bacon, 1/2 cup	1	
Blackeye peas with bacon & jalapeño, 1/2 cup	1	
Blackeye peas with snaps, 1/2 cup	1	
Crowder peas, 1/2 cup	1	
Field peas with snaps, 1/2 cup	1	
Purple hull peas, 1/2 cup	1	

	POINTS VALUE	
Cascadian Farm		
◆ Peas (garden), 2/3 cup	1	(6)
◆ Peas (petite sweet), 2/3 cup	0	(6)
◆ Peas (sweet), 2/3 cup	1	(6)
Del Monte		
◆ Organic peas, 1/2 cup	0	(6)
◆ Peas, sweet, no salt added, 1/2 cup	0	(6)
◆ Peas, sweet, very young small, 1/2 cup	0	(6)
Dole		
◆ Sugar peas, 1/2 cup	0	(6)
Faraon		
◆ Black eye peas, uncooked, 1/4 cup	1	(5)
◆ Split peas, uncooked, 1/4 cup	2	(5)
◆ Whole green peas, uncooked, 1/4 cup	2	(6)
Glory		
Blackeye peas, 1/2 cup	1	
Blackeye peas/rice, 1/2 cup	1	
Field peas with snaps, 1/2 cup	1	
Glory Seasoned		
Field peas, 1/2 cup	1	
Glory Sensibly Seasoned		
Blackeye peas, 1/2 cup	1	
Goya		
◆ Blackeye peas, 1/2 cup	1	(5)
◆ Whole green peas, 1/2 cup	1	(6)
Green Giant		
◆ Select sugar snap peas, frozen, 3/4 cup	0	(6)
◆ Sweet peas, 50% less sodium, 1/2 cup	1	(6)
◆ Sweet peas, 50% less sodium, young tender, canned, 1/2 cup	1	(6)

	POINTS VALUE	
◆ Sweet peas, frozen, 2/3 cup	1	(6)
◆ Sweet peas, very young small early, canned, 1/2 cup	1	(6)
◆ Sweet peas, young tender, canned, 1/2 cup	1	(6)
Green Giant Simply Steam		
◆ Baby sweet peas, 2/3 cup	0	(6)
◆ Sugar snap peas, 2/3 cup	0	(6)
Hanover		
◆ Blackeye peas in brine, 1/2 cup	1	(5)
◆ Sweet peas, 2/3 cup	0	(6)
Hanover The Gold Line		
◆ Petite peas, 1/2 cup	1	(6)
◆ Snow peas, 1 cup	0	(6)
◆ Sugar snap peas, 3/4 cup	0	(6)
Kounty Kist		
◆ Very young small early June peas, 1/2 cup	1	(6)
LeSueur		
◆ 50% less sodium very young small early peas, canned, 1/2 cup	0	(6)
Baby sweet peas & butter sauce, frozen, 3/4 cup	1	
◆ Baby sweet peas, frozen, 2/3 cup	0	(6)
Early June peas & butter sauce, frozen, 3/4 cup	1	
◆ Peas small early June, 1/2 cup	1	(6)
◆ Very young small early peas, canned, 1/2 cup	1	(6)
Market Day		
◆ Extra young tiny peas, 2/3 cup	0	(6)

Vegetables

	POINTS VALUE
Minnesota Valley	
Small early June peas, 1/2 cup	1 (6)
Tree of Life	
Organic green peas, 2/3 cup	1 (6)
Organic green peas, 2/3 cup	1 (6)

Peppers

B&G

	POINTS VALUE
Hot cherry peppers, 1 piece	0
Hot chopped peppers, 1 tsp	0
Hot pepper ring, 7 pieces	0
Jalapeno slices, 7 pieces	0
Pepperoncini, 3 pieces	0
Real chopped jalapenos, 2 Tbsp	0
Roasted peppers with imported balsamic vinegar, 1/2 piece	0
Roasted peppers with oregano & garlic, 1/2 piece	0
Sliced hot cherry peppers in oil, 7 pieces	1
Sweet bell pepper topper, 8 pieces	0
Sweet cherry peppers, 1 piece	0
Sweet fried peppers, 1 oz	0
Sweet pepper strips, 8 pieces	0
Sweet salad peppers with oregano & garlic, 8 pieces	0

B&G Sandwich Toppers

Hot peppers, 7 pieces (1 oz)	0

Cherchies

Pretty hot peppers, 2 Tbsp	1
Pretty peppers, 2 Tbsp	1
Roasted peppers 'n garlic, 2 Tbsp	1

CHI-CHI'S

	POINTS VALUE
Green chilies diced, 2 Tbsp	0
Green chilies whole, 1	0
Green jalapeno wheels, 1/4 cup	0
Green jalapenos whole peppers, 2	0
Red jalapeno wheels, 1/4 cup	0

Dole

Bell pepper, 1 medium	0

Faraon

Chipotles peppers, 1 oz	0
Nacho sliced jalapeño peppers, 3 tsp	0
Serrano peppers, 4 pieces	0
Sliced jalapeño peppers, 3 tsp	0
Whole jalapenos, 3 pieces	0
Yellow chiles, 2 Tbsp	0

Hanover

Diced green peppers, 3/4 cup	0

Herdez

Serranos, 4 pieces	0
Sliced jalapenos, 1/4 cup	0
Whole jalapenos, 3 pieces	0

La Rosa D'oro

Cherry peppers stuffed with prosciutto & provolone cheese, 1 oz	2

Las Palmas

Diced green chiles, 2 Tbsp	0
Green chile strips, 1	0
Sliced jalapenos, 3 Tbsp (drained)	0
Whole green chile, 1	0
Whole jalapenos, 2	0

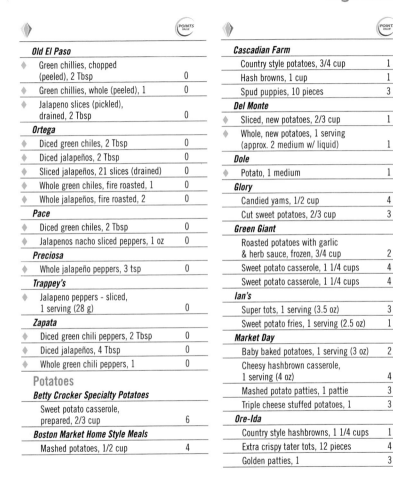

Old El Paso

Green chillies, chopped (peeled), 2 Tbsp	0
Green chillies, whole (peeled), 1	0
Jalapeno slices (pickled), drained, 2 Tbsp	0

Ortega

Diced green chiles, 2 Tbsp	0
Diced jalapeños, 2 Tbsp	0
Sliced jalapeños, 21 slices (drained)	0
Whole green chiles, fire roasted, 1	0
Whole jalapeños, fire roasted, 2	0

Pace

Diced green chiles, 2 Tbsp	0
Jalapenos nacho sliced peppers, 1 oz	0

Preciosa

Whole jalapeño peppers, 3 tsp	0

Trappey's

Jalapeno peppers - sliced, 1 serving (28 g)	0

Zapata

Diced green chili peppers, 2 Tbsp	0
Diced jalapeños, 4 Tbsp	0
Whole green chili peppers, 1	0

Potatoes

Betty Crocker Specialty Potatoes

Sweet potato casserole, prepared, 2/3 cup	6

Boston Market Home Style Meals

Mashed potatoes, 1/2 cup	4

Cascadian Farm

Country style potatoes, 3/4 cup	1
Hash browns, 1 cup	1
Spud puppies, 10 pieces	3

Del Monte

Sliced, new potatoes, 2/3 cup	1	(6)
Whole, new potatoes, 1 serving (approx. 2 medium w/ liquid)	1	(6)

Dole

Potato, 1 medium	1	(6)

Glory

Candied yams, 1/2 cup	4
Cut sweet potatoes, 2/3 cup	3

Green Giant

Roasted potatoes with garlic & herb sauce, frozen, 3/4 cup	2
Sweet potato casserole, 1 1/4 cups	4
Sweet potato casserole, 1 1/4 cups	4

Ian's

Super tots, 1 serving (3.5 oz)	3
Sweet potato fries, 1 serving (2.5 oz)	1

Market Day

Baby baked potatoes, 1 serving (3 oz)	2
Cheesy hashbrown casserole, 1 serving (4 oz)	4
Mashed potato patties, 1 pattie	3
Triple cheese stuffed potatoes, 1	3

Ore-Ida

Country style hashbrowns, 1 1/4 cups	1
Extra crispy tater tots, 12 pieces	4
Golden patties, 1	3

Vegetables

Ore-Ida (cont'd)

	POINTS VALUE
Hash browns, 1 pattie	1
Mashed potatoes, prepared, 2/3 cup	2
Mini tater tots, 19 pieces	4
Onion tater tots, 9 pieces	3
Potato wedges with skin, 9 pieces	2
Potatoes O'Brien, 3/4 cup	1
Southern style hashbrowns, 3/4 cup	1
Tater tots, 9 pieces	3
Toaster hash browns, 2 patties	5
Twice baked potatoes, butter, 1 piece	4
Twice baked potatoes, Cheddar cheese, 1 piece	4
Twice baked potatoes, sour cream & chives, 1 piece	4
Tree of Life	
Organic sweet potato puree, 1/2 cup	2

Pumpkin
Libby's

Solid pack pumpkin, 1/2 cup	0
Tree of Life	
Organic pumpkin puree, 1/2 cup	0

Radishes
Del Monte

Sliced beets, 1/2 cup	0
Sliced, pickled beets, 1/2 cup	1
Dole	
Red radishes, 7	0
Eden	
Daikon - dried & shredded, 2 Tbsp	0
Pickled daikon radish, 2 slices	0
Market Day	
Sweet potato medley, 1 serving (3 oz)	2

Spinach
Birds Eye

	POINTS VALUE
Chopped spinach, 1 cup	0
Creamed spinach with a real cream sauce, frozen, 1/2 cup	1
Cut leaf spinach, 1 cup	0
Boston Market Home Style Meals	
Creamed spinach, 1/2 cup	4
Cascadian Farm	
Spinach (cut), 1/3 cup	0
Del Monte	
Chopped spinach, 1/2 cup	0
Spinach, no salt added, 1/2 cup	0
Spinach, organic baby leaf, 1/2 cup	0
Dole	
Spinach, 1 1/2 cups (shredded)	0
Glory	
Spinach, 1/2 cup	0
Green Giant	
Creamed spinach, frozen, 1/2 cup	1
Cut leaf spinach & butter sauce, frozen, 1/2 cup	0
Green Giant Harvest Fresh	
Spinach, frozen, 1/2 cup	0
Hanover The Gold Line	
Spinach, 1 cup	0
Tree of Life	
Organic chopped spinach, 1 cup	0
Organic chopped spinach, 1 cup	0
Veggie Patch	
Bistro au naturel - spinach & three cheese bites, 3	3
Spinach bites with three cheese, 3	3

	POINTS VALUE
Squash & Zucchini	
Birds Eye	
Cooked winter squash, 1/2 cup	1
Cascadian Farm	
Winter squash, 1/2 cup	1
Del Monte	
Zucchini with Italian style tomato sauce, 1/2 cup	0
Sabra	
Classic babaganoush, 1 oz	2
Tomatoes	
Contadina	
Crushed tomatoes in tomato puree, 1/4 cup	0
Crushed tomatoes with Italian herbs, 1/4 cup	0
Crushed tomatoes with roasted garlic, 1/4 cup	0
Diced tomatoes, 1/2 cup	0
Diced tomatoes - Italian, 1/2 cup	1
Diced tomatoes with roasted garlic, 1/2 cup	1
Diced tomatoes with sauteed onions, 1/2 cup	1
Peeled whole tomatoes, 1/2 cup	0
Stewed tomatoes, 1/2 cup	1
Stewed tomatoes - Italian style, 1/2 cup	1
Del Monte	
Chunky tomatoes, chili style, 1/2 cup	0
Chunky tomatoes, pasta style, 1/2 cup	1
Diced tomatoes in brine, 1/2 cup	0

	POINTS VALUE
Diced tomatoes in brine, seasoned with basil, garlic & oregano, 1/2 cup	0
Diced, tomatoes with garlic & onion, 1/2 cup	1
Diced, tomatoes with green pepper & onion, 1/2 cup	0
Diced, tomatoes with jalapenos, 1/2 cup	0
Organic crushed tomatoes in rich, thick puree, 1/4 cup	0
Organic diced tomatoes seasoned with basil, garlic & oregano, 1/2 cup	1
Organic diced tomatoes, in tomato juice, no salt added, 1/2 cup	0
Organic peeled diced tomatoes in tomato juice, 1/2 cup	0
Organic whole peeled tomatoes, 1/2 cup	0
Petite diced tomatoes in brine, 1/2 cup	0
Petite diced tomatoes in brine, seasoned with basil, garlic & oregano, 1/2 cup	0
Sliced tomatoes in brine, 1/2 cup	0
Stewed, Cajun recipe, 1/2 cup	0
Stewed, Italian recipe, 1/2 cup	0
Stewed, Mexican recipe, 1/2 cup	0
Stewed, original recipe, 1/2 cup	0
Stewed, original recipe, no salt added, 1/2 cup	0
Tomato wedges, 1/2 cup	0
Eden Organic	
Crushed tomatoes, 1/4 cup	0
Crushed tomatoes with basil, 1/4 cup	0

Vegetables

	POINTS VALUE
Eden Organic (cont'd)	
◆ Crushed tomatoes with onion & garlic, 1/4 cup	0
◆ Diced tomatoes, 1/2 cup	0
◆ Diced tomatoes with basil, 1/2 cup	0
◆ Diced tomatoes with green chilies, 1/2 cup	0
◆ Diced tomatoes with roasted onion, 1/2 cup	0
◆ Whole roma tomatoes with basil, peeled, 1/2 cup	0
◆ Whole roma tomatoes, peeled, 1/2 cup	0
Fanci Food	
◆ Diced Italian tomatoes, 1/2 cup	0
Las Palmas	
◆ Crushed tomatillos, 1/2 cup	1
Lucini	
Tuscan marinara with roasted garlic sauce, 1/2 cup	1
Muir Glen Organic	
◆ Diced tomatoes with basil & garlic, 1/2 cup	0
◆ Diced tomatoes with garlic & onion, 1/2 cup	0
◆ Diced tomatoes with Italian herbs, 1/2 cup	0
◆ Premium diced tomatoes, 1/2 cup	0
◆ Premium diced tomatoes no salt added, 1/2 cup	0
◆ Premium ground peeled tomatoes, 1/4 cup	0
◆ Premium stewed tomatoes, 1/2 cup	0
◆ Premium whole peeled tomatoes, 1/2 cup	0

	POINTS VALUE
◆ Premium whole peeled tomatoes with basil, 1/2 cup	0
◆ Whole peeled plum tomatoes, 1/2 cup	0
◆ Whole peeled tomatoes, 1/2 cup	0
Muir Glen Organic Farm Select	
◆ Fire roasted crushed tomatoes, 1/4 cup	0
◆ Fire roasted diced tomatoes, 1/2 cup	0
◆ Fire roasted diced tomatoes with medium green chilies, 1/2 cup	0
◆ Fire roasted whole tomatoes, 1/2 cup	0
Progresso	
◆ Crushed tomatoes with added puree, 1/4 cup	0
◆ Diced tomatoes, 1/2 cup	0
Diced tomatoes with Italian herbs, 1/2 cup	1
◆ Whole tomatoes peeled with basil, 1/2 cup	0
Sardo	
Sundried tomatoes, 1 oz	2

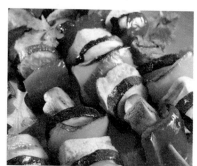

Weight Watchers®
Food Products

Find **POINTS**® values for all your
favorite Weight Watchers food products
right here, in one convenient place!

With Weight Watchers food products
you can count on great taste, quality, and value.

Weight Watchers® Food Products Listing

BEVERAGES

Smoothies
Weight Watchers Smoothie Drink Mix

	POINTS VALUE
Smoothie - creamy chocolate, 1 packet	1
Smoothie - French vanilla, 1 packet	1
Smoothie - white chocolate peppermint, 1 packet	1
Smoothie - wild berry, 1 packet	1

BREAD & BAKED GOODS

Bagels
Weight Watchers

Original bagel, 1	2
Petite bagels, 1	1

Bread
Weight Watchers

100% whole wheat bread, 2 slices	1
English muffin, 1	1
Multi-grain bread, 2 slices	1
Seedless rye, 2 slices	1
Wheat English muffin, 1	1
Wheat sandwich roll, 1	2

Brownies
Weight Watchers

Chocolate brownie, 1	2

Cakes
Weight Watchers

Carrot cake with cream cheese icing, 1 cake	1
Chocolate cake with chocolate icing, 1 cake	1
Golden sponge cake with creamy filling, 1 cake	1
Lemon cake with lemon icing, 1 cake	1

Weight Watchers Smart Ones

Double fudge cake, 1	4
Strawberry shortcake, 1	4

Danish/Sweet Rolls/Pastries
Weight Watchers Smart Ones

Chocolate eclair, 1	3

Flatbread/Pita/Wraps
Weight Watchers

Pita pocket bread, 1	1

Muffins
Weight Watchers

Banana nut muffin, 1	3
Blueberry muffin, 1	3
Double chocolate muffin, 1	3

BREAKFAST, CEREALS & CEREAL BARS

Cereal Bars
Weight Watchers Snack Bars

Baked apple 'n cinnamon 1 bar	2
Banana nut bread, 1 bar	2
Chocolate chip brownie, 1 bar	2
Double chocolate delight, 1 bar	2
Fruity nutty madness, 1 bar	2
Sweet & salty, 1 bar	2

Weight Watchers Mini Bars

Chocolate caramel mini bars, 1 bar	1
Cookies & cream mini bars, 1 bar	1

Weight Watchers® Food Products Listing

	POINTS VALUE
Dark chocolate raspberry mini bars, 1 bar	1
Mint cookie crisp mini bars, 1 bar	1
Peanut butter bliss mini bars, 1 bar	1
Red velvet mini bars, 1 bar	1

Cereal, Hot
Weight Watchers

Oatmeal – blueberry harvest, 1 cup	2
Oatmeal - maple brown sugar, 1 cup	2

CANDY, COOKIES & DESSERTS

Candy
Weight Watchers

Cappuccino cream melts, 2 pieces	0

Weight Watchers by Whitman's

Almond nougat, 3 pieces	3
Caramel medallions, 3 pieces	3
Coconut, 3 pieces	3
Crispy butter cream caramel, 3 pieces	3
Double chocolate mousse, 3 pieces	3
English toffee squares, 3 pieces	3
Mint patties, 3 pieces	3
Nougie nutty chew, 3 pieces	3
Peanut butter crunch, 4 pieces	3
Peanut butter cups, 2 pieces	4
Pecan crowns, 3 pieces	3

Weight Watchers Fruities

Blackberry, 3 pieces	0
Cherry, 3 pieces	0
Strawberry, 3 pieces	0

Cookies
Weight Watchers

	POINTS VALUE
Chocolate chip soft cookie, 1 cookie	1
Oatmeal raisin soft cookie, 1 cookie	1
Peanut butter soft cookie, 1 cookie	1

Ice Cream
Weight Watchers

Candy bar ice cream bar, 1 bar	3
Chocolate chip cookie dough cup, 1 cup	2
Chocolate fudge brownie cup, 1 cup	2
Chocolate round ice cream sandwich, 1 sandwich	2
Cookies and cream cup, 1 cup	2
Chocolate mousse bars, 2 bars	2
English toffee crunch bar, 2 bars	2
Giant chocolate cookies 'n cream bar, 1 bar	2
Giant chocolate fudge sundae cone, 1 cone	2
Giant cookies 'n chocolate cream bar, 1 bar	2
Giant fudge bar, 1 bar	1
Giant latte bar, 1 bar	1
Giant mint fudge cone, 1 cone	2
Giant orange sorbet & ice cream bar, 1 bar	2
Giant vanilla fudge sundae cone, 1 cone	2
Giant wildberry sorbet & ice cream bar, 1 bar	2
Key lime sherbet & ice cream bar, 2 bars	2

Weight Watchers® Food Products Listing

Ice Cream, Weight Watchers (cont'd)

POINTS VALUE

Mint ice cream sandwich, 1 sandwich	2
Mint chocolate chip cup, 1 cup	2
Passion fruit sherbet & ice cream bar, 2 bars	2
Peanut butter delight cup, 1 cup	3
Strawberry sherbet & ice cream bar, 2 bars	2
Turtle sundae cup, 1 cup	3
Vanilla ice cream sandwich, 1 sandwich	2
Vanilla round ice cream sandwich, 1 sandwich	2

Weight Watchers Smart Ones

Brownie a la mode, 1	4
Chocolate chip cookie dough sundae, 1	3
Mint chocolate chip sundae, 1	3
Mocha fudge sundae, 1	3
Peanut butter cup sundae, 1	3

Mousses
Weight Watchers Smart Ones

Chocolate mousse, 1	3

Pies
Weight Watchers Smart Ones

Key lime pie, 1	4

DAIRY & EGGS

Cheese
Weight Watchers

Light string cheese, 1 piece	1
Natural reduced fat Cheddar cheese snacks, 2 pieces	2
Natural reduced fat medium Cheddar, 2 slices	2
Natural reduced fat pepper Jack, 2 slices	2
Natural reduced fat shredded Cheddar cheese, 1 pouch	2
Natural reduced fat shredded Mexican style blend, 1/3 cup	2
Natural reduced fat shredded mozzarella cheese, 1/3 cup	2
Natural reduced fat Swiss cheese, 2 slices	2
Pepper Jack singles, 1 slice	1
Reduced fat cream cheese spread, 1 oz	1
Reduced fat singles, 1 slice	1
Reduced fat whipped cream cheese, 2 Tbsp	1

Yogurt & Yogurt Drinks
Weight Watchers

Amaretto cheesecake nonfat yogurt, 6 oz	1
Berries 'n cream nonfat yogurt, 6 oz	1
Black cherry fat free yogurt, 4 oz	1
Black cherry nonfat yogurt, 6 oz	1
Boston cream pie nonfat yogurt, 6 oz	1
Cherry cheesecake nonfat yogurt, 6 oz	1

	POINTS VALUE
Key lime pie nonfat yogurt, 6 oz	1
Lemon cream pie fat free yogurt, 4 oz	1
Lemon cream pie nonfat yogurt, 6 oz	1
Peach fat free yogurt, 4 oz	1
Peach nonfat yogurt, 6 oz	1
Raspberry nonfat yogurt, 6 oz	1
Smooth & creamy strawberry shortcake fat free yogurt, 4 oz	1
Smooth & creamy white chocolate cheesecake fat free yogurt, 4 oz	1
Strawberry banana nonfat yogurt, 6 oz	1
Strawberry fat free yogurt, 4 oz	1
Strawberry nonfat yogurt, 6 oz	1
Vanilla fat free yogurt, 4 oz	1
Vanilla nonfat yogurt, 6 oz	1
White chocolate raspberry nonfat yogurt, 6 oz	1

PASTA, RICE & GRAINS

Pasta
Weight Watchers

Sides - chicken herb whole grain pasta, 1 cup	3
Sides - tomato parmesan whole grain pasta, 1 cup	4

Rice
Weight Watchers

Sides - wild mushroom brown & wild rice, 1 cup	3

	POINTS VALUE

PREPARED FOODS
Weight Watchers Smart Ones

Angel hair marinara, 1	4
Broccoli & Cheddar roasted potatoes, 1	5
Chicken enchilada Suiza, 1	6
Chicken mirabella, 1	4
Chicken oriental, 1	4
Creamy rigatoni with broccoli & chicken, 1	6
Fettucini alfredo, 1	4
Fiesta chicken, 1	5
Honey dijon chicken, 1	4
Lasagna bolognese, 1	5
Lasagna florentine, 1	6
Lemon herb chicken piccata, 1	4
Macaroni & cheese, 1	5
Pasta primavera, 1	5
Ravioli florentine, 1	5
Roast turkey medallions, 1	4
Salisbury steak with macaroni & cheese, 1	6
Salisbury steak, 1 (9 oz)	4
Santa Fe style rice & beans, 1	6
Shrimp marinara with linguini, 1	3
Spaghetti bolognese, 1	6
Spicy Szechuan style vegetables & chicken, 1	4
Swedish meatballs, 1	5
Three cheese macaroni, 1	6
Three cheese ziti marinara, 1	6
Traditional lasagna with meat sauce, 1	6
Tuna noodle gratin, 1	5

Weight Watchers® Food Products Listing

	POINTS VALUE
Weight Watchers Smart Ones Anytime Selections	
Calzone Italiano, 1	6
Chicken and cheese quesadilla, 1	4
Fiesta quesadilla, 1	4
Cheese pizza minis, 1 tray	5
Pepperoni pizza minis, 1 tray	5
Vegetable pizza minis, 1 tray	5
Weight Watchers Smart Ones Artisan Creations	
Grilled flatbread Chicken bruschetta, 1 piece	6
Grilled flatbread chicken marinara with mozzarella cheese, 1 piece	6
Grilled flatbread savory steak and ranch, 1 piece	6
Grilled flatbread southwestern style chicken fiesta, 1 piece	6
Fajita chicken pizza, 1	7
Weight Watchers Smart Ones Bistro Selections	
Beef pot roast, 1	3
Chicken carbonara, 1	5
Chicken enchiladas Monterey, 1	6
Chicken fettucini, 1	7
Chicken marsala with broccoli, 1	4
Chicken parmesan, 1	5
Chicken Santa Fe, 1	2
Creamy chicken Tuscan with zucchini, 1	4
Creamy parmesan chicken, 1	5
Dragon shrimp lo mein, 1	5
Fire-grilled chicken & vegetables, 1	6

	POINTS VALUE
Grilled chicken in garlic herb sauce with zucchini, 1	4
Grilled mandarin chicken, 1	6
Home-style chicken, 1	5
Meatloaf with mashed potatoes, 1	5
Penne pollo, 1	6
Pepper steak, 1	5
Picante chicken and pasta, 1	5
Roast beef with gravy, 1	5
Roast beef with portabello gravy, 1	4
Roasted chicken with sour cream & chive mashed potatoes, 1	4
Salisbury steak and asparagus, 1	4
Sirloin beef and Asian style vegetables, 1	4
Slow-roasted turkey breast, 1	4
Southwest style adobo chicken, 1	5
Stuffed turkey breast, 1	6
Sweet & sour chicken, 1	4
Teriyaki chicken & vegetables, 1	4
Thai style chicken & rice noodles, 1	5
Turkey medallions with mushroom gravy and green beans, 1	4
Weight Watchers Fresh Ready Meals	
Baked ziti, 1	6
Oriental style chicken, 1	6
Chicken cacciatore, 1	4
Fettuccini primavera, 1	4
Lasagna with meat sauce, 1	6
Meatloaf with garlic mashed potatoes, 1	6
Roast turkey with cranberry stuffing, 1	5

Weight Watchers® Food Products Listing

	POINTS VALUE
Shrimp fettuccini with vegetables, 1	5
Three cheese macaroni, 1	4
Turkey meatballs with pasta & sauce, 1	6
Turkey meatloaf with garlic mashed potatoes, 1	6
Vegetable lasagna, 1	5

Weight Watchers Smart Ones
Fruit Inspirations

Cranberry turkey medallions, 1	7
Honey mango barbeque chicken, 1	5
Orange sesame chicken, 1	7
Pineapple beef teriyaki, 1	6

Weight Watchers Smart Ones
Pizzas Bistro Selections

Four cheese pizza, 1	7
Pepperoni pizza, 1	8

Weight Watchers Smart Ones
Morning Express

Breakfast quesadilla, 1	4
Canadian style bacon English muffin sandwich, 1	4
English muffin sandwich, 1	4
Stuffed breakfast sandwich, 1	5

SNACKS

Cheese Snacks
Weight Watchers

	POINTS VALUE
Cheddar twists, 1 pouch	2

Crackers
Weight Watchers

Multigrain crisps - original, 1 pouch	2

Pretzels
Weight Watchers

Pizza pretzel thins, 1 pouch	2

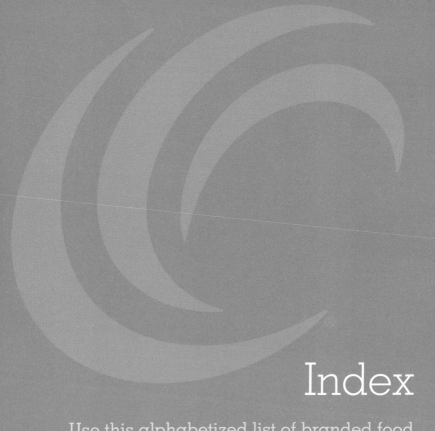

Index

Use this alphabetized list of branded food categories to help you find just what you want.

Page numbers are listed for each product category.

Index

A

Anchovies 314
Appetizers 397
Apples 319
Applesauce 319
Apricots 320
Artichokes 518
Asian Sauces 261
Asparagus 518
Avocado 320

B

Bacon 345
Bagels 146
Baking Powders 96
Bananas 321
Barbecue Sauces 262
Beans 519
Beef 346
Beef Soups 495
Beer 108
Berries 321
Beverage Mixes 111
Biscuit Mixes 96
Biscuits 147
Bouillon, Broth & Stocks 498
Bran 182, 385
Bread 148
Bread Crumbs 96
Bread Dough 96

Breadsticks 158
Breath Mints 204
Broccoli 523
Broth 498
Brownies 158
Brussels Sprouts 524
Butter 281
Butter Substitutes 281

C

Cabbage 524
Cakes 160
Cakes, corn 482
Cakes, rice 482
Candy 204
Carrots 526
Cauliflower 523
Celery 526
Cereal, hot 182
Cereal, ready to eat 184
Cereal Bars 192
Chai Drinks 133
Cheese 281
Cheese Snacks 443
Cherries 322
Chicken 346
Chicken Soups 499
Chili 494
Chips, corn 444
Chips, other 465
Chips, pita 465

Chips, potato 470
Chips, soy 491
Chips, tortilla 488
Chips, vegetable 491
Chocolate 96
Chocolate Drinks 111
Clams 314
Cocoa 111
Coconut 97
Coffee 112
Cookies 216
Cooking Spray 368
Corn 526
Corn Cakes 482
Corn Chips 444
Crab 314
Crackers 445
Cream/Creamers 298
Croutons 166
Crusts, pie/pastry 103

D

Danish 166
Dessert Mix 97
Dips 331
Dips, other 341
Dough, bread 96
Dough, pie/pastry 103
Doughnuts 169
Dressings, salad 370
Dried Fruit 322, 456

Drinks, fruit 113
Drinks, meal replacement 126
Drinks, milk & milk based 127, 305
Drinks, vegetable 142
Drinks, yogurt 306

E

Egg 302
Egg Entrees 398
Egg Substitutes 302
Entrees, egg 398
Entrees, ethnic 398
Entrees, fish & seafood 404
Entrees, meat substitutes 412
Entrees, meat 406
Entrees, pasta 416
Entrees, poultry 406
Entrees, vegetable 438
Ethnic Entrees 398
Extracts 98

F

Fish Entrees 404
Fish Products, other 318
Flatbread 170
Flavorings for Milk 305
Flounder 314
Flour 98
French Toast 200
Frosting 99
Frozen Fruit Bars 254

Index

Frozen Yogurt 236
Fruit, dried 322, 456
Fruit Bars, frozen 254
Fruit Cobblers/Crisps 238
Fruit Cocktail/Salad 325
Fruit Juices & Drinks 113
Fruit Parfait 326
Fruit Snacks 457

G

Game Birds 351
Gefilte Fish 314
Gelatins 238
Grain Sides 432
Grains 385
Grapefruit 327
Grapes 327
Gravies 264
Greens, leafy 528
Grilling Sauces 262
Ground Meat 351
Gum, chewing 240

H

Haddock 314
Ham 358
Herring 315
Honey 100
Horseradish/Horseradish Sauce 265
Hot Sauces 266
Hummus 334

I

Ice Cream 243
Ice Cream Cones 252
Iced Tea 137
Ices 254
Icing 99

J

Jam 335
Jelly 335
Jerky 351
Juices, fruit 113
Juices, vegetable 142

K

Ketchup 267
Kiwifruit 327

L

Lard 104
Latin Sauces 266
Leafy Greens 528
Lentils 528
Lettuce 528
Luncheon/Deli Lunches 304, 352

M

Mangoes 327
Margarine 304

Index

Marinades 267
Marmalade 336
Mayonnaise 269
Meal Replacement Drinks 126
Meat & Poultry Entrees 406
Meat Sauces 279
Meat Soups, other 502
Meat Substitutes 511
Meat Substitutes Entrees 412
Meats, other 366
Melons 327
Milk, flavorings for 305
Milk & Milk Based Drinks 127, 305
Molasses 100
Mousses 256
Muffins 171
Mushrooms 528
Mustard 269

N

Nectarines 328
Noodles 386
Nori 175
Nuts 457

O

Oils 368
Olives 270
Omelets 200
Onions 528
Oranges 327
Oysters 315

P

Pancakes 200
Papayas 328
Pasta 386
Pasta Entrees 416
Pasta Salads 414
Pasta Sauces 272
Pastes 98
Pastries 166
Peaches 328
Peanut Butter 336
Pears 329
Peas 532
Peppers 534
Pickles 276
Pie Filling 101
Pie Mixes 101
Pie/Pastry Dough & Crusts 103
Pies 256
Pineapples 329
Pita 170
Pita Chips 465
Pizza 425
Plums 330
Popcorn 466
Popover Mixes 96
Pork 358
Potato Chips 470
Potato Sides 432
Potatoes 535
Preserves 337

Index

Pretzels 478
Puddings 257
Pumpkin 536

R

Radishes 536
Relish 278
Rice 390
Rice & Corn Cakes 482
Rice Drinks 133
Rice Sides 432
Rolls 175

S

Salad Dressings 370
Salads, pasta & vegetable 414
Salmon 315
Salsa 338
Sandwiches 436
Sardines 315
Sauce, horseradish 265
Sauces, Asian 261
Sauces, barbecue/grilling 262
Sauces, hot & Latin 266
Sauces, other 270
Sauces, pasta 272
Sauces, seafood 278
Sauces, steak & meat 279
Sausage 362
Scallops 316
Seafood Entrees 404

Seafood Sauces 278
Seafood Soups 502
Seasonings 380
Seeds, Snack & Trail Mixes 482
Sherbets 254
Shortening 104
Shrimp 316
Sides, potato, rice & grain 432
Sides, vegetable 438
Smoothies 127
Snack Mixes 482
Snacks, cheese 443
Snacks, fruit 457
Soft Drinks 129
Sorbets 254
Soups, beef 495
Soups, chicken 499
Soups, other 504
Soups, other meat 502
Soups, seafood 502
Soups, turkey 504
Soups, vegetable 504
Soy 516
Soy Drinks 133
Specialty Fruits 330
Spices 104
Spinach 536
Sports Drinks 135
Spreads 341
Spreads, other 341
Squash 537
Steak Sauces 279

Index

Stews 503
Stocks 498
Stuffing Mix 177
Sugar 106
Sugar Substitutes 106
Sweet Rolls 166
Syrups 100

T

Taco Shells 178
Tangerines 330
Tea 137
Tilapia 317
Tomatoes 537
Toppings 252
Tortilla Chips 488
Tortillas 179
Trail Mixes 482
Tuna 317
Turkey 364
Turkey Soups 504

V

Vegetable & Soy Chips 491
Vegetable Entrees 438
Vegetable Juices & Drinks 142
Vegetable Salads 414
Vegetable Sides 438
Vegetable Soups 504
Vegetables, other 529
Vinegars 383

W

Waffles 202
Water 142
Wheat Germ 182
Whitefish 318
Wine & Wine Coolers 144
Wraps 170

Y

Yeast 106
Yogurt, frozen 236
Yogurt & Yogurt Drinks 306

Z

Zucchini 537

Trademark Acknowledgments

Aroastica, Blazing Buffalo, Bar B Q Sauce Basted, Bianco D'Oro, Custom Cut, Cracked Pepper Mill, Honey Coat, Golden Classic Oven Roasted Chicken Breast, Maple Glazed Honey Coat, Londonport, Mesquite Wood Smoked, Ovengold, Salsalito, Sweet Slice, Deli Dinners and Hans Jurgen are trademarks of Boar's Head Provision Co., Inc., used with permission.

Bac*Os, Basic 4, Betty Crocker, Big Deluxe Classics, Bisquick, Bisquick Shake 'N Pour, Boo Berry, Bowl Appétit!, Bugles, Butter Tastin, Cascadian Farm, Cheerios, Chef Inspirations, Chex, Chicken Helper, Cinnamon Toast Crunch, Cocoa Puffs, Colombo, Complete Desserts, Betty Crocker Complete Meals, Cookbook Favorites, Cookie Crisp, Count Chocula, Country Corn Flakes, Create a Meal!, Create 'n Bake, Dunkaroos, Fiber One, Frankenberry, French Toast Crunch, Fruit by the Foot, Fruit Gushers, Fruit Roll-Ups, Gardetto's, Gold Medal, Golden Grahams, Golden Homestyle, Golden Layers, Grands!, Great Measure, Green Giant, Green Giant Select, Hamburger Helper, Hearty Morning, Honey Nut Clusters, Jeno's Crisp 'n Tasty, Jumbo Pop, Just For One!, Kaboom, Kix, LeSueur, Kountry Kist, Lucky Charms, Mexicorn, Mini Feet, Muir Glen, Nature Valley, Niblets, Oatmeal Crisp, Old El Paso, Peanut Butter Toast Crunch, Perfect Portions, Pillsbury, Pizza Rolls, Pop-Secret, Potato Buds, Progresso, Purely O's, Ready To Bake!, Seasoned Skillets, Simply Bake, Simply Steam, Slow Cooker Helper, Spud Puppies, Stand 'n Stuff, Suddenly Salad, SuperMoist, Toaster Scrambles, Toaster Strudel, Total, Totino's Crisp Crust Party Pizza, Trix, Tuna Helper, Warm Delights, Wanchai Ferry, Wheaties, and Wondra are trademarks of General Mills, Inc. and its affiliates, used with permission.

5th Avenue, Almond Joy Bites, Almond Joy, Breath Savers, Bubble Yum with Hershey's, Bubble Yum, Cacao Reserve, Cadbury Crème Eggs, Cadbury Dairy Milk, Cadbury Fruit & Nut, Cadbury Mini Eggs, Cadbury Roast Almond, Cadbury Royal Dark, Cadbury, Caramello, Carefree Koolerz, Carefree, Dagoba Organic, Dagoba, Del Puesto, Fast Break, Giant Hershey's Kiss, Good & Fruity, Good & Plenty, Heath Bites, Heath, Hershey's, Hershey's Bites, Hershey's Chocolate Shoppe, Hershey's Cookies 'N' Crème, Hershey's Goodnight Hugs, Hershey's Goodnight Kisses, Hershey's Hot Cocoa Dutch Collection, Hershey's Hugs, Hershey's Hugs, Hershey's Kisses, Hershey's Mini Kisses, Hershey's Miniatures, Hershey's Nuggets Cookies 'N' Crème, Hershey's Nuggets, Hershey's Pot of Gold, Hershey's Pot of Gold, Hershey-ets, Hershey's Bake Shoppe, Hershey's Bliss, Hershey's Extra Dark Sticks, Hershey's Extra Dark, Hershey's Golden Almond, Hershey's Hugs & Kisses, Hershey's Kissables Special Dark, Hershey's Kissables, Hershey's Kisses Snacksters, Hershey's Kisses Special Dark, Hershey's Nuggets Special Dark, Hershey's S'mores, Hershey's Snacksters, Hershey's Special Dark Sticks, Hershey's Sugar Free, Hershey's Sweet & Salty, Hershey's Take5, Ice Breakers Center Ice, Ice Breakers Chewy Sours, Ice Breakers Ice Cubes, Ice Breakers Sours, Ice Breakers Cool Blasts, Ice Breakers, Jolly Rancher Crayon, Jolly Rancher Double Blasts, Jolly Rancher Rocks, Jolly Rancher Screaming Sours, Jolly

Trademark Acknowledgments

Rancher Sour Blasts, Jolly Rancher Stix, Jolly Rancher Sugar Free, Jolly Rancher, Joseph Schmidt, Kissmobile, Kit Kat Big Kat, Kit Kat, Krackel, Lorena Picositos, Lorena, Malteser, Mauna Loa Mountains, Mauna Loa, Milk Duds, Mounds, Mr. Goodbar, Nibs, Payday Pro, Payday, Pelon Pelo Rico, Reese's Bites, Reese's Nutrageous, Reese's Pieces, Reese's, Reese's Snack Barz, Reese's Snacksters, Reese's Sugar Free, Reese's Sweet & Salty, Reese's Whipps, Reesesticks, Rolo, Scharffen Berger, Skor, Special Dark, Stick Free, Symphony, Tu-Box, Twizzlers Pull-N-Peel, Twizzlers Rainbow Twists, Twizzlers Sourz, Twizzlers Strawz, Twizzlers Tweeterz candy coated Twizzlers Bits, Twizzlers Twerpz, Twizzlers Twist-n-Fill, Twizzlers, Whatchamacallit, Whoppers, York Bites, York Sugar FreeYork, Zagnut, and Zero, are trademarks and service marks owned by or licensed to Hershey Foods Corporation.

Always Tender, Chi-Chi's, Black Label, Compleats, Cure 81, Curemaster, Dona Maria, Bufalo, El Torito, Herdez, Red Label, Old Smokehouse, Wranglers, Hormel, House of Tsang, Pillow Pack, Herb-Ox, Marrakesh Express, Dinty Moore, Kid's Kitchen, SPAM, Saigon Sizzle, Bangkok Padang, Little Sizzlers, Natural Choice, Manny's, Not-So-Sloppy-Joe, Szechuan Spicy, Mongolian Fire, Hibachi Grill, Hunan Smokehut, Simply Tsang, Stagg, Chili Laredo, Classic, Country Brand, Dynamite Hot, Ranch House, Silverado, Steak House, Vegetable Garden and Turkey Ranchero are trademarks owned or licensed by Hormel Foods, LLC or Hormel Foods Corporation and used with permission.

Jennie-O Turkey Store, Jennie-O, Breakfast Lover's and So Easy are trademarks owned or licensed by Jennie-O Turkey Store, LLC and used with permission.

Drenchers and Sun Shower Brands are produced and distributed by NBI Juiceworks.

Tribe is a trademark of Tribe Mediterranean Foods, Inc.

Notes

Notes

Notes

Notes